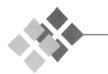

MW01234203

Practical
Health Care
Simulations

Practical Health Care Simulations

Gary E. Loyd, MD, MMM
Clinical Director, Simulations Center
University of Louisville School of Medicine
Department of Anesthesiology
University of Louisville Hospital
Louisville, Kentucky

Carol L. Lake, MD, MBA, MPH
Professor and Chair
Department of Anesthesiology and Perioperative Medicine
University of Louisville School of Medicine
University of Louisville Hospital
Louisville, Kentucky

Ruth B. Greenberg, PhD
Director for Health Sciences Center Academic Programs
University of Louisville School of Medicine
Louisville, Kentucky

ELSEVIER
MOSBY

ELSEVIER
MOSBY

The Curtis Center
170 S Independence Mall W 300E
Philadelphia, Pennsylvania 19106

PRACTICAL HEALTH CARE SIMULATIONS   ISBN 1-56053-625-X

Library of Congress Control Number: 2004103678

Printed in the United States of America

Last digit is the print number: 9 8 7 6 5 4 3 2 1

Contents

Contributors

Gina L. Adrales, MD
Assistant Professor, Department of Surgery, Gastrointestinal Surgery, Medical College of Georgia, Augusta, Georgia

Gary L. Anderson, PhD
Associate Professor of Physiology, Physiology and Biophysics, University of Louisville, School of Medicine, Louisville, Kentucky

Lorena E. Beeman, RN, BSN, MS, CCVT
Adult Cardiopulmonary Critical Care, Clinical Education, Community Training Center and Human Simulation Lab, University of New Mexico Hospitals, Albuquerque, New Mexico

William F. Bond, MD
Clinical Assistant Professor, Emergency Medicine, Penn State University College of Medicine, Hershey, Pennsylvania; Leigh Valley Hospital, Allentown, Pennsylvania

Brigitte Bonin, MD, FRCSCC
Associate Professor, Department of Obstetrics, Gynecology and Newborn Care, University of Ottawa, Member of the Division of Maternal Fetal Medicine, Active Staff of the Ottawa Hospital-General Campus, Ottawa, Ontario, Canada

Judith A. Buchanan, PhD, DMD
Associate Dean for Academic Affairs, School of Dental Medicine, University of Pennsylvania, Philadelphia, Pennsylvania

Clinton O. Chichester, PhD
Chairman and Professor, Biomedical Sciences, University of Rhode Island, Kingston, Rhode Island; Scientific Staff, Department of Medicine, Rhode Island Hospital, Providence, Rhode Island

J. J. M. C. H. de la Rosette, MD, PhD
Professor and Chairman in Urology, Academisch Medisch Centrum, University of Amsterdam, Amsterdam, The Netherlands

Susan L. DeSousa, BSc, RRCP/RRT
Coordinator, The Canadian Simulation Centre, Anesthesia, Respiratory Therapy, Sunnybrook and Women's College Health Sciences Centre, Toronto, Ontario, Canada

Mary L. Eichorn, MSN, RN, CNS, CEN
ACLS Coordinator, Clinical Education, University of New Mexico Hospitals, Albuquerque, New Mexico

Martin P. Eason, MD, JD
Assistant Professor, Director Simulation Laboratory, Office of Academic Affairs, Quillen College of Medicine, East Tennessee State University, Johnson City, Tennessee

Brian R. Felice, PhD, MBA
Biomedical Sciences, University of Rhode Island, Kingston, Rhode Island

Sheena M. Ferguson, MSN, RN, CCRN
Director, B*A*T*C*A*V*E*, Clinical Education, Community Training Center and Human Simulation Lab, University of New Mexico Hospitals, Albuquerque, New Mexico

Glen A. Franklin, MD
Assistant Professor of Surgery, Department of Surgery, University of Louisville, University Hospital, Louisville, Kentucky

Alejandro Gandsas, MD, FACS
Head, Division Bariatric and Minimally Invasive Surgery, Sinai Hospital, Baltimore, Maryland

Michael S. Goodrow
Director of Operations, Patient Simulation Center, Office of Curriculum Development and Evaluation, University of Louisville School of Medicine, Louisville, Kentucky

James A. Gordon, MD, MPA
Director, G. S. Beckwith Gilbert and Katherine S. Gilbert Medical Education Program in Medical Simulation, Assistant Professor of Medicine, Emergency Medicine, Harvard Medical School, Attending Physician, Department of Emergency Medicine, Massachusetts General Hospital, Boston, Massachusetts

Ruth B. Greenberg, PhD
Director for Health Sciences Center Academic Programs, University of Louisville School of Medicine, Louisville, Kentucky

Ronald W. Holder, Jr., MHA, CMPE
Administrator, Department of Anesthesiology and Perioperative Medicine, University of Louisville, Louisville, Kentucky

S. Barry Issenberg, MD
Associate Professor of Medicine, Assistant Dean, Research in Medical Education, Director, Educational Research and Technology, Center for Research in Medicine Education, University of Miami School of Medicine, Jackson Memorial Hospital, University of Miami Hospital and Clinics, Miami, Florida

Yolanda Jaramillo, BSN, MPH, RN
Women's Health Care, Clinical Education, Community Training Center and Human Simulation Lab, University of New Mexico Hospitals, Albuquerque, New Mexico

M. P. Laguna, MD, PhD
Urology, Academisch Medisch Centrum, University of Amsterdam, Amsterdam, The Netherlands

Carol L. Lake, MD, MBA, MPH
Professor and Chair, Department of Anesthesiology and Perioperative Medicine, University of Louisville, University of Louisville Hospital, Louisville, Kentucky

Adam I. Levine, MD
Assistant Professor of Anesthesiology, Physiology and Biophysics, Program Director, Anesthesiology, Residence Training Program, Director of Simulation, Mount Sinai School of Medicine, Mount Sinai Hospital, New York, New York

Michelle T. Lewis
University of Louisville School of Medicine, Louisville, Kentucky

Gary E. Loyd, MD, MMM
Clinical Director, Simulations Center, University of Louisville School of Medicine, Department of Anesthesiology, University of Louisville Hospital, Louisville, Kentucky

Alfred E. Lupien, PhD, CRNA
Chairman and Associate Professor, Department of Nursing Anesthesia, Medical College of Georgia, Augusta, Georgia

Steven A. McLaughlin, MD
Assistant Professor, Emergency Medicine, University of New Mexico, Albuquerque, New Mexico

D. N. Mitropoulos, MD, FEBU
Assistant Professor, Urology, University of Athens, Urology, Laiko General Hospital, Athens, Greece

Pamela J. Morgan, MD, CCFP, FRCPC
Associate Professor, Anesthesia, University of Toronto, Sunnybrook's Women's
College Health Sciences Centre, Toronto, Ontario, Canada

Michael A. Olympio, MD
Professor, Anesthesiology, Wake Forest University School of Medicine, Wake Forest
University Baptist Medical Center, Winston-Salem, North Carolina

Joseph A. O'Daniel, BS
Orthopaedic Surgery, University of Louisville School of Medicine, Louisville, Kentucky

David Ost, MD
Assistant Professor of Medicine, Pulmonary and Critical Care Medicine, New York
University School of Medicine, New York, New York North Shore University
Hospital, Manhasset, New York

Adrian E. Park, MD
Professor of Surgery, Department of Surgery, University of Maryland, University of
Maryland Medical Center, Baltimore, Maryland

Glenn D. Posner, MDCM
Senior Resident, Obstetrics, Gynecology and Newborn Care, University of Ottawa,
Ottawa, Ontario, Canada

Martin A. Reznek, MD
Chief Resident, Steering Committee, Department of Emergency Medicine, Detroit
Receiving Hospital & Wayne State University School of Medicine, Human Patient
Simulation Center, Eugene Applebaum College of Pharmacy and Health Sciences,
Wayne State University, Detroit, Michigan

Craig S. Roberts, MD
Associate Professor, Department of Orthopaedic Surgery, University of Louisville
School of Medicine, Orthopaedic Clinic, University of Louisville Hospital,
Louisville, Kentucky

Kathleen R. Rosen, MD
Associate Professor, Anesthesiology, West Virginia University, West Virginia
University Hospital, Morgantown, West Virginia

Brian K. Ross, PhD, MD
Professor of Anesthesiology, Department of Anesthesiology, University of
Washington, University of Washington Medical Center, Seattle, Washington

Lori Schumacher, RN, MS, CCRN
Assistant Professor, Advanced Practice Nursing, Medical College of Georgia,
Augusta, Georgia

Howard A. Schwid, MD
Professor of Anesthesiology, Department of Anesthesiology, University of
Washington, VA Puget Sound Health Care System, Seattle, Washington

Robert E. Sedlack, MD
Assistant Professor of Medicine, Mayo Clinic College of Medicine, Mayo Clinic,
Division of Gastroenterology and Hepatology, Rochester, Minnesota

David Seligson, MD
Professor and Vice Chair, Department of Orthopaedic Surgery, University of
Louisville School of Medicine, Orthopaedic Clinic, University of Louisville
Hospital, Louisville, Kentucky

Marc J. Shapiro, MD
Assistant Professor of Medicine, Brown University School of Medicine, Director,
Rhode Island Hospital Medical Simulation Center, Attending Physician,
Emergency Department, Providence, Rhode Island

Viva Jo Siddall, MS, RRT, RCP, CCRC
Assistant Professor, Clinical Anesthesiology, Feinberg School of Medicine,
Northwestern University, Chicago, Illinois

Elizabeth H. Sinz, MD
Associate Professor of Anesthesiology and Critical Care Medicine, Anesthesiology,
West Virginia University, West Virginia University Hospital, Morgantown, West
Virginia

Linda L. Spillane, MD
Associate Professor, Emergency Medicine, University of Rochester, Strong Memorial
Hospital, Rochester, New York

Alicia C. Vogt
University of Louisville School of Medicine, Louisville, Kentucky

John N. Williams, DMD, MBA
Professor and Dean, Periodontics, Endodontics and Dental Hygiene, University of
Louisville School of Dentistry, University of Louisville Hospital, Louisville,
Kentucky

Mary Wright, MSN, RNC, CNS
Instructor, Maternity Nursing, College of Nursing, University of New Mexico,
Albuquerque, New Mexico

Preface

As postsecondary institutions throughout the country begin the twenty-first century, they are responding to changes in the health care environment and industry with changes in their health care education programs. From the community college that prepares associate degree nurses and allied health professions to the medical school that prepares primary care and subspecialty physicians, the need to change what and how students learn has emerged as the primary challenge in clinical education. We wrote *Practical Health Care Simulations* in response to one of those changes—the development of simulation as an educational tool.

High-fidelity simulation is a relatively new tool for health education, training, and research. In the past ten years, however, the availability of computer-driven patient simulators—lifelike, risk-free, and available 24/7—has grown. Patient simulators, which began as a tool to train anesthesiologists and other critical care professionals, are moving out of departments of anesthesiology and into community college health care programs, undergraduate medical education programs, and community agencies. Although the costs involved in building a simulation center are high and the training required to run a simulation center is labor-intensive and steep, more institutions are choosing to invest in simulation-enhanced education. When we began to design the Paris Simulation Center at the University of Louisville, we relied on telephone conversations and national meetings to guide our decision making process, for we could not find a single book that could serve as a "how-to" resource. Now, four years later, we have learned a lot, both from our own experiences and from our colleagues around the country.

Because the number of institutions investing in simulation-enhanced education continues to grow, we wanted to create a resource that would provide useful guidance for the new or soon-to-be simulation educator. A great deal of knowledge is shared in *Practical Health Care Simulations,* as exemplified by the contributions of both pioneers in medical simulation and recent innovators. We also wanted to include information about some of the less costly types of simulation that are used to enhanced health care education and training.

Practical Health Care Simulations presents this growing wealth of knowledge about medical simulation in a format that both novice and experienced health care educator can understand and use. The format is diverse, reflecting the diverse paradigms from which different health care workers approach their work with simulation. Some of the work is based in published studies, while other work is a description of actual simulations or anecdotal experiences. Our goal was to bring together the different approaches to using medical simulation in educational settings in a single resource—a resource that covers both the basic and more advanced aspects of medical simulation and appeals to all educations seeking to improve their teaching, training, and research.

We thank our authors for their contributions. They provide insights and advice about medical simulation that has not yet been described in published studies. We also thank Mike Goodrow and John Gillespie, our colleagues in the Paris Simulation Center, for their supporting roles in testing simulations and Mary Beth Titsworth and Steffany Barnes, who helped with our research and manuscript preparation. Special thanks to Mike Goodrow for refining the details of several of the simulation examples.

Gary E. Loyd, MD, MMM
Carol L. Lake, MD, MBA, MPH
Ruth Greenberg, PhD

❖ SIMULATION: THE BASICS

Chapter 1

THE HISTORY OF MEDICAL SIMULATION

Kathleen R. Rosen, MD

The introduction of human patient simulation (HPS) is a major step in the evolution of health sciences education. Progress in diverse fields over the past century has had an impact on the development of HPS in its current forms:

1. Human flight, on earth and in space, is no longer just a fantasy. The aviation industry is commonly described as the model for medical simulation.

2. Knowledge increased about the structure and function of the human body and its response to disease, drugs, the environment, and aging.

3. Another significant factor is the evolution of medical technology and acute care specialties: anesthesiology, resuscitation, emergency medicine, trauma, and critical care. Training in acute care was enhanced through the creation of education and certification courses such as basic life support (BLS), advanced cardiac life support (ACLS), pediatric advanced life support (PALS), advanced trauma life support (ATLS), and fundamentals of critical care support (FCCS).

4. The process of health science education and evaluation evolved to a student-centered, competency-based method.

5. The manufacturing industry produced many revolutionary synthetic materials that allowed the construction of modern computers and medical mannequins.

6. The final step in the development of HPS is the phenomenal growth of computer hardware and software. Computers facilitated the mathematic description of human physiology and pharmacology, worldwide communication, and the design of virtual worlds.[1]

Early Simulation History

The history of technologic innovation is the history of tortuous paths which advances often take to acceptance.
S.B. Harris, *The Society for the Recovery of Persons Apparently Dead*[2a]

Many great ideas are ignored or dismissed only to be rediscovered at a future date with better understanding and acceptance. There are three major reasons for slow historical progress: skepticism, lack of communication, and burden of proof. Many of the advances in medicine, education, technology, and resuscitation during the late 20th century have a basis in historical events. It is hard to define the point in time when rehearsal and repetition were recognized as essential to memory and learning or when humans first tried to reverse death. The Torah documents, in detail, the resuscitation of a child by the prophet Elijah using mouth-to-mouth breathing.[2a] The earliest primitive medical simulations were simple anatomic reproductions, designed for practice of skills. Crude obstetric mannequins were described as early as the 17th century.[2]

3

The early 20th century was marked by several significant and seemingly unrelated events. In the early 1900s an anonymous young girl was pulled from the River Seine, an apparent victim of suicide. Stories about her death and her traditional death mask were legendary.[3] In 1910 a report produced by Flexner revolutionized the course of medical education. Edwin Link took 1.5 years to build the prototype for flight simulation in 1928–1929. Asmund Laerdal founded a house for children's books in 1940.[4] World War II stimulated creativity and technology. By mid-century interest in resuscitation was renewed. Anesthesiology grew and matured as an independent and pioneering medical specialty. These historical threads have woven together in the development of 21st century medical simulation.

Historical Landmarks in the Evolution of Medical Simulation
Before 1950

c. 3000 BC	Egyptian mythology: story of Isis saving husband with mouth-to-mouth resuscitation.[5]
1300 BC	Hebrew midwives in Egypt revive newborns.[5]
800 BC	First recorded resuscitations in the Bible: prophet Elijah gives mouth-to-mouth resuscitation; midwife in Exodus.[5,7]
200 BC–500 AD	Scholars advise mouth-to-mouth for newborns. Description of sheep tracheostomy.[6]
175 AD	Galen uses bellows to re-expand lungs of dead animal.[5]
960 AD	Avicenna describes intubation.[5]
Early ages	Heat method to reverse body cooling with death; flagellation method to elicit a response.[7]
1400s	Italian midwives use mouth-to-mouth to revive newborns.[2a]
1530	Fireplace bellows inserted in mouth of men and animals: "Inflate with moderation and gentleness" (Paracelsus, Basel).[2a,7,5,8]
1543	Vesalius (Belgium) reports pig tracheostomy; watches lungs inflate as he blows through a straw.[5]
1667	Hooke (England) proves in a dog experiment that a supply of fresh air is essential to life, not simply lung motion.[5]
1711	Fumigation method: insufflate smoke into animal bladder and then patient rectum.[7]
1744	Tossach (England) reports resuscitation of a coal miner with mouth-to-mouth.[2a]
1745	Fothergill (England) advocates mouth-to-mouth as safer alternative for lung inflation than bellows for three reasons: bellows availability, mouth moisture and heat, and risk of bellows trauma.[5]
1754	Pugh designs homemade endotracheal tubes for newborn resuscitation; tubes placed by palpation. Black (Scotland) discovers carbon dioxide.[5]
1766	Swiss government recommends attempted resuscitation of drowned persons.[2a]
1767	Dutch Society for the Recovery of Drowned Persons offers 5-step revival program: (1) warming, (2) removal of swallowed water, (3) general stimulation, (4) bellows breathing, and (5) bloodletting.[2a]
1770	Inversion: Revival from drowning by hanging upside down with chest compressions.[2a,7]
1773	Fothergill (England) recommends barrel method: lay patient either on top or inside large wine barrel.[2a,7]
1774	Society for the Recovery of Persons Apparently Drowned formed in London. It is later called the Humane Society, then the Royal Humane Society. Society member uses shock on 4-year-old Catherine Greenhill; member Hunter makes

dual bellow device and uses combined positive- and negative-pressure ventilation (PPV and NPV).

1775 Discovery of oxygen by Priestly (England).[5]

1776 Hunter (England) proposes use of oxygen for artificial ventilation.[5]

1782 Royal Humane Society recommends use of bellows in resuscitation and develops several devices that deliver both PPV and NPV.[5]

1786 Hunter (England) tests intravenous opium or gin as cardiac stimulants.[5]

1788 "An Essay on the Recovery of the Apparently Dead" by Kite reviews 442 attempted resuscitations. Kite identifies that the time delay to delivery of treatment is critical to resuscitation success. He develops his own portable "defibrillator" as well as metal endotracheal tube.[5,7,2a]

1799 Reece reanimation chair combined artificial respiration and invasive electricity.[5]

1803 Russian method: bury the body in snow.[7]

1806 Chaussier (France) devises metal endotracheal tube.[5]

1811 Fumigation abandoned as lethal dose of tobacco discovered.[7]

1812 Trotting horse revival method: remove victim from wate, lay across horse's back, and run horse on beach.[2a,7]

1815 Trotting revival nixed by citizens for clean beaches.[7]

1818 Mary Shelley writes *Frankenstein,* which proposes a dark side to reanimation and stokes societal fears over these new techniques.[2a]

1829 Report by LeRoy (France) documents pneumatic trauma and death from mechanical PPV. Bellows abandoned because of risk of overinflation.[5,7]

1831 Side-to-side compression of chest for artificial breathing.[7]

1838 Dalziel (England) describes tank-style negative pressure ventilation.[5]

1846 First public demonstration of general anesthetic in the "Etherdome."[9,10]

1854 First indirect laryngoscopy by music teacher.[8a]

1856 Hall proposes rolling for ventilation: changing position from prone (with back compression) to side to deliver a tidal volume of 300–500 ml, 16 times/minute.[2a,5]

1858 Ribemont (France) uses metal endotracheal tube.
  Silvester (England) devises arm lift maneuver that uses pectoral muscles for respiration.[5]
  Balassi (Hungary) employs first successful closed-chest massage.[5]

1868 Hill (England) uses closed-chest massage for arrest during chloroform anesthesia.[5]

1870 McClellan (England) devises portable pocket-size bellows.[5]

1871 Trendelenberg (Germany) devises tube with inflatable cuff to prevent aspiration.[5]

1874 Schiff (Germany) performs dog experiment: chloroform overdose was reversed by combination of artificial respiration, open cardiac massage, and continuous abdominal compression.

1878 Macewer (Scotland) uses first endotracheal anesthetic.[5]
  Boehm studies resuscitation by killing cats and measuring intra-abdominal pressure during chest compression.[5]

1880 Waldenburg (Germany) devises cuirass ventilator (small, portable suction applied to chest).[5]

1885 O'Dwyer uses intubation for patients with diphtheria.[8a]
  Koenig uses one-handed external compression.[5]

1892 Tongue stretching used or respiratory resuscitation.[2a]

1893 Eisenmenger (Austria) uses endotracheal tube with inflatable cuff for airway surgery.[5]

1895 First direct laryngoscopy.[8a]
  Schafer and Oliver experiment with adrenal extracts.

1899	Prevost and Batelli show that low-voltage current induces ventricular fibrillation that can be reversed by application of additional current.[5]
1900	Kuhn (Germany) devises flexible metal endotracheal tube.[8a]
	Pruss uses direct cardiac massage effect for chloroform, asphyxia, and electric shock.[5]
1900s	Herlitzka studies adrenaline in the isolated rabbit heart and injects Locke's solution (potassium, sodium, calcium, bicarbonate, and dextrose) via carotid artery into the aorta to restart the heart.[5]
1901	Ingelsrud (Norway) uses open massage to revive arrest during hysterectomy. It becomes the prevailing human technique until 1960.[5]
1903–1904	Schafer (U.S.) develops completely prone method of respiration that is adopted by the American Red Cross.[5]
1905	Floresco revives dog from ether overdose by ventilation through phrenic nerve stimulation and electrodes placed in the right ventricle through the jugular system.[5]
	Long Island Society of Anesthetists founded (precursor to the American Society of Anesthesiologist).[9]
1908	Machine devised for compression of dog chest that was less efficient than manual method.[5]
	Locke resuscitates intact animals with his solution and describes effects of excessive adrenaline administration.[5]
1910	New York Society of Anesthetists founded.[9]
1914	First report of use of epinephrine during resuscitation.[6]
1918–1919	First modern tank respirators at Case Western Reserve and Harvard for treatment of polio.[5]
1920	Edwin Link takes his first flying lesson.[11]
1920s	Jackson and Jackson make improved scope for direct laryngoscopy.[8a,5]
	Magill advocates inhalation anesthesia and cocaine for blind nasal intubation. He makes his own endotracheal tube with inflatable cuff.[8a,5]
	Hooker and Kouwenhoven convert ventricular fibrillation with external current.[6]
1922	*Current Research in Anesthesia and Analgesia* (*Anesthesia and Analgesia* currently) first published.[9]
1927	Ralph M. Waters, MD, establishes the first academic department of anesthesia at the University of Wisconsin, Madison.[10,10a]
1928–1929	Link builds first "blue box" in basement of father's piano and organ factory, Binghamton, NY.
	Majority of early Link simulators sold to amusement parks.[11]
1931	Link becomes full-time flight instructor. His school offered both trainer and actual flight time.[11,11a]
1932	Gale and Waters (U.S.) describe one-lung anesthesia.[5]
	MacIntosch sand Leatherdale (England) use endobronchial intubation.[5]
	Nielsen (Denmark) uses artificial respiration that combined prone chest compression with lifting of arms.[5]
	Eve and Killick (England) technique of artificial respiration: place patient prone on tilt table and use gravity to move diaphragm.[5]
1933	Hooker uses dogs to quantify electricity needed to induce and reverse fibrillation.[5]
1933	Calcium increases contractility after defibrillation.[5]
1934	Army buys 6 Link trainers.[11,11a]
	Thiopental appears in clinical anesthesia practice.[10]

1935	Rovenstein establishes second academic department of anesthesia at Belleview Hospital.[9]
	American Society of Anesthesiologists established.[9]
1935–1940	Link Celestial Trainer used for training of Great Britain's Air Force.[15]
1938	Military purchases 10,000 blue box trainers.[11,11a]
	Military uses mouth-to-mouth in WW II.[7]
	First plastic skeleton made by founders of Medical Plastics.[12]
	American Board of Anesthesiology founded.[10]
1939	First American Board of Anesthesiology written examination.[9]
1940	*Anesthesiology* first published.[10]
1941	Rocket flight simulator completed.[13]
1942	Curare introduced.[8a]
	Case report of procainamide reversal of ventricular fibrillation.[5]
1946	Mendelson syndrome report.[8a]
1947	Beck (U.S.) reports first successful AC defbrillation during adolescent pectus excavatum surgery.[5,14]
	Gurich and Yuniev (Russian physicians) report results from work done a decade earlier. They showed that DC charge was more effective than AC for resuscitation and that chest compressions should be given if there is a > 2-minute delay to accessing electricity.[5]

EDWIN A. LINK: Pioneer and Visionary

Edwin Link was born on July 26, 1904 in Indiana. In 1910 his family moved to the site of his legacy, Binghamton, NY, where his father started Link Piano and Organ Company. Link was not a stellar student. He attended five different high schools before leaving to work in his father's business in 1922. During that time he became interested in flying and took his first lesson in Los Angeles during 1920. At Link Piano and Organ Company, he showed a mechanical aptitude and talent for organ repair but held onto his love of flight. He bought his first airplane, a Cessna AA, in 1928 and began a career as a pilot. He also began working on the prototype of his flight trainer because he believed that there must be an easier, safer, and less expensive way to learn how to fly. In 1929, he patented the flight trainer based on pneumatic principles and formed Link Aeronautical Corporation. Initially, the Link trainer was a popular amusement park ride. Link opened his own flying school in 1930 to demonstrate the educational value of his trainer.

Link married Marion Clayton in 1931. She was a reporter assigned to interview Link about his invention. She helped Link's operations through her business management skills, including using her writing talents to publicize his inventions. The Great Depression forced Link to work at local airports in the early 1930s. He invented an electric billboard for display from an airplane at night. In the pursuit of this new business, he perfected his skill at instrument flying. In 1934, the U.S. Army Air Corps began delivery of mail with several catastrophic and fatal results due to poor visibility. The Army purchased six Link trainers after Link arrived for a meeting by air in thick fog. In 1935 Link trainers were purchased by Japan and the Soviet Union. By the time European nations desired Link trainers for military preparation for World War II (WW II), two upgrades had occurred. Link opened a Canadian plant in 1937 because Britain required that the trainers be manufactured on British soil. These early trainers were generic.

Military needs during WW II spurred many Link inventions: Celestial Navigation Trainer, a bomber crew trainer, and the first airplane-specific model.

Events following WW II, trainer glut, and market competition threatened the health of Link Corporation, but by the early 1950s military and commercial aviation showed a renewed interest in simulation training. Computers and electronics were incorporated into flight simulation. Edwin Link stepped down as president of Link Aviation in 1953, when the job offered limited creativity and intense business management demands. In 1954, Link merged his company with the larger General Precision Equipment Corporation. He was then able to pursue his new passion for underwater exploration.

1950s

This decade was characterized by tremendous strides in the fields of medicine and surgery and the introduction of pioneering technologic innovations to come in the 1960s. Anesthesia matured as a medical specialty. Surgeons advanced the science of resuscitation through development of cardiothoracic surgery, teaching the techniques of open cardiac massage, direct application of electricity to the heart, and use of pharmacology (calcium, lidocaine, epinephrine, THAM) as a resuscitation adjunct.[5,5a,8,15] Defibrillation was described as ineffective after 3 minutes, and use of chest compressions was recommended if electricity was not immediately available.

Anesthesia and medicine specialists made tremendous progress in respiratory knowledge and management. In 1950, the currently available techniques of artificial respiration were compared. The Nielson method (alternation compression of the chest in the prone position with lifting of the arms) was clearly superior to all other forms.[5] The American Red Cross championed this technique until mouth-to-mouth breathing was shown to be a superior option.[5] Safar verified the efficacy of mouth-to-mouth breathing, recommended the head tilt-jaw lift maneuver to clear the airway, and devised an oral airway.[5,5a] Endotracheal intubation became routine in anesthesia, and rapid-sequence induction was devised to minimize aspiration risk.

Advances in medical science were accompanied by developments in medical technology. Collaboration of medical teams at Johns Hopkins University produced the first external defibrillator. Pacemaker technology introduced the first implantable transvenous electrodes and battery-operated generator. Polio epidemics stimulated the development of long-term ventilation methods, including the positive pressure ventilator. A self-inflating resuscitation bag was invented. Asmund Laerdal revolutionized the doll industry with the discovery of new soft plastics. Believing that use of a lifelike doll would motivate students to learn mouth-to-mouth resuscitation, he commissioned sculptress Emma Mathiasson to make a three-dimensional head based on the death mask of the girl from the River Seine.[3,4]

Simulation in the aerospace industry recovered from a post-WW II slump. The birth of analog computers facilitated increase in flight simulation complexity and realism in the replica cockpits.[11,24a] Link Aviation merged with General Precision Equipment to maintain their position in the simulation industry as competition grew. In 1955, civil aviation embraced simulation technology as the FAA required simulation recertification to maintain commercial pilots' licenses. NASA developed biotelemetry to monitor astronauts.[20a] Analog computers were used in the Mercury program flight simulator.[19a]

Historical Landmarks in the Evolution of Medical Simulation: 1950s

1950   Gordon (U.S.) compares tidal volumes produced by various methods of artificial
              respiration in healthy volunteers. Nielsen's mouth-to-mouth technique proves
              far superior to Eve's rocking method, which, in turn, proves superior to
              Schaefer's arm lift. The Silvester method proves to be the least effective; it is
              the only method in which the patient is not prone.[5]
              American Red Cross adopts Nielsen method and begins instruction in mouth-to-
              mouth breathing as preferred method of artificial respiration.[5]
              Beck begins to teach physicians the technique of open cardiac resuscitation.[5]
              Case report of lidocaine reversal of ventricular fibrillation.[5]
1950s   Routine use of endotracheal tubes for anesthesia.
              Cardiac massage is performed by directly massaging the heart.[8]
              Improvement of Link simulator with use of analog computers.[11]
              Polio epidemics: Ibsen (Scandinavia) and Safar (U.S.) demonstrate benefits of
              PPV compared with tank ventilation in polio victims.[5]
1953   Intracardiac calcium proves effective for cardiac standstill (either spontaneous or
              due to defibrillation) during pediatric heart surgery.[5]
1954   J.O. Elam proves superiority and simplicity of mouth-to-mask ventilation
              compared with arm lift.[8]
              Link Aviation merges with General Precision Equipment Corporation (GPE).
              Link remains president.
1956   Zoll reports his resuscitation series using external current and epinephrine.[5,15]
1957   First successful external defibrillation with Johns Hopkin's equipment.[20a]
              Peleska (Prague) states that defibrillation is ineffective after 3 minutes.
              Combination of compression and electricity is optimal.[5]
1958   Peter Safar verifies benefits of mouth-to-mouth resuscitation and the need for
              head tilt/jaw lift to clear airway obstruction by tongue. He introduces S-shaped
              oral airway (one end, adult size; one end, pediatric size) for facilitation of
              mouth-to-mouth technique.[5,5a]
              Ruben introduces self-inflating bag.[5]
              Laerdal begins research and development for mouth-to-mouth mannequin.[20a]
              NASA develops biotelemetry.[20a]
1959   Link retires to pursue interest in underwater research.[11]
              THAM buffer is used to treat acidosis after cardiac arrest.[5]

1960s

The physiologic effects and benefits of chest compression were discovered serendip-
itously during early trials of the Hopkins defibrillator.[7,5a] Sodium bicarbonate was introduced for the buffering of acidosis, and bretyllium was used for ventricular arrhythmias. Demonstrations of chest compression that failed to produce adequate ventilation
instigated the implementation of modern forms of cardiopulmonary resuscitation
(CPR).[5] The safety of rapid-sequence inductions was improved with the addition of Sel-
lick's maneuver.[9] DC was found to be superior to AC for defibrillation.[5] Anesthesiologists established the first intensive care units. The National Academy of Science held a
conference to standardize resuscitation protocols.

Medical science resuscitation advances were overshadowed by technology enhancements during the 1960s. Medical electronics was improved with defibrillators, DC
counter-shock, patient monitors, and EKG telemetry. Early defibrillators weighed 100

lb and required an AC source. These pioneers would frequently topple off rolling carts en route to a code; hence, the nickname "crash cart," which endures today.[5] Respiratory care was facilitated by numerous developments: the Robertshaw double-lumen endotracheal tube, Brook resuscitation airway, and the Elder system that allowed the delivery of oxygen and PPV by mask.[5,9] The birth of Resusci Annie in 1960 was the first of three significant events in the history of medical simulation. The device was initially designed for the practice of mouth-to-mouth breathing. Harvey, the simulator of cardiology patients, debuted at the University of Miami. "Simulation in anesthesia was first demonstrated in the late 1960s, when "neither the technology nor the profession was ready for it."[16] The first primitive full-scale human patient anesthesia simulator was constructed at the University of Southern California.[17,18] The product, designated Sim 1, included a rudimentary patient mannequin and anesthesia workstation. Only six drugs were programmed, and monitoring was not integrated.

Advances in resuscitation created a major dilemma. The medical community was convinced of the efficacy of modern techniques but did not have the resources to deliver these procedures outside the hospital. An ambulance with coronary care equipment was introduced in Belfast in 1963. In the U.S., however, resuscitation was designated as a medical procedure and limited to practice by physicians or under their direct supervision. Governor Ronald Reagan of California was the first to authorize resuscitation by physician delegates.[20a] Subsequently, the first paramedic training programs were launched, and ATT designates 911 as the national emergency notification number.[20a]

Health sciences education was at the brink of a revolution. A classic apprenticeship model had not changed significantly since the incorporation of Flexner's suggestions in 1910. Although Bloom's taxonomy was published in 1956, it would be years before his principles were integrated into medical education. The initial reports of the use of standardized patients appeared.[19] Problem-based learning was developed at McMaster University.[20]

Analog computers flourished with plentiful software and hardware developments. Gordon Moore of IBM predicted increases in computer power. Moore's law envisioned a doubling of power and halving of price every 18 months. Computer games with joysticks, word-processing, three-dimensional images, and computer-aided design were early developments. Researchers at MIT and Stanford accelerated computer growth through introduction of the mouse and windows concept. Sketchpad by Sutherland introduced manipulation of objects on the screen by pointing.[21] Sutherland then turned his talents to the initial development of virtual reality. Replacement of analog computer systems by digital computers allowed improved flight modeling. Mixed analog and digital computer systems were used in the development of Gemini simulators by the collaboration of General Precision Equipment with NASA.[19a] The Apollo simulators were the first fully digital products.[19a] Computer milestones in the later 1960s included hypertext, linking of nonvideo multimedia, and electronic mail. Computer innovations continued into the next decade.

Historical Landmarks in the Evolution of Medical Simulation: 1960s

1960s   Safar and Harris note that closed chest compression does not produce adequate ventilation of the lungs.[5]

Mouth-to-mouth breathing and massage are combined to form CPR.

Electronic monitors are used.[8a]

Physician-delivered anesthesia triples compared with era before WW II.[10]

1960	"Resusci Annie" born.
	Kowenhoven, electrical engineer at Hopkins, introduces closed chest massage.[7,5a]
1961	First primitive use of computer-assisted learning in medicine is recorded.[22]
1962	First use of RSI and Sellick's maneuver.
	Brook introduces airway with exhalation valve for mouth-to-mouth rsuscitatin.[5]
	Lown shows superiority of DC shock and describes synchronized cardioversion of atrial dysthrhythmias.[5]
	Biarbonate is introduced for the treatment of acidosis.[5]
1963	Belfast rescue vehicle is equipped with coronary care equipment.[5a]
	Sutherland produces his MIT doctoral thesis for manipulation of objects on a computer screen with a pointing device.[21]
1964	GPE works with NASA to develop simulators for the Gemini program.[19a]
	Elder demand-valve resuscitator delivers compressed oxygen via face mask.[5]
1965	Governor Reagan authorizes the use of physician delegates.[20a]
	DC shock is developed.[20a]
1967	First report of ventricular fibrillation resuscitation outside the hospital.[6]
	Ohio State University produces on-line tutorial for basic sciences.[22]
1968	Motorola launches EKG telemetry system: APCOR.[20a]
	ATT designates 911 as national emergency number.[20a]
	First paramedic programs appear.
	General Precision Equipment Corporation merges with Singer Company.[11]
	Cardiology patient simulator debuts from University of Miami; named "Harvey."[23]
	Bretyllium is shown effective in the management of ventricular fibrillation.[5]

1970s

Resuscitation medicine was advanced through the sharing of knowledge and development of training aids. The National Academy of Science reviewed the status of resuscitation in a second conference. It endorsed a program of community education facilitated by the Red Cross and the American Heart Association (AHA).[5,7] The first AHA guidelines for CPR and its instruction were published in 1974 with generous financial support from Laerdal. Rosen, as a fourth-year medical student, produced an interactive, multiple-choice questionnaire program with feedback for the practice of these guidelines. The fate of this primitive product is unknown. Laerdal also introduced its first mannequin for endotracheal intubation.[24] Heimlich described and crusaded for emergency help for choking victims with his abdominal thrust maneuver. Cooper began to study the occurrence of anesthesia-related critical events.[25] Objective Scale Clinical Examinations (OSCEs) were first used in medical education.[26] Smaller portable, battery-operated defibrillators were produced by Physiocontrol.[20a] Evolution of equipment and technology guided simulation milestones of this decade. The University of Vermont used hypertext to link patient data.[21] Nursing and allied health discovered the benefit of standardized patients, clinical simulations, and competency-based learning.

Computing matured with the incorporation of widgets, the first spreadsheet program, and expansion of computer drawing and painting programs.[21] Pong debuted as the first commercial computer game. Singer-Link expanded its focus and manufactured power plant simulators in addition to aeronautic models. The company revolutionized the field of computer imaging with its digital image generator (DIG).[11] Visual and hydraulic motion systems improved and brought full-flight simulation (FFS) to aviation. Research in the field of haptics began at the University of North Carolina. The Apollo 13 module was brought home safely with the help of extensive problem-solving using NASA's aeronautic simulators. Ground simulation was also essential to repairs during the Skylab 2 mission. FFS was a reality by the end of the decade.[24a] The first use of a computer to facilitate visualization of anatomy in facial fractures was described in 1974.[27]

Historical Landmarks in the Evolution of Medical Simulation: 1970s

1970s	Link begins to manufacture power plant simulators.
	Massachusetts General Hospital produces computerized clinical encounter simulations.[22]
	University of Illinois develops MERIT simulations for recertification in internal medicine.
	Effectiveness of computer-assisted instruction (CAI) is shown in nonhealth disciplines.[22]
1970	Smaller portable defibrillator, Lifepak 4, is introduced by Physiocontrol.
1972	National Library of Medicine provides sponsorship and free access to medical simulations from Ohio State University, Michigan, and University of Illinois. [22]
1973	CPR is introduced with instruction by AHA and Red Cross.[7]
	University of Wisconsin develops patient encounter simulation prototype that is basis for future NBME computerized examinations.
	Computer-aided modeling of medical physiology is first reported.[28]
	Biomedical computer (BMC) is one of the first medical microcomputers.[28]
1974	AHA publishes first guidelines with support from Laerdal.
1975	Smaller portable defibrillator, Lifepak 5, is produced by Physiocontrol.[20a]
	Standardized patients in medical education is first reported.[29]
	Objective Structured Clinical Examination (OSCE) is first reported.[29]
1978	Singer-Link's DIG (digital image generator) pioneers computer imaging.

1980s

Anesthesiology efforts in this decade focused on patient safety and education. There was increased interest in characterization of medical errors.[30] Cooper founded the Anesthesia Patient Safety Foundation (APSF), the world's first patient safety organization.[31] The International Society for Quality in Health Care (ISQUA) was formed the next year.[32] The APSF was a model for the future development of the National Patient Safety Foundation (NPSF).[33] The ASPF helped to fund the development of the two original full-scale anesthesia patient simulators, and medical education began to explore competency measurement through use of OSCE tests.

Computers continued to grow and prosper. User interfaces matured to resemble those in use today. Meshing of computer text with graphics and video became facile. Medical education was invaded by computer-based simulation, which made irreversible changes. N. Ty Smith used 20 years of experience in cardiovascular physiology and anesthesia to develop the first digital precursor to the current BodySim.[34] It was based on sophisticated multicompartment modeling of physiology and pharmacology. Gas-Man soon followed with its classic computer-based tutorials about anesthetic gas uptake and distribution.[35,36] The first resuscitation-specific software was introduced in 1983. Madscientist software incorporated in 1986 and continued with a variety of acute care products and a unique sense of humor.[37] The Anesthesia Simulator-Recorder, precursor to the Anesoft product line, appeared.[38,39] The first program capable of three-dimensional modeling and manipulation of anatomy was developed as an adjunct to surgery.[40] The value of computers in medical education was realized, and a challenge for efficiency in education through cooperation was proposed.[22] The efficient transfer of diagnostic cardiology skills practiced with simulation to the clinical environment was demonstrated in a multicenter trial using Harvey.[41]

In 1986, Gaba pioneered the construction of C.A.S.E. (Comprehensive Anesthesia Simulation Environment) at Stanford. Gaba partnered with CAE-Link and the full-scale mannequin system was born in 1988. It was a combination of the C.A.S.E. system, the anesthesia simulator-recorder mathematical models, and CAE-link simulation technology.[42] Good and Loral Aviation partnered in a similar but independent effort at the University of Florida in Gainesville that same year. The philosophy and mission of these two simulation groups was distinct and different. The Stanford team was focused on team performance during critical events. They patterned their program after Crew Resource Management from flight simulation and titled it Anesthesia Crisis Resource Management (ACRM).[43] Good and colleagues at Gainesville used their simulator to introduce residents to anesthesia techniques, common errors, and machine failures.

The majority of flight simulation news in the 1980s was related to business and/or government. After the death of founder Edwin Link in 1981, Singer separated Link's general and flight simulation divisions. The company survived to design and produce a fleet of military flight simulators. It also produced its first naval and submarine simulators. In 1988 CAE purchased the flight division from Singer. A report by the FAA covering the period 1962–1972 disclosed horrifying statistics: FAA-required training flights were responsible for eight crashes and 41 deaths. The National Transportation and Safety Board was ordered to find a better solution. Simulation technology advanced sufficiently for U.S. and international aviation regulatory groups to adopt the "zero flight time rules" (ZFT). ZFT authorized the use of high-fidelity simulators for training and evaluation of aviation personnel.[24a] NASA researchers invented modern virtual reality (VR). Members of this development team used the technology to make the first VR surgical simulator that explored the technique of tendon transfer and resultant limb function.[44]

Historical Landmarks in the Evolution of Medical Simulation: 1980s

1980s	Link makes a fleet of military flight simulators as well as naval models for ships and submarines.
	Interactive video files add dimension to patient encounter simulations.[22]
	Personal computers relate to expansion of interest in medical simulation.[22]
1980	First voice recognition computer software research appears.[28]
1981	Edwin Link dies.[11]
	Singer divides simulation into flight and general divisions.[11]
1983	Initial development of automated record keeping.[28]
1984	Utilizing digital computing, the first precursor to Body software is constructed.[28]
1985	First PALS course is given.[6]
	University of Michigan publishes first catalog of patient simulations.[22]
	Effectiveness of computer simulations in medical practice demonstrated.[22]
	Sleeper appears as an early anesthesia software simulator.[28]
1986	C.A.S.E.(Comprehensive Anesthesia Simulation Environment) Standard becomes the precursor of CAE-Link simulator.

CD ROM systems revolutionize medical information storage and retrieval.[22]
CAE-Link patient simulator is born in Palo Alto.
The precursor to METI HPS is born in Gainesville.

1989   Sleeper is adapted for the PC.[28]

1990s

Medical simulation experienced rapid growth in many directions during this decade. General development in computer science and nonmedical simulation produced an indirect effect on medical simulation. In 1990, the world wide web was born, and there was no looking back. The term *virtual reality* was introduced to describe immersive environments. Colonel Satava returned from the Gulf War convinced that there must be a better way to train reservist medical personnel for combat triage readiness.[44] The military was a major impetus in the transfer of modeling and simulation technology to medicine.[45] The military still accounted for 80% of all modeling and simulation work.[46] However, the gaming industry surpassed the military as the driving force in the development of high-resolution graphics.[24a] There was an increase in the diversity (> 140 types) and realism of motion platforms.[24a] Jane's simulation and training system and advanced helicopter simulators were the result. There was a proven savings in terms of both cost and lives for helicopters and military simulators.[47] The three branches of the armed forces established simulation training programs near Orlando.[48–50] An inexpensive modification of the Microsoft Flight Simulator game was adopted for preflight training.[49]

Medical milestones included the first Virtual Human Project and a global interest in patient safety issues. In the Virtual Human Project, the national library of medicine employed imaging data from actual human cadavers to develop anatomic models that allow three-dimensional viewing and manipulation of anatomic structures. These images were the basis for much of the work in surgical simulation, medical virtual reality, and internet-based simulation.[44,48] The U.S. Institute of Medicine focused global attention on medical safety with the release of its report, "To Err is Human." This report estimated that as many as 98,000 patients die annually from medical errors. Quality and safety agencies multiplied. The Japan and Australian Councils for Quality Health Care (JCQHC) were established.[51,52]

The potential for simulation to counteract the dwindling resources for practice of medical skills was recognized. The traditional resources included animals, cadavers, and patients without consent.[53,54] Worldwide acceptance of this type of training grew.[55,56] The endorsement of simulation technology can be summarized by the news headline: "Medical simulation is the wave of the future, U of O doctors say."[57] Institutional, regional, and national simulation centers were established. The Harvard hospitals founded the first large center (Boston Center for Medical Simulation) in 1994. Simulation centers spread throughout the world. The U.S., Europe, and Japan developed dozens of facilities. Collaborative groups and scientific meetings (International Meeting on Medical Simulation and Medicine Meets Virtual Reality) emerged for the exchange of scientific, educational, and administrative ideas.

By the end of the decade, human patient simulation and crisis management began to invade other medical disciplines: military medicine, intensive care medicine, pediatrics, emergency medicine, surgery, trauma, cardiology, and even dentistry.[58a,59a] Emergency medicine and military medicine triage and team-training exercises used multiple simultaneous mannequins.[59] Immersive environments were constructed. The CAVE at the University of Michigan broke new ground with the triage and management of patients in a virtual environment.[60] SimSuite refined its haptic interface and patented its virtual reality interventional cardiology simulator in 1998.[61] A vocabulary was proposed for describing this expanding area of technology.[62]

Computer-based Simulation: Laptop and Internet

A proliferation of PC-based simulation software was stimulated by the increase in power and decrease in cost of the personal computer. Anesoft and its precursors were some of the most prolific developers of acute care simulation software. This effort began at the University of Washington in the 1980s. In the early 1990s, this group produced the Anesthesia Simulator Consultant (1990) and two versions of Rhythm & Pulse (1992–1993) before its incorporation as Anesoft in 1995. Further improvements in the ASC became the Anesthesia Simulator. The ACLS simulator grew from the early versions of Rhythm & Pulse and included automated debriefing.[63] Three additional Anesoft products were introduced in the second half of the decade: Critical Care Simulator (1995), Hemodynamics Simulator (1998), and Sedation Simulator (1998). Body Simulation software was launched in 1992.[28] This DOS-based product was converted to a Windows platform and renamed BODYWIN in 1998.[28]

Many products with a narrower focus were also developed. RELAX, a screen-based simulator from the University of Florida, taught the science of neuromuscular blockade and its monitoring.[64] The Virtual Anesthesia Machine was an on-line tutorial from the same institution.[65] The utilization of pulmonary artery catheters was hotly debated because of the potential for iatrogenic injury and limited efficacy data. The Pulmonary Artery Catheter Education Project (PACEP) was a unique collaboration between several medical and health sciences organizations that attempted to address this controversy through improved, standardized, and free on-line education.[66] Critical Concepts, Inc. offered physiology learning, single-task lessons (ECG, pulmonary function tests. artrial blood gases) and integrated patient care modules (ACLS and clinics) in its software product line.[67] The Physiology Labs integrated traditional text, self-assessment questionnaires, animations, and laboratory exercises.

Computerized Mannequins

The prototypes developed in California and Florida became commercial products during this decade. Growth of the human patient simulation industry was slow at first but accelerated into the next millennium. In 1991–1992, collaboration between Gaba and the Boston Simulation group spurred the development of centers for ARCM training on both coasts.[68a] The CAE-Link simulator was the early leader but began to falter during sequential ownership changes to Eagle and finally MedSim. The only portion of the product to remain in manufacture and sales was Ultrasim. This ultrasound simulation mannequin originated in 1995 and was based on real U.S. patient data sets. It initially replicated abdominal pathology relevant to obstetrics and gynecology but soon expanded to the representation of diverse intra-abdominal problems. It was one of the first mannequin products to include education adjuncts such as course syllabus, instruction manuals, and clinical case presentations.

The Loral-Gainesville simulator showed slower growth than CAE-Link in the first part of the decade but weathered its administrative turnover to Medical Education Technologies (METI) much better. Significant armed forces contracts and the debut of the first full-body pediatric simulator (PediaSim) propelled METI into the role of industry leader by the end of the decade.

As with other innovations in technology, the cost of these new modalities limited the purchase of mannequins to only a small portion of medical centers. Several European centers developed their own computerized simulation mannequins. The University of Basel pioneered Team Oriented Medical Simulation (TOMS) in 1994.[68] TOMS integrated surgical and anesthesia simulation in the simultaneous training of entire operating room teams. PatSim presented several unique features: lip color changes, rashes, sweat, tears, oral secretions, vomit, and bleeding. Less complete or intricate simulators earned the designation of moderate or intermediate fidelity. The ACCESS and Leiden simulators are two examples of economical design.[69,70] Alternatively, sharing of simulation resources through telemedicine was described later in the decade.[71,72]

Several simulators with a much narrower focus were also introduced. Although the Harvey cardiology simulator was a pioneer product, the first full-body version was not launched until the 1990s.[73] In 1992, physicians from Australia recognized the importance of rehearsing the confrontation of critical events during cardiopulmonary bypass and developed the Manbit's perfusion simulator.[74] Gaumard medical pursued an interest in perinatal critical events and developed a birthing simulator that included a newborn mannequin capable of central and peripheral cyanosis.[75]

Surgical Simulation

Two major forces propelled the development of computerized surgical simulation during the 1990s. The adoption of minimally invasive procedures as alternatives to traditional open operations was hampered by an extended long learning curve for these complex technical skills. The Society of American Gastrointestinal Endoscopic Surgeons (SAGES) was the first group to develop guidelines for laparoscopy training in 1991. Lanier created the first simplified vision of intra-abdominal anatomy that allowed the operater to perform a cholecystectomy.[44] Organ elasticity and separation of tissues with cutting appeared next. The KISMET simulator (1993) even incorporated telesurgery. Fidelity and variety of the early surgical simulations were poor but improved rapidly in parallel with technology and computer power. In the early simulators, a choice was made between visual representation and tissue realism. The Limb Trauma Simulator designed for the military is an example. The Minimal Access Therapy Training Unit Scotland (MATTUS) was the first effort at national coordination of training in these procedures.[76]

The second critical event was the completion of the first Visible Human Project by the National Library of Medicine in 1994. This dataset, based on radiologic images from actual patients, enabled accurate three-dimensional reconstruction of anatomy. The Visible Human was available via the internet. Anatomic data files were the basis for later (1996) simulations of the liver and gynecologic organs. Preoperative planning was a prime purpose of these simulations.

Some simulators emphasized the development of eye-hand coordination in a laparoscopic environment. The simple Laparoscopic Training Box (Laptrainer) by U.S. Surgical Corporation facilitated practice of precision pointing, peeling grape or chicken skin, knot tying, and precise movement of objects. The Sinus Surgery Simulator focused on the efficient flight path through navigational guides.[77] The Anastomoses Simulator assessed skills performance through analysis of hand motions for accuracy and pressure. Several centers have developed Objective Assessment of Technical Skills (OSATS) training programs. Laparoscopic trainers have been shown to be an effective training method for the acquisition of skills. Unfortunately, the training transfer from simulated environment has been reported to be only 25%.

Surgical subspecialties also accepted the simulation challenge. An ophthamology simulator (SimEdge) integrated manipulation of haptic instruments with visualization of ophthalmic anatomy through a microscope.[78,79] Two different orthopedic arthroscopy simulators were introduced. The Prosolvia shoulder simulator employed on-line manipulation of instruments by a mouse. The American Board of Orthopedics sponsored the development of a knee arthroscopy simulator by Boston Dynamics for education and certification.

Education

A major shift in the philosophy of medical education occurred during the 1990s. The new theories acknowledged that effective medical management merged knowledge, skills, behavior, and attitudes.[81-83] The traditional apprenticeship model tested only knowledge milestones. Brown University was the first U.S. school to revise its curriculum around the concept of competencies.[80] The Accreditation Council for Graduate Medical Education adopted the six core competencies.[81] Methods for evaluation of physicians expanded to include standardized patients,[19] Objective Scores Clinical Evaluation (OSCE),[82,83] and even computerized simulation.[84] Many of these methods have been time-intensive. The Team OSCE (TOSCE) has been shown to be an efficient and valid method to streamline competency-based testing.[85]

No one has ever proved the validity or value of simulation education and training in any other industry.[86] In fact, David Gaba asserted, "No industry in which human lives depend on the skilled performance of responsible operators has waited for the unequivocal proof of the benefit of simulation before embracing it."[87] Several studies attempted to provide some of these data for medical simulation. On a simple level, students have enjoyed medical simulation exercises.[88] Performance has been shown to be enhanced through simulation.[89] The discovery that residents achieved initial anesthesia skills more rapidly with simulation stimulated many programs to use this technology for orientation.[90] Practice of ACLS algorithms with software-based simulation resulted in greater retention of information than traditional textbook study.[91,92]

Attempts to document validity and reliability of simulation were only partially successful. In one study, agreement was shown for technical but not behavioral ratings.[93] Discriminant or construct validity was demonstrated easily.[94,95] The debate over the use of mannequin-based simulation for competency testing became heated.[96,97] It was suggested that validity will always be elusive and that medicine must ultimately accept simulation on the basis of faith or common sense similar to the aviation industry.[98]

Simulation growth during this decade was sufficient to generate forums for the exchange of techniques, education methods, and research. The first HPS meeting was sponsored by the University of Rochester in 1995. This group partnered with both the Society for Education in Anesthesia and the Society for Technology in Anesthesia to sponsor programs before the International Meeting on Medical Simulation was proposed in 1999. European simulation groups joined together to form a Society for Simulation in Europe (SESAM) that sponsors annual continuing education programs. The Medicine Meets Virtual Reality meeting and *Virtual Medical Worlds* journal were created to share ideas in the domain of medical virtual reality and telemedicine. The journal *Simulation and Gaming* devoted an issue to medical simulation.

Historical Landmarks in the Evolution of Medical Simulation: 1990s

1990	Anesthesia Simulator Consultant (pre-Anesoft anesthesia simulator) appears.
1991	Studies appear in *Health Technology and Infomatics* journal.
1992	Rhythm & Pulse (pre-Anesoft ACLS simulator) appears.
1993	Inaugural Medicine Meets Virtual Reality Conference (MMVR).
	Rhythm & Pulse 2.0 is updated.
	Medical Council of Canada uses standardized patients for assessments.[29]
	Immersion Medical (formerly HT Medical) patents Touchsens technology.
1994	Netscape appears.
1995	Hughes Aircraft buys CAE-Link.[11]
	First University of Rochester Human Patient Simulation Conference.
	Wright's Anesthesia & Critical Care Resources started on the Internet.[99]
	Anesoft founded and releases Anesthesia Simulator 2.0, ACLS Simulator 3.0, and Critical Care Simulator.
1996	Robert Wood Johnson Medical School introduces self-directed computer-based pathology course.[29]
	The Visible Human Initiative is envisioned.[100]
1997	Sophus medical, acute care PC-based simulation, is founded.
	Anesoft Anesthesia and ACLS Simulators are updated.
	MIST VR Trainer is introduced.[101]
1998	Hughes Aircraft Defense Electronics is purchased by Raytheon.[11]
	Medical Simulation Corporation is founded.
	Medical School Objectives Project originated by AAMC.
	Anesoft Hemodynamic and Sedation Simulators are introduced.
	Education Commission for Foreign Medical Graduates (ECFMG) implements clinical skills assessment with standardized patients.[29]
1999	Link facility in Binghampton is closed.[102]
	Pediasim is created by METI.
	UMedic provides a 4-year multimedia computer instruction for cardiology.[29]
	Denx simulator appears for dentistry.[47]

Twenty-first Century: World of Simulation

Military flight simulators are expensive but have proved cost-effective.[24a] Simulation in the civilian transportation industry focused for the first time on events on the ground. Future Flight Central (FFC) is to be the first air traffic control simulation. It will be a full-size control tower with radar and 360° windows. The University of Iowa is working with the National Highway Safety Administration to develop the National Advanced Driving Simulator.

World events are shaping the direction for future simulation growth. The global threat of terrorism brings new initiatives for military training and civilian preparedness for chemical and biological warfare.[103] Medical casualty rates have not improved since introduction of the helicopter to military triage.[104] It is challenging to maintain adequate military readiness during peace time.[105] Future training will employ multimodal simulation, including PC-based exercises, digital mannequins, virtual workbenches, and Total Immersive Virtual Reality (TIVR). The validation of HPS for trauma training of inexperienced military personnel was reported.[106] The military is a major force and source of money for the development of virtual reality in medicine.[107] Even NASA will use medical mannequins to train astronaut flight crews for medical emergencies.[108]

Several key events relevant to the world of medical simulation have already occurred. The 2000 revision of ACLS guidelines was the culmination of attempts to standardize resuscitation training worldwide.[109] One university risk management plan offers decreased insurance premiums for anesthesiologists who take ACRM training.[25] A study describing the current usage of medical simulation reports underutilization of this technology and blames cost as the primary problem.[110] Companies strive to offer lower-price alternatives to full-scale simulation.

Computer-based Simulation: Laptop and Internet

Anesoft updates its five previously introduced products with Browser-applet versions in 2000 and again in 2002. Anesoft launches its sixth product, the Bioterrorism Simulator, in 2002. Automatic online updates will become available to registered Anesoft software users during 2003. A study shows that practice with screen–based simulation improves performance during HPS crisis challenge.[111] The internet is integrated with onsite haptic tools to deliver interactive education in gross anatomy.[112] There is renewed interest in software simulation as a cost-efficient alternative to full-scale or immersive environment simulation.

Mannequin-based Techniques

Cost conservation is also the prime directive for mannequin-based simulation. Expansion of simulation opportunities through interactive teleconferencing continues.[72] Groups collaborate and share resources in multidisciplinary simulation centers. Commercial manufacturers finally offer mid-fidelity simulators at a fraction of the cost of full-scale high-fidelity models. Laerdal introduces the first SimMan mannequin. METI launches its ECS mannequin. SIMA takes a new approach and packages a personal computer, software, monitor interface, eight training scenarios, and simulation training but no mannequin. The delivery room sees the development of another neonatal resuscitation simulator for perinatal crisis intervention.[25,113] Neosim facilitates neonatal CRM despite low mannequin fidelity.[129]

Surgical Simulation

The current progress in surgical simulation is compared with Edwin Link's flight simulator.[44] Unfortunately, fidelity is the inverse of complexity.[44] Experience with endoscopy simulators grows. Preparatory training on the Endoscopic Surgical Simulator (ESS) improves operating room performance for junior otolaryngology residents. The bronchoscopy trainer advances skills in the removal of foreign bodies.[114] The National Capital Area Medical Simulation Center envisions virtual environment triage simulation and the introduction of a surgical airway simulator in the future.[115,116] An immersive virtual reality for laparoscopic cholecystectomy, designated REMIS, is introduced.[117] HT Medical refines its intravenous catheter simulator and predicts the development of similar simulators for peritoneal lavage and pericardiocentesis.[115]

Virtual Reality

As Satava observes, "The greatest power of virtual reality is the ability to try and fail without consequence to animal or patient. It is only through failure—and learning the cause of failure—that the true pathway to success lies." There is a proliferation of commercial virtual medical environments. SimSuite by Medical Simulation Corporation (MSC) is the first interventional cardiology training system. MSC gains support from the American College of Cardiology. Together they outfit a mobile SimSuite training unit. Seattle's Swedish Heart Institute and Geisinger Health System in Pennsylvania are the first fixed installations. MSC anticipates an additional 12–15 SimSuite centers in 2003. A second interventional system is developed at Mitsubishi Electric. The simulated factors include fluoroscopy, catheter physics, hemodynamics, haptics, and fluid flow.[118]

Modern Education

Human patient simulation (HPS) becomes accepted in undergraduate medical education. Even some medical licensing exams have evolved to include standardized patient and computerized simulations.[119] Italian medical license exams use a combination of computer-based simulation and standardized patients.[120] Harvey simulator teaches introduction to physical diagnosis and clinical skills.[121] HPS replaces animal exercises and demonstrates physiology at some institutions.[122,123] HPS is validated and used to evaluate medical students' acute care airway skills.[124,124a,125a] A unique program of on-demand multidisciplinary simulation debuts for medical student training in Boston.[125] Simulators are used to present abnormal physical findings during a standardized patient exam.[126] Communication skills are assessed during wound suturing or urinary catheterization through use of standardized patients and a lower-body mannequin.[127] The value of real-life scenarios in problem- and case-based learning is demonstrated.[128] Difficulty of learning cases and task trainers in medical education are assessed and compared.[129,129a,130a] Research describes simulation training lasting over 90 minutes as too fatiguing. The optimal duration for a simulation training session is 75–90 min.[149]

Medical educators acknowledge that simulation is the future of medical education.[130a] They recommend that we embrace the technology and control its evolution in medical education before business and government seize the opportunity. Critical thinking is essential in acute health care. Simulation offers the best hope for teaching and evaluating medical problem solving.[130] Several surgical groups propose the integration of simulation technology into surgical education and evaluation. Advanced Trauma Life Support courses, which employ HPS, show an enhancement of the acquisition of trauma management skills, with residents describing an increase in confidence.[131] Anesthetists from New Zealand value ACRM and recommend a review every two years.[132] Evidence accumulates for the validity and reliability of simulation assessment.[133,134] Data about the expected learning curves for anesthesia skills in clinical practice provide a basis for training with simulation.[135]

The imperative to collaborate and exchange ideas continues to grow.[136] Multiple meetings are held each year. Journals devoted to the topics of health informatics and simulation multiply. The *Journal for Education in Perioperative Medicine* and the *Human Simulation Web Community*, two internet-based resources, offer peer-reviewed publication for simulation education materials.[137,138]

The Future

The U.S. government is currently funding several efforts in the fields of medical simulation and patient safety.[139] One group will explore the question, "Does simulation reduce the time to learn clinical skills?," using one of the new interventional cardiology systems. Hardware and software or internet simulations will measure the training of surgeons, anesthesiologists, and other health care personnel about patient safety in diverse projects. One broad project will explore the construction of a national web-based morbidity and mortality conference to discuss near-misses in an anonymous, blame-free environment. Development of neonatal/pediatric simulation training program is in progress. The Visible Human Initiative, a complex integrated multimodal project, is predicted to be the future of simulation.[56]

In a 2003 keynote address, Loftin summarized the challenges for the future of medical simulation. Some challenges are common to many worlds of simulation. The most familiar is fidelity. Other common problems are human-simulator interfaces, interoperability of simulators, curriculum integration, embedded feedback, data representation, and cost. The grand challenges are unique to the world of medical modeling and simulation. The overwhelming difficulty is the representation of human tissues and their physiology by physics-based and mathematical formulas in real time. Integration of simulation modalities including standardized patients in a seamless manner is another key concern. The final question addresses the clinical relevance of simulation both in terms of transfer of training to the patient care environment and assessment of competency.[140]

Historical Landmarks in the Evolution of Medical Simulation: 2000 and After

2000   L3 communications purchases flight simulation and training from Raytheon.[11]
         Inaugural International Meeting on Medical Simulation takes place.
         Laerdal SimMan begins beta testing.
2001   METI releases the Emergency Care Simulator (ECS).
         Sophus partners with Laerdal.
2002   Medical Simulation Corporation's SimSuite opens first two centers. Seattle's
         Swedish heart Institute and Geisinger Health System in Pennsylvania.
         Anesoft creates Bioterrorism Simulator.
2003   David Gaba receives the Society for Education in Anesthesia's Duke Prize for
         innovation in anesthesia education.

References

1. Smith C, Daniel P: Simulation technology: A strategy for implementation in surgical education and certification. Presence: Tele-operators and Virtual Environments 2000;9(6).
2. Buck GH: Development of simulators in medical education. Gesnerus 1991;48(Pt 1):7–28.
2a. Harris SB: The Society for the Recovery of Persons Apparently Dead. Skeptic 1992;1:24–31. *http://www.skeptic.com/01.2.harris-dead.html* [accessed 2-2-2004].
3. Laerdal. The girl from the river seine. *http://www.laerdal.no/preview.asp?docID=1117082* [last accessed 5-30-2003].
4. Laerdal History. *http://www.laerdal.com/document.asp?docID=1117121* [last accessed 5-30-2003].
5. Thangam S, Weil MH, Rackow EC: Cardiopulmonary resuscitation: A historical review. Acute Care 1986;12:63–94.
5a. Hart First Response: A History of Resuscitation: *http://www.hartfirstresponse.org.uk/CPRhistory.html* [accessed 2-2-2004].
6. Fischer J: Pre-hospital pediatric cardiac arrest: What affects outcome? *http://pediatric-emergency.com/Arreslx4.htm* [last accessed 5-30-2003].

7. History of CPR: *http://www.ukdivers.net/history/cpr.htm* [last accessed 5-30-2003].
8. Mackie I: The history of resuscitation in Australia. *http://slsa.asn.au/upload/documents/s10159712328559_ SLSA_CPR_History.pdf* [last accessed 5-30-2003].
8a. Doyle DJ: Airway management in the electronic age. Am J Anesthesiol 2001;28(3):124–127.
9. Stoller JK: The history of intubation, tracheotomy, and airway appliances. Respir Care 1999;44:595–601.
10. Waisel DB: The role of World War II and the European theater of operations in the development of anesthesiology as a physician specialty in the USA. Anesthesia 2001;94:907–914.
10a. University of Wisconsin, Department of Anesthesiology, Department of History: *http://www.anesthesia.wisc.edu/history.html* [accessed 2-24-2004].
11. Alaniz M: Life after link: A brief history and lineage of our CAE_Link Silver Spring Operation. *http://www.grinet.com/LAL/linkstory.htm* [last accessed 5-30-2003].
11a. L3 Communications. Link simulation and training: Setting the standard for over 70 years. *http://www.link.com/history* [accessed 2-24-2004].
12. Corporate Info: *http://www.medicalplastics.com/corporate-info.html* [last accessed 5-30-2003].
13. Tomayko JE: Computers in spaceflight: The NASA Experience. (Kent A, Williams JG. eds): http://www.hq.nasa.gov/pao/History/computers/Ch9–2.html [last accessed 5-30-2003].
14. History of paramedics. Nov 20, 1986. http://www.monroecc.edu/depts/pstc/parashis.htm [last accessed 5-30-2003].
15. Zoll PM, Linenthal AJ, Norman LR, et al: Treatment of unexpected cardiac arrest by external electrical stimulation of the heart. N Engl J Med 1956;254:541–546.
16. Gravenstein JS: Simulation for training, learning, and testing in anesthesia. *http://www.anaesthesiologie.med.uni-erlangen.de/esctaic97/a_graven.htm* [last accessed 5-30-2003].
17. Abrahamson S, Denson JS, Wolf RM: Effectiveness of a simulator in training anesthesiology residents. J Med Educ 1969;44:515–519.
18. Denson JS, Abrahamson A: Computer-controlled patient simulator. JAMA 1969;208:504–508.
19. Barrows HS: An overview of the uses of standardized patients for teaching and evaluating clinical skills. Acad Med 1993 68:443–453.
19a. Computers in spaceflight: The NASA experience: *http://www.hq.nasa.gov/pao/History/computers/Ch9-2.html* [accessed 2-26-2004].
20. Hay PJ, Katsikitis M: The 'expert' in problem-based and case-based learning: Necessary or not? Med Educ 2001;35:22–26.
20a. Bonadonna P. History of paramedics: *http://www.monroecc.edu/depts./pstc/parashis.htm* [accessed 2-25-2004].
21. Myers BA: A brief history of human computer interaction technology. ACM Interact 1998;5:44–54.
22. Piemme TE: Computer-assisted learning and evaluation in medicine. JAMA 1988;260:367–372.
23. Center for Research in Medical Education at University of Miami, *http://www.crme.med.miami.edu/harvey_about.html* [accessed 2-26-2004].
24. Howells TH, Emery FM, Twentyman JEC: Endotracheal intubation using a simulator: An evaluation of the laerdal adult intubation model in the teaching of endotracheal intubation. Br J Anaesth 1973;45:400–402.
24a. Strachan IW: Leaps all around propel advances in simulators. Nat Defense Mag Nov: 2000. Available at *http://www.nationaldefensemagazine.org/index.cfm.*
25. Friedrich MJ: Practice makes perfect: Risk-free medical training with patient simulation. JAMA 2002;288:2808–2812.
26. Hardin RM, Gleeson PA: Assessment of clinical competence using an objective scaled clinical examination (OSCE) Med Educ 1979;13:41–54.
27. Fujino T, Calderhead RG: Historical overview. In Advances in Simulation and Computer-aided Surgery. Sussex, John Wiley & Sons, 1994, pp 11–16.
28. Smith NT: Thirty-five years with a computer. Personal communication, Febuary 25 2003
29. Lane JL, Slavin S, Ziv A: Simulation in medical education: A review. Simulat Gam 2001;32:297–314.
30. Cooper JB, Newbower R, Kitz R: An analysis of major errors and equipment failures in anesthesia management: Considerations for prevention and detection. Anesthesiology 1984;60:34–42.
31. Cooper JB, Pierce EC: Safety foundation organized: http://www.gasnet.org/societies/apsf/newsletter/1986/spring/#article%201 [last accessed 5-30-2003].
32. General Information: *http://www.isqua.org.au/isquaPages/General.html* [last accessed 5-30-2003].
33. About the foundation: *http://www.npsf.org/html/about_npsf.html* [last accessed 5-30-2003].
34. Advanced Simulation Corporation: http://www.advsim.com/BodySim/index.htm [last accessed 5-30-2003].
35. Philip JH: Understanding anesthesia inhalation uptake and distribution. *http://www.gasmanweb.com* [last accessed 5-30-2003].
36. Phillip JH: GASMAN: An example of goal oriented computer-assisted teaching which results in learning. Int J Clin Monit Comput 1986;69:387–394.

37. Mad Scientist Software, Inc: *http://www.madsci.com* [last accessed 5-30-2003].
38. Schwid HA: The anesthesia simulator-recorder: A device to train and evaluate anesthesiologists' responses to critical incidents. Anesthesiology 1990;72:191–197.
39. Schwid HA: A flight simulator for general anesthesia. Comput Biomed Res 1987;20:64–75.
40. Marsh JL, Vannier MW: The "third" dimension in craniofacial surgery. Plast Reconst Surg 1983;71:759–767.
41. Ewy, GA, Felner JM, Juul D, et al: Test of a cardiology patient simulator with students in fourth year electives. J Med Educ 1987;62:738–743.
42. Gaba DM: Simulator training in anesthesia growing rapidly, CAE model born at Stanford. J Clin Monit 1996;12:195–198.
43. Anesthesia Crisis Resource Management of the Simulation Center for Crisis Management Training in Health Care (Gaba D, director). *http://anesthesia.stanford.edu/VASimulator/acrm.htm* [last accessed 5-30-2003].
44. Satava RM: Accomplishments and challenges of surgical simulation: Dawning of the next-generation surgical education. Surg Endosc 2001;15:232–241.
45. Loftin B: Med School 1.0: Can computer simulation aid physician training? Quest 5: 2002;5:16–19.
46. Drake J: Commercial simulaton market drives industry's future growth. National Defense Magazine Nov. 1998. *http://www.nationaldefensemagazine.org/index.cfm* [last accessed 5-30-2003].
47. Ziv A, Small SD, Wolpe PR: Patient safety and simulation-based medical education. Med Teacher 2000;22:489–495.
48. U.S. ARMY PEO STRI: *http://www.stricom.army.mil/* [last accessed 5-30-2003].
49. Kennedy H: Simulation reshaping military training: Technology jumping from teenagers' computers to pilots' cockpits. National Defense Magazine Nov. 1999. *http://www.nationaldefensemagazine.org/article.cfm?Id=113* [last accessed 5-30-2003].
50. Ackerman JM: The visible human project 1992. Proc IEEE 1992;86:504–511.
51. About the Japan Council for Quality Health Care. *http://jcqhc.or.jp/html/english/about_jcqhc.htm* [last accessed 5-30-2003].
52. Australian Council for Safety and Quality in Health Care: About us. http://www.safetyandquality.org/index.cfm?page=About [last accessed 5-30-2003].
53. Feldman DS, Novack DH, Farber NJ, Fleetwood J: The ethical dilemma of students learning to perform procedures on non-consenting patients. Acad Med 1999;74:79.
54. Ardagh M: May we practice endotracheal intubation on the newly dead? J Med Ethics 1997;23:289–294.
55. Riley RH, Wilks DH, Freeman JA: Anaesthetists attitudes toward an anesthesia simulator. A comparative survey: USA and Australia. Anaesth Intens Care 1997;25:514–519.
56. Kurrek MM, Fish KJ: Anaesthesia risis management training: An intimidating concept, a rewarding experience. Can J Anaesth 1996;43:430–434.
57. Cohen L: Medical simulation is the wave of the future, U of O doctors say. Can Med Assoc J 1999;160:557.
58. Arne R, Stale F, Ragna K, Petter L: PatSim—Simulator for practicing anaesthesia and intensive care. Development and observations. Int J Clin Monit Comput 1996;13:147–152.
58a. Watterson L, Flanagan B, Donovan B, Robinson B: Anaesthetic simulator: Training for the broader health-care profession. Aust NZ J Surg. 2000;70(10): 735–737. PMID: 11021488 [PubMed—indexed for MEDLINE].
59. Small SD, Wuerz RC, Simon R, et al: Demonstration of high-fidelity simulation team training for emergency medicine. Acad Emerg Med 1996;4:3123.
59a. Ellis C, Hughes G: Use of human patient simulation to teach emergency medicine trainees advanced airway skills. J Accid Emerg Med 1999;16:395–399.
60. Medical Readiness Trainer at the University of Michigan. Dec 20, 2002. *http://www-vrl.umich.edu/mrt/index.html* [last accessed 5-30-2003].
61. SimSuite Education Centers of the Medical Simulation Corporation: *http://www.simsuiteed.com/ReadArticle.asp?articleId=206* [last accessed 5-30-2003].
62. Meller G: A topology of simulators for medical education. J Dig Imaging 1997.
63. Schwid HA: Components of an effective medical simulation software solution. Simulat Gaming 2001;32(2):240–249.
64. Ohrn MAK, van Oostrom JH, van Meurs WI: A comparison of traditional textbook and interactive computer teaching of neuromuscular block. Anesth Analg 1997;84:657–661.
65. Lampotang S, Dobbins W, Good ML, et al: *http://www.anest.ufl.edu/~eduweb/vam* [last accessed 5-30-2003].
66. Pulmonary Artery Catheter Education Project: http://www.pacep.org [last accessed 5-30-2003].
67. Critical Concepts, Inc: http://www.critcon.com/ccionline/php/main.php3?SID=&UID=-1&Action=100&CID=0 [last accessed 5-30-200].

68. Team Oriented Medical Simulation (TOMS) in Switzerland: *http://www.gasnet.org/societies/apsf/newsletter/1996/spring/apsfled_betzen.html* [last accessed 5-30-2003].
68a. Gaba D: Simulation training growing rapidly. CAE Model born at Stanford. APSF Newslett *http://www.apsf.org/loadurl/loadurl.php?www.gasnet.org/societies/apsf/newsletter/1995/fall/simulator.html* [accessed 2-26-2004].
69. Byrne AJ, Hilton PJ, Lunn J: Basic simulations in anaesthesia: A pilot study of the ACCESS system. Anaesthesia 1994;49:376–381.
70. Chopra V, Engbers FH, Geerts MJ, et al: The Leiden anaesthesia simulator. Br J Anaesth 1994;73:287–292.
71. Tooley MA, Forrest FC, Mantripp DR: MultiMed-remote interactive medical simulation. J TeleMed Telecare 1999;5(Suppl 1):S119-S121.
72. Cooper JB, Barron D, Blum R: Video teleconferencing with realistic simulation for medical education. J Clin Anesth 2000;12:256–261.
73. St. Clair EW, Oddone EZ, Waugh RA, et al: Assessing housestaff diagnostic skills using a cardiology patient simulator. Ann Intern Med 1992;117:751–756.
74. Sydney Perfusion Simulator: http://www.manbit.com/SPS.htm [last accessed 5-30-2003].
75. Obstetrics/childbirth simulators. Gaumard Scientific Company, Inc: *http://www.gaumard.com/html/oci.html* [last accessed 5-30-2003].
76. Cuschieri A, Wilson RG, Sunderland G: Training initiative list scheme (TILS) for minimal access therapy: The MATTUS experience. J R Coll Surg Edinb 1997;42(5):295–302.
77. Edmond CV: Impact of endoscopic sinus surgical simulator on operating room performance. Laryngoscope 2002;112:1148–1158.
78. SimEdge SA: *http://perso.wanadoo.fr/simedge/flash/english* [last accessed 5-30-2003].
79. Sinclair MJ, Peifer JW, Haleblian R, et al: Computer-simulated eye surgery: A novel teaching method for residents and practitioners. Ophthalmology 1995;102:517–521.
80. Smith SR, Dollase RH, Boss JA: Assessing students' performances in a competency-based curriculum. Acad Med 2003;78(1):97–107.
81. Core Competencies of the ACGME: http://www.acgme.org/outcome/comp/compMin.asp [last accessed 5-30-2003].
82. Roberts J, Norman G: Reliability and learning from the objective structured clinical exam. Med Educ 1990;24:219–223.
83. Matsell DG, Wolfish NM, Hau E: Reliability and validity of the objective structured clinical exam in paediatrics. Med Educ 1991;25;293–299.
84. Stevens RH, Kwak AR, McCoy JM: Evaluating preclinical medical students by using computer-based problem-solving examinations. Acad Med 1989;64 685–687.
85. Singleton A, Smith F, Harris T, et al: An evaluation of the Team Objective Structured Clinical Examination (TOSCE). Med Educ 1999;33:34–41.
86. Rall M: Editorial: Symposium: Simulation in anaesthesia and intensive care medicine 2000. Annual Meeting of the Society in Europe for Simulation Applied to Medicine (SESAM). Eur J Anaesthesiol 2000;515–516.
87. Gaba DM: Improving anesthesiologist's performance by simulating reality. Anesth 1992;76:491–494.
88. Holzman RS, Cooper JB, Gaba DM, et al: Anesthesia crisis resource management: real-life simulation training in operating room crises. J Clin Anesth 1995;7:675–687.
89. Chopra V, Gesink BJ, de Jong J, et al: Does training on an anaesthesia simulator lead to improvement in performance? Br J Anaesth 1994;73:293–297.
90. Good et al: Can simulation accelerate the learning of basic anesthesia skills by beginning anesthesia residents? Anesthesiology 1992;77:A1133.
91. Schwid HA, O'Donnel D: Anesthesiologists' Management of simulated critical incidents. Anesthesiology 1992;76:495–501.
92. Schwid HA, Rooke GA, Ross BK, Sivarajan M: Use of a computerized advanced cardiac life support simulator improves retention of advanced cardiac life support guidelines better than a textbook review. Crit Care Med 1999;27:821–824.
93. Gaba DM, Howard SK, Flanagan B, ET AL: Assessment of clinical performance during simulated crises using both technical and behavioral ratings. Anesthesiology 1998;89:8–18.
94. Devitt JH, Kurrek MM, Cohen MM, et al: Testing the raters: inter-rater reliability of standardized anaesthesia simulator performance. Can J Anaesth 1997;44:924–928.
95. Devitt JH, Kurrek MM, Cohen MM, et al; Testing internal consistency and construct validity of during evaluation of performance in a patent simulator. Anesth Analg 1998;86:1160–1164.
96. Kapur PA, Steadman RH: Patient simulator competency testing: Ready for take-off? Anesth Analg 1998;86:1157–1159.

97. Forrest F, Taylor M: High level simulators in medical education. Hosp Med 1998;59:653–655.
98. Tarver S: Anesthesia simulators: Concepts and applications. Am J Anesthesiol 1999;26:393–396.
99. Wright AJ: Wright's Anesthesia and Critical Care Resources on the Internet, 1995: *http://www.eur.nl/FGG/ANEST/wright/contents.html* [last accessed 5-30-2003].
100. Ward RC: The virtual human project, 1996: *http://www.ornl.gov/~rwd/info.html* [last accessed 5-30-2003].
101. Haluck RS, Webster RW, Snyder AJ, et al: A virtual reality surgical trainer for navigation in laparoscopic surgery. Medicine Meets Virtual Reality 2001;171–177.
102. Latham :. Facility in Binghamton, once Link's, to close. CGSD Newslett 1999: *http://www.cgsd.com/CGSDnews/CGSDnews10.html* [last accessed 5-30-2003].
103. Vardi A, Levin I, Berkenstadt H, et al: Simulation-based training of medical teams to manage chemical warfare casualities. Isr Med Assoc J 2002 4:540–544.
104. Myjak MD, Rosen J: MEDNET: A medical simulation network grand challenge. Stud Health Technol Inform 2001;81:341–347.
105. Moses G, Magee JH, Bauer JJ, Leitch R: Military medical modeling in the 21st century. Stud Health Technol Inform 2001;81:322–328.
106. Holcomb JB, et al: Evaluation of trauma team performance using an advanced human patient simulator for resuscitation training. J Trauma 2002;52:1078–1085.
107. Leitch RA, Moses GR, Magee H: Simulation and the future of military medicine. Mil Med 2002;167:350–354.
108. Dawson DL, Billica RD, McDonald PV. Modeling and simulation for space medicine operations: preliminary requirements considered. Stud Health Technol Inform 2001;81:106–112.
109. American Heart Association in collaboration with the International Liaison Committee on Resuscitation: Guidelines 2000 for Cardiopulmonary Resuscitation and Emergency Cardiovascular Care. Circulation 2000;22;102
110. Morgan PJ, Cleave-Hogg D: A worldwide survey of the use of simulation in anesthesia. Can J Anaesth 2002;49:659–662.
111. Schwid HA, Rooke GA, Michalowski P, Ross BK: Screen-based anesthesia simulation with debriefing improves performance in a mannequin-based anesthesia simulator. Teach Learn Med 2001;13(2):92–96.
112. Dev P, Montgomery K, Senger S, et al: Simulated medical learning on the internet. J Am Med Inform Assoc 2002;9(5):437–447.
113. Halamek LP, Kaegi DM, Gaba DM, et al: Time for a new paradigm in pediatric medical education: Teaching neonatal resuscitation in a simulated delivery room environment. Pediatrics 2000;106(4):E45.
114. Hilmi OJ, White PS, McGurty DW, Oluwole M: Bronchoscopy training: Is simulated surgery effective? Clin Otolaryngol 2002;27:267–269.
115. Kaufmann C, Liu A. Trauma training: Virtual reality applications. Stud Health Technol Inform 2001;81:236–241.
116. Surgical Simulation Laboratory of NCA Medical Simulation Center. Uniformed Services University of the Health Sciences: *http://www.simcen.org/surgery/* [last accessed 5-30-2003].
117. Witzke DB, Hoskins JD, Mastrangelo MJ, et al: Immersive virtual reality used as a platform for perioperative training for surgical residents. Stud Health Technol Inform 2001;81:577–583.
118. Cotin S, Dawson SL, Meglan D, et al: ICTS, an Interventional Cardiology Training System. Stud Health Technol Inform 2000;70;59–65.
119. Helwig D: Memorial's dramatic Dean: Can drama help medical students learn? Can Med Assoc J 1989;140:1364–1365.
120. Guagnano MT, Merlitti D, Manigrasso MR, et al: New medical licensing exam using computer-based case simulations and standardized patients. Acad Med 2002;77:87–90.
121. Karnath B, Frye AW, Holden MD: Teaching and testing physical examination skills without the use of patients. Acad Med 2002;77:753.
122. Euliano TY, Good ML: Simulator training in anesthesia growing rapidly, Loral model born in Florida. J Clin Monit 1997;13:53–57.
123. Zvara DA, Olympio MA, MacGregor DA: Teaching cardiovascular physiology using patient simulation. Acad Med 2001;76:534.
124. Rogers PL, Jacob H, Thomas EA, et al: Medical students can learn the basic application, analytic, evaluative and psychomotor skills of critical care medicine. Crit Care Med 2000; 28:550–554.
124a. Morgan PJ, Cleave-Hogg DM, Guest CB, Herold J: Validity and reliability of undergraduate performance assessments in an anesthesia simulator. Can J Anaesth 2001;48:225–233.
125. Gordon JA, Pawlowski J: Education on-demand: The development of a simulator-based medical education service. Acad Med 2002;77:751–752

125a. Murray D, Boulet J, Ziv A, et al: An acute care skills evaluation for graduating medical students: a pilot study using clinical simulation. Med Educ 2002;36(9):833–841. PMID:12354246 [PubMed—indexed for MEDLINE].
126. Karanth B, Frye AW, Holden MD: Incorporating simulators in a standardized patient exam. Acad Med 2002;77:754–755.
127. Kneebone R, Kidd J, Nestel D, et al: An Innovative model for teaching and learning clinical procedures. Med Educ 2002;36:628–634.
128. Dammers J, Spencer J, Thomas M.: Using real patients in problem-based learning: Students' coments on the value of using real, as opposed to paper cases, in a problem-based learning module in general practice. Med Educ 2001;35:27–34.
129. Gercama AJ, de Haan M, van der Vleuten CPM: Reliability of the Amsterdam Clinical Challenge Scale (ACCS), a new Instrument to assess level of difficulty of patient cases in medical education. Med Educ 2000;43:519–524.
129a. Stringer KR, Bajenov S, Yentis SM: Training in airway management. Anaesthesia 2002;57:967–983.
130. Rauen CA: Using simulation to teach critical thinking skills: You can't just throw the book at them. Crit Care Nurs Clin North Ame 2001;93–103.
130a. Owen H, Plummer JL: Improved learning of a clinical skill: The first year's experience of teaching endotracheal intubation in a clinical simulation facility. Med Educ 2002;36:635–642.
131. Marshall RL, Smith JS, Gorman PJ, et al: Use of a human patient simulator in the development of resident trauma management skills. J Trauma 2001;51:17–21.
132. Garden A, Robinson B, Weller J, et al: Education to address medical error: A role for high fidelity patient simulation. N Z Med J 2002;115:133–134.
133. Schwid HA, Rooke GA, Carline J, et al. Evaluation of anesthesia residents using mannequin-based simulation. Anesthesiology 2002;97:1434–1444.
134. Faulkner H, Regehr G, Martin J, Reznick R: Validation of an objective structured assessment of technical skills for surgical residents. Acad Med 1996;71(12):1363–1365.
135. Filho GRO: The construction of learning curves for basic skills in anesthetic procedures: An application for the cumulative sum method. Anesth Analg 2002;95:411–416.
136. Girard M, Drolet P: Anesthesiology simulators: Networking is the key. Can J Anaesth 2002;49:647–649.
137. Journal of Education in Perioperative Medicine. Schubert A (ed): *http://www.jepmadmin.org* [last accessed 5-30-2003].
138. Simdot: Human Simulation Web Community. Taekmon JM (ed): *http://www.simdot.org/simcenter/libSim/simdot* [last accessed 5-30-200].
139. Disseminating research results. In Agency for Healthcare Research and Quality: *http://www.ahcpr.gov/qual/newgrants/dissem.htm* [last accessed 5-30-2003].
140. Loftin RB: Grand challenges in medical modeling and simulation [to appear in the Proceedings from the Western Multiconference 2003].

Chapter 2

CURRENT STATUS OF SIMULATION IN EDUCATION AND RESEARCH

Martin A. Reznek, MD

In the traditional model of health care education, the patient remains the cornerstone of teaching. Since the earliest days of medicine, students have relied on live patients to acquire and hone their diagnostic, therapeutic, and procedural skills. Through the years, many health care educators have found serious ethical and practical flaws in the live patient-based system and have searched for alternatives with little success; investigations of mock patients, plastic models, cadavers, and animals have found them to be inferior teaching modalities.[1,2] Due to this historic lack of acceptable alternatives, health care educators have continued to rely on the live patient-based training system despite its significant flaws.

Recently, however, advances in computer technology over the past two decades have enabled the introduction of two new, highly promising teaching applications for health care: high-fidelity computer-enhanced mannequin simulation (CEMS) and virtual reality (VR). Because computer simulation technology is in the early stages of development, its merits in health care education have yet to be proved. However, as this technology develops further and becomes more widely accepted, many health care educators believe that CEMS and VR will prove to be ethically, fiscally, practically, and educationally more sound than live patient training.[3–6] As simulation technology in general advances and as more health care applications are developed, this technology stands to augment the current system of health care education and eventually may even replace it.

Despite the fact that health care-related computer simulation technology is only in its infancy, numerous applications already have been developed, and many are currently being used or tested in health care training. This chapter provides an overview of the current status of CEMS and VR in health care education.

Simulation: Definition and Rationale

Simulation is the act of mimicking a real object, event, or process by assuming its appearance or outward qualities.[3] To be an effective teaching tool, a simulator must provide realistic and educationally sound feedback to a user's questions, decisions, and actions.[7] Sufficient realism should be present for the user to suspend disbelief; however, a simulator does not need to be identical to real life to accomplish this goal.[8]

In the arena of health care education, simulation has many potential benefits over live patient training. From an ethical standpoint, simulation is much more sound. The existence of learning curves in medicine has been well demonstrated.[9–16] For this reason, patients experience additional risks when students are learning and practicing their skills.

In addition to its ethical merits, simulation also is likely to prove educationally superior to live patient-based education for several reasons. First, the clinical setting is not an optimal arena for learning because it is specifically designed for patient care and safety and not necessarily for student education. Because simulation involves no risk to patients, the training scenarios and the simulators themselves can be designed solely with the goal of optimizing the educational experience. With simulation-based training, students also have the opportunity to repeat lessons as many times as necessary to achieve success and proficiency. But probably even more important is the fact that, when training with simulation, students have the opportunity to learn from their mistakes. In the real world, supervisors are obligated to intervene before students make a mistake on a live patient; thus, the students often miss experiencing the negative outcomes of their actions. Learning from one's errors is reported to be highly effective and possibly even superior to standard methods of learning.[17–19]

Simulation-based education is also potentially more efficient than live patient-based teaching. When relying on real patients for teaching opportunities, students become dependent on random chance. They must wait for the arrival of patients with specific issues that need to be learned; therefore, there is no guarantee that they will learn all of the lessons that they require. In fact, the majority of students will not have the opportunity to experience rare diseases or procedures even once during their training. With simulation, however, learning opportunities can be guaranteed and even repeated multiple times. Furthermore, lessons can take place at times that are convenient for both students and educators because they are not constrained by financial or safety concerns inherent in the clinical setting. With simulation, teachers and students can focus all of their attention on the learning tasks at hand. In addition, simulation lends itself easily to recording; thus, students and teachers can review the students' performances as many times as necessary. Finally, simulation has the potential to be more cost-efficient than live patient-based training because the instruments are reusable, fewer iatrogenic injuries are likely to occur, and live patient care is more efficient when less constrained by teaching requirements.[4]

Computer-enhanced Mannequin Simulation: Background and Current Technology

The birth of modern simulation as well as the majority of advances in the field can be credited to the aerospace industry. Flight simulation was conceived in 1929 when Edwin Link designed an amusement park ride that gave the sensation of flying a plane; he later modified the design into the Link Flight Simulator.[6] Training with this primitive simulator was associated with a 90% reduction in nighttime and bad-weather accidents.[4] The modern flight simulator incorporates computer-generated displays and is much more realistic; however, the original principles remain the same today. The success of this type of training and its cost-effectiveness in the aerospace sector are well documented.[20,21] Other industries as diverse as the military, business management, transportation, and nuclear power followed the aerospace industry and also found success with computer-based simulation.[3,7,22]

In medicine, anesthesiologists were the first to explore this technology. The earliest computer-enhanced patient simulator, Sim One, was introduced in 1967 at the University of Southern California. This simulator consisted of a life-sized mannequin connected to a computer, an instructor's console, an interfacing unit, and an anesthesia machine. Sim One was able to simulate blood pressure abnormalities, several cardiac arrhythmias, airway compromise, and cardiac arrest.[23] Advances in computer and simulation technology have allowed major improvements in patient simulators since Sim One; however, the original concept and general design endure today.

At present, several different patient simulators of varying complexity and realism are in existence. The most advanced and comprehensive of these simulators is the Human Patient Simulator (HPS) (Medical Education Technologies, Inc. [METI], Sarasota, FL).[24] The HPS has more than 40 realistic findings in seven anatomic areas.[7] Anatomically correct clinical signs include breath sounds associated with chest rise, heart sounds, palpable pulses (carotid, brachial, femoral, radial, and pedal), peripheral blood pressure, pupillary reflexes, muscle twitch from nerve stimulation, and urine output. In addition, the mannequin is able to speak by way of a microphone from the operator. Each of these clinical signs is physiologically appropriate and dynamic during simulation. For example, during an asthma exacerbation the mannequin wheezes, and during hypotension the radial, femoral, brachial, and carotid pulses disappear at pressures of 90, 80, 70, and 60 mmHg, respectively. In addition, the HPS can simulate extremity, intrathoracic, and intrabdominal bleeding as well as increased salivation and lacrimation. The HPS includes its own real-time monitoring system that provides the simulated patient's electrocardiogram, respired carbon dioxide levels, pulse oximetry signal, invasive pressures (arterial, central venous, and pulmonary artery), cardiac output, and temperature. If desired, the simulator can also be set up to interface with conventional monitoring devices. All physical findings of the HPS, as well as the signals to the monitoring devices, can be modified by the operator as needed or automatically by the computer during a scenario. The simulator is programmed to respond appropriately to more than 50 medications and several physical interventions, including intubation (accidental endobronchial or esophageal intubation are possible), chest compression, ventilation, electrocardioversion, cricothyroidotomy (the airway can be automatically altered to make intubation difficult or impossible), needle decompression of the chest, chest tube thoracostomy, pericardiocentesis, peritoneal lavage, and insertion of peripheral venous and arterial catheters as well as central venous lines. The HPS has approximately 25 preprogrammed patients; each has a unique base-line physiology reflecting the simulated patient's age, gender, and medical history. In addition, more than 40 different preprogrammed medical scenarios can be simulated on these patients. If additional patients or scenarios are desired, they are easy to design and program. A few examples of possible scenarios include myocardial ischemia/infarction, asthma exacerbation, pneumothorax, pericardial tamponade, hypotension, hypertension, diabetic ketoacidosis, brain injury, hypothermia, blood loss, anaphylaxis, and multiple electrolyte abnormalities. METI also has also created a pediatric version of HPS, PediaSim, that uses a pediatric mannequin based on the anatomy of a 20-kg ,6-year old child. This simulator has all the capabilities of the HPS with the exception of the trauma procedures.[24]

The capabilities of the Eagle Patient Simulator (Medsim Eagle Simulation, Inc., Binghamton, NY) are similar to those of HPS and PediaSim. Physical findings, monitoring systems, drug recognition systems, scenarios, and overall realism are comparable. The Eagle Patient Simulator, however, does not have active bleeding, salivation, or lacrimation and is more limited than HPS in the number of procedures that can be performed.[25] The Eagle Patient Simulator is no longer produced, but several centers throughout the country and the world still use this system. Two other comparable simulators have been made in Europe (the Anesthesia Simulator SOPHUS and the Leiden Anesthesia Simulator), but they are believed to be less comprehensive than the HPS and Eagle Patient Simulator.[25] To the best of the author's knowledge, they are no longer in production.

The HPS is highly sophisticated and comprehensive and, accordingly, has a price tag greater than $150,000.[26] For many types of training in health care, this high level of simulation may not be necessary, and simpler simulators would be adequate. Recognizing this fact, METI and other companies are producing less complex and less expensive computer-enhanced patient simulators. METI makes a portable simulator called the Emergency Care Simulator (ECS).[24] This simulator has a less complex respiratory system and computer than the HPS. It does not have an internal gas analyzer or an automatic drug recognition system, and many interventions are not automatically sensed by ECS. Instead, the instructor must enter the gases, medications, and procedural interventions as they are given or performed by trainees. In addition, ECS has fewer preprogrammed patients and scenarios than HPS, and it does not have dynamically reacting pupils, a thumb twitch reflex, or a pulmonary artery catheter. ECS includes its own monitoring system, but unlike HPS, conventional monitoring devices and conventional defibrillators are not compatible with ECS. The advantages of this simulator are that it can be moved into various environments (useful for emergency medical service, military, police, and wilderness training) and that it costs less than $40,000.[24,27]

Laerdal (Stavanger, Norway), the company that makes Resusci Anne, also makes two computer-enhanced simulators.[28] SimMan costs less than $30,000 and is designed for training in advanced airway skills. SimMan can be used for advanced cardiac life support (ACLS) and advanced trauma life support (ATLS) training. It has an anatomically correct airway, peripheral pulses, pulse oximetry, and ECG readings. The airway is dynamic, as with HPS, and can be made difficult or impossible to intubate. Sim Man can be used to practice intubation, peripheral venipuncture, cricothyroidotomy, needle decompression, and tube thoracostomy. SimMan also has an optional trauma package upgrade that includes moulage accessories for greater realism. Laerdal also makes AirMan™, an even simpler and less expensive simulator. This simulator comes only with a head and torso and is designed for airway management and ACLS-like training. Intubation and cricothyroidotomy can be performed on this simulator, but the other procedures included in SimMan are not available. AirMan costs less than $15,000.[28,29]

The patient simulators mentioned above are the most advanced of the computer-enhanced medical simulators and have potential applications in nearly every area of health care. However, two other simpler and more focused simulators also fit into the category of CEMS. The first is Harvey, a cardiology mannequin simulator released in 1976. Harvey is able to simulate the arterial pulse, blood pressure, jugular venous wave, precordial movements, and heart sounds in normal and diseased states.[30] The simulator is designed for training in physical diagnosis only. Unlike the previously described simulators, it is not designed to be interactive; therefore, trainees cannot perform interventions on the mannequin. Harvey was created by cardiologists for their field, but it has also been found to be useful in other fields, such as emergency medicine, to determine possible areas of insufficient training in the cardiovascular examination.[31] The second simulator is a pelvic examination simulator that was recently developed at Stanford University. This pelvis-only mannequin is equipped with internal devices that sense students' palpations and movements during a simulated pelvic exam. By interpreting the sensors' readings, the simulator's computer is able to provide the user with visual feedback about which structures they are palpating and how much pressure they are applying.[32] According to the creator of this simulator, it is likely to become commercially available in the near future.[33]

Computer-enhanced Mannequin Simulation: Current Applications

Although many health care fields recently have begun to use CEMS in their training, the field of anesthesia historically has been the most active and progressive in this area. The popularity of this training modality in anesthesia is mainly due to the work of Gaba, Fish, and Howard, which began in the late 1980s. At that time, it was recognized that 65–70% of all incidents and accidents in anesthesia could be attributed to human error. In an attempt to gain better insight into this problem, anesthesiologists came across extensive research in the aerospace sector. The airlines and NASA had begun to address human error in their profession and developed a simulation-based curriculum, called Crew Resource Management (CRM), to educate pilots in avoiding human error. Gaba, Fish, and Howard adapted the principles of CRM to anesthesia and developed a program called Anesthesia Crisis Resource Management (ACRM).[34,35]

The ACRM course has been well received. Students find the mannequin and scenarios very realistic and believe that they benefit from the crisis resource management and teamwork discussions.[26,36,37] More than 100 simulator centers are in operation throughout the world, and ACRM or similar courses are used at many of these centers as part of anesthesia trainee education or continued medical education for anesthesiologists and nurse anesthetists.[25] In fact, in Denmark, Rational Anesthesia, a variant of ACRM, is now required for certification, and the Harvard Risk Management Foundation (the insurer of hospitals affiliated with Harvard) has established a rate structure for its malpractice insurance that differentiates between simulation-trained and non-simulation-trained anesthesiologists.[38]

Other fields in medicine also have begun to adopt crisis management training. In emergency medicine, two different crisis management courses have been created. Emergency Medicine Crisis Resource Management (EMCRM) was created using ACRM as a template.[39,40] The overall design is similar to ACRM, but the crisis management principles and the learning scenarios are tailored to cover unique issues encountered in emergency medicine. The course is designed mainly for resident training; however, attending physicians, nurses, and medical students also have found the course useful. A similar course was designed by adding computer-enhanced mannequin simulation to MedTeams' Emergency Team Coordination Course (Dynamics Research Corporation, Andover, MA), a commercially available crisis management course for emergency medicine.[41] In addition to emergency medicine, ACRM-like courses also have been developed for perinatal care and intensive care.[42,43]

The proponents of ACRM and other anesthesia crisis management courses historically have been the driving force behind computer-enhanced simulation in health care. However, educators from other fields have begun to show increasing interest in this training modality, and, as a result of their growing involvement, new, highly diverse applications of this technology are being discovered and implemented. Computer-enhanced mannequin simulators now are used for training in nearly every health care field to teach lessons that vary over a broad spectrum of complexity.

Some institutions are exploring the utility of computer-enhanced mannequin simulators in teaching focused tasks. In New Zealand, a group has developed a course to teach "advanced airway skills."[44] Trainees are able to practice airway skills as well as hone their general management of an emergency. The course creators believed that the patient simulator in conjunction with their curriculum was a highly effective teaching tool and reported their intent to develop the course further. Although this project involved emergency medicine trainees, it clearly is applicable also to training for anesthesiologists, anesthetists, EMS/paramedic personnel, and military medics. Other individual tasks as varied as basic physical examination skills, patient transportation, and conscious sedation are also being explored as potential areas of training that may benefit from CEMS; to the author's knowledge, however, no formal assessments of this work have been published to date.

In addition to specific task training, some centers are exploring the use of CEMS in ACLS and ATLS training. Officially, computer-enhanced simulators are not accepted by the American Heart Association or the American College of Surgeons; however, some institutions currently use CEMS to augment their courses and have found favorable results. For ACLS, validation studies are currently in progress, and for ATLS, two studies have been published. Marshall et al. found that ATLS training augmented with CEMS appeared to improve the development of trauma management skills and that training with the simulator significantly improved team behavior and individual self-confidence.[45] A second study is currently ongoing, but the initial results have been comparable.[46]

Many health care training programs across the country also use CEMS-based teaching as a standard part of their general curricula. At our institution, as well as others, CEMS technology is a standard part of the nurse anesthetist training program. It is used during the first year of training to enhance the traditional didactic curriculum by reinforcing lessons learned in the classroom with clinical applications. Several institutions across the country also have begun to add CEMS into the nursing, physician assistant, and pharmacy training programs. Educators at our center have even used the simulator to introduce physical therapy students to the intensive care setting. To the author's knowledge, no formal evaluations of CEMS training in these fields have been performed, but according to many program directors, the subjective responses from the students and educators have been overwhelmingly positive.

CEMS training also has been widely used in prehospital personnel education. Many programs in America use simulators for training EMS and paramedic students as well as for refresher courses in both groups. In Canada, the Shock Trauma Air Rescue Society (STARS) has even built a mobile simulation center that allows access to a greater number of EMS personnel in the country. The STARS "Emergency Medical Education Unit" program is well accepted; the program directors report an extremely high demand for this type of training.[47]

The military also has found success in using CEMS technology to train its field medics and other medical personnel.[48] Computer-enhanced simulators have been field-tested with favorable results and now are used at several military facilities. The armed forces and several other government institutions have found CEMS highly useful for bioterrorism and weapons of mass destruction training.[49,50]

In medical schools, CEMS is used at every educational level. Some institutions have incorporated computer-enhanced simulators into the basic science portion of medical education. Basic science students have found CEMS to be highly enjoyable and beneficial when used to teach cardiac and respiratory physiology.[51] Some centers also use this technology to augment pharmacology courses.

A number of medical schools now use CEMS as a standard portion of the curriculum during clinical rotations such as anesthesia and emergency medicine.[52,53] In addition, a group at Harvard University has proposed a system in which clinical students can call the simulation center at any time to experience a simulation of a medical event or procedure that they may have seen but did not have the opportunity to practice first-hand.[54] In standard medical training, it is clear that students, in most instances, must learn mainly through observation because more senior trainees take precedence for the hands-on training opportunities. With the interesting pilot program at Harvard, students will have the opportunity to get more hands-on training earlier in their medical education.

CEMS technology is also being explored in resident training. In addition to the crisis management courses mentioned earlier, residency programs are adding simulation to many other facets of their curricula. One general surgery program has designed a three-day orientation course that uses simulation to introduce interns to several common clinical scenarios.[55] The interns believed that the course was beneficial and that their self-confidence improved significantly as a result. Although the initial program, as reported in the literature, did not involve CEMS, this technology was subsequently added to the program with even better results.[56] In many emergency medicine training programs, interns undergo a month of orientation. In our program, like many others, the orientation period includes lectures, procedure training using plastic and animal models, and a limited amount of clinical exposure. At this early stage of training, for the safety of patients, the interns can only take a secondary role during the most challenging procedures and cases. In response, we are currently designing a CEMS portion of the orientation program that will give interns the valuable experience of being the primary physician in highly challenging clinical scenarios. At the University of New Mexico, CEMS recently was incorporated as a standard portion of the entire three-year emergency medicine residency curriculum. The creators of this program are also currently exploring the possibility of using CEMS as a tool for resident evaluation.[57]

Although simulation training is logistically and financially feasible at most medical centers large enough to support medical student and residency training programs, this may not be the case for remote or smaller medical centers. For this reason, the use of CEMS in distance learning is also being explored. One group actively performing research in this area believes that for lower levels of training, such as students, CEMS may not be optimal because more basic skills cannot be practiced with the currently available distance-learning technology. However, they believe that when cognitive training is the main goal, as is the case at more advanced levels of training, distance simulation with CEMS may be highly beneficial.[58]

Virtual Reality: Background and Current Technology

The term *virtual reality* was first used by Jaron Lanier in the late 1980s; however, the origin of this technology began with the work of Ivan Sutherland at MIT and Harvard University during the mid 1960s. In a groundbreaking presentation, entitled "The Ultimate Display," Sutherland introduced an entirely new concept for computer-human interaction. He proposed a model for a computer display that would simulate the physical world and allow the user to interact directly with the computer within that simulated world. Within five years, Sutherland produced the first head-mounted display, and VR became a reality.[59]

Today VR applications are often classified by the level of computer-user interaction. A classification system proposed by Voelter and Kraemer divides VR technology into four categories: immersive VR, desktop VR, pseudo VR, and inverse VR. **Immersive VR** completely integrates the user into the world of the computer. Modern flight simulators can be classified as highly immersive. Pilots physically sit inside the simulators and are surrounded by realistic visual displays and sounds. These simulators can even move to reproduce the motion of flight. Similar flight simulation programs are available for use on personal computers. In this case, however, the programs would be classified as **Desktop VR** because the simulation occurs entirely on a computer screen (the user is less "immersed" in the simulation). **Pseudo VR** refers to a program with even more limited computer-user interaction. In pseudo VR applications, users mainly observe the virtual environment and have little ability to manipulate or affect it. For example, in some VR anatomy programs, users can control the rotation of the three-dimensional anatomic models to facilitate learning, but they cannot deform the models or virtually dissect them. Finally, **inverse VR** describes the integration of a computer into the user's world, as opposed to the reverse in standard VR. An example of this technology is a program that enables quadriplegics to use eye movements to control a computer that facilitates communication or other tasks in the real world.[60]

Augmented reality is a fifth category of VR that has been described by other groups in the literature and should be added to complete Voelter and Kraemer's classification.[61,62] In augmented reality, the virtual world is superimposed on the real one so that both can be experienced simultaneously. This goal can be achieved by presenting virtual images on see-through, head-mounted displays or mobile screens. For example, a program has been created to aid facial surgeons during operations by allowing them to see the internal anatomic structures (based on data from the patient's radiographic studies) superimposed on the surface anatomy. In effect, this method allows the surgeon to "virtually" see through the patient's skin.[61]

All virtual reality programs have four essential components: software, hardware, input devices, and output devices.[62] The software defines the virtual environment using mathematical algorithms and equations, and the hardware performs the calculations required by the software to produce the environment. The equations and algorithms used to define the virtual environment can be derived from data from photographs, pathology sections, plain radiographs, computed tomography, magnetic resonance, or ultrasound. Computer-aided design (CAD) programs are used to convert the real-world image data into wire-frame surface models consisting of polygons. Texture and coloring are added to the surface models through a process called rendering to give the final virtual images.[63] The resolution of the surface models depends on the number and size of polygons. To improve resolution, the size of the polygons must be decreased and their number increased. This approach causes the number of necessary calculations to multiply and therefore increases the demands on the software and hardware. The result is a trade-off between image quality and speed of image updating.[64] Both factors are important contributors to the realism of the virtual environment. Ideally, image frames should be refreshed from 24 to 30 times a second for the human eye not to notice the updating.[65]

The computer-generated environment can be presented to the user via one or more output devices. Generally, virtual images are projected either on high-resolution monitors (with or without three-dimensional capability) or on head-mounted displays. In the case of augmented reality, the displays are semitransparent. Speakers can be added for audio output, and devices have been created to give haptic feedback (including force feedback and tactile touch). To date, haptic feedback has been the most difficult portion of the virtual environment to simulate. The current tactile touch simulation devices are limited in their realism. Pneumatic bladders, vibrating transducers, electrical stimulation, and current-sensitive shape memory alloys are being explored, but to date these efforts have had limited success.[63] Work in the area of force feedback devices, however, has been more productive. For simple force feedback simulation tasks, such as simulating resistance in two dimensions, relatively basic pulley systems can produce highly realistic results. For complex simulation in three dimensions, more elaborate feedback devices have been created. To date, the most widely used device in medical VR is the PHANToM (SensAble Technologies, Woburn, MA). The PHANToM is composed of a multijointed mechanical arm with a "wand" extension or thimble at its end that the user can hold and manipulate to "feel" the position, orientation, shape, and compliance of a virtual object shown on a computer screen.

In both the real and the virtual worlds, a person relies on six degrees of freedom of movement around an object to determine the object's orientation and position in space. The first three degrees of freedom are the Cartesian coordinates "X," "Y," and "Z." Movement within these axes is necessary to establish an object's position. The remaining three degrees of freedom, called "pitch," "yaw," and "roll," refer to the possible directions of rotation about a point or an object.[6] Pitch, yaw, and roll are needed to determine an object's orientation in space.

The PHANToM realistically conveys a virtual object's position and orientation using all six degrees of freedom. Simulation of an object's compliance, however, is limited to three degrees of freedom. This limitation occurs because force feedback information at any given instant can be conveyed only for a single point on the surface of a virtual object. This sensation is similar to probing an orange with a pencil; you gain a good idea of the compliance of the orange at any point you touch, but you cannot gain compliance information from multiple points simultaneously. Despite this limitation, the force feedback simulation is highly realistic when combined with the visual simulation of a virtual object. The PHANToM has been used to simulate the shape and compliance of many anatomic structures, and some programs can even simulate puncturing and cutting.

In VR, the computer output determines the realism of the user's experience, but it is the input from the user to the computer that makes VR truly interactive. Conventional computer input tools, such as the mouse, keyboard, and voice recognition, can also be used in VR applications, but other more advanced devices have been designed specifically for VR purposes. Tracking devices have been created to detect the position and movement of the user's head, body, and limbs. Full body suits exist, but, for most applications, tracking just the user's head and hand(s) is sufficient. Currently, VR tracking devices employ electromagnetic, mechanical, and gyroscopic sensors. "Biosensors" that track muscle and neuronal activity are also under development.[63]

VR technology is only in its infancy, but it is already impressive and certainly advanced enough to be used in many areas of health care education. When VR programs are used, it is important to recognize the limits of existing VR technology. If one expects perfect realism, the current VR applications might be disappointing. That being said, computing and electronics technology are advancing at an exponential rate, and the overall realism of VR applications promises to improve rapidly.[22]

Virtual Reality: Current Applications

Virtual reality programs are used for all levels of training. To date, the majority of the available VR applications were designed mainly for physician education; however, many of the applications and concepts also apply to other areas of health care. Current medical VR applications can be classified by the type of instruction that they provide: basic science education, clinical education, and medical procedures training.

In the category of basic science, a few VR programs have been designed to improve anatomy education. The Anatomic VisualizeR was developed at the University of California, San Diego. This VR program includes several three-dimensional (3-D) anatomic models derived from data from the Visible Human Project. When using this program, students can virtually dissect the 3-D models and simultaneously use conventional two-dimensional (2-D) resources, such as diagrams, text, and videos. Students are able to adjust the size, opacity, and orientation of the various 3-D organs to improve their understanding of the spatial relationships between adjacent and deeper structures. This function of the program is thought to be an extremely effective method for learning anatomic relationships.[5,66,67]

The 3D Human Atlas has been developed in Japan. This program is designed to help students understand anatomic cross-sections and how they relate to the anatomy of the entire body. MRI scans of a live model were used to make the cross-sections. These MRI-derived sections are presented one at a time along with a 3-D computer rendering of the entire body of the live model. An opaque plane through the 3-D model shows the student where the cross-section that is being viewed would be situated on the model. Like the Anatomic VisualizeR, the 3D Human Atlas has variable opacities for the external and internal structures of the 3D whole-body rendering.[68] A similar program is used at the University of Kentucky to assist in teaching medical students to read CT scans.[69]

The VOXEL-MAN 3D Navigator is another recently created VR anatomy program. This program also uses images from the Visible Human Project to generate 3-D anatomy models. It is unique in that its images have extremely high resolution. One can see detail as fine as small nerves and vessels.[70]

VR programs also have been designed for teaching brain anatomy. One program includes conventional teaching modules of gross brain sections, histology, and neuroradiology but adds a 3-D anatomic model of the brain. Like previously discussed VR anatomy-training programs, this program allows users to adjust the views of the brain; variable opacities facilitate the learning of various brain structures and their anatomic relationships.[5,71]

Some of the VR applications designed for procedural training (discussed below) also include anatomy lessons related to the procedures that they simulate. Although it was not their intended purpose, in most cases these simulators certainly could be used at the basic science level for more focused anatomy lessons.

To date, the number of VR programs created for basic science education is relatively small, but many more applications have been produced for more advanced clinical training. The military, most likely due to the success of VR in combat and aviation training, also is exploring VR for educating medical personnel. One military group has developed a desktop VR program for medic training in casualty triage, resuscitation, and evacuation.[72] Thirty different injuries can be simulated, several interventions can be performed, and the virtual patient's condition and vital signs respond appropriately to the simulated injuries and interventions. This program has an educational module as well as practice modules and a testing module for each simulated injury. Audio, textual, and graphic feedback are employed, but there is no haptic feedback. Similar VR medic trainers also have been designed by other groups.[73,74] One of these simulators is unique in that a virtual medic has been added to the animation. The user can watch the virtual medic perform examinations and procedures that the user selects during the simulation.[73]

Similar programs are also used for EMS and nursing training. RTI International (Research Triangle Park, NC), has designed VR programs for EMS trauma training, bioterrorism response, and critical care nursing.[75] In the domestic terrorism-related training programs, the simulated patients show the physical and physiologic signs of various chemical and biologic agent exposures.[76,77] RTI has also begun work on a VR program to educate health care personnel about overcoming difficulties specific to examining pediatric patients.[77]

A VR emergency department program, created recently in Norway, is designed for trauma team training and distance learning. From remote locations, multiple participants can play different roles (e.g., surgeon, nurse) and simultaneously participate in the care of simulated trauma patients in the virtual emergency department. The trauma bay includes all equipment needed for trauma resuscitation, there are multiple simulated patients with various injuries, and several interventions can be performed.[78–80] Although more clinical scenarios are still under development, a pilot study of this program has shown that it is feasible for multiple users in remote locations to work simultaneously in the same simulated environment. Users enjoyed this program and believed that it was instructive.[79]

A similar project in neonatology also has shown initial success in multiple, remote user interaction in a single virtual environment. A virtual newborn has variable breathing, movement, crying, heart rate, and skin color. These five parameters can be controlled from a command computer that can be networked to other computers by local cables or an internet connection. Multiple users simultaneously can observe the changing condition of the virtual neonate, and users are able to communicate with each other in real time through headphones and a microphone at each console.[81] To the best of the author's knowledge, at this time users can only observe the virtual neonate; however, further development of the software will allow users to perform virtual medical interventions on the baby as well.

The greatest amount of work in VR for health care education has come in the category of medical procedure training; simulators have been developed for many different examinations, invasive procedures, and surgeries. The VR simulators described below are in various stages of development, but all have been well received and several are commercially available.

VR simulators have been created for facial surgery, neurosurgery, robotic-assisted cardiac surgery, abdominal trauma surgery, laparoscopic cholecystectomy, endoscopic sinus surgery, temporal bone dissection, arthroscopic surgery of the knee and shoulder, vascular anastamosis, cardiac catheterization, inferior vena cava filter placement, prostate radioactive seed placement, and transurethral resection of the prostate.[82–98] In general, minimally invasive surgeries are easier to simulate realistically due to the limited visual and haptic feedback inherent in such procedures. During minimally invasive surgery, the surgical field is viewed on a computer or TV monitor, away from the patient, and the haptic feedback is transmitted through the surgical instruments. Several of the simulators mentioned above have multiple interactive modules, including those for teaching, practicing, and testing.

In addition to the operating room (OR) procedures in the previous paragraph, several non-OR invasive procedures also have been simulated. Like the OR procedure simulators, most have haptic feedback capabilities, and the more advanced programs have modules for education, practice, and testing. Simulators have been developed or are currently under development for IV catheter insertion, acupuncture, skin suturing, lumbar puncture, epidural anesthesia, bone marrow biopsy, leg trauma assessment and treatment, pericardiocentesis, cricothyroidotomy, diagnostic peritoneal lavage, and emergency thoracotomy.[99–111]

Finally, a number of VR programs simulate minimally invasive or noninvasive procedures and examinations. Examples include occular examination, ultrasound, hysteroscopy, sigmoidoscopy, ureteroscopy, bronchoscopy, upper GI endoscopy, lower GI endoscopy, and endotracheal intubation.[112–121] The intubation simulator is in an early stage of development, but it is unique because, to the best of the author's knowledge, it is the only educational VR simulator to date to use augmented reality. This simulator, when completed, will allow students to see "through" the "skin" of a METI HPS so that they can see the internal anatomy while they learn to intubate.[121] Also of note, Immersion Medical (Gaithersburg, MD) currently produces a single system that simulates multiple procedures, including bronchoscopy and upper and lower GI endoscopy.[122]

Simulator Evaluation: Current Research and Future Challenges

CEMS and VR in general have been well received in the health care community. Subjective studies of nearly every simulator report that both novices and experts find them enjoyable to use and, in most cases, valuable educational tools. To date, however, relatively few well-designed, objective studies of simulators have been performed. The reason is probably two-fold: (1) because the technology is relatively new, experience in this area is limited, and (2) objective evaluation of human performance in any setting is difficult.

In the area of CEMS, only two objective studies, to the best of the author's knowledge, have been published in the English-language medical literature. One study showed that the patient simulator could be used to discriminate the performance of resident and staff anesthesiologists during certain scenarios; in other words, the simulator showed construct validity (called "discriminant validity" by the authors).[123] The other study reported improvement in performance during emergencies after training with the simulator.[124] The second study was limited by the fact that the simulator was also used as the testing tool for performance evaluation. In regard to future evaluation efforts, it is the author's strong belief that objective assessment of any computer-enhanced mannequin simulator as a whole will be extremely difficult to perform. However, evaluation of specific components of a simulator and individual simulation scenarios will probably prove to be more feasible and much more meaningful.

A slightly greater number of objective studies have been published for various VR applications. The number of these studies is still limited, however, and they vary greatly in quality of experimental design. Unlike CEMS, individual VR applications usually are designed to simulate a single task or scenario; therefore, objective evaluation may prove to be somewhat easier than with CEMS technology.

To the best of the author's knowledge, only 19 studies evaluating VR applications with objective study designs have been published to date in the English-language medical literature.[125–143] These studies address various issues, including validation, performance improvement, and comparison of simulators with other teaching modalities. Although all these studies have provided useful information, several are unfortunately flawed due to issues such as using the simulator under investigation as the subject performance assessment tool. Overstating the conclusions that can be drawn from the results has also been an issue in several studies. For example, demonstration of one type of validity does not necessarily mean that the simulator is valid as a whole.

Although the positive subjective responses to the simulation applications that have been tested to date may be sufficient to show that simulation technology promises to play an important role in health care education, the proper evaluation of each individual computer-enhanced mannequin simulator and VR simulator is essential before it can be accepted into general use. Well-designed objective research will also provide valuable information that can be used to improve individual simulators and simulation technology as a whole. A few individuals and groups across the country have begun to recognize that it will be vital to develop and use standardized templates to ensure proper and efficient evaluation of current and future simulators.[141,142,144,145] Ideally, proper evaluation of any simulator should include tests of the following: usability, validity, reliability, skills transfer, comparison with other teaching modalities, and cost analysis.

Testing for usability is an essential first step. As with any computer program, a simulator must be intuitive, easy to use, enjoyable, and easily accessible. If it does not have these qualities, people will not be inclined to use the simulator, and it will not be an effective teaching tool.

A simulator must also be tested for validity. It is generally accepted that five levels of validity are important in simulation testing: face, content, construct, concurrent, and predictive. To test face and content validity, experts in the simulated task give feedback about the realism of the simulator. **Face validity** relates to the overall realism of the simulation, and **content validity** relates to the realism of more specific, individual components of the simulator. Subjective data are sufficient to show face and concurrent validity; for the remaining three types of validity, however, objective data are required. **Construct validity** is assessed by evaluating the performance of experts and novices on the simulator. If the performance of experts and novices on the simulator can be discriminated, the simulator shows construct validity. In other words, experts in the simulated task should be more efficient and make fewer mistakes than novices. Concurrent validity is evaluated by testing subject performance first in the real setting and then on the simulator. For a simulator to show **concurrent validity,** the performances of individuals in the two settings should correlate. **Predictive validity** testing also requires performance evaluations in both real and simulated settings. In this case, however, individual subject performances are first evaluated on the simulator and then during the real task. The performance during simulation must be predictive of the real task performance for the simulator to show predictive validity. Testing for concurrent and predictive validity ideally requires that novices perform tasks on live patients. This method, of course, raises significant ethical concerns and places major constraints on evaluation of predictive validity. In the coming years, the health care simulation community will have to address this issue seriously and determine whether there are acceptable compromises or alternatives for such levels of testing. Potential solutions may include animal models, novice testing compromised by supervisor intervention, or acceptance of face, content, and construct validity as sufficient.

A third facet of simulator testing is reliability. This type of testing is more important if a simulator is assessed for use as an evaluation tool. Two types of reliability are important: **interrater reliability** and **test-retest reliability**. To show interrater reliability, independent evaluators must have a high level of agreement in assessing individual user performances on a simulator. In addition, individual users must also show consistent performances on the simulator to establish test-retest reliability.[145]

The forth element of simulator evaluation is skills transfer testing. If a simulator has shown acceptable validity and usability, it is likely but not certain that practice with that simulator will improve user performance in the real task. It must be shown definitively that the specific tasks that the simulator is designed to teach are being learned by the users.

Once usability, validity, reliability, and skills transfer have been shown, it can be concluded that the simulator is an effective teaching tool. However, before the simulator will be widely accepted by health care educators, it must also be assessed for cost-effectiveness and objectively compared with other available teaching modalities. If the simulator is shown to be an effective teaching tool and to be more cost-effective than other modalities that teach the same task, health care educators will readily adopt it.

Conclusion

This is an exciting time in health care education. VR and CEMS have the potential to improve health care training significantly and may even revolutionize our traditional teaching systems. Already many VR and CEMS applications are highly impressive. It is remarkable to consider that this technology is only in its infancy. But even more remarkable is the fact that, as more health care educators become involved and as computer chips continue to double in power every 18–24 months,[22] this technology promises to advance at an exponential rate. The theoretical benefits of CEMS and VR over live-patient training, coupled with the overwhelmingly positive response to the current technology, warrants serious, well-designed, objective investigation of individual simulators so that they can be widely adopted in health care training.

References
1. Nelson MS: Models for teaching emergency medicine skills. Ann Emerg Med 1990;9: 333–335.
2. Totten VY: Ethics and teaching the art of emergency medicine. Ethical Issues Clin Emerg Med 1999;17:429–439.
3. Gorman PJ, Meier AH, Krummel TM: Simulation and virtual reality in surgical education: Real or unreal? Arch Surg 1999;134:1203–1208.

4. Haluck RS, Krummel TM: Simulation and virtual reality for surgical education. Surg Technol Int 1999;8:59–63.
5. Hoffman H, Vu D: Virtual reality: teaching tool of the twenty-first century? Acad Med 1997;72:1076–1081.
6. Ahmed M, Meech JF, Timoney A: Virtual reality in medicine. Br J Urol 1997;80(Suppl 3):46–52.
7. Issenberg SB, McGaghie WC, Hart IR, et al: Simulation technology for health care professional skills training and assessment. JAMA 1999;282:861–866.
8. Jones K: Simulators: A Handbook for Teachers. New York, Nichols Publishing, 1980.
9. Shackford SR, Rogers FB, Osler TM, et al: Focused abdominal sonogram for trauma: The learning curve of nonradiologist clinicians in detecting hemoperitoneum. J Trauma 1999;46:553–562.
10. Delaney KA, Hessler R: Emergency flexible fiberoptic nasotracheal intubation: A report of 60 cases. Ann Emerg Med 1988;17:919–926.
11. Smith JE, Jackson AP, Hurdley J, Clifton PJ: Learning curves for fiberoptic nasotracheal intubation when using the endoscopic video camera. Anaesthesia 1997;52:101–106.
12. Watson DI, Baigrie RJ, Jamieson GG: A learning curve for laparoscopic fundoplication. Ann Surg 1996;224:198–203.
13. Martin KR, Burton RL: The phacoemulsification learning curve: perioperative complications in the first 3000 cases of an experienced surgeon. Eye 2000;14:190–195.
14. Carmody BJ, Otchy DP: Learning curve of transrectal ultrasound. Dis Colon Rectum 2000;43:193–197.
15. Vrancic JM, Piccinini F, Vaccarino G, et al: Endoscopic saphenous vein harvesting: Initial experience and learning curve. Ann Thorac Surg 2000;70:1086–1099.
16. Gates E: New surgical procedures: Can our patients benefit while we learn? Am J Obstet Gynecol 1997;176:1293–1298.
17. Wu AW, Folkman S, McPHee SJ, Lo B: Do house officers learn from their mistakes? JAMA 1991;265:2089–2094.
18. Short D: Learning from our mistakes. Br J Hosp Med 1994;51(5):250–252.
19. McIntyre N, Popper K: The critical attitude in medicine: The need for a new ethics. Br Med J 1983;287:1919–1924.
20. Lessons learned. Army devises systems to decide what does, and does not, work: The real value of experience. Wall Street J May 23, 1997.
21. Goldiez BF: History of networked simulators. In Clarke TL (ed): Distributed Interactive Simulation Systems for Simulation and Training in the Aerospace Environment. Bellingham, WA, SPIE Optical Engineering Press, 1995, pp 39–58.
22. Krummel TM: Surgical simulation and VR: The coming revolution. Ann Surg 1998;228:635–637.
23. Abrahamson S: Sim One: A patient simulator ahead of its time. Caduceus 1997; 13(2):29–41.
24. Available at http://www.meti.com.
25. Gaba DM: Human work environment and simulators. In Miller RD (ed): Anesthesia. Philadelphia, Churchill Livingstone, 2000.
26. Forrest F, Taylor M: High level simulators in medical education. Hosp Med 1998;59:653–655.
27. Personal and e-mail conversation with METI sales representative, Torroni S. January 20, 2003.
28. Available at http://www.laerdal.com.
29. Personal conversation with Laerdal customer support representative, name unknown. January 20, 2003.
30. Gordon MS, Ewy GA, DeLeon AC, et al: "Harvey," the cardiology patient simulator: Pilot studies on teaching effectiveness. Am J Cardiol 1980;45:791–796.
31. Jones JS, Hunt SJ, Carlson SA, Seamon JP: Assessing bedside examination skills using "Harvey," a cardiology patient simulator. Acad Emerg Med 1997;4:980–985.
32. Pugh CM, Srivastava S, Shavelson R, et al: The effect of simulator use on learning and self-assessment: The case of Stanford University's E-pelvis simulator. In Medicine Meets Virtual

Reality 2001: Outer Space, Inner Space, Virtual Space. Amsterdam, IOS Press and Ohmsha, 2001, pp 396–400.

33. Personal conversation with Pugh CM, January 23, 2003.
34. Gaba DM, Fish KJ, Howard SK: Crisis Management in Anesthesiology. New York, Churchill Livingstone, 1994.
35. Howard SK, Gaba DM, Fish KJ, et al: Anesthesia crisis resource management training: Teaching anesthesiologists to handle critical incidents. Aviat Space Environ Med 1992; 63:763–769.
36. Doyle DJ, Arellano R: The Virtual Anesthesiology™ training simulation system. Can J Anaesth 1995;42:267–273.
37. Gaba DM, DeAnda A: A comprehensive anesthesia simulation environment. Anesthesiology 1988;69:387–394.
38. Gaba DM, Howard SK, Fish KJ, et al: Simulation-based training in anesthesia crisis resource management (ACRM): A decade of experience. Simul Gaming 2001;32:175–193.
39. Reznek M, Smith-Coggins R, Howard S, et al: Emergency Medicine Crisis Resource Management (EMCRM): Pilot study of a simulation-based crisis management course for emergency medicine. Acad Emerg Med [in press 2003].
40. Available at http://anesthesia.stanford.edu/vasimulator/emedicine.htm.
41. Small SD, Wuerz RC, Simon R, et al: Demonstration of high fidelity simulation team training for emergency medicine. Acad Emerg Med 1999;6:312–323.
42. Available at http://anesthesia.stanford.edu/vasimulator/sdre.htm.
43. Available at http://anesthesia.stanford.edu/vasimulator/icu.htm.
44. Ellis C, Hughes G: Use of human patient simulator to teach emergency medicine trainees advanced airway skills. J Accid Emerg Med 1999;16:395–369.
45. Marshall RL, Smith JS, Gorman PJ, et al: Use of a human patient simulator in the development of resident trauma management skills. J Trauma 2000;51:17–21.
46. Knudson MM: Trauma training in simulation. Proceedings of the 50th Annual Detroit Trauma Symposium, November 14–15, 2002, Detroit, MI.
47. Kiriaka JL: EMS roadshow. J Emerg Med Serv 2000;25(9 Suppl):1–6.
48. Available at www.afams.af.mil/programs/projects/lftt/projects/com_tra.htm.
49. Kyle RR, Lowry RJ, Mahy AM, et al: A multiple disciplinary approach to teach weapons of mass destruction and terrorist crises management using patient simulation. Proceedings of the International Meeting on Medical Simulation, January 10–13, 2002, Santa Clara, CA.
50. Templeton L: Life-like simulators give a dose of reality training. Teexan 2000;20(3):1–2.
51. Moral ID, Diaz de Teran C, Gonzalez JM, Rabanal A: Using a full patient simulator for teaching physiology. Proceedings of the International Meeting on Medical Simulation, January 10–13, 2002, Santa Clara, CA.
52. Takayesu JK, Gordon JA, Farrell SE, et al: Learning emergency and critical care medicine: What does high-fidelity patient simulation teach? Acad Emerg Med 2002;9:476–477
53. Noonan D: Wiring the new docs. Newsweek June 24, 2002, pp 58–62.
54. Gordon JA, Wilkerson WM, Shaffer DW, Armstrong EG: "Practicing" medicine without risk: Students' and educators' responses to high-fidelity patient simulation. Acad Med 2001; 76:469–472.
55. Marshall RL, Gorman PJ, Verne D, et al: Practical training for postgraduate year 1 surgery residents. Am J Surg 2000;179:194–196.
56. Personal conversation with Marshall RL and Gorman PJ.
57. McLaughlin SA, Doezema D, Sklar DP: Human simulation in emergency medicine training: A model curriculum. Acad Emerg Med 2002;9:1310–1318.
58. von Lubitz DKJE, Carrasco B, Gabbrielli F, et al: Transatlantic medical education: preliminary data on distance-based high-fidelity human patient simulation training. In Westwood JD, Hoffman HM, Mogel GT, et al (eds): Medicine Meets Virtual Reality 11: NextMed: Health Horizon. Amsterdam, IOS Press and Ohmsha, 2003, pp 379–385.
59. Schroeder R: Virtual reality in the real world. Futures 1993;Nov:963–972.
60. Voelter S, Kraemer KL: Virtual reality in medicine: A functional classification. In Lemke

HV, Inamura K, Jaffe CC, Vannier MW (eds): Computer Assisted Radiology. New York, Springer, 1995, pp 1297–1298.
61. Wagner A, Rasse M, Millesi W, Ewers R: Virtual reality for orthognathic surgery: The augmented reality environment concept. J Oral Maxillofacial Surg 1997;55:456–462.
62. Raposio E, DiSomma C, Fato M, et al: An "augmented-reality" aid for plastic and reconstructive surgeons. In Morgan KS, Hoffman HM, Stredney D, Weghorst SJ (eds): Medicine Meets Virtual Reality: Global Healthcare Grid. Amsterdam, IOS Press and Ohmsha; 1997, pp 232–235.
63. Burt DER: Virtual reality in anesthesia. Br J Anaesth 1995;75:472–480.
64. Rawn CL, Gorman PJ, Graham WP, et al: Virtual reality becomes reality in plastic surgery. Perspect Plast Surg 2000;14:105–118.
65. Edmond CV, Jr., Wiet GJ, Bolger B: Virtual environments. Surgical simulation in otolaryngology. Otolaryngol Clin North Am 1998;31:369–381.
66. Hoffman H, Murray M, Danks M, et al: A flexible and extensible object-oriented 3D architecture: Application in the development of virtual anatomy lessons. In: Morgan KS, Hoffman HM, Stredney D, Weghorst SJ (eds): Medicine Meets Virtual Reality: Global Healthcare Grid. Amsterdam, IOS Press and Ohmsha, 1997, pp 461–466.
67. Hoffman HM, Colt HG, Haas A: Development of an experimental paradigm in which to examine human learning using two computer-based format. In Westwood JD, Hoffman HM, Mogel GT, et al (eds) Medicine Meets Virtual Reality 2001: Outer Space, Inner Space, Virtual Space. Amsterdam, IOS Press and Ohmsha, 2001, pp 187–191.
68. Suzuki N, Takatsu A, Hattori A, et al: 3D and 4D atlas system of living human body structure. In Westwood JD, Hoffman HM, Stredney D, Weghorst SJ (eds): Medicine Meets Virtual Reality: Art, Science, Technology: Healthcare (R)evolution™. Amsterdam, IOS Press and Ohmsha, 1998, pp 131–136.
69. Mastrangelo MJ, Adrales G, McKinlay R, et al: Inclusion of 3-D computed tomography rendering and immersive VR in a third year medical student surgery curriculum. In Westwood JD, Hoffman HM, Mogel GT, et al (ed): Medicine Meets Virtual Reality 11: NextMed: Health Horizon. Amsterdam, IOS Press and Ohmsha, 2003, pp 199–203.
70. Pflesser B, Petersik A, Pommert A, et al: Exploring the visable human's inner organs with the VOXEL_MAN 3D Navigator. In Westwood JD, Hoffman HM, Mogel GT, et al (eds): Medicine Meets Virtual Reality 2001: Outer Space, Inner Space, Virtual Space. Amsterdam, IOS Press and Ohmsha, 2001, pp 379–385.
71. Kling-Petersen T, Rydmark M: The brain project: an interactive learning tool using desktop virtual reality on personal computers. In Morgan KS, Hoffman HM, Stredney D, Weghorst SJ (eds): Medicine Meets Virtual Reality: Global HealthCare Grid. Amsterdam, IOS Press and Ohmsha, 1997, pp 529–538.
72. Willy C, Sterk J, Schwarz W, Gerngross H: Computer-assisted training program for simulation of triage, resuscitation, and evacuation of casualties. Mil Med 1998;163:234–238.
73. Chi DM, Kokkevis E, Ogunyemi O, et al: Simulated casualties and medics for emergency training. In Morgan KS, Hoffman HM, Stredney D, Weghorst SJ (eds): Medicine Meets Virtual Reality: Global health Care Grid. Amsterdam, IOS Press and Ohmsha, 1997, pp 486–494.
74. Kizakevich PN, McCartney ML, Nissman DB, Starko K: Virtual medical trainer: Patient assessment and trauma care simulator. In:Westwood JD, Hoffman HM, Stredney D, Weghorst SJ (eds): Medicine Meets Virtual Reality: Art, Science, Technology: Healthcare (R)evolution™. Amsterdam, IOS Press and Ohmsha, 1998, pp 309–315.
75. Available at http://www.rti.org/vr.
76. Kizakevich PN, Lux L, Duncan S, Guinn C: Virtual simulated patients for bioterrorism preparedness training. In Westwood JD, Hoffman HM, Mogel GT, et al (eds): Medicine Meets Virtual Reality 11: NextMed: Health Horizon. Amsterdam, IOS Press and Ohmsha, 2003, pp 165–167.
77. Hubal RC, Deterding RR, Frank GA, et al: Lessons learned in modeling virtual pediatric patients. In Westwood JD, Hoffman HM, Mogel GT, et al (eds): Medicine Meets Virtual Reality 11: NextMed: Health Horizon. Amsterdam, IOS Press and Ohmsha, 2003, pp 127–130.

78. Available at *http://www.telenor.no/fou/prosjekter/matador/*.
79. Halvorsrud R: The MATADOR project: A novel simulator in emergency medicine. Proceedings of the Medicine Meets Virtual Reality, January 24–27, 2001, Newport Beach, CA.
80. Halvorsrud R, Hagen S, Fagernes S, et al: Trauma team training in a distributed virtual emergency room. In Westwood JD, Hoffman HM, Mogel GT, et al (eds): Medicine Meets Virtual Reality 11: NextMed: Health Horizon. Amsterdam, IOS Press and Ohmsha, 2003, pp 100–102.
81. Divjak M, Holobar A, Prelog I, Zazula D: VIDERO: Virtual delivery room. Proceedings of the Slovenian Electro-technical and Computer Science Conference, September 2000, Portoroz, Slovenia.
82. Montgomery K, Sorokin A, Lionetti G, Schendel S: A surgical simulator for cleft lip planning and repair. In Westwood JD, Hoffman HM, Mogel GT, et al (eds): Medicine Meets Virtual Reality 11: NextMed: Health Horizon. Amsterdam, IOS Press and Ohmsha, 2003, pp 204–209.
83. Larsen OV, Haase J, Østergaard LR, et al: The virtual brain project- development of a neurosurgical brain simulator. In: Westwood JD, Hoffman HM, Mogel GT, et al (eds): Medicine Meets Virtual Reality 2001: Outer Space, Inner Space, Virtual Space. Amsterdam, IOS Press and Ohmsha, 2001, pp 379–385.
84. Goncharenko I, Emoto H, Matsumoto S, et al: Realistic virtual endoscopy of the ventricle system and haptic-based surgical simulator of hydrocephalus treatment. In Westwood JD, Hoffman HM, Mogel GT, et al (eds): Medicine Meets Virtual Reality 11: NextMed: Health Horizon. Amsterdam, IOS Press and Ohmsha, 2003, pp 93–95.
85. Larsen OV, Haase J, Hansen KV, et al: Training brain retraction in a virtual reality environment. In Westwood JD, Hoffman HM, Mogel GT, et al (eds): Medicine Meets Virtual Reality 11: NextMed: Health Horizon. Amsterdam, IOS Press and Ohmsha, 2003, pp 174–180.
86. Tanaka H, et al: Brain surgery simulation system using VR technique and improvement of presence. In Westwood JD, Hoffman HM, Stredney D, Weghorst SJ (eds): Medicine Meets Virtual Reality: Art, Science, Technology: Healthcare (R)evolution™. Amsterdam, IOS Press and Ohmsha, 1998, pp 150–154.
87. Røtnes JS, Kaasa J, Westergaard G, et al: Digital trainer developed for robotic assisted cardiac surgery. In Westwood JD, Hoffman HM, Mogel GT, et al (eds): Medicine Meets Virtual Reality 11: NextMed: Health Horizon. Amsterdam, IOS Press and Ohmsha, 2003, pp 424–430.
88. Bro-Nielsen M, Helfrick D, Glass B, et al: VR simulation of abdominal trauma surgery. In Westwood JD, Hoffman HM, Stredney D, Weghorst SJ (eds): Medicine Meets Virtual Reality: Art, Science, Technology: Healthcare (R)evolution™. Amsterdam, IOS Press and Ohmsha, 1998, pp 117–123.
89. Tseng CS, Lee YY, Chan YP, et al: A PC-based surgical simulator for laparoscopic surgery. In Westwood JD, Hoffman HM, Stredney D, Weghorst SJ (eds): Proceedings of Medicine Meets Virtual Reality: Art, Science, Technology: Healthcare (R)evolution™. Amsterdam, IOS Press and Ohmsha, 1998, pp 155–160.
90. Weghorst S, Airola C, Oppenheimer P, et al: Validation of the Madigan ESS simulator. In Westwood JD, Hoffman HM, Stredney D, Weghorst SJ (eds): Medicine Meets Virtual Reality: Art, Science, Technology: Healthcare (R)evolution™. Amsterdam, IOS Press and Ohmsha, 1998, pp 399–405.
91. Wiet GJ, Bryan J, Dodson E, et al: Virtual temporal bone dissection simulation. In Westwood JD, Hoffman HM, Mogel GT, et al (eds): Medicne Meets Virtual Reality 2000: Envisioning Healing: Interactive Technology and the Patient-Practitioner Dialogue. Amsterdam, IOS Press and Ohmsha, 2000, pp 378–384.
92. Muller W, Bockholt U: The virtual reality arthroscopy training simulator. In Westwood JD, Hoffman HM, Stredney D, Weghorst SJ (eds): Medicine Meets Virtual Reality: Art, Science, Technology: Healthcare (R)evolution™. Amsterdam, IOS Press and Ohmsha, 1998, pp 13–19.
93. Smith S, Wan A, Taffinder N, et al: Early experience and validation work with Procedicus VA: The Prosolvia virtual reality shoulder arthroscopy trainer. In Westwood JD, Hoffman HM, Robb RA, Stredney D (eds): Medicine Meets Virtual Reality: The Convergence of Physical & Informational Technologies: Options for a New Era in Healthcare. Amsterdam, IOS Press an Ohmsha, 1999, pp 337–343.

94. O'Toole RV, Playter RR, Krummel TM, et al: Measuring and developing suturing technique with a virtual reality surgical simulator. J Am Coll Surg 1999;189:114–128.
95. Medical devices on parade. St. Paul Pioneer Press, St. Paul, MN, May 20, 2000.
96. Hahn JK, Kaufman R, Winick AB, et al: Training environment for inferior vena caval filter placement. In Westwood JD, Hoffman HM, Stredney D, Weghorst SJ (eds): Medicine Meets Virtual Reality: Art, Science, Technology: Healthcare (R)evolution™. Amsterdam, IOS Press and Ohmsha, 1998, pp 291–297.
97. Alterovitz RA, Pouliot J, Taschereau R, et al: Simulating needle insertion and radioactive seed implantation for prostate brachytherapy. In Westwood JD, Hoffman HM, Mogel GT, et al (eds): Medicine Meets Virtual Reality 11: NextMed: Health Horizon. Amsterdam, IOS Press and Ohmsha, 2003, pp 19–25.
98. Oppenheimer P, Gupta A, Weghorst S, et al: The representation of blood flow in endourologic surgical simulators. In Westwood JD, Hoffman HM, Mogel GT, et al (eds): Medicine Meets Virtual Reality 2001: Outer Space, Inner Space, Virtual Space. Amsterdam, IOS Press and Ohmsha, 2001, pp 365–371.
99. Ursino M, Tasto JL, Nguyen BH, et al: CathSim: An intravascular catheterization simulator on a PC. Stud Health Technol Inform 1999;62:360–366.
100. Leung K, Heng P, Sun H, Wong T: A haptic needle manipulation simulator for Chinese acupuncture. In Westwood JD, Hoffman HM, Mogel GT, et al (eds): Medicine Meets Virtual Reality 11: NextMed: Health Horizon. Amsterdam, IOS Press and Ohmsha, 2003, pp 187–189.
101. Webster RW, Zimmerman DI, Mohler BJ, et al: A prototype haptic suturing simulator. In Westwood JD, Hoffman HM, Mogel GT, et al (eds): Medicine Meets Virtual Reality 2001: Outer Space, Inner Space, Virtual Space. Amsterdam, IOS Press and Ohmsha, 2001, pp 567–569.
102. Gorman P, Krummel T, Webster R, et al: A prototype haptic lumbar puncture simulator. In Westwood JD, Hoffman HM, Mogel GT, et al (eds): Medicne Meets Virtual Reality 2000: Envisioning Healing: Interactive Technology and the Patient-Practitioner Dialogue. Amsterdam, IOS Press and Ohmsha, 2000, pp 106–109.
103. Hiemenz L, Stredney D, Schmalbrock P.: Development of the force-feedback model for an epidural needle insertion simulator. In Westwood JD, Hoffman HM, Stredney D, Weghorst SJ (eds): Medicine Meets Virtual Reality: Art, Science, Technology: Healthcare (R)evolution™. Amsterdam, IOS Press and Ohmsha, 1998, pp 272–277.
104. Dang T, Annaswamy TM, Srinivasan MA: Development and evaluation of an epidural injection simulator with force feedback for medical training. In Westwood JD, Hoffman HM, Mogel GT, et al (eds): Medicine Meets Virtual Reality 2001: Outer Space, Inner Space, Virtual Space. Amsterdam, IOS Press and Ohmsha, 2001, pp 97–102.
105. Machado LdS, de Mello AN, Lopes RdD, et al: A virtual reality simulator for bone marrow harvest for pediatric transplant. In Westwood JD, Hoffman HM, Mogel GT, et al (eds): Medicine Meets Virtual Reality 2001: Outer Space, Inner Space, Virtual Space. Amsterdam, IOS Press and Ohmsha, 2001, pp 293–297.
106. Delp SL, Loan P, Basdogan C, Rosen JM: Surgical simulation: An emerging technology for training in emergency medicine. Presence 1997;6:147–159.
107. Kaufmann C, Liu A: Trauma training: virtual reality applications. In:Westwood JD, Hoffman HM, Mogel GT, et al (eds): Medicine Meets Virtual Reality 2001: Outer Space, Inner Space, Virtual Space. Amsterdam, IOS Press and Ohmsha, 2001, pp 236–241.
108. Thurfjell L, Lundin A, McLaughlin J: A medical platform for simulation of surgical procedures. In Westwood JD, Hoffman HM, Mogel GT, et al (eds): Medicine Meets Virtual Reality 2001: Outer Space, Inner Space, Virtual Space. Amsterdam, IOS Press and Ohmsha, 2001, pp 509–514.
109. Liu A, Kaufmann C, Ritchie T: A computer-based simulator for diagnostic peritoneal lavage. In Westwood JD, Hoffman HM, Mogel GT, et al (eds): Medicine Meets Virtual Reality 2001: Outer Space, Inner Space, Virtual Space. Amsterdam, IOS Press and Ohmsha, 2001, pp 279–285.
110. Chapman DM, Marx JA, Honigman B, et al: Emergency thoracotomy: Comparison of med-

ical student, resident and faculty performances on written, computer and animal-model assessments. Acad Emerg Med 1994;1:373–381.

111. Chapman DM, Rhee KR, Marx JA, et al: Open thoracotomy procedural competency: Validity study of teaching and assessment modalities. Ann Emerg Med 1996;28:641–647.

112. Kaufman DM, Bell W: Teaching and assessing clinical skills using virtual reality. In Morgan KS, Hoffman HM, Stredney D, Weghorst SJ (eds): Medicine Meets Virtual Reality: Global Healthcare Grid. Amsterdam, IOS Press and Ohmsha, 1997, pp 467–472.

113. Stallkamp J, Walper M: UltraTrainer: A training system for medical ultrasound examination. In Westwood JD, Hoffman HM, Stredney D, Weghorst SJ (eds): Medicine Meets Virtual Reality: Art, Science, Technology: Healthcare (R)evolution™. Amsterdam, IOS Press and Ohmsha, 1998, pp 298–301.

114. Knudson MM, Sisley AC. Training residents using simulation technology: experience with ultrasound for trauma. J Trauma 2000;48(4):659–665.

115. Vanchieri C: Virtual reality: Will practice make perfect? J Natl Cancer Institute 1999;91: 207–209.

116. Muller-Witting WK, Bisler A, Bockholt U, et al: Development and evaluation of a complex training system for hysteroscopy. In: Westwood JD, Hoffman HM, Mogel GT, Stredney D, Robb RA, eds. Medicine Meets Virtual Reality 2001: Outer Space, Inner Space, Virtual Space. Amsterdam, IOS Press and Ohmsha, 2001, pp 336–339.

117. Tuggy ML: Virtual reality flexible sigmoidoscopy simulator training: Impact on resident performance. JAPBF 1998;11:426–433.

118. Merril J, Millman A, Walderman T, Merril G: Kidney stones and virtual reality. Virtual Reality Special Report Nov/Dec 1995:44–46.

119. Bro-Nielsen M, Tasto JL, Cunningham R, Merril GL: PreOp_ endoscopic simulator: A PC-based immersive training system for bronchoscopy. In Westwood JD, Hoffman HM, Robb RA, Stredney D (eds): Medicine Meets Virtual Reality: The Convergence of Physical & Informational Technologies: Options for a New Era in Healthcare. Amsterdam, IOS Press and Ohmsha, 1999, pp 76–82.

120. 5DT releases world's first virtual reality esophago-gastro-duodeno (EGD) scope training simulator. Pract Gastroenterol 2000;14(7):54,57.

121. Rolland J, Davis L, Hamza-Lup F, et al: Development of a training tool for endotracheal intubation: distributed augmented reality. In Westwood JD, Hoffman HM, Mogel GT, et al (eds): Medicine Meets Virtual Reality 11: NextMed: Health Horizon. Amsterdam, IOS Press and Ohmsha, 2003, pp 288–294.

122. Available at *http://www.immersion.com*.

123. Devitt JH, Kurrek MM, Cohen MM, et al: Testing internal consistency and construct validity during evaluation of performance in a patient simulator. Econ Health Systems Res1998; 86:1160–1164.

124. Chorpra V, Gesnik BJ, de Jong J, et al: Does training on an anesthesia simulator lead to improvement in performance? Br J Anaesthesia 1994;73:293–297.

125. Chapman DM, Marx JA, Honigman B, et al: Emergency thoracotomy: Comparison of medical student, resident and faculty performances on written, computer and animal-model assessments. Acad Emerg Med 1994,1.373–381.

126. Chapman DM, Rhee KR, Marx JA, et al: Open thoracotomy procedural competency: validity study of teaching and assessment modalities. Ann Emerg Med 1996; 8:641–647.

127. Tuggy ML. Virtual reality flexible sigmoidoscopy simulator training: impact on resident performance. JAPBF 1998;11:426–433.

128. Knudson MM, Sisley AC. Training residents using simulation technology: experience with ultrasound for trauma. J Trauma 2000;48:659–665.

129. Torkington J, Smith SG, Rees BI, Darzi A. Skills transfer from virtual reality to a real laparoscopic task. Surg Endosc 2001;15:1076–1079.

130. Torkington J, Smith SG, Rees BI, Darzi A: The role of the basic surgical skills course in the acquisition and retention of laparoscopic skill. Surg Endosc 2001;15:1071–1075.

131. Jordan JA, Gallagher AG, McGuigan J, McClure N: Virtual reality training leads to faster

adaptation to the novel psychomotor restrictions encountered by laparoscopic surgeons. Surg Endosc 2001;15:1080–1084.

132. Ahlberg G, Heikkinen T, Iselius L, et al: Does training in a virtual reality simulator improve surgical performance? Surg Endosc 2002;16:126–129.

133. Rowe R, Cohen RA: An evaluation of a virtual reality airway simulator. Anesth Analg 2002; 95:62–66.

134. Pedowitz RA, Esch J, Snyder S: Evaluation of a virtual reality simulator for arthroscopy skills development. Arthroscopy 2002;18(6):E29.

135. Ferlitsch A, Glauninger P, Gupper A, et al: Evaluation of a virtual endoscopy simulator for training in gastrointestinal endoscopy. Endoscopy 2002;34:698–702.

136. Seymour NE, Gallagher AG, Roman SA, et al: Virtual reality training improves operating room performance: Results of a randomized, double-blinded study.

137. Watterson JD, Beiko DT, Kuan JK, Denstedt JD: Randomized prospective blinded study validating acquisition of ureteroscopy using computer based virtual reality endourologic simulator. J Urol 2002;168:1928–1932.

138. Strom P, Kjellin A, Hedman L, et al: Validation and learning in the Procedicus KSA virtual reality surgical simulator. Surg Endosc 2002 Oct 29(online publication).

139. Wilhelm DM, Ogan K, Roehrborn CG, et al: Assessment of basic endoscopic performance using a virtual reality simulator. J Am Coll Surg 2002;195:675–681.

140. Shah J, Montgomery B, Langley S, Darzi A: Validation of a flexible cystoscopy course. BJU Int 2002;90:833–835.

141. Rawn CL, Reznek MA, Pugh CM, et al: Validation of a shoulder arthroscopy and IV insertion simulator: establishing a standard simulation evaluation protocol. Proceedings of the Tenth Annual Medicine Meets Virtual Reality Conference: Digital Upgrades: Applying Moore's Law to Health. January 23–26, 2002, Newport Beach, CA.

142. Reznek MA. Rawn CL, Krummel TK: Evaluation of the educational effectiveness of a virtual reality intravenous insertion simulator. Acad Emerg Med 2002;9:1319–1325.

143. Moorthy K, Jiwanji M, Shah J, et al: Validation of a web-based training tool for lumbar puncture. In Westwood JD, Hoffman HM, Mogel GT, et al (eds): Medicine Meets Virtual Reality 11: NextMed: Health Horizon. Amsterdam, IOS Press and Ohmsha, 2003, pp 219–225.

144. Berg D, Berkley J, Weghorst S, et al: Issues in validation of a dermatologic surgery simulator. I: Westwood JD, Hoffman HM, Mogel GT, et al (eds): Medicine Meets Virtual Reality 2001: Outer Space, Inner Space, Virtual Space. Amsterdam, IOS Press and Ohmsha, 2001, pp 60–65.

145. Satava RM: Report on the metrics for objective assessment of surgical skills workshop. Proceedings of the Telemedicine and Advanced Technology Research Center (TATRC) Third Annual Advanced Technology Portfolio Review, January 22, 2003, Newport Beach, CA. Available at *www.tatrc.org/website_mmvr2003/presentations/satava_files/frame.htm.*

Chapter 3

SPACE CONSIDERATIONS IN HEALTH CARE SIMULATION

Michael A. Olympio, MD

Space considerations in the design and construction of a simulation center can be one of the most exciting and demanding phases of the initial project. Contracting your own home, if you have ever had the experience, is a suitable analogy. A creative, organized, and prepared mind helps alleviate many of the pitfalls encountered by those less prepared. Financial partners and administrators appreciate a thoroughly planned and cost-accounted design, because it facilitates the timely and sequential process to completion without cost overruns. The reward is a handsome facility, suited for and unique to the institution, designed to meet the functional requirements of the simulation curriculum at an affordable price.

Certain aspects of space considerations are primary, whereas others are secondary. This chapter explores variations in form vs. function, organized in such a manner as to give initial considerations to essential space requirements. All simulation centers require a minimal amount of space to accommodate the mannequin or several mannequins and part-task trainers. The mannequins are life-size and heavy and must be placed on a firm surface. They are connected via thick, heavy cables to a rack of computer, pneumatic, hydraulic, and electronic equipment. Large H-cylinders are typically used instead of pipeline supplies, and they require significant additional space. The equipment is operated by a controller who is ideally seated at a keyboard and computer terminal. Additional mannequins, therefore, will determine the amount of space required for additional racks, gurneys, and control stations, particularly if the mannequins will be operated concurrently.

Many simulation centers replicate at least the anesthesia and operating room environment and therefore require space for the anesthesia machine, drug and supply cart, cardiovascular monitor, and some type of surgical simulation equipment. An intensive care (ICU) ventilator may require 20 square feet (sf) alone. Some highly effective simulation centers cannot physically contain more that 3 or 4 students at a time, yet they provide an important element of the curriculum.

Aside from the mannequin and associated equipment, additional space is required for interaction with the students, whether on or off site. This space is typically designated as a briefing and/or debriefing room. If the center intends to utilize part-task trainers such as intubating heads, bronchoscopic lungs, and laparoscopic or ultrasound simulators, countertop space should be included. An office for the simulation center and a separate control room are desirable but not essential in the local design.

As the simulation curriculum expands, so will the need for cabinet space. In addition to the usual storage of office and computer supplies, the cabinets will soon fill with videotapes, spare parts, electronic headsets, tools, disposable medical supplies and fluids, teaching files, and, of course, the essential coffee supplies, food, beverages, and snacks.

Other large items are considered essential by most teams, but they do not have to be located immediately within the simulation suite. Examples include an advanced cardiac life support (ACLS) standardized code cart, difficult intubation cart, and a gurney for storage or transfer of the mannequin. More realistic (and functional) centers may include a refrigerator, scrub sink, surgical tables, and linen bins.

Once the essential components and floor space requirements are determined, consider professional architectural assistance. Typically, the institution will utilize experienced and knowledgeable contractors who retain structural drawings of all available pre-existing space. Their immediate concerns include standard building and fire codes, pedestrian traffic and egress to safety, location of restrooms, and specifically the structural components of the area in question, delineating load-bearing walls and columns and firewalls, which for practical purposes should not be altered. The locality of medical gas supplies determines the need for cylinder storage and ventilation. Structural components in the ceilings and floors determine the potential for overhead lighting, gas columns, and underground floor cabling. Distance considerations between computer and simulator components are absolutely critical in initiating a floor plan, and remember the potential for noise pollution between rooms and adjacent facilities.

Once the concepts of space have materialized, it is time to convince the financial investors. Each financial model of support differs in some way. One must understand *why* the investors are paying for the simulation center. Their rationale determines the amount of space to develop as well as what space not to include. Look beyond the initial estimate for construction, because cost overruns are common and maintenance, faculty, and operational expenses must be considered. Convince the investors that the overall look and size of the facility will include such intangible benefits as recruitment, publicity, and revenues, or it might lead to competition and power struggles between users. Negotiations to obtain win-win contracts with industry should not be neglected, because they may provide attractive new and essential pieces of equipment for the facility.

Form is a statement of function, and the facility will be designed to meet the functional requirements of the simulation curriculum. What students? Visitors? Dignitaries? How many at a time? What setting? Where will the center be located? How will they enter the facility? Where and how will they be taught? Will there be a videotape review session, slide presentations, or access to clinical laboratory data? What teaching methods will be used at the facility—bedside lecturing, full-scale, small group, didactic, or observational? And, most importantly, how will the simulation encounter be recorded in the context of viewing angles?

Finally, this chapter includes representations and floor plans of several distinctly different, yet successful simulation centers. Featured are the Canadian Simulation Center in Toronto and the centers at the University of California, Los Angeles and San Francisco; the University of Louisville; the University of Texas Medical Branch in Galveston; and Wake Forest University in Winston-Salem.

ESSENTIAL AND SUPPLEMENTAL SPACE

Simulator Mannequins

The simulator mannequin is the centerpiece of the simulation center, occupying at least 6 feet in length and 2 feet in width. The actual dimensions are determined by the bed, gurney, or operating table that you choose for support. Obviously, if a hospital bed is used, the footprint will nearly double or triple. Most surgical simulations require outstretched arms on adjustable arm boards, which conveniently provide standing room for students both above the torso and beside the chest. Access to outstretched arms is critical, particularly if intravenous or arterial lines are to be placed or if pulses are to be checked and for monitoring peripheral nerve stimulation. Outstretched arms provide more convenient access to chest tube insertion, needle decompression of a tension pneumothorax, electrocardiograph (ECG) lead placement, and auscultation of lung and heart sounds. Furthermore, the T-shaped orientation provides a natural and typical physical barrier between primary and adjunct caregivers. The outstretched arms mandate an additional footprint of approximately 4 sf. Table 1 summarizes the space requirements for simulation centers.

The pediatric mannequin is the size of a 12-year old child (approximately 4 feet in height); however, the gurney, bed, or operating table required to store the pediatric mannequin is no smaller than the size required for an adult. Some centers have a minimum of one adult and one pediatric mannequin. Whether or not a center intends to operate both mannequins at the same time, storage space is still required for the additional mannequin. We find that a substitution of the adult for the child mannequin (using the same control systems) requires only 20 minutes. It is convenient to maintain the second mannequin on site to expedite the substitution.

The mannequin requires some type of control system. At present the two popular vendors are Medical Education Technologies, Inc. (METI, Sarasota, FL) and Laerdal Medical Corporation (Wappingers Falls, NY). These control systems may contain a combination of pneumatic, fluidic, electronic, and computer control systems. The Laerdal control system consists of a compressor/pneumatic system with a footprint of 2 sf, and a Link Box of 1 sf, which can be located on top of the pneumatic system. The METI system is a larger, vertical cabinet with a footprint of 9 sf, including clearance for the rear hoses, and more to accommodate the front door opening, which swings out about 2 feet. Access is required on all four sides for maintenance purposes, but the rack can be rolled about on its wheels. The noise from the METI control rack varies in amplitude and may be disruptive to an audio taping. Special consideration should be given to the construction or installation of a sound barrier or even a closet to house the rack. Particularly after recording sessions, the noise can diminish the quality of the debriefing. While considering the space required for these controllers, also note the approximate 6-foot maximal separation from the mannequin, depending on the location of the controller relative to the mannequin. The METI umbilical cord, for example, emanates from the groin, thus allowing less separation if the controller is placed at the foot of the table.

Additional components accompany the mannequin. Included is the controlling interface: a computer of some type, with monitor, mouse, and keyboard. The processor may be contained within the rack and does not require additional space, or a laptop computer can be used with the Laerdal system. In limited space applications, the instructor

Table 1.
Estimate of Space Requirements for a Single-Mannequin Facility

	Length*		Width*		Square Feet	
	Min	Max	Min	Max	Min	Max
Primary space requirements						
Mannequin	6	7	2	4	12.0	28.0
Mannequin arms	1	2	0.5	1	0.5	2.0
Mannequin controllers	1	4.5	2	2	2.0	9.0
Control interface	1	2	1	2	1.0	4.0
Gas cylinders	4	5	1	2	4.0	10.0
Drug and supplies cart	2	3	1.5	2	3.0	6.0
Trash can	1.5	2	1.5	2	2.3	4.0
IV Pole	1.5	2	1.5	2	2.3	4.0
Oxygen transport	1	1.5	1	1.5	1.0	2.3
Oxygen cylinder	0.5	0.5	0.5	0.5	0.3	0.3
Coordinator's desk	3	4	2	2	6.0	8.0
Administrative computer	2	3	2	2	4.0	6.0
Printer	1	2	1	2	1.0	4.0
Fax machine	1.5	2	1.5	2	2.3	4.0
Cardiovascular monitor	1	2	1	2	1.0	4.0
Audio communications	1.5	2	1.5	2	2.3	4.0
Video recorders	1.5	2	1.5	2	2.3	4.0
TV monitors	1.5	2	1.5	2	2.3	4.0
Subtotal					49.6	107.6
Separation factor: 30% of subtotal					14.9	32.3
Students (1 to 3 zones of six)	7.5	22.5	5	5	37.5	112.5
Students (1 or 2 at the head)	2.5	5	2.5	2.5	6.2	12.5
Total for primary space requirements					108.2	264.9
Secondary space requirements						
Anesthesia machine	3	5	4	5	12.0	25.0
Mechanical ventilator	1.5	2.5	1.5	2.5	2.3	6.3
Gas column	2	3	2	3	4	9
ACLS code-blue cart	1.5	2	2.5	3	3.8	6.0
Difficult intubation cart	1	2	2	3	2	6
Fluid warmer	1.5	2	2	2	3	4
Convection warmer	1.5	2	1	1.5	1.5	3
Mayo stand	1	1.5	2	2	2.0	3.0
Sharps container	1	2	1	2	1	4
Linen bin	1.5	2	1.5	2	2.3	4
Cautery unit	2	2.3	1.2	1.5	2.4	3.5
Basin holder	2	2	2	4	4	8
Gurney	7	8	2	2.5	14	20
Refrigerator	2	3	2	3	4	9
Scrub sink	1.5	2	1.5	2.5	2.3	5
Scanner	1.5	1.8	1	1.2	1.5	2.2
Academic computer	2	3	2	2	4	6
Camera controllers	0.5	1	0.5	1	0.3	1.0
TV monitors	1.5	2	1.5	2	2.3	4.0
Video mixers	1.5	2	1.5	2	2.3	4.0
Countertop and drawers	4	40	2	2	8.0	80.0
Briefing room	9	16	12	19	108.0	304.0
Director's office	7	10	9	16	63.0	160.0
Control room	9	25	7	12	63.0	300.0
Total for secondary space requirments					313.0	977.0
GRAND TOTAL for single mannequin facility					421	1242

*(All measurements are estimates measured in feet.)

may find it convenient to stand next to the controller, with the operating interface placed directly on it (METI) or nearby in the case of the laptop system for Laerdal. With both systems, it is possible to separate the computer interface from the controller, typically within a separate control room. We learned, however, that if the mouse is significantly separated from the processor, it may require a signal booster to function properly.

The Laerdal system provides a dedicated cardiovascular monitor that does not interface with other monitoring equipment. This type of setup requires the monitor to remain with the students, and its 1.5-sf footprint allows it to be placed at the foot of the bed or on any adjacent surface.

If the compressed medical gasses (air, oxygen, carbon dioxide, and vacuum) are required for complete functionality of the center, a ventilated cabinet (12 sf) offers the most convenient setup. In this manner, the user can purchase H-cylinders that last a suitable length of time. Local safety regulations may require that such cabinets be negatively ventilated to prevent the risk of flammable or hypoxic environments if a leak occurs. A broken valve on an H-cylinder of nitrogen or carbon dioxide, of course, can be fatal to the occupants in the room. By placing these cylinders in a cabinet, one also has the option of hard-piping the gas throughout the facility and into medical gas wall outlets. This approach contributes to realism and convenience and removes hoses from the floor. It also allows the piping to be run through the control room to simulate an oxygen failure, and it may be less expensive than extending pre-existing medical piping into the facility. Alternatively, significant reductions in space can be accomplished by piping in medical air (the largest consumption) and using smaller E-cylinders for carbon dioxide and nitrous oxide. These gasses are the least consumed, and the cylinders can be located adjacent to the rack.

Adjunct Equipment

With the mannequin and control system in place, the issue of floor space surrounding the mannequin is a matter of individual application of primary and secondary equipment. The smallest simulation center that the author has seen was no larger than a storeroom closet, approximating 80 sf. However, with a little creativity (and ventilation!) the simulation room was used quite effectively for part-task training and for anesthesia and critical care training. Thus, floor space requirements are a function of (1) the amount and size of adjunct equipment and (2) the number of students that you intend to teach around the mannequin.

Certain pieces of adjunct equipment are quite common; examples include an anesthesia machine, mechanical ventilator, IV pole, chair, and whatever surgical props may be chosen. Anesthesia machines are generally large and cumbersome devices, particularly the older models, which are more likely to find a rest home in the simulation lab. They can occupy from a minimum of 12 to a maximum of 25 sf and are associated with medical gas hoses and power cords that require an additional amount of space and restrict the flow of traffic behind the machine. Consideration should be given to the location of the medical gas supplies, whether from the ceiling or the side wall. Typically, the ceiling-mounted medical gas column cannot occupy the same space (above) as the anesthesia machine because of vertical clearance problems and the need to drape the hoses to the back of the machine. Therefore, the ceiling column can occupy another 4–9 sf. Fortunately, the anesthesia machine is mobile, and movement can be facilitated with Cast-r-Guards, which push the floor hoses out of the way.

If an anesthesia machine is available, it can substitute for a mechanical ventilator but is not as sophisticated as an ICU ventilator. These devices can be used quite effectively as training adjuncts for respiratory therapy, physicians, and ICU nurses alike. They typically offer pressure-controlled ventilation, electronic positive end-expiratory pressure (PEEP), and various spontaneous and mandatory modes of ventilation as well as various weaning strategies. Therefore, a dramatic increase in teaching capacity can be accomplished by keeping an ICU ventilator nearby. Since the setting may be changed from an operating room (OR), emergency room (ER), or floor bed to an ICU setting, adequate space must be allowed for removal of the anesthesia machine and insertion of the ICU ventilator. These ventilators vary in footprint, ranging from 2.3 to 6.3 sf. Remember to allow additional room for the gas hose connections behind the ventilator.

Other adjuncts include a drug and supplies cart, an ACLS code-blue cart, a trash can, IV poles, fluid warmer, convection warmer, and a Mayo stand, all of which are considered standard pieces of equipment in most operating rooms. The drug and supplies and ACLS carts are typically constructed of commercially available wheeled tool chests, each about 3.8 sf. Smaller stainless steel carts with a single drawer may serve as a difficult intubation (DI) cart, with a light-source on top, but these carts vary in size. A trash can requires 4 sf, whereas the base of an IV pole occupies about 3 sf. A pressure-infusion fluid warmer system, a free-standing convection warmer, and a Mayo stand also require 3 sf each. Although these items are nonessential, they offer a great deal of realism in full-scale simulation; therefore, their space requirements should be considered. If you have the luxury of retaining rather than borrowing your own ICU ventilator, add at least another 2.25 sf. This valuable piece of equipment allows the center to become a critical care unit and allows the removal of the anesthesia machine.

E-cylinders of oxygen are required in some simulations, representing transport or back-up oxygen systems. They are typically stored in a wheeled carrying device and require room for storage. It is also convenient to store a second empty oxygen transport cylinder in simulating an equipment crisis. Each wheeled cylinder requires a minimum of 1 sf of space, and additional cylinder refills require half that amount.

Other large, nonessential equipment includes a sharps container (4 sf, floor-type), a linen bin (4 sf), a cautery (3 sf), and a basin holder (4 sf). A gurney may be essential in some settings but is included within the list of secondary items in Table 1. It is a large item, occupying at least 14 sf. For nursing training, the issue of patient transfer and positioning is quite relevant; for anesthesia and surgery, the methods of returning a prone patient to the supine position during a crisis can be taught; and for advanced cardiac life support, transfer from a bed to a hard surface may be critical for cardiopulmonary resuscitation (CPR). The gurney is also used to facilitate transfer of the mannequin to other physical locations. The main operating table is too heavy to transport through a hospital, particularly with carpeted flooring.

A refrigerator and scrub sink are well worth the space that they occupy. The refrigerator contains iced and frozen saline for malignant hyperthermia scenarios in anesthesia—and certainly food and drink items if the center happens to be distant from the cafeteria or if you plan to provide refreshments during longer sessions or receptions. A medium-sized refrigerator occupies 4 sf. The scrub sink is a convenient wet area for preparing and servicing the mannequin; for preparing IV fluids, pleural evacuation containers, and urine bags; and for cleaning reusable equipment and hands. If you have the room and the money, install a genuine scrub sink for only 5 sf.

Personnel

Student groups of various sizes might also determine the need for open floor space, but the distance from the mannequin becomes a limiting factor. Larger groups tend to include visitors (10–50), primary and secondary school groups (15–40), medical students (15–25), and nursing classes (5–20). Full-scale crisis resource management scenarios might include 5–10 different students and actors. Consider the degree of interaction that people need to have with the mannequin itself before apportioning floor space. Typically students in the third row distant from the mannequin become only superficially involved and cannot examine or observe the mannequin's respiration, pulses, breath sounds, or eye signs; nor can they place needles, monitors, or tubes. Generally speaking, three groups of six at most can occupy each of three zones (left, right, foot) around the mannequin, with two additional students at the head. Each of the three zones should contain a minimum of 2.5 × 2.5 ft per person and 37.5 sf. (7.5 × 5 ft) for each group of six. An additional two students can fit at the head for an additional 12.5 sf. Crowding 20 people around the mannequin is difficult and not highly productive, but it is done frequently.

Additional students or observers are best distributed to other parts of the simulation suite, if this option is available. For example, in centers with an observation room (which might contain a slave monitor, sound, and visual image of the mannequin), it would be much better to locate the additional students here. Although they may not have hands-on capability, they may serve as assessors or consultants and may communicate with the students around the mannequin. Observation rooms are described below under "Facilities."

Significant consideration should be given to space requirements for an eventual full-time lab coordinator, if not an adjacent office for the simulation center director. The coordinator assumes responsibility for the day-to-day operations of the lab and at a minimum requires counter space for a computer, printer, scanner, and fax machine. File cabinets quickly fill with student files, research protocols, curricula, instruction manuals, warranties, and other supplies. An absolute minimum of 14 sf is required for this administrative space, which is described in greater detail below. A separate office for the director, located adjacent to the simulation center, represents the institutional significance of the simulation center. It is discussed under "Facilities" below.

Shelf and Countertop Equipment

Just as floor space is critical to the location of the mannequin and personnel, the countertop is an often-overlooked space that can be critical to the mission of the simulation facility. Monitoring devices are an essential part of the simulation suite, but they may be portable and carried onto the scene. They guide the management of an otherwise plastic and rigid mannequin and provide realistic sound effects. Cardiovascular monitors can be integrated and supply all of the essential monitoring needs (noninvasive blood pressure, electrocardiogram, invasive blood pressure, temperature, pulse oximetry, respiratory gas monitoring, and oxygen concentration), or separate modules and boxes may be used. Fortunately, these devices stack nicely on top of one another and are typically placed on top of the anesthesia machine for operating room settings. However, nearby shelf space or wall brackets can be used to secure these devices if no anesthesia machine is used. Again, the cable connections to the mannequin and to the control rack restrict the amount of separation between the monitor, mannequin, and control rack and the flow of traffic around the mannequin. An additional 1–4 sf should be allowed for these monitors.

Within the control area, a whole host of electronic equipment may be a part of the facility, particularly if extensive sound and recording systems are installed. Typically separate computers are required for operation of the mannequin and for general teaching purposes. First, the mannequin control interface can be located on top of the mannequin controller rack, but if a separate control room is built, the monitor, keyboard, and mouse will consume about 3 linear feet. (All countertops are typically 2 feet in depth). Remember to leave at least 2 linear feet for simulator operation or scenario notes. In addition, adequate space for a legal pad facilitates note-taking during development of a simulation or during the simulation itself.

The simulation lab coordinator requires an administrative desktop computer (or laptop with docking station), printer, fax, and scanner to conduct essential administrative tasks in the center. Together with telephone, keyboard, monitor, and mouse, this equipment requires approximately 6 linear feet. The third ("academic") computer is dedicated to the briefing/debriefing room via an electronic link to an LCD projector and Smart-Board (Smart Technologies, Inc., Calgary, Alberta, Canada). This combination of equipment has dramatically facilitated our teaching efforts, primarily because of the distant and interactive nature of the SmartBoard. This technology allows the teacher to control the computer from within the briefing/debriefing room, showing slide presentations or writing notes on the board with electronic pens and subsequently saving or printing the documents. The computer link to the SmartBoard can also be used with live, interactive web-based applications such as the Virtual Anesthesia Machine created at the University of Florida Department of Anesthesiology.[1] Thus, a separate academic computer for this function enables the three computers to operate the simulator concurrently, to conduct academic courses in the briefing room, and to provide administrative functions by the lab coordinator at the same time. The space requirements are the standard ones for any computer set-up, but consider adequate linear footage (7 ft) for the printer, monitor and keyboard, mouse, scanner, and enough room again for note-taking. Image processing from digital cameras or recorders mandates an additional linear foot for serial port connectors.

Sound transmission throughout the lab must be considered as well. Carefully consider the directionality and privacy of communications in planning countertop space requirements. Communications experts can save a lot of time and money by designing the system correctly the first time and by planning within your budget. They can also suggest which equipment can or should be stacked together to facilitate connections and to save space. Theoretically, an electronic rack, 2 feet in width, can house all of the following equipment, thus minimizing linear space.

Consider which of the following communications functions must be performed, and remember that each of these functions requires a separate electronic "box," which is probably stackable. Examples include the following: (1) sound/voice headset from controller broadcast to simulation room or from controller to briefing room; (2) sound/voice microphone from controller to participants wearing headsets; (3) voice microphone from controller to mannequin's voice; and (4) sound from the computer, videocassette recorder (VCR), or simulation room into the briefing room. Allow two linear feet for the stack or for each individual component. Other electronic "boxes" also require linear countertop space.

Video recording of the simulation is required for detailed debriefing, research efforts, or subsequent teaching of a prior lesson. Consider recording the actions around the mannequin as well as the data from the monitors and perhaps from the group discussions that precede or follow the simulation. To blend these various images into a single tape or digital video disc (DVD), a recording mixer is required. This multi-button controller, about 1 foot in width, is connected to another electronic box and fed into a preview monitor. Each of these devices requires about 1 linear foot. Another full-size television monitor requires 2–3 additional feet. These devices send the image to the DVD recorder or VCR (additional 2 feet). A second VCR deck may be considered for dubbing from the first, or a third deck may be needed for playback into the briefing room during concurrent teaching lessons. The VCRs can be stacked. A sound amplifier is used to balance the inputs into the final recording. Since the images are derived from a single or multiple cameras, each is best manipulated through the remote pan/tilt/zoom/focus controller. These small devices can also be stacked or placed side by side in a single layer, 2 feet wide. The images must be sent to the LCD projector for display in the briefing/debriefing room. Therefore, an input selector at the television monitor is required; no separate device is needed. However, multiple computer inputs into the LCD projector do require another electronic selector box, approximately 2 feet in width, and it is also stackable. Additional countertop space within the control room may be consumed by academic working surfaces, situated above chair inserts.

Countertops may well be considered essential within the simulation suite itself. Certainly, if cabinets are designed into the suite, the combination of floor and wall systems determines the number of linear feet of available countertop. These surfaces have a number of uses, not the least of which is to display some or all of the medical equipment that may be used in the simulation. Multiple airway devices, breathing circuits, monitors, drug infusion pumps, catheters, intravenous fluids, defibrillators, chest tube evacuation systems, and surgical instruments occupy space. During class instruction, the countertop may be needed for course syllabi and handouts. Part-task trainers (such as airway mannequins), laptop PC-based programs, or surgical virtual reality trainers for laparoscopy can occupy a dozen or more linear feet, depending on the number of installations.

Simulation centers that serve large groups of students or commercial accounts and centers that conduct full-day sessions may find it convenient to have a food-service area with enough room for a microwave oven and coffee pot. Even more realistic is consideration of retaining a work surface for making repairs to the simulator.

Supplemental Trainers

A number of supplemental simulation trainers and facilities should be considered in the design of the simulation center. Numerous part-task trainers are available and can be positioned around the facility to complement the full-scale mannequin. These part-task trainers are either software/computer-based systems or actual pieces of hardware that can be placed on top of the counter (as mentioned in the previous section) or on small, but firm tables. For example, most health care professionals are quite familiar with all of the ACLS training models, including the head/airway simulator, the upper torso with arms, the neonatal models, and all of the associated electronic boxes, monitors, and defibrillators. These devices, along with the large storage cases, may consume a significant amount of linear space. Volumes as much as $2 \times 2 \times 4$ feet for each of the adult cases, $1 \times 1 \times 1$ feet for each monitor, and $2 \times 2 \times 0.5$ feet for each controller should be allowed. Other sophisticated and interactive lung and airway models can also be permanently positioned along the countertops for fiberoptic training, but they may be more accessible if they are placed on small, wheeled carts (8 sf) at a suitable height.

Surgical simulators vary in size. They may be simple, homemade devices for tying sutures or highly expensive haptic devices that require a dedicated workstation and chair. The seated trainee visualizes a full-scale monitor atop a rack of video recording equipment, similar in magnitude to the intraoperative systems. More sophisticated centers may use the simulation lab to install a full-scale mock-up of the digital endoscopic recording equipment that is now used for minimally invasive surgery. These systems can occupy large volumes of space, depending on the features of the rack and the manner in which it is maneuvered around the operative table. For example, a ceiling-mounted boom and docking station may consume large amounts of ceiling space, with a volume of $6 \times 6 \times 3$ feet above the operating table. This boom is connected to the rack, which might be $2.5 \times 2.5 \times 6$ feet in volume.

Similarly, the simulation center may be used to train people in using the automated information management (AIM) systems for anesthesiologists and operating room nurses. These anesthesia systems, which are modifications of PC-based computers, are typically stacked or connected to the anesthesia machine, whereas the OR station is placed on top of a work surface, measuring about 1.5×1.5 feet. Room must be allowed for the monitor, keyboard, mouse, and processor.

Facilities

Additional facilities may or may not have to be located immediately within the simulation area. The control room must be located at some distance, whereas the briefing/debriefing room, lecture hall, and office for the director of medical simulation may be located at some distance. Five of the six centers described below have the luxury of attached facilities. For those with large enough control rooms, it is quite enlightening for groups of visitors or students to occupy the control room during a simulated crisis. Observers are not only able to witness the complexities of crisis simulation, but more importantly, they gain an appreciation for the interval between onset of a problem and recognition by the student. They can also appreciate various hemodynamic changes resulting from physiologic alterations. As many as 4–8 students can occupy a modest control room.

Distance learning has become a more integral component of some academic centers.[2] Relaying video images and bidirectional sound to distant and pre-existing conference facilities can greatly reduce the size requirement of the simulation center. One discreet advantage of locating the briefing/debriefing room in the simulation center is that it can be used for live viewing by another audience. Examples may include a group of spectators or a group directly involved in the simulation, such as a group of consultants. In such cases, direct visualization and audio monitoring may be essential. More sophisticated centers may choose to send the video and audio signals to a more distant location for viewing and monitoring. Consider, however, that a distant arrangement does not facilitate movement of large groups through the area. For example, a preprofessional class of 30 students may conveniently be split into three groups, one in simulation, one in the control center, and one in the briefing room. Then, as the scenario develops, the groups can rotate through the three areas. In this manner, larger groups can experience the full nature of simulation.

Separation of the simulation office may be a necessity, but there are several means of justifying an attached facility. As the program develops, walk-in visitors arrive on a weekly, if not daily basis. They may include other health care professionals who want to begin their own simulation curricula. The adjacent office facilitates discussion with these health care professionals as well as with industry representatives, hospital and medical school executives, and medical school alumni.

The size of the briefing and office facilities can vary significantly and is determined by availability and intended use. A briefing room of 11×17 feet, for example, can comfortably fit 12 chairs and a simple lectern; leaving approximately 6 feet between the screen and front row of seats (see details of the Wake Forest schematic). If a more complicated podium is needed for electronic control systems, allow a volume of $2 \times 2 \times 4$ feet. Rather than using mobile chairs, a large rectangular or oval table can be used to facilitate group discussion before and after the simulation. This set-up may require a larger room, depending on the size of the table. If a 35-mm slide projector is mounted on the back wall of the briefing room, adequate clearance must be allowed for seating beneath or next to the projector. An LCD projector can be more easily mounted on the ceiling in the center of the room. This arrangement is essential if the SmartBoard technology is used. If a television monitor and VCR combination is used within the briefing room, a larger area must be allowed to accommodate the system. Stationary or mobile carts typically consume $3 \times 3 \times 6$ feet in volume. Also consider locating a cardiovascular slave monitor in the room. It can be mounted on the wall using an inexpensive television wall platform sold at most electronic stores.

The size of the adjacent office may be determined by local restrictions or customs regarding academic office space. Ample filing cabinets and book shelves should be installed as well as extra chairs for visitors, as mentioned above. There are no other special considerations regarding the office space, and its size and design are typically left to the resources of the institution.

Storage Cabinets

The need for storage cabinets becomes overwhelming as the simulation center grows. One cannot have too many. Therefore, in planning space requirements, consider four different types of cabinets: (1) vertical cabinets, (2) file (deep) drawer cabinets, (3) overhead adjustable shelf cabinets, and (4) small drawer cabinets. Table 2 lists items likely to be stored in these cabinets.

Consider building custom cabinets. Typically, a large institution has its own cabinet maker, and custom cabinets give the advantage of using space most efficiently. With the need for countertop area, it is helpful to fill the space beneath with various types of

Table 2.
Listing of Simulation Center Supplies Requiring Storage Cabinets

Service manuals	Mannequin supplies	Masks, caps, booties
Product manuals	Central line kits	Surgical gloves
Reference books	Airway intervention kits	Defibrillator supplies
Medical textbooks	Storage boxes for mailing	Automated defibrillators
Warranties	Anesthesia machine parts	Drug infusion pumps
Computer reference books	Suction apparatus	Volatile agents
Printer paper	Monitoring devices	IV fluids and infusion sets
Letterhead stationary	Storage cases for scopes	Malignant hyperthermia supplies
Curriculum syllabi	Medical gas hoses	Syringes
ACLS instruction kits	Gas hose fittings	Needles
ACLS hardware and materials	Medical gas gauges	Intravenous catheters
Videotapes	Surgical instruments	Carbon dioxide absorbent
Office supplies	Foam	Light bulbs
Head sets	Head cradles	Non-rebreathing bags
Batteries	Cervical collars	Corrugated hose
Cables	Mock drug vials	Emergency airway devices
Kitchen items	Electronic equipment	Medical gas cylinders
Food	Various types of tape	Gas cylinder transport dolly
Cleaning supplies	Pillows	Hanging files
Telephone books	Warming blankets	Journals
Cassette tapes	Blood coolers	Surgical gowns
Instructional DVDs	Costumes for mannequin	Surgical sheets
Tools		

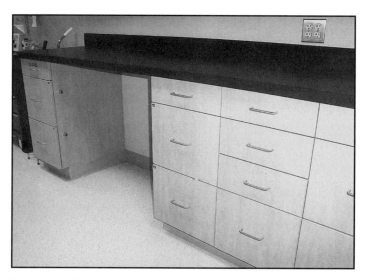

Figure 1. Example of a 36-inch surface height workbench with underlying drawers. This elevation is convenient for part-task simulators, such as intubating mannequins. The 12-inch tall drawers can accommodate standard hanging files. A 5-inch drawer sits above the 24-inch combination of units. In this example, two 6-inch drawers can replace the 12-inch file drawer. (Photo taken from the WFUBMC PSL shown in Fig. 9).

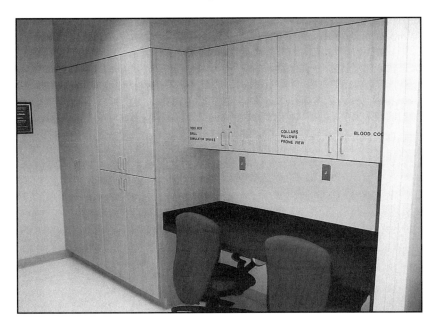

Figure 2. Example of a 29-inch surface height seated desk and workspace, which conveniently allow a computer workstation. Each station is 36 inches in width and allows an 18-inch door width on the overhead cabinets. (Photo taken from the WFUBMC PSL shown in Fig. 9).

drawer systems. These stacks and rows of drawers support the countertop and can be spaced such that openings provide room for a chair and workbench (Fig. 1).

Office cabinet systems typically have standard, repeatable dimensions. The typical depth for drawers and countertops is 24 inches, whereas the standard width of a hanging-file drawer is 16 inches. All of the sections and overhead units repeat this 16-inch unit of measure. The surface height of a "seated" workbench is typically 29 inches (Fig. 2). Optimal front panel heights for the hanging file drawers measure 14 inches. Two 5-inch drawers can then be stacked above the file drawer for a total of 24 vertical inches, above a 4-inch toe board. Alternatively, a pair of 12-inch drawers can fill the space and provide ample storage for much of the equipment listed in Table 2. The 12-inch drawers can also accommodate the hanging files, but they rub against the upper edge.

The surface of the "standing" workbench is 36 inches above the floor. It also provides room for standard drawer systems, but now the total height of the drawers will be 29 vertical inches instead of 24. Figure 1 displays the combinations of two 12-inch drawers with an additional 5-inch drawer. It also displays the combination of a single 12-inch drawer with two 6-inch, and one 5-inch drawer. Thus, any combination of 14-, 12-, 6-, and 5-inch drawers that total 29 inches in height can be located beneath the 36-inch workbench. These standard, repetitive units make the design simple, easy to build in subunits, and extremely functional.

Above these work surfaces, one can add wall cabinets that are 14 inches in depth and 30 inches tall (Fig. 3). Their width matches the bottom units, with a 16-inch pattern. Cabinets above can be fitted with adjustable shelves, typically containing 2 shelves (3

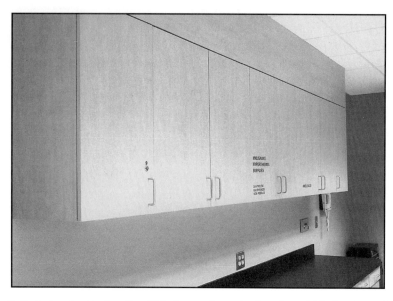

Figure 3. Typical wall cabinets with a 16-inch repeating subunit and two 18-inch units overlying the workbench. These cabinets are 14 inches in depth and 30 inches tall. (Photo taken from the WFUBMC PSL shown in Fig. 9).

surfaces) in each 30-inch tall cabinet. Tall cabinets are useful for larger objects and storage boxes. They might have doors that are 7 feet tall, and the cabinet may be 3 feet wide with a double door, each measuring 16 inches in width (see Fig. 2). Tall cabinets should be deeper than other units, perhaps 28 inches compared with the 24 inches beneath a work surface. Adjustable shelving is possible, and the height of the cabinet can also be split vertically with double upper/lower doors.

Alternatively, one can install premanufactured plastic cabinetry, an example of which stands at 6.5 × 3.5 × 2 feet in dimension (Fig. 4). This particular cabinet is specifically designed for medical supplies and has 12 drawers in combinations of 3, 6, or 9 inches deep. An upper cabinet has doors opening to a number of adjustable shelves between 4 and 8 feet. These types of cabinets are superb for disposable medical supplies, and many operating rooms use wheeled carts for ease of restocking their supplies. Metal file cabinets are also commonly in use and can store many supplies because of their open, lateral file design. These systems offer the most flexibility because the drawers allow a combination of hanging files and supplies in the same drawer.

Consider open floor shelving to hold the surgical linens and personal protective gear. These shelves may be a standard 14 inches deep and 36 inches tall, suited for any length of wall. This dimension accommodates 2 shelves and 3 surfaces.

As one example of the amount of storage cabinetry in a full-scale facility, the Wake Forest University Patient Simulation Laboratory contains 21 hanging file drawers, 20 shallow drawers, 25 overhead cabinets with shelves, 2 tall cabinets (one of which is split vertically in two), and 1 open floor shelf-cabinet. The total volume of all lower cabinets is 192 cubic feet, and the total volume of the upper cabinets is 103 cubic feet. (see Fig. 9).

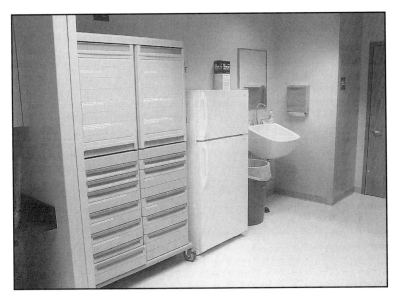

Figure 4. Premanufactured cabinet unit on wheels, next to a small refrigerator and scrub sink. See text for details. (Photo taken from the WFUBMC PSL shown in Fig. 9).

MECHANICAL/CONTRACTOR FACTORS

Architectural and Building Code Mandates

The simulation center will almost certainly be limited by existing building codes and local facility constraints. Few centers have the luxury of designing their simulation center to fit within new construction and must retrofit the center into existing space. Frequently, an optimal space is the decommissioned operating room or acute care facility. Because the simulation facility replicates the same facility that is decommissioned, the required infrastructure is already present, and the center will teach students who are already located nearby. If you must retrofit the facility into a nonclinical area, other challenges exist.

First, locate the hallways and thoroughfares leading to the center. One of the most respected simulation centers in the United States is located in downtown Cambridge, MA, within an office building![3] Thus, the choice for location is wide open, but you should consider your clients and their ability to find the center. Hallways determine the type of entrance and the flow of traffic through the facility. Consider one entrance for routine presimulation briefings, one for visitors, and another entrance for the "urgent" arrival of caregivers. The flow of personnel through the center should not disrupt an ongoing simulation, since visitors frequently arrive unannounced. Some simulation centers are located at the end of a hallway, which may or may not be conducive to your simulation objectives.

Existing Structures

One of the most expensive—and unexpected—findings in the construction of the Wake Forest Simulation Laboratory was the need for relocation of fiberoptic cable

($7,000). A vertical drop, such as ours, may necessitate the cutting and resplicing of the cable. The simulation space may need to be redesigned if such cables exist or if their location does not allow a structural redesign. In our situation, the cable was directly in the center of the simulated operating table, and we could not work around it.

A second consideration includes the pre-existence of lead-lined walls, which might simply be drawn into the plan without relocation. If they must be relocated, be certain to estimate the cost of removal or even the potential gain of utilizing the lead elsewhere. Traffic flow and wall design may further be determined by pre-existing structural components, such as load-bearing walls, columns, and firewalls, that cannot be easily relocated. Ventilation shafts are more easily rerouted horizontally in the ceilings and then dropped vertically along a wall. Restroom facilities are typically mandated on a regional square-footage basis.

Medical Gas Piping

Medical gas supplies do not influence the space requirements for a simulation facility, but they may influence its location and layout. Full-scale human patient simulators generally require compressed gases to operate, including air, oxygen, and carbon dioxide. The cost and convenience of using the central supply of piped-in gas determine the type of supply that you choose. Even with the use of larger H-cylinders, the issues of medical gas piping are still relevant. You may wish to hard-pipe the walls of the facility, originating from the cylinder supply cabinet. The installation, rerouting, or extension of existing pipelines can be quite expensive and is regulated by multiple agencies such as the Compressed Gas Association[4] (CGA @ *www.cganet.com*). The CGA publishes numerous books, pamphlets, periodicals, and guidelines for the safe handling of medical gases, and these regulations must be followed by the experts responsible for the design and construction of the facility. Additional regulations regarding the safe handling of medical gasses are also published by the American National Standards Institute[5] (ANSI @ *www.ansi.org*) and the National Fire Protection Association[6] (NFPA @ *www.nfpa.org/Home/index.asp*). Readers are referred to their own physical plant engineering office for details about the enforcement of national and local codes.

Computer and Technical Component Separation

Computer, video, and sound cables will be routed throughout the facility, and space limitations may be determined by maximum allowable separations of this equipment. For example, the computer monitor, keyboard, and mouse for the simulator may be located in another room, distant from the mannequin itself. Some cables do not have significant limitations in separation, whereas others do. The mouse cable, for example, requires a signal amplifier for distances greater than approximately 20 feet. These separation limits may affect the design of the facility. Large bundles of cables may be difficult to route inside a particular wall. Remote operation of the videocassette recorder (VCR) can be accomplished through the use of a remote infrared sensor, installed to the wall of the lecture room and connected by hard wire to the distant VCR. High-quality radio transmitters will have no problem reaching the head-set receivers of the participants. Larger simulation rooms may be enhanced through the use of mounted video cameras with high-quality zoom lenses. These lenses are capable of reading the fine print on medicine vials at a distance of 20 feet or more. The camera is operated remotely with a pan/tilt/zoom/focus controller.

Noise Insulation

A factor often overlooked in commercial construction is sound insulation. The highest-quality sound recordings are obtained only when the background noise is significantly less than the student's voices. Noise pollution results from surrounding clinical or research units, and a significant degree of noise can emanate from the simulator's pneumatic and electronic controllers. Nearby construction and jackhammer noise will paralyze the facility. Proper planning may also include an insulated closet for the noisy mannequin controller. This closet requires ventilation to avoid overheating of electronic components and consumes approximately 50% more floor space than the controlling rack itself. One must allow clearance for door and panel openings and for cable connections. Relatively inexpensive foam wall insulation can be purchased in large sheets from commercial vendors. It has the perceived effect of reducing the internal space of the simulation room but can be highly effective in suppressing noise.

FINANCIAL SUPPORT

Funding

Obviously, the more money that you have to construct the simulation center, the more elegant and larger it will be. Funding is determined at the local level, either through obvious sources or more creative ones. Creative funding is limited only by the imagination, talent, and time resources of the developer. Although not the subject of this chapter, amounts of funding from different sources vary by large magnitudes. Regardless of funding sources and the limits thereof, one should not create a center any larger than what can be realistically filled with teachers and students at any given time. Functional considerations, discussed below, should dictate the overall size of the facility, if funding is available. Some institutions charge rent based on square footage. This practice alone should warrant a limitation in space.

Ownership

Ownership determines who has the most pride in the simulation facility and usually dictates the character of the facility. Do not assume that various types of owners have the same goals for the facility. These goals vary as much as the personalities of individuals. Some may care only about teaching and learning. Others are motivated by commercialism and potential profits from industry. Still others are motivated by accreditation. Many see these centers as focal points of the institution and use them for as many media presentations as possible. Invariably, the simulation center will be used as a recruiting tool by administrators and program directors. Still others are motivated strictly by the research potential of such centers and care little about other factors. Thus, in determining space requirements, take an honest accounting of the primary function of the lab and what kind of space is required to develop that particular "image."

Revenues

Building a simulation center and purchasing the mannequin and equipment should be considered as start-up costs only. Annual expenses include disposable items, faculty salary support, technical coordinator salary, rent, depreciation, upgrades, service policies, additional equipment, and repairs. If the center is not supported by a stream of revenues and depends on hospital, medical school, or institutional support, it is certain that the size and visibility of the center will come under tighter scrutiny as the years go by. Many simulation directors have taught under adverse, temporary, and cramped conditions for prolonged periods before construction of a new facility. Many will tell you that size and elegance did not primarily determine the quality of learning or the capacity for teaching. These elements are found in the imagination of the students and teachers. Thus, if your revenue stream is restricted or nonexistent, a modest facility is the easiest to justify and maintain into the future.

FUNCTIONAL CONSIDERATIONS

Medical Students

Beginning with medical students, one must consider the size of the individual groups that will use the facility. Larger groups require more space and a little creativity. The number of students around the mannequin is generally limited not by the size of the room but rather by the ability to see and interact with the mannequin. Since the concept of simulation is predominantly interactive, consider how additional rooms within the facility might become interactive, thus increasing student capacity. For example, a well-designed debriefing/observation room should include a live audio and video feed from the simulation room and the ability to interact verbally with the active students and/or instructors in the control room. Properly positioned cameras with zoom/pan/tilt features can provide an impressive amount of feedback to a second student group unlimited in size. In fact, an instructor can use the camera controls to pinpoint observations for the second group, thus facilitating their assessment of the simulation. This focused feedback promotes small group discussions in the debriefing room, led by the observers. In this manner, a small simulation room with a larger observation room greatly enhances the numbers of students who can "actively" participate in a simulation. These observers can actually serve as a "panel of experts" for the active clinicians. Indeed, researchers from the Center for Medical Simulation[3] have demonstrated much longer distance interactive learning through a live connection to Rochester, New York at the 2000 annual meeting of the Society for Education in Anesthesia. A distant intrainstitutional lecture hall can serve as a second learning site.

Another location for students to learn is located within the control room of the simulation center. Here the students can observe the selection and activation of physiologic variables that are required to emulate a patient. As a learning experience, they can be subjected to Socratic-type questioning from the instructor as she or he conducts the scenario. With a large number of students in three separate rooms, the ability to educate the masses becomes a reality.

Resident Physicians

In general, resident physicians will not be available in groups as large as medical students. In fact, our experience has shown that groups of 2–4 students are much more common, and residents tend to have the greatest degree of primary interaction with the simulator. Space is a consideration only when ancillary equipment is intended for use.

Nurses, Paramedics, and Technicians

More curriculum-based bedside teaching is conducted with these groups, which generally consist of 4–10 students per session. Sessions include a significant amount of demonstration and lecturing by the instructor. In such environments, as ridiculous as it may sound, one ought to consider the installation of retractable bleachers that can be drawn out, when needed, to provide seating for a dozen students or more, all of whom are within 15 feet of the mannequin. The retracted bleachers might only consume 3 feet in depth against a wall.

Visitors

Various types of visitors have similar requirements. They include institutional tour groups, student applicants, industry representatives, dignitaries, donors, academic visitors, and, indeed, television recording crews. It is fair to say that the more elegant the center, the more visitors you will have. Plan accordingly. If negotiations are to be conducted, ample room for chairs and a working surface is required. This goal is best accomplished with an attached director's office, but such a layout is not required. A pathway that allows intrusion of visitors during the conduct of a simulation is required. Providing that pathway can be a dilemma if space is not planned anew. Large groups may be facilitated with refreshments, luncheons, or drinks, all of which require countertop space or tables. A sink and refrigerator are convenient for clean-up and storage.

Visitors do not always announce their arrival, and of course they want to witness the facility in action without interfering. They should be able to see and hear the intensity of the event without disrupting the students. Therefore, an observation room with one-way glass, audio-visual feeds, and a separate entrance works very well. Instructors in the control room should be able to see people arriving and to communicate with them from the control room. In addition, there should be enough room in the control area to accommodate a small group of people who want to observe the operations or talk with the instructor during the simulation.

CLINICAL SETTINGS

Because simulation centers are used for a variety of different students, the clinical settings will vary. One might consider adapting the simulation room to the size of a hospital room, operating room, intensive care unit, emergency room, or labor suite. Alternatively, a mass casualty area, for example, may be of any size and have any number of mannequins on the floor. Regardless of which setting is most commonly used, arrangements should be made to store the various pieces of clinical equipment required for diverse groups that use the simulation center. Large pieces of equipment, such as operating tables, hospital beds, ventilators, anesthesia machines, and surgical tables, generally have wheels and can be rolled into an adjacent storage room when necessary. If the simulation center is a single large room, temporary wall partitions, vertical drapes, or drape coverings can be used to hide unnecessary equipment.

It may not be necessary to dedicate all of this equipment to the simulation facility. One can borrow equipment from the clinical facility if needed. This arrangement certainly reduces expenses, capital equipment, and the need for storage space. In borrowing such equipment, it helps to involve relevant clinical specialists in the simulation scenario. A floor nurse who rolls an extra bed to the suite may well appreciate participating in a "code-blue." Respiratory therapists who lend an ICU ventilator can describe their favorite ventilator complications for simulation and then respond to the call for help. And who does not need surgical nurses in OR scenarios?

FLOW PATTERN

The physical location of the simulation center and the flow of visitors through the center dictate special considerations for space. Some centers are located separately from the health care facility and require space for transportation facilities, be it bicycles, automobiles, or access to public transportation. Are there places to park a vehicle? Where will the school bus park after it delivers a group of medical explorers? Are there convenient locations for distant travelers to congregate prior to the simulation episode? Inclement weather requires space for additional clothing, heavy coats, umbrellas, and other winter gear. Students frequently bring heavy back-packs to the simulation facility. Is there a place to store them securely?

On arrival at the simulation center, where will the students initiate the experience? Will it be a lecture hall, conference room, briefing room, or the simulation room itself? A good understanding of intent leads to good planning of the facility. For example, if a lecture hall or conference room is used for assembly, it may not need to be adjacent to or even a part of the simulation center. If the students or a second group of students are to respond emergently, is there an appropriate entrance for their arrival that does not interfere with the control center or with a third group of observers? Will any of these people need to pass through a private office or supply area, or is there enough space for a separate entrance or hallway?

TEACHING METHODS

Various styles of teaching are common in simulation centers and influence space requirements. Styles may include (1) an instructor who teaches at the bedside, (2) students in self-study groups at part-task trainers, (3) an instructor who monitors two or three students in full-scale, crisis simulation, (4) multiple people responding in crisis and practicing team interaction skills, (5) observational learning, (6) distance or classroom education, and (7) bedside demonstrations for large groups. Each of these styles has a different requirement for space, as discussed above. Flexibility and prioritization are key. If the predominant form of teaching is done at the bedside with larger groups of students, a larger simulation room may be constructed instead of a briefing room. A control room may be eliminated as well. Storage and filing cabinets are necessary if you educate multiple types of health care professionals and if you have an active research program.

RECORDING METHODS

Many simulation centers use a home movie camera and tripod to record the simulation events. Some may have taken written notes of the session and never used cameras. Although the particular recording method will not determine the size of your center, it may well influence the design. For example, if high-quality recording equipment is installed to capture multiple views, it becomes advantageous to move the masses of observational students into a more comfortable, seated environment such as a classroom or debriefing room. Recording angles should visualize all of the dynamic components of simulation: (1) overhead view of the patient and students; (2) tangential view of the equipment, monitors, and students; and (3) detailed and dedicated view of the cardio-vascular and respiratory monitor, which may be obtained from a secondary video card. Distance of the camera from the point of action should be minimized, and many find it quite valuable to spend the extra money for a high-quality camera lens with zoom, pan, and tilt. It is amazing how such a lens can record the most intricate details. Although usually not an issue, consider on which wall and ceiling area the cameras will be mounted. An optimal tangential angle extends about 120 degrees from the head, below the left arm, particularly for the standard operating room configuration.

DESCRIPTIONS OF ESTABLISHED SIMULATION CENTERS

Canadian Simulation Center, Toronto

The Canadian Simulation Center in Toronto (Fig. 5) totals 1,262 square feet, ex-cluding the main hallway. It consists of five rooms, including two seminar rooms, one simulation room, a combined control room and office, and a storage closet. The large (149-sf) storage room houses the H-cylinders of air, oxygen, and nitrous oxide, along with smaller cylinders of oxygen, carbon dioxide, and nitrous oxide. There is also room for a refrigerator and multiple pieces of medical equipment, including fiberoptic scopes, IV infusion pumps, and a cardiotocograph. The control room (70 sf) contains all of the necessary electronic, computer, and audiovisual equipment. It has a one-way window looking into the single, 400-sf simulation room, which has another one-way window at

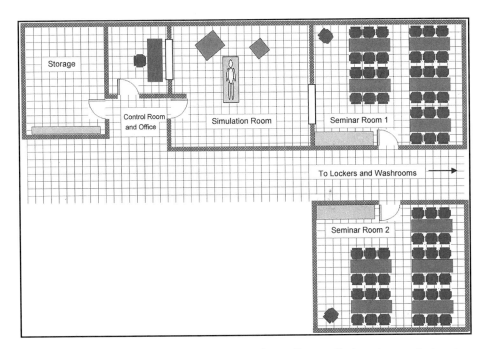

Figure 5. Floor diagram of the Canadian Simulation Center, Toronto. Scale = 1 square foot per box. See text for a complete description.

the other end for viewing from the adjacent 326-sf seminar room. A second seminar room across the hall has the same dimensions. Within each seminar room is a VCR, a 32-inch television monitor, coffee maker, microwave oven, projector with screen, five tables, and 31 chairs. Lockers and washrooms are nearby along the same hallway.

University of California, Los Angeles (UCLA)

The simulation center at UCLA (Fig. 6) consists of 504 sf, excluding the main hallway, and contains four rooms. It is used predominantly for the training of small groups of students. The simulator is moved to another location in the physiology department, when necessary (e.g., for training larger groups of medical students). The largest room and simulation suite is a long rectangle, 23 × 10 ft. This room contains the mannequin, anesthesia machine and equipment, H-cylinders of gas, storage cabinets, and a separate area at the far end that is used for part-task training. This area has the equipment for IV and arterial puncture training, intubation stations, and endoscopy simulators. The control room (80 sf) is located at the far "anesthesia" end of the simulation suite. It contains the control desk with all of the mannequin controls, the audiovisual recording equipment, cabinets for simulation files, and a few chairs. The center has a dedicated 76-sf office for the simulation coordinator, containing an L-shaped desk, credenza, and chairs. Within the 112-sf de-

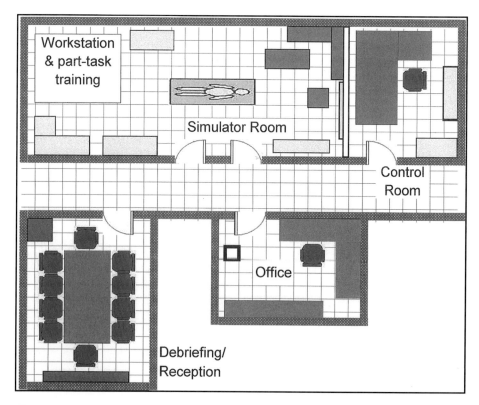

Figure 6. Floor diagram of the University of California, Los Angeles simulation center. Scale = 1 square foot per box. See text for a complete description.

briefing room is a rectangular table with 10 chairs, and the TV/VCR combination is located on a desk at the end of the room. The office and debriefing room are separated from the control and simulation room by a 30-foot hallway. Access to any of the four rooms is gained via the hallway. Within the 1120 sf debriefing room is a rectangular table with 10 chairs, and the TV/VCR combination is located on a desk at the end of the room.

University of California, San Francisco

The simulation center at the University of California, San Francisco, occupies a single, unused but licensed operating room at San Francisco General Hospital. It is rectangular in shape, and the control room is segregated from the simulation area by portable room dividers, standing 5.5 feet tall. The hospital building authorities would not allow the construction of a divided wall within an existing operating room, and they closely regulate the use of the facility. For example, special approval was required before installation of a mounted video camera. The conference room for the simulation center is detached, located some 40 yards from the simulation room. This arrangement creates problems in teaching an audience at a distance or retaining observational students on stand-by for participation. There is neither a waiting room nor proximity of a debriefing area to accommodate exchange between the simulation and didactic areas. The director of the center considers it to be the smallest possible space for effective simulation; however, the author has seen even smaller (storage) rooms in use. Such small centers limit the amount of on-site equipment and storage, but with a bit of imagination, cooperation, and struggle, equipment can be relocated to the facility as needed. On the other hand, surgical and anesthesia simulations provide all of the real ancillary equipment and medical supplies to which one normally has access, since the simulation room is located immediately adjacent to the actual operating room. Furthermore, under flexible contractual agreements, disposable medical supplies are also readily available, and the simulation suite can be stocked in identical fashion as the operating room. Medical gases are readily available and do not consume what is otherwise a major building expense. Perhaps even more importantly, the faculty and students who might be called upon as participants are readily available as a captive audience. Students can be assigned to the simulation center during a regularly scheduled work day for a single simulated case and then immediately return to clinical duty. Faculty can assume teaching responsibilities within the simulated environment, consistent with their routine cross-coverage of other sites. Thus, the simulation suite is a "real" facility. It can easily be converted to any of the other venues. Neither rent nor utilities are paid, and the physical plant maintenance remains a part of the operating room responsibility.

University of Louisville

The Louisville simulation center (Fig. 7) is the largest of these examples and accommodates four simulation mannequins in separate rooms at the same time. The facility was constructed through the generosity of a single individual grant and spans nearly 2,500 sf with outer dimensions of 70 × 35 feet. It was designed with the intent of balancing the lab and classroom space. Each of the four simulation rooms is roughly 320 sf (20 × 16), providing sufficient space for 10–12 students and 1–2 instructors per room. The four simulation rooms also provide space for storage of additional equipment, stretchers, and teaching tools. Each pair of labs has a 26 × 8 ft. control room, enabling one controller to run two simulations simultaneously. Two groups of students can

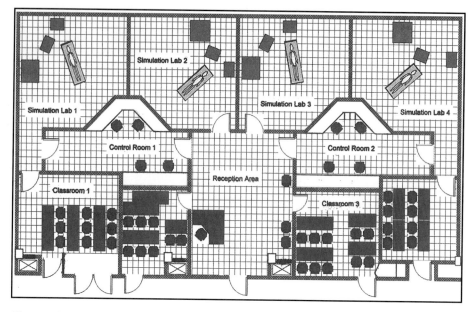

Figure 7. Floor diagram of the University of Louisville simulation center. Scale = 1 square foot per box. See text for a complete description.

also be observed concurrently. The generous reception area is 20 × 18 ft., and four classrooms make up the remaining space. The classrooms vary in size and seat between 8 and 10 students, depending on the configuration of the room. Particularly large groups occasionally attend the facility, and as many as 31 students have been squeezed into a single classroom. Although the lobby area is quite large, it follows the function of the lab and accommodates a number of annual public-relations events. The lobby is also used as a staging and exchange area for larger sequential groups of students.

University of Texas Medical Branch, Galveston

The new simulation center at the University of Texas Medical Branch in Galveston (Fig. 8) approximates 1,119 sf and was created from two pre-existing operating rooms with a shared storage area. It contains adequate facilities for two concurrent simulation programs. The two simulation rooms are each 280 sf with a convenient shared connection to the control room, measuring 8 × 9 ft. This room conveniently contains 16 linear feet of counter surface with overhead cabinet space. One-way windows allow a view to the side of each mannequin within the simulation rooms. The 12 × 16 ft. foyer entrance to the simulation suite conveniently serves the dual purpose of an observation room and entry way, again with one-way windows looking into the two simulation rooms. One of the simulation rooms contains a permanently located simulator, whereas the other contains a portable mannequin and movable overhead camera. This allows optimal flexibility in changing the simulation setting. The L-shaped arrangement provides an adjacent conference room, which does not allow a direct view into the simulation room but does contain all of the electronic audio/video reception equipment to view live or videotaped presentations. The conference room is generous at 19 × 12 ft. and contains a rec-

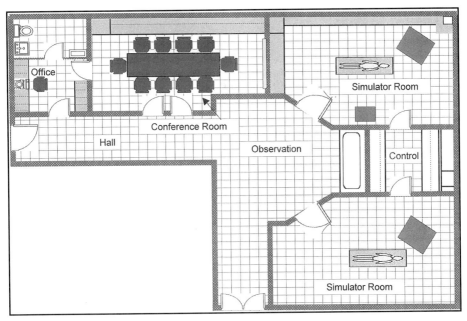

Figure 8. Floor diagram of the University of Texas Medical Branch, Galveston simulation center. Scale = 1 square foot per box. See text for a complete description.

tangular table seating 10 persons. The conference and simulation rooms also contain 47 linear feet of counter surface and floor cabinets and an additional 38 linear feet of overhead cabinets. The far end of the conference room enters into the 56-sf simulation office, containing 13 linear feet of work and desk surface. The office is even attached to a private, 40-sf lavatory.

Wake Forest University, Winston-Salem

The simulation center at Wake Forest University (Fig. 9) is part of the medical center, detached from the department of anesthesiology. As such, it was designed to accommodate a director of simulation with an attached 152-sf office and a simulation center totaling 1,247 sf. The center consists of five rooms, including the office, briefing room, large simulation room, panoramic control room, and utility closet. Although the 67-sf closet is outside the doors of the facility, it is isolated enough to provide storage of bulky items, such as an ICU ventilator and fluid warming poles. Access to the center is gained either through the briefing room, simulation room, or director's office, depending on the type of scenario and visitors. Most scenarios begin in the 175-sf briefing room, with students arriving through its main entry. The instructor can remain within the 190-sf control room before and during the students' arrival, utilizing the one-way view through and into the briefing room. Self-taught scenarios are initiated electronically from the control room by the simulation coordinator, who can speak into the briefing room and initiate a computer slide presentation on the SmartBoard. The operator also has the ability to initiate a videotaped preview for the students in the briefing room or to videocast a live scene from the simulation room. There is ample space in the

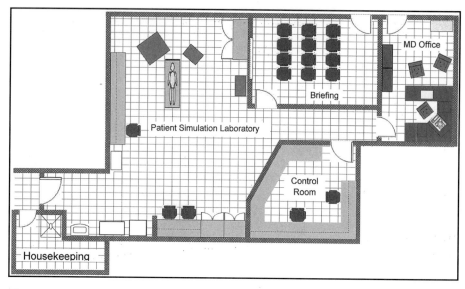

Figure 9. Floor diagram of the Wake Forest University Baptist Medical Center, Winston-Salem simulation center. Scale = 1 square foot per box. See text for a complete description.

18 × 28 ft. simulation room to accommodate large groups of visitors (20 or so) comfortably. The room serves not only as the main simulation area but also as a computer workspace and desk for two seated chairs with workbench space for an additional chair.

Storage within the simulation center is generous, with 45 linear feet of overhead cabinets, 26 linear feet of floor mounted files and drawers, 6 linear feet of tall cabinets, 6 linear feet of bookshelves and 5 feet of standing file cabinets (see Figs. 1–4). The center also contains 72 linear feet of countertop and desktop space. The center does not have separate storage for extra gurneys or mannequins or larger pieces of equipment, which are frequently placed beneath the control room window. A 5 × 2 ft. ventilated closet in the simulation room houses all medical gas cylinders. It would have been advantageous to extend the closet for housing the simulator rack to achieve better sound insulation. Finally, a scrub sink and refrigerator are located by the clinical "emergency" entrance (see Fig. 4).

References

1. Lampotang S, Lixdas D, Liem EB: The Virtual Anesthesia Machine, 2000. Available at *http://www.anest.ufl.edu/~eduweb/vam/* (free access).
2. Via DK, Kyle RR, Trask JD, et al: Using high-fidelity patient simulation and advanced distance education network to teach pharmacology to second-year medical students. J Educ Perioperat Med 2003 [in press].
3. Center for Medical Simulation. 65 Landsdowne Street, Cambridge, MA. Available at *www.harvardmedsim.org/index.html.*
4. Compressed Gas Association, 4221 Walney Road, 5th Floor, Chantilly, VA 20151-2923; telephone, 703-788-2700.
5. National Fire Protection Association, 1 Batterymarch Park, P.O. Box 9101, Quincy, MA, 02269-9101; telephone, 617-770-3000.
6. American National Standards Institute, 1819 L Street, NW, Washington, DC, 20036; telephone, 202-293-8020.

Chapter 4

HUMAN CONSIDERATIONS IN HEALTH CARE SIMULATION

Pamela J. Morgan, MD, CCFP, FRCPC, and
Susan L DeSousa, BSc, RRCP

Simulation Center Coordinator/Manager

The role of the simulation center coordinator is challenging to define (for simplicity, the term *coordinator* is used to reflect both titles: coordinator and manager). The person filling this role assumes several important and key responsibilities. Most importantly, this person acts as the primary liaison between the center and its users.

Job Description

The job description for the coordinator depends on the needs and objectives of each individual center. Despite the differences among centers, several responsibilities commonly belong to the coordinator. He or she is responsible for the daily maintenance of the center. Duties include answering phones, responding to all inquiries about the center, and maintenance of supplies and cleaning. As the primary liaison for the center, the coordinator must identify, contact, and meet with potential or existing users both within the institution and in the outside community. Facility tours and marketing of the center are key responsibilities.

Scenario development is also a significant role of the coordinator. The coordinator must be able to conduct needs assessments for users to ensure that the learning objectives of each user group are met. The coordinator or the user may be the primary scenario developer, or the coordinator may work in conjunction with the user to develop and script scenarios.[1] In either case, the coordinator must be able to advise about the scenario content to ensure that it works within the capabilities of the simulator and related equipment. Scenario programming, testing, and troubleshooting are vital roles. Scenario development also includes setting up the room appropriately and ensuring the availability of all necessary equipment, props, and actors (if needed) for each scenario. The coordinator works to ensure the smooth operation of every aspect of each scenario from start to finish.

Equipment purchase, maintenance, repair, and troubleshooting are often the responsibility of the coordinator. The coordinator may need to advise about the use of equipment and equipment purchases and serve as liaison with equipment manufacturers. Regular maintenance of the simulator(s) and associated equipment is essential for quality assurance and quality control.

Program and course development may be shared among several members of the center staff, including the simulation coordinator. The coordinator helps to develop programs necessary for the success of the center. The coordinator must be able to advise about the applicability of each program with regard to the curriculum, simulator equipment, center resources, staff, and availability. The coordinator may be responsible for developing and circulating course material as well as overseeing course registration and course planning (e.g., catering, space allocation). The coordinator may be expected to approach different professional organizations and prepare the necessary documentation for continuing education course credits for participants.[2]

For centers involved in simulation research, the coordinator may assume the role of research assistant, again depending on availability of staff in the specific center. The coordinator may be involved to various degrees in study design, participant recruitment, data collection, input, and much more.

Training of team members may also be part of the coordinator's job description. Some center coordinators train other members of the simulation team to run the simulator(s) in high-volume centers, including scenario programming. For example, the Ontario Air Ambulance Base Hospital mobile simulation program in Toronto, Canada (www.basehospital.com/index.asp) has trained seven team members in the complete operation of the simulator(s) to assist and/or perform off-site training programs.

The coordinator may also be expected to manage the center's finances. Duties may include collecting and processing all monies pertaining to the center, such as course registration fees, user fees, and grant awards. Preparing and maintaining a budget as well as fund raising may also fall within the coordinator's responsibilities.

Every component of the coordinator's job description noted above may not be necessary for every center. The coordinator's job description is summarized in Table 1.

Time Commitment

A full-time equivalent (FTE) is the ideal time commitment for a simulation center coordinator due to the extensive job description outlined above. In a survey of simulation centers worldwide, 82% reported having dedicated personnel for the operation of the simulator.[3] It is important to have a dedicated person available as often as possible to answer inquiries related to the center, to market the center to interested user groups, and to establish a continuous presence within the simulation center's institution. Courses and/or training sessions may need to be scheduled on evenings and weekends

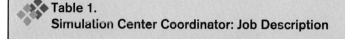

Table 1.
Simulation Center Coordinator: Job Description

1. Secretarial duties
2. Scheduling and operation of simulator sessions
3. Scenario development, programming, and testing
4. Maintenance and ordering of supplies
5. Equipment purchasing, maintenance, troubleshooting, and repair
6. Assistance with ongoing research
7. Budget management
8. Marketing and client outreach
9. Course and program development
10. Team training

to accommodate the user. A flexible schedule for coordinators is necessary to accommodate the various user groups.

Qualifications

The qualifications of a simulation center coordinator vary considerably among centers and should reflect the needs and goals of each center. The educational qualifications described are just a guideline and should be used as a starting point. The list is by no means inclusive.

◆ A postsecondary education in a science or health-related field
◆ Clinical experience in a medical field and/or experience working in an acute-care setting
◆ Teaching and/or research experience
◆ Skills in oral/written communication
◆ Excellent computer skills
◆ Good technical skills
◆ Experience working with different types of medical equipment

The clinical experience in health care and/or an acute-care setting is helpful for curriculum development, designing scenarios, and ensuring realism during scenario programming and execution. It is also beneficial for equipment preparation and troubleshooting. Clinical experience is vital if the coordinator is to be involved in program development and teaching within the center.

Technical and computer skills are essential due to the many pieces of equipment within a simulation center, including but not limited to the simulator(s) and the computer(s) that operate them. Other types of equipment may include intensive care unit (ICU) ventilators, anesthesia gas machines, defibrillators, intravenous (IV) pumps, computer-based simulation, and much more.

Equally important for the success of the center, are the coordinator's personality traits. First and foremost, the person must have an interest in medical simulation. The person must be a self-directed learner and independent, with the ability to solve problems. He or she must also be energetic, eager to learn, and approachable. It is also important that the candidate have an active interest in teaching, willingness to accept challenges, and ability to exhibit leadership qualities. The field of medical simulation is constantly changing and progressing. It is important for the coordinator to stay up to date with the latest developments in the field of simulation, from both technical and educational standpoints. All of these characteristics are important and reflect the coordinator's job description outlined above.

Secretary/Receptionist

In some centers it may be possible to hire a secretary/receptionist who can help download work from the simulation coordinator. He or she may be responsible for answering telephones, sending and receiving faxes, organizing times for educational and research events, ensuring catering for such events, and sending out reminders to participants about the time and place of each scheduled session. In addition, the secretary may perform the usual secretarial duties, such as word processing, filing, copying materials, and taking minutes at meetings. It may be possible to obtain some financial support for a secretary/receptionist through the center's institution.

Simulation Center Medical Director

Job Description

The job description for a simulation center medical director varies considerably among centers and depends on the time commitment of each director and the needs of each center. The medical director oversees the operation of the center as a whole. He or she may not necessarily be responsible for the day-to-day operation of the center. Again, the job description depends on the amount of faculty and additional staff available to the center.

The medical director is responsible for recruiting staff and faculty for the center. He or she also participates in teaching sessions and is invaluable as a course instructor; however, the teaching role within the center can be quite time-consuming. The director must advocate the center and encourage others to become involved in simulation teaching. This goal involves interacting with other health care program educators in medicine, nursing, respiratory therapy, paramedicine, and other allied health professions.

The medical director is also responsible for aiding in the development of programs and curriculum for the center. He or she must promote teaching and education at all levels, including undergraduate and resident education, continuing medical education (CME), and education for allied health professionals. The medical director oversees or supervises all members of the simulation team.

The medical director is a vital liaison between the simulation center and its users. This role requires participation in fund raising and marketing of the center to help ensure its success. He or she must act as a liaison with departments and administration within the institution and be a strong advocate for the center and simulation in education. The director should interact with other members of the simulation community on a local, national, and international level. He or she is the contact person for issues relating to simulation within the institution, including media relations and institutional public relations.

If research is a focus of the center, the director may be responsible for the promotion and development of research proposals, including recruitment of a research team to implement a research program. The director should encourage grant submission to secure research funding. Other roles may include implementation of projects, participant recruitment, program evaluation, and publication. Such duties vary according to the size of the research team. It is important for the director, along with other members of the research team, to interact with other researchers in the field.

The director oversees the financial aspects of the center, including budget creation, fund allocation and disbursement, development of user fees, and much more. Depending on the center, some of the financial responsibilities may be delegated to other members of the simulation team.

Time Commitment

The time commitment for a medical director varies depending on the extent of the center's activities and additional available staff. It also depends on the amount of time he or she is relieved of other duties, such as clinical and/or administrative responsibilities. It may not be necessary for the director to be available on a day-to-day basis; however, it is important that he or she be available for consultation when appropriate.

Qualifications

The qualifications of the medical director depend on the directive and focus of each center. For example, a surgical skills simulation center may require a director to have a surgical specialty. The director's qualifications should directly reflect the needs of each center.

The director should have extensive experience with medical simulation and its application to education. He or she must be familiar with the strengths as well as the limitations of simulation, the obstacles that simulation training faces in evaluation and certification, and the cost versus benefit of simulation.

The director must be familiar with the technical aspects of simulation, including scenario development and operation of the simulator(s) and related equipment. The director must be familiar with all branches of medical simulation including but not limited to computer-based simulation, part-task trainers, and high-fidelity simulation.

The director must exhibit excellence in patient care and teaching. This trait ensures excellence in program development, implementation, and course instruction. The director should have interest and experience in patient safety and human factors, including crisis management training and debriefing.

Educational Consultant: The Role of the Professional Educator

Job Description

The professional educator has a valuable role in health care simulation. He or she provides input from an academic background centered on educational and evaluation methodologies and can add interesting and insightful information to the simulation programs. The professional educator is an expert in the understanding of how to develop educational programs from both theoretical and practical bases. In addition, the educator's expertise in educational measurement and evaluation can greatly assist simulation programs as they begin work in these areas. Finally, the professional educator has the expertise to determine the outcome of both learning and assessment programs that have been developed.

At the University of Toronto, the vast majority of undergraduate and postgraduate programs in medicine have educational consultants whose role has become an integral part of the courses. Each undergraduate course in the Faculty of Medicine is required to produce both qualitative and quantitative data, which demonstrate that the course is providing the educational experience that the institution expects. It is the job of the professional educator to ensure, in conjunction with course directors, that the educational and evaluative processes are valid and reliable tools in the learning process. It seems logical, therefore, that any developing educational program, including those developed in human simulation, should consider the integration of a professional educator in personnel considerations.

Human simulation programs are rapidly developing as the availability of high-fidelity simulation increases worldwide.[3] However, few studies in the literature have critically evaluated the educational and evaluation processes using high-fidelity patient simulation. As research into this area develops, the role of the professional educator in the educational processes becomes exceedingly important in considerations such as of the use of simulation for performance assessment or maintenance of certification. Indeed, few centers are using simulation for this purpose—and many cite as the reason the lack of valid and reliable testing methods.[3]

In many centers, physicians are responsible for the educational input and evaluation of learning and assessment methods using simulation. Some of these physicians may have expertise in the area of educational programs, but many do not. Consultation with an expert educator can only strengthen the simulation programs and should be considered by all centers hoping to establish research and educational curricula.

Time Commitment

The amount of commitment from the professional educator obviously differs among simulation centers. For simulation programs that are just beginning to develop educational programs, the commitment may be greater at the outset, but taper as the programs get under way. It is important, however, to ensure ongoing qualitative and quantitative analyses of the simulation programs. In our center, the professional educator's commitment is in the order of 0.05 FTE for contribution to simulation-based education and evaluation. Financial compensation comes from the university department.

Qualifications

The expertise of the individual educator may differ from person to person. Some will have expertise in educational methodologies and curriculum and others in measurement and evaluation. Although not critical in the process, it may be useful to match the simulation program's needs with the qualifications of the educator consulted. For example, if the research directive of the simulation program is to develop valid and reliable testing methods using simulation, a professional educator with expertise in this area may be preferred. Most professional educators associated with our university programs have a minimum of a masters' level degree in education, and many consultants have doctorate-level degrees in education.

Research Director

Job Description

The simulation center research director is an important and pivotal position; he or she should be responsible for the overall research program in simulation. The research director may provide not only leadership guiding the research program, but also support and advice to new investigators interested in a career in simulation-based research. This advice may extend beyond the director's area of medical training, but he or she should have the skills to provide an appropriate template that any medical, surgical, or paramedical discipline can follow in order to succeed.

The research director should also be responsible for the accountability of the research output of the center and should regularly review the ongoing studies, including their progress and success. The research director should be a consultant to new investigators to help them obtain funding and to ensure the viability of their studies. Often the research director provides scholarly review of peer-reviewed articles being prepared for submission.

As a simulation center becomes recognized as a research center, the director may initiate a program designed to offer research training for postgraduate trainees or fellows. This involvement helps to supply high-quality researchers who can continue the established research program in the center or encourage the development of other research programs in other areas of the country.

Another critical role of the research director, in conjunction with the medical director, is to provide solid evidence of the scientific viability of the simulation center. This type of feedback is critical to demonstrate that monetary support from the university, individual institution, or public sector has resulted in high-quality productivity as evidenced by peer-reviewed grants, publications, and scholarly presentations.

Finally, the research director should provide an annual written report to the medical director, outlining the research activities of the center.

Time Commitment

As with other personnel considerations, the time commitment for the research director is directly proportional to the ongoing research activity in the center. If a center is at the beginning stages of research activity, the research director may need to be on site to establish the initial research program. Although this commitment is necessarily guided by financial support, it is reasonable to consider a 0.2 FTE commitment in the initial stages. As the research program becomes more established and self-supporting, the simulation center coordinator may be able to handle the operation of the research program in conjunction with the research associate. At that point, the research director may have a smaller time commitment while continuing consultative and administrative roles in the simulation center.

Qualifications

The research director should have a background in research with an established reputation and evidence of productivity, including authorship of peer-reviewed papers and knowledge and success in obtaining peer-reviewed funding.

Research Associate

The research associate is a valuable member of the simulation team. He or she should provide the expertise needed to facilitate ongoing research activity. This expertise includes a sound knowledge of how to conduct clinical research studies. He or she should have experience in the preparation of study proposals for funding requests and the ability to search and access the ongoing available funding agencies to download application forms. The research associate's expertise will be extremely useful in helping new investigators learn the requirements and process of obtaining non-peer-reviewed and peer-reviewed funding.

The research associate should have advanced computer skills. Facility with database set-ups, database entries, and Excel spreadsheets is invaluable. Although not crucial, the ability to do basic statistical analyses facilitates the timely interpretation of study results.

Often the research associate can contribute to the success of research studies by participation in the scenarios presented in the simulation center. Since the research associate has an integral knowledge of the study proposal, he or she can role-play various personnel who may be involved in the simulation sequence.

The research associate can also provide information about timelines and applications for research presentations at local, national, and international meetings. He or she can provide assistance in the preparation of abstracts for these presentations as well as the final poster or oral presentation. With respect to publications, the research associate can provide literature searches for background preparation of publications.

In summary, the research associate should have expertise in (1) literature searches, (2) the conduct of clinical studies, (3) database formation and data entry, (4) spreadsheet entries, (5) basic statistical analyses, and (6) preparation of research presentations, including abstracts and poster presentations.

Faculty Facilitators

Faculty participation in a simulation program is essential. In a worldwide survey of simulation centers, all centers reported faculty involvement.[3] For centers with a multidisciplinary focus, it is important to acquire faculty from each of the participating disciplines. For example, the simulation center at Stanford University (http://anesthesia.stanford.edu/VASimulator/Simulator.htm) utilizes two to four faculty members from each of the relevant domains, mainly emergency medicine, ICU, and anesthesia. Faculty facilitators from the various disciplines help to ensure expertise, course relevancy, and accuracy of information.

Faculty facilitators are largely responsible for course development and implementation. Faculty play a major role in scenario development and, depending on the resources of the center, scenario programming. Ideally, faculty should be trained in all aspects of simulation, including operation of the simulator(s) and scenario programming. For example, the University of New Mexico School of Medicine simulator program offers a full body simulation program.[4] This program was designed to prepare faculty/educators from multiple disciplines to use simulation for education. The University of Maryland simulation program also conducts a faculty training program, consisting of workshops and hands-on experiences.[5] It is not necessarily the role of faculty members to operate the simulator(s) or program scenarios; however, knowledge of what is involved in these essential tasks assists them in developing and running courses and integrating simulation into their curriculum.

One of the major advantages to simulation training is the opportunity for debriefing after a scenario or teaching session. It is important for faculty facilitators to be trained in the debriefing process and to be familiar with the basic principles of crisis management.[6] The Center for Medical Simulation at Harvard (www.harvardmedsim.org) currently offers an extensive 2-day course in simulation debriefing for simulation instructors.

Faculty must have an interest in simulation and its importance in education. Faculty facilitators are also course instructors; therefore, excellence in teaching and patient care must be a requirement. It is not always necessary for the course instructor to be a physician. Any person with expertise in the required field will be beneficial in the facilitator role. It is important to tailor the instructor to the course participants. For example, the Canadian Simulation Centre for Human Performance and Crisis Management Training utilize nurse educators as course instructors when running courses for various nursing groups (e.g., cardiovascular ICU nurses, critical care nurses, postanesthetic care unit nurses).

Actors, Role Players

Critical event occurrence, recognition, management, and resolution can be affected by the participant's interaction with other members of the team. High-fidelity simulations are unique in that they force the learner to interact both physically and psychologically with both material and personnel. In contrast, in computer-based simulations the actions, emotions, and perceptions of others are not a concern and do not impact the outcome. During critical events in real-life situations, interactions with and management of others in the room often affect the outcome of the event. It is crucial for clinicians to be aware of the importance of managing human performance and stress to ensure positive outcomes during crisis management. For these reasons and many others, actors are an essential component of simulation training.

Actors provide a sense of realism to a scenario, when relevant. For example, an actor playing the part of a surgeon adds realism to a scenario with an anesthesiologist managing hypotension due to acute blood loss during a surgical procedure. One of the hurdles to simulation training is accomplishing a sense of realism for participants. Actors must be familiar to some extent with the role that they are playing. Actors are not required to be experts, but they should have some sense of the character's role. For example, an anesthesiologist is capable of role-playing a surgeon because they work closely in an operating room, giving each knowledge of the other's role.

If familiarity with a role is not possible, this problem can be overcome through the use of headsets. Outfitting actors with wireless headsets allows the instructor and/or operator to communicate with the actors and to direct their responses and actions. If headsets are not available, phone calls from the instructor to the actor can be made into the simulator room and worked into the scenario. For example, in an operating room setting, the instructor can make a call to the circulating nurse and pretend to be the laboratory calling with blood results. It is important to plan for communication with the actors, even with scripted scenarios, to deal promptly with unexpected turns.

The actors participating in the scenario may or may not be briefed ahead of time about their role in the scenario. When actors are not briefed about the scenario content, the simulation can result in a learning experience for the actor as well. Lack of briefing also provides an enhanced level of realism because very little "acting" occurs and the responses are often more realistic. This approach is beneficial if the actor is also a course participant. For example, if you are teaching communication skills during a medical emergency, the actor may be asked afterward if he or she truly appreciated the extent of the emergency from the communication among team members. Actors who are not briefed about the scenario content should not be forced to play a role that is vital to the scenario outcome.

If actors are briefed ahead of time, they have the opportunity to ensure that the scenario stays on track and that all learning objectives are met within the scenario. A

Table 2. Summary of the Human Considerations in Health Care Simulation Centers

Title	Role	Qualifications
Simulation center coordinator/manager	To facilitate the day-to-day operation of the simulation center	Clinical experience in an acute care setting, technical/computer skills, and an interest in simulation, teaching, and education
Medical director	To oversee the entire operation of the simulation center	Medical degree with a special interest in simulation-based education
Professional educator	To provide expert input into simulation education and evaluation programs and their outcomes	Masters degree or higher in an educational field
Research director	To provide the expertise to oversee a structured research program in simulation	Medical degree with research experience and achievement with a special interest in simulation
Research associate	To provide support for the research director as well as coordinating ongoing studies, grant applications, and publications	Experience in the performance of clinical studies, grant applications, database formation, and entry
Faculty facilitators	To assist in the development of scenarios and educational programs	Medical degree and experience in simulation-based education
Actors/role players	To participate in educational programs to promote realism	Interest in simulation

prescenario actor team briefing should always occur in these instances. Briefing sessions should review scenario content, prop locations, key plots, and expected outcomes.[7] Actors should be briefed ahead of time about the "boundaries" of their assigned role and instructed not to offer help or information outside of their role's area of expertise.[7] It is common for actors to assume their real-life role during a scenario and stray from their assigned role. For example, a resident physician role-playing a nurse may leave the role of nurse and offer to help out in a resident capacity. This behavior should be discouraged.

The number of actors needed depends on each individual scenario. Scenarios should be tailored to accommodate the number of actors that are available to help maintain realism.

Putting it All Together

There is no overall formula to calculate the personnel considerations for every simulation center. As is obvious from the discussion in this chapter, each simulation center may have individual needs, strengths, and aspirations. These directives drive the requirements for personnel. Table 2 summarizes the basic concepts of human considerations in medical simulation centers addressed in this chapter. As technology develops over the next decade, it is likely that more personnel with more advanced roles may enter the world of health care simulation.

References

1. Henry J, Murray WB: Expanding operator role to minimize faculty expense in the simulation laboratory. International Meeting on Medical Simulation, San Diego, California, 2003, abstract 45.
2. Tarshis J, DeSousa S, Brown R, et al: Simulator CME for family practice anesthetists: A nationwide program. Can J Anesth 2003;50:A110.
3. Morgan PJ, Cleave-Hogg D: A worldwide survey of simulation in anesthesia. Can J Anesth 2002;49:659–662.
4. Skartwed R, Ferguson S, Hansbarger C, Wilks D: Training program designed to prepare educators from multiple disciplines to use simulation as an educational tool. International Meeting on Medical Simulation, Santa Clara, California, 2002, abstract 34.
5. Schaivone K, et al: Development of a comprehensive simulation experience: A faculty training project. International Meeting on Medical Simulation, San Diego, California. 2003, abstract 41.
6. Gaba D, Fish K, Howard S: Crisis Management in Anesthesiology. Philadelphia, Churchill Livingstone, 1994.
7. Small S, Gaba D: Directing actors. In Gaba DM, Kurrek MM, Small SD (eds): Advanced Crisis Management Instructor Course Manual, 1995.

Chapter 5

STRATEGIC AND BUSINESS PLANNING FOR A HUMAN PATIENT SIMULATOR CENTER

Ronald W. Holder, Jr., MHA, CMPE

Over recent years, a major paradigm shift has been occurring within the field of medicine. Physicians are acknowledging that medicine is a business, albeit begrudgingly. The number of physicians who have or are pursuing business degrees is on the rise. Similar increases in the recognition of medicine as a business are occurring in academic medicine as well.

A recent study by Warters et al. has shown that medical school deans are now valuing business education to a much greater extent than in the past when they evaluate candidates for department chair positions.[1] Likewise, with the recognition that medicine is a business, the percent of department administrators with post-baccalaureate degrees has increased substantially in recent years. Between 1999 and 2002, the percent of academic department administrators with advanced degrees increased from 66% to 71% nationally.[2,3]

At all levels, academic medical centers are continuing to realize the importance of business skills and business planning as a way to compete in times of decreasing governmental funding and increasing reliance on revenue from other sources to make ends meet. Whether you are interested in creating a world-class human patient simulator center or plan to supplement the academic mission of your department with a much smaller simulation program, viewing your project as a business and planning for your new program on the front end can save significant time, money, and headaches further down the road. The dean, the sponsors, the university administration, the director, the department chair, and most notably whoever is responsible for the budget are likely to be highly interested in the degree to which a simulator program enriches the educational and research missions of the medical school, university, or department. However, many of the same people will inevitably want to know the return on investment: "Are we making money or losing money on the simulator program?"

The goal of this chapter is to give you the tools to be able to understand the finances and project planning behind a simulator center project and the financial framework to argue the worth of the project.

Why Plan?

The well-known cliché, "If you fail to plan, you plan to fail," is as applicable to a patient simulator project as any other proposed venture. What is the relevance of this cliché as it pertains to the development of a human patient simulation project? While failing to meet goals is usually not viewed as positive, success or failure, when viewed in the light of the size of your proposed simulator project, can:

1. Enrich or dilute the educational experience of the students or residents.

2. Affect your ability to attract and retain quality students or residents.

3. Attract or discourage philanthropy.

4. Affect your ability to obtain grants or publish papers on the subject.

5. Increase or decrease your school, department, or division's local, regional, or national image.

6. Accelerate or retard your career path.

These success-dependent effects can be gainful or costly, but the extent of the effect is difficult to quantify.

The problems encountered in quantifying the extent to which any academic enrichment initiative improves medical education complicates allocation of the cost of such initiatives to various revenue sources. If you cannot prove that a patient simulator program improves medical student examination results, increases medical student acceptance to high-quality residency programs, or improves the quality of applicants to the medical school by x percent, a request that a significant portion of medical school tuition dollars be used to fund the patient simulator project is illegitimate. Likewise, the inability to quantify the impact of a simulator program on the health of the constituents of a city, county, or state certainly does not aid in the argument that tax or state dollars should support the initiative.

Without a written plan, how do you convince philanthropists that your cause is just? What reason do vendors have to believe that your project merits financial consideration? How do contributors know what they are getting for their investment?

How do faculty not involved with the simulator project feel about using clinical income, limited investment income, or endowment income to fund your pet simulator project over their own research or educational project? The days of business on a handshake are long gone; if you seek someone else to provide funds for your business venture, you need more than a verbal sales pitch.

A simple plan is often sufficient in most academic settings. Without a written business plan, your simulator project is really no more than an idea or a dream. A complicated plan breeds rigidity in thought and action. When a plan is complicated and compliance to the plan is rigidly followed, planning becomes the focus and successfully "doing" takes a back seat.[4]

Initially, your simulator center is not likely to be self-funded. Grants may be funded, paying customers may come, but in the beginning, a simulator center, like any other business venture, requires a venture capitalist or at least an "angel" to provide start-up funding for your project. Regardless of the nature of the contributor, ultimately you are trying to romance money away from someone else who may already have very different ideas about what to do with it. Unless your simulator project has a benefactor with an open checkbook, a business plan forces those planning the project to take a realistic look at the project from the standpoint of the customer, the contributor, the student, and the manager—not just the biased dreamer.

At that point, you may already know the scope of your simulator project. Maybe a large surplus in the university coffers resulted in your being asked to lead a simulator project as a way to spend the reserves. Perhaps you already have qualified faculty and staff and beautiful space waiting to accommodate your project. Perhaps the chair of the department is begging you to take additional time away from revenue-producing clinical work to start this project. Perhaps you will wake up soon.

Planning is not as important in the fantasyland of plenty, but how many universities have the luxury of infinitely deep pockets? Higher education in many states is far from the land of plenty. With many states rapidly approaching financial ruin, higher education continues to take financial hits for the sake of other public programs. Within higher education, public funding for medical education is often targeted as a way to save money for other university programs because clinical faculty have a means to obtain funding for education by seeing patients and billing for services.

Academic medicine itself is on the verge of financial disaster. How long can we continue the trend of academic physicians approaching the clinical workload of private practice physicians without the pay for said work approaching the pay of private practice physicians? Academic days for faculty continue to dwindle, and academic salaries do not keep pace with private industry. The percent of publications in peer-reviewed journals by American authors decreases annually, due in part to the reduced time that academic clinicians have for nonclinical work. In times of clinical days by financial necessity, a written business plan for the simulator project will keep all parties educated about the financial commitments required to keep the simulators operating when external forces might encourage otherwise.

If you are to have a successful simulator program, you will need to secure adequate resources for your simulator project from people or organizations that are being solicited by many others for the same scarce resources. A simple, straightforward business plan will give your project competitive advantage over others seeking funds with only a dream.

The Planning Process

In war, as in business, the difference between strategy and tactics is contact.[5] Strategy is planning. Tactics is implementation. Strategy is the game plan for the championship game. Tactics are decisions made after the coin is tossed. Strategy may be as simple as the goal, "We're going to have the best human patient simulator center in the state/region/nation." Tactics are hiring the right staff, ordering supplies, marketing, training, securing additional funding, ongoing negotiations, and day-to-day operations of your established simulator project. The tactics will be different for every simulator center. An entire book could be (and probably has been) written about the different business tactics required for different situations that may be encountered. Conversely, many strategies for simulator project development that provide the skeleton for tactical decisions will remain constant, regardless of the specific environment. These strategies are addressed here.

Strategic planning answers the questions, "What are we going to do and how are we going to get there?" While the business plan and financial considerations are the main foci of this chapter, financial planning does not exist in a vacuum. Much must be decided before the planner of a successful simulator center can begin putting price tags on the project, write the business plan, and build a budget.

The eight steps of the planning process are listed in Table 1. Many view strategic planning and business planning as interchangeable terms, but they are different. Business planning starts after the strategic planning is completed[7] and often focuses more on how the chosen alternative will be accomplished—not on which alternative will be pursued.

```
❖❖ Table 1.
    The Strategic Planning Process*
```

Strategic planning	1. Identifying the organization's current position including present mission, long-term objectives, strategies and policies. 2. Analyzing the environment. 3. Conducting an organizational audit. 4. Identifying the various alternatives strategies based on relevant data. 5. Selecting the best alternative.
Business planning and ongoing assessment	6. Gaining acceptance of the chosen strategy. 7. Preparing long-range and short-range plans to support and carry out the strategy. 8. Implementing the plan and conducting ongoing evaluation.

* Simyar and associates[6] define the entire planning process as eight steps of strategic planning. The planning process should be viewed as three separate processes: strategic planning, business planning, and ongoing assessment.

Simyar's eight steps should be viewed as three distinct elements of planning: strategic planning, business planning, and ongoing assessment. In his model for the planning process, steps one through five constitute strategic planning. Step seven and implementation from step eight constitute business planning, and the remainder of step eight constitutes ongoing assessment. Step six, gaining acceptance of the strategy, cannot be placed with any one element, because the quest for acceptance is present throughout the process. When the project is just a dream, you have to sell it. When you are investigating various alternatives, you have to consider how you can sell the idea; when an alternative has been selected, your sales pitch will need to be more refined (the business plan); and as the purse strings continue to tighten on medical education, your salesmanship may keep the doors of your simulator lab open.

Strategic Planning

Within the strategic planning process are three distinct phases. Strategic planning consists of the environmental assessment, identifying possible alternatives, and selecting the best alternative. As you proceed through the planning process, keep the stakeholders of the project in the loop because Simyar's "gaining acceptance" should occur throughout. At every point in the strategic planning process, you will be acquiring information to use later for the written business plan.

Once you have the go-ahead to develop a plan to sell to the organization, but before you begin analyzing the environment, you should make a point of visiting some human patient simulators at other facilities to see the varying levels of interaction with other entities within and outside the organization.

Assess the Environment. The first step of strategic planning is the environmental assessment. The environment that you want to assess at this point is twofold: the internal environment and the external environment. Simyar's steps 1 and 3, identifying the organization's current position and conducting an organizational audit, are internal environment assessments.

You know that you want to have a simulator project. Does the chair of your department? Does the dean of the school of medicine? The university president? Whether your dream (and it is still a dream at this point) is to have a very large patient simulator center that will be used by many departments throughout the medical school as well as to train paraprofessionals throughout the community as revenue-producing encounters or whether your dream is to have a simulator in the conference room closet, many of the questions will be the same:

◆ In the organization, who are the stakeholders that stand to benefit from having a patient simulator program? Who are the ones that would be threatened?
◆ Would the stakeholders be supportive of the initiative? To what extent?
◆ Is a patient simulation center in line with the organization's mission statement? Is it in line with the organization's education goals? Clinical goals? Research goals?
◆ Are there currently underutilized endowment funds waiting for the right project? Is there a school benefactor wanting to leave a legacy that might match well with this new educational opportunity?
◆ Are funds available within the organization for start-up?
◆ What is the organization's stance on contributions from industry and/or philanthropists?
◆ Are there individuals or groups that will be barriers to progress? Can their attitude be changed? What will it take?
◆ Will you and other contributing faculty have nonclinical time to devote to the effort?
◆ What is the infrastructure of the organization? Is capable information technology support available? Grants management? Accounting? Purchasing? Marketing? How much will you and your own staff have to do yourself?

These questions are far from exhaustive, but an assessment of the organizational environment is important. If you do not know where the barriers to progress are until you reach them, your downhill road to failure will be bumpy and steep.

The Internal Environment. When you initially try to assess the willingness of the organization to support the development of a human patient project, nine times out of ten the chief executive will ask for a proposal or a business plan. Anything other than a resolute "no" is positive. At first, think big. Overshoot your desire for the size of your simulator project. As you begin to sort through more concrete data and the financial figures, scaling back the size of the project due to constraints in the system will be easier than to inflate figures for an even larger simulator project. Once the chief stakeholder, whether he or she is the dean, chair, or director of education, asks for additional information about your simulator project, the real planning begins and the questions become more detailed.

You can now start identifying parts of the existing infrastructure that can help or detract from your effort. Identify champions for the cause. Can individual faculty within your specialty or in other specialties benefit from a simulator center? Would they use it? Will they spend the time to develop scenarios for their specialty? How much funding is currently available? Are matching funds programs available? Can the grants staff research and help write grant proposals? What are the requirements for capital equipment purchases? What types of information technology support do you have within your organization?

Now that you have approval to pursue a simulator project, keep the key stakeholders in the loop. Invite the dean to one of your planning meetings. Send minutes from the meeting and updated plans to the department chair. Do not waste large amounts of time on stakeholder and opponent management, but sell the benefits of your project to those who would be barriers within the organization, as new and improved information about your project comes to light.

In assessing the internal environment, you will want to ask yourself, "What does our organization do? Who are we?" A key element in strategic planning is understanding who you are, what you do well, what you do not do well, what the roles of the various individuals that encompass "us" do, and how they all fit within the mission of the organization. By taking a step back to look at the organization as it is, you will better be able to plan how to get from point A (no simulator program) to point B (the chosen simulator program alternative) and to determine who else needs to be involved to get there.[8]

When you write your business plan, you will need to describe in one of the first sections what Peter Drucker called "the business of the business."[9] Describing the business of the business in the written business plan is not as easy as it sounds. A good way to conduct the organizational audit is via a **S**trengths, **W**eaknesses, **O**pportunities, and **T**hreats[10] (SWOT) analysis of your organization. With the SWOT analysis, you have a tool to assess your organization now and a tool you can use intermittently to assess progress. Ideally, if your organization is progressing in accordance with its well-defined mission, Strengths will increase, Weaknesses will decrease, different items will be listed as Opportunities, and Threats will always be around, although the sources or magnitudes may alter over time.

The External Environment. Once you have assessed the internal environment, you will want to conduct an external environmental assessment or market analysis. In health care administration, a market analysis is often described as assessing whether or not there is competition for your proposed service and whether or not there is room for growth within your market. Although this definition is far from complete, it does apply to human patient simulators. Further down the road you will look into sources of revenue for your simulators. Integral to knowing the extent to which your simulator can begin to pay for itself is knowing whether or not any other organizations can perform the same functions within your market area.

Is there room in the market for medical education courses provided in the human patient simulators to physicians, nurses, or paraprofessionals locally? Regionally? Nationally? Is there competition for the types of courses that you can offer, or would you have the market cornered? If you plan to offer a course to emergency medical technicians, you might want to know how many of them are in your hospital's catchment area. Would other small medical colleges, nursing schools, or paraprofessional schools be interested in purchasing time or classes but unable to financially justify a simulator of their own? Such an analysis is often called a needs assessment and, unlike health care, the demographics of such utilization will fit the normal economic supply-and-demand curve. Figure 1 shows that the demand for your simulator services in the market will decrease as you increase the price of services. If you charge seven hundred dollars per conference registration, only fifty professionals are interested in using your center for training. If the charge is three hundred, perhaps the market will provide one hundred seventy-five customers interested in purchasing the service.

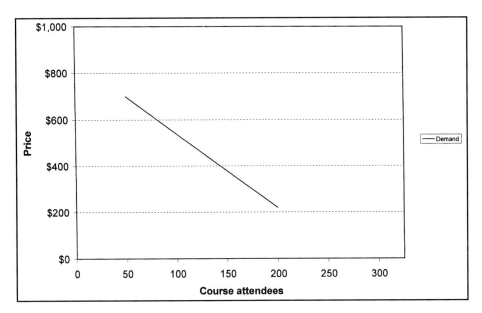

Figure 1. The demand curve slopes downward to illustrate the increasing number of customers willing to purchase the service as the price decreases. At higher prices, fewer customers are willing to purchase it. At lower prices, potential customers increase. The figures in these and subsequent graphs and tables are for illustration purposes only and do not represent actual market, cost, or revenue data for simulator projects.

Conversely, as Figure 2 shows, the director of a simulator center will almost always be able to offer more hours of continuing medical education to the community if the price received for services is higher. Perhaps if you can get seven hundred dollars per registration, you can afford to offer (or your chair will let you offer) education to two hundred fifty attendees annually, but if you can only receive three hundred dollars per registration, you can offer education to only one hundred twenty-five attendees.

Where the demand curve and the supply curve intersect (Fig. 3) is called the equilibrium price. In this case, the equilibrium price of $380 would result in 150 attendees. If your courses are priced at or around the equilibrium price and your market data are correct, you should have very few empty seats in your simulator course and receive the best possible price for all of those seats to be filled. At the equilibrium price, the market is at its most efficient point, because little waste is produced. For the purposes of this example, empty seats in the simulator sessions or customers wanting the training at the chosen price but unable to get it constitute waste.

Both supply-and-demand curves can be shifted by any number of economic events. Both curves need not be affected for a resultant change to the equilibrium price. Consider the effects to the equilibrium price if the director of the simulator center loses days to work in the simulator center due to increases in clinical demands (Fig. 4). Perhaps, to continue to supply the same amount of courses from the simulator lab, the director must conduct more of them on weekends. In order to keep the center director happy, the price required to offer any number of sessions from the center increased; as a result, the

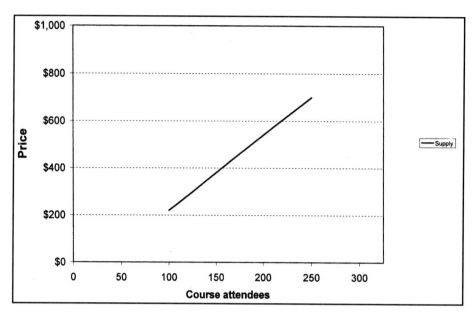

Figure 2. The supply curve slopes upward to illustrate the willingness of the seller of the service to provide courses for more attendees as the price received for services sold increases. If the seller can receive a higher price, more courses can be provided; if the price received is low, the seller will provide fewer courses.

equilibrium price is now $460 for 125 attendees (Supply2), compared to $380 for 150 attendees in the first example (Supply1). Whereas after the adverse event (additional clinical responsibilities) the director could accommodate the same number of attendees (150) for $540 dollars, according to the demand curve, only 100 attendees would be interested in the services for that price. With the new supply curve and the existing demand curve, 150 attendees would represent market inefficiency, in that the supplier would need $540 to accommodate it, but the market needs a price of $380 to provide that many attendees.

In general terms, if the demand for the services that you provide is high and no one else (or few others) can provide it, the supply is low; therefore, the price can be high. However, if the demand is low and the supply is high, the price that you can expect to receive for any courses that you might offer will be much lower. You can get a rough idea of what type of volume and pricing the market will support by looking at the marketing materials for the competition for the types of training that you will be offering both in and out of your market and during your visits to other simulator centers.

Unfortunately, assessing the external environment must also include the extent to which your medical school or department is "keeping up with the Joneses." Medical schools are in constant competition for high-quality medical students, and academic departments likewise compete for high-quality residency applicants. What are the schools or departments comparable to your own doing in terms of human patient simulator projects? Has their commitment to having a human patient simulator lab affected the qual-

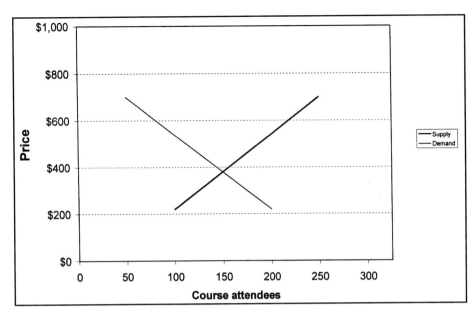

Figure 3. Market efficiency. The point at which the supply and demand curves intersect represents the price at which the market is efficient. At that price, both seller and customer will produce and consume the same amount of services or product—in this case, simulator course registrations. There should be no empty seats at the conferences, nor should there be customers willing to purchase the course at that price but excluded due to the inability of the seller to offer enough courses at that price.

ity of the incoming classes? Has your school or department lost high-quality students to other organizations who may possess a competitive advantage by having a three mannequin human patient simulator lab while your school or department has none?

Whereas revenue and cost are easier to define when developing a budget for the various continuing education sessions that you plan to offer to the public, costs associated with the inability to recruit quality medical students due to your school's lack of cutting-edge educational methods are hard to quantify and are called opportunity costs. Are mediocre students more expensive to educate than excellent ones? What costs does the medical school incur trying to keep up with other programs or schools who recruit the same caliber of students? Can some of these costs be eliminated in favor of the simulator program and allocated to the new simulator project?

Identify Alternatives. After the environmental assessment, including visiting human patient simulator centers of various sizes and talking to the directors of such centers, the stakeholders in the project will need to discuss viable alternative methods to accomplish the dream. The alternatives will be many. The viable alternatives will be few. Some of the stakeholders will not be knowledgeable about all of the potential means to accomplish the end; therefore, the knowledgeable facilitator will have researched human patient simulator configurations in existence in other departments or medical schools and vendors that offer human patient simulators before convening the first meeting to discuss possible alternatives as a group. The list of alternatives for a simulation center is likely to include:

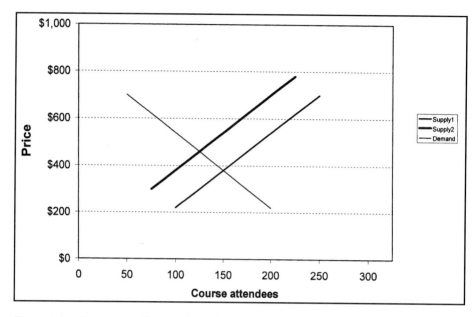

Figure 4. An adverse event effects market efficiency. Adverse effects can happen to the supply curve, demand curve, or both. In this example, the supply curve is shifted because the director of the center is not getting enough academic time to provide the courses due to increased clinical demands. Therefore, the cost to produce the courses is higher. The adverse event moves the supply curve, causing it to intersect with the demand curve at a different point and hence results in a different price at which the market is efficient.

◆ No human patient simulation project.
◆ Defer/table the project.
◆ Mannequin(s) from Vendor A and no dedicated space.
◆ Mannequin(s) from Vendor B and no dedicated space.
◆ Mannequin(s) from Vendor A with a dedicated suite.
◆ Mannequins(s) from Vendor B with a dedicated suite.
◆ A new building with several simulation suites, a classroom, every type of mannequin in existence, and research space to partner with industry to develop new ones.

There are two different schools of thought with regard to generating alternatives for the stakeholders to consider before selecting the alternative to pursue: (1) the facilitator walks into the meeting with a long list and lets the group pare it down to a list of favorites to investigate further, or (2) you start with a blank piece of paper and generate alternatives as a group during the meeting. The former alternative is often quicker, but the latter is usually better for the purpose of building support for the endeavor. The more the stakeholders participate in generating ideas and in the strategic planning process, the more the stakeholders will feel ownership for the project and provide support for the project to reach fruition.

One might think that, for the purposes of brainstorming, think tank, or generating creative ideas, the more people seated around the table discussing ideas, the merrier. Although this assumption is true to a certain extent, eight seems to be the critical mass at which point the number of people generating ideas begins to become counterproductive. Try to keep the group of stakeholders or committee members between four and eight. The exception to getting more people involved in the process of generating alternatives for any decision is solicitation of alternatives from a larger group of people before the initial meeting of stakeholders. Then you can either start with this list for the stakeholders to pare down, as described above, or use the list as facilitator-provided alternatives to keep the creative juices flowing if the stakeholders hit a mental road block while generating ideas.

Regardless of which option you choose for generating alternatives for the stakeholders to consider, do not squash creativity by not including a suggested alternative on the list for discussion. If the group decides to remove it later because it is impossible to achieve, then the group can decide to do so. If you as the facilitator refuse to include it during the alternative generation phase because it is fantastical, you could breed resentment when you are seeking support. Both computers and televisions were envisioned by dreamers in early phases of development as eventually being in every home. At the time, executives in both fields thought that the markets were much smaller and that the very idea of such a large market was ridiculous! Once a robust list of alternatives has been generated, the group can pare the list down to a small few for more intense deliberation.

Select the Best Alternative. Several methods are available for paring the list down to only a few alternatives. One method used to narrow down a lengthy list of alternatives to a select few is multivoting. Each committee member uses the same multiple number of votes to weight the extent to which each option is favored. Each person can be provided with a number of beans equal to the number of alternatives under consideration. The facilitator or process owner (in this case, you, the hopeful simulator project director) labels a series of paper or plastic cups with numbers that correspond to the various alternatives. The committee members are then encouraged to place their allocated beans into the numbered cups corresponding to the degree to which the person likes each alternative.

Each voting member is likely to have varying degrees of preference for each of the alternatives. One member may put all beans in one cup, whereas another may spread the beans across several cups. The facilitator can blind the voting process by keeping the cups in a different room and allowing each voter to vote in turn. The facilitator would then mark down the results and give the beans to the next voter. Once all participants have voted, the alternatives that received the highest votes should be considered for further analysis. Most votes will result in an obvious "break point" between the alternatives for consideration and those to be discarded. Now that the field of alternatives has been narrowed somewhat, a great way to dig deep into comparative advantages and disadvantages of the various alternatives is the SWOT analysis. At this point, hopefully, firing the faculty member who wants to start a human patient simulator center is not still on the list as an alternative for further consideration.

The group will want to discuss each alternative at length while completing the SWOT analysis of each. If the number of alternatives is lengthy, the stakeholders should be provided with copies of the SWOTs for all alternatives. The stakeholders should be provided with ample time (but not so much as to lose focus) to consider each SWOT and reconvene to vote on which alternative to pursue. Once the committee or stakeholders have had sufficient time to digest the SWOT analyses for all of the alternatives under consideration, another vote needs to take place to select the alternative to pursue. Multivoting can be used again, or even a show of hands. Use your best judgment given the interpersonal dynamics of the group of decision makers.

Once you have chosen your idea, you should consider creating a mission statement for selected goals, such as the following: "The mission of the State University Human Patient Simulation Center is to enrich the education of the University's medical, nursing and dental students by providing them with scenarios designed to improve each student's clinical skills, training, and judgment in a highly variable but safe environment." The mission statement should not be overly lengthy but complete enough to give the reader a good overview of the organization's *raison d'être*. If you need an easy starting point for crafting a mission statement for your simulator project, look to your department, school, or university mission statement and plug the simulator project into it to describe how it will advance that organization toward its goals.

A line without a defined beginning or end is a circle. Any attempt at planning the trip from point A to point B without identifying said points is likely to result in a lost traveler. The choice to move in any particular direction is a guess.[11] Despite your best managerial efforts, writing a business plan without knowing the current state of affairs and what you intend to accomplish is folly. If your strategic planning efforts have been successful, you should have a good grasp not only of where your organization is, what the organization does well, and what it does not do so well but also of what you plan to achieve. Knowing these elements after a completed strategic planning process, you are ready to write your business plan.

The Business Plan

Writing a business plan is a necessary step to initiate any new business endeavor. In the private sector, a business plan is required by most lending organizations before they will consider letting your organization borrow money. As expressed previously, even in academic circles, where seeking financial support from an external lender is not often a part of the process, a written business plan is a good idea, because in almost every case you will be spending someone else's money.

Although every business plan will not conform to the same structure or contain the same elements, almost every business plan will contain a lot of the information that you discovered or developed during the strategic planning phase. The sections contained in any business plan should include a table of contents, executive summary, description of the business, description of the product, definition of organizational structure, environmental or market data (including competition), opportunities for growth, potential threats, productivity goals, financial estimates (budget), and any appendices.

Executive Summary. The first section of any business plan should be the executive summary. The summary should contain the vital pieces of information from each of the other sections that can be used by those not knowledgeable with the details of your type of business to come up to speed quickly. For this part of the business plan, a good guide is the first rule of journalism: specify who, what, when, where, why, and how. Keep it to 1–2 pages. The details will follow in subsequent sections of your plan.

Who? Be brief but informative. Who is planning the simulator effort? Is this a medical school-wide project? Is it to be conducted solely within one department? Perhaps several schools will use it as well. Provide the reader with the answer to three specific "who" questions: (1) Who is in charge? (2) Who is involved? and (3) Who will benefit?

What? We know who you are now. What is it exactly that you propose to do? This section is a good place to put a mission statement if you have drafted one. By the time you explain "what" in a brief paragraph or two, you will have essentially created a mission statement for your project.

When? When do you intend to start this project? Is there a ramp-up phase, or will all facilities and mannequins come online at the same time? Is there an end to a trial period built into the project? How long will it take from acquisition of the funding and required approval before the project can host the first simulation encounter? Are there any contingencies built into the "when" such as the availability and acquisition of appropriate space for the new center?

Where? Where will the simulator project be located? If the space requirements are a small closet, say so. If the proposal will call for a dedicated suite or building, describe the main parts of the dedicated area, such as the number of suites, classrooms, offices, and observation areas. Do you already have the space, or is the success of the project contingent on obtaining funding for the space as well?

Why? Why do you want a human patient simulator? Do data support your organization's decision to have one? Can you reference educational outcome data? Are students making medical school or residency program preferences based on the extent to which the school or department has embraced human patient simulation?

How? The "how" portion of the executive summary is perhaps the hardest portion to limit to one or two paragraphs. The majority of the pages that follow the executive summary will focus on the "how." You will want to mention here any funding already secured, whether it be from industry or philanthropy. Leon Festinger's theory of cognitive dissonance and Mancuso's primary law of small business point out that the best time to raise money is when you do not need it.[12] Investors want to invest in a winner, and any stress encountered by the decision of whether or not to invest in a business venture is diluted by knowledge that someone else already has as much or more to lose, yet chose to invest in the business. If someone else believes in the undertaking enough to provide five hundred thousand dollars worth of start-up, another philanthropist or investor may not worry as much about his one hundred thousand dollar contribution, because he is not the one with the most to lose.

Description of the Business. If the person reading your business plan has made it this far, he or she is at least somewhat interested in the concept of your human patient simulator project. Now you need to give the details. In this section you should spend time describing not only what a human patient simulator is, but also the advantages to using one for medical education. Include in the description of the business a brief history of human patient simulation. Reference relevant literature as it pertains to the advantages of your specific course of action. If you encountered a human patient simulator project of comparable size and scope while visiting other institutions, sing the praises of their program in this section.

If you have selected a vendor and/or specific mannequin models, describe their features, focusing on the main selling points. The patient simulator vendor should be more than helpful with this part of your plan, because the vendor's success at selling the mannequins to your organization depends solely on your ability to obtain the financing.

You will want to describe the product, the mannequin vendor, price ranges, assessment of the quality of the vendor's product, and the quality of the vendor's business practices. An important decision factor in purchasing such an expensive piece of equipment as the human patient simulators will be whether or not the company will still be around in one, three, or five years to provide support. Although a company's past success or failure is not a 100% indicator of future success or failure, knowing the company's past performance provides you with better information to use than knowing nothing about the company at all. Successful companies will continue to enjoy success and unsuccessful ones will continue to struggle, more often than not.

Describe any trends in human patient simulation at comparable organizations. Is every medical school hopping on board with patient simulation? What is the trend? Perhaps you want to chart the number of medical schools with human patient simulator labs over the past five years.

Will the simulator project be used exclusively for the educational benefit of your organization, or will you offer educational courses to professionals in the community in order to finance the effort or build the organization's local image? Have you figured out from your environmental/market analysis the appropriate price at which you can offer courses offered to local physicians, emergency medicine technicians, and nurses? The annual number of courses that the patient simulator project can provide to the students of the organization as well as an estimate of the number of courses that can be provided externally to bring in revenue should be estimated. If you can estimate the current cost of providing similar coursework to the students of your organization, state it in this section. If the cost for the simulator is greater, discuss the justification for the additional cost.

Do your plans for your simulator project include research? Do you have examples of other simulator programs that have been successful in securing either private or public funding for the development of patient simulator based teaching? Are you going to develop new scenarios within your organization or will you contract with outside entities to write the programming for new simulations as needed?

All of the major technologic purchases, including the simulators, must be listed with the number of each and the expected costs. How many adult mannequins will you have? Will you have pediatric manikins? Will you have any computerized simulators or adjunct mannequins? How many computers will you need? Projectors? Additional monitors or televisions in the classrooms or viewing areas? Cameras? Video- and audio-conferencing equipment? What is the window for technologic obsolescence? How often do you expect the simulators or other expensive peripheral technology to require upgrades or replacement?

Where will the simulator center be housed? Describe the facilities and the associated cost. Are the costs for renovation included in the total facilities costs for the start-up? Does the organization own the property, or will it be leased? What infrastructural requirements must be met, and what are their costs? Does the project need additional high-bandwidth data lines, phones, and other information technology accommodation?

What are the costs for furniture and other furnishings? You can be as detailed or as brief as you like about facility and start-up costs in this section of your business plan. You may want to break out some of the big-ticket items and group together a lot of the smaller-ticket items. Use your best judgment in the context of your audience. Details about expenditures should be included in the budget section toward the end of your business plan, regardless of whether you are specific in the body of the plan.

As of the time of this chapter, medicine is experiencing a malpractice crisis. Malpractice rates are driving some practitioners to other states or out of medicine entirely. Will using human patient simulators for some of the teaching affect malpractice costs for the organization? Will simulation help to defend health care professionals accused of malpractice? If any of the above is true and you have data to support it, tell the reader about it.

Description of the Product. What is it exactly that you will be doing once you have all those bright, shiny simulators and wonderful new space to keep them? What is the extent of the teaching that you will do? Do you plan to apply for teaching and research grants? Will you be developing scenarios for other simulator labs? Will teaching be limited to your own students, or do you intend to offer continuing medical education courses to faculty from other schools? What about doctors, nurses, and paraprofessionals?

A good piece of information to include in this section of your business plan is a sample calendar of events. Include a calendar of one month, or if you expect that your activities will vary by season, provide the reader with a couple of sample months. Other than the obvious reason of forcing you, as the director of the simulator center, to plan your calendar in advance, the advantages of including one or two months worth of simulator center activities are threefold:

1. First and foremost, you are providing the reader with an organized visual aid to describe the total amount of activities you plan to conduct throughout the course of the year. Is it reasonable to ask for 50% faculty time and salary support if your expected timeline includes only two or three classes in a given month and no plans for research?

2. A calendar with delineated class topics and expected attendance will give the reader just enough detail to assist with financial decision making further down the road. Are two of the courses provided exclusively to the surgery department residents? Perhaps the surgery department needs to dedicate some line-item financial support to the center. Is the nursing school using it as much as the medical school? If so, it should pay part of the ongoing operational expenses. The same applies to the school of dentistry or any allied health programs that may use the simulator for education. Are as many classes being provided to professionals and paraprofessionals outside the organization as to your own students and faculty? If so, then university officials will certainly expect that the simulation center will be able to provide much more revenue toward its own operation than otherwise.

3. It never hurts to break up a large amount of text with a graph, table, or chart. If the information can be expressed with a graphic, then express it with one periodically. Remember, you are trying to convince someone else to spend money on your project. In addition to fighting economic inertia (i.e., "I'll keep my money where it is and not spend it on your new project, thank you very much"), you do not want to find yourself combating reader boredom as well. Your potential investors may not read all thousand words, but they will certainly look at the picture.

In this section you also want to walk the reader through a scenario or two to illustrate what a class with your simulator will entail. Do not describe more than three, and one may be good enough if it is a good example. Optimally, you should include an example of a class that might be offered to students of the school and an example of a revenue-producing class that will be offered to those outside the school. A simple paragraph or two about each will work. Once written, the paragraph can be used as the short course description in your marketing brochure (if external) or course catalog (if internal).

Each short description should focus on the basics. Who will be teaching the course? Who should attend, and how many attendees do you expect? How long is the course? Describe the educational goals of the course and what knowledge should be gained after successful completion of the course. If the course is offered to the public, what is the charge per attendee?

In planning for any large project, every question seems to lead to two or three more questions that need to be answered before you have the answer you seek. On a detailed scale, writing a plan for a couple of scenarios may lead you to whole new questions that you need to answer. Perhaps at this point you realize that you do not yet know how to get the registration fees for your course into an account at your university that you can use to buy the supplies you need. Is the yet unrealized important function one that can be accommodated within the new staffing plan or existing organizational staff?

The purpose of including brief course synopses is not to describe every course that will be offered in the Simulation Center but to give the reader a good idea of what a simulator course is and the reason for doing it. Many of the readers of your business plan will have no medical training, much less be able to understand your specific specialty, yet the success of your project depends on convincing them that the simulator project is worth the investment. Keep it simple.

Definition of Organizational Structure. In the first year of operation, the simulators are likely to be the most expensive part of the budget for your center. After the first year, the most expensive line item of the budget will be labor; therefore, the reader of a business plan will definitely want to know "who's going to be running this thing."

The easiest way to quickly describe the personnel involved with your simulator project is to include an organizational chart in this portion of your business plan. Since you do not want full-page graphics interrupting your text, a small one may be inserted in this section and the full organizational chart provided in the Appendices (referenced here).

Although an organizational chart has some of the same benefits as using a calendar instead of a paragraph to provide a brief summary of planned events, all of the pertinent information relevant to staffing your simulation center should not be conveyed within the confines of an organizational chart (see Chapter 4). Immediately after the chart should be a brief description of each position. More complete job descriptions should be provided in the Appendices. If any of the staff are already identified, you want to include a brief biographical paragraph about them, similar to those found in conference brochures for featured speakers. More detail needs to be provided for the director than for any other position, but a brief paragraph about each employee adds a personal touch to the plan in addition to providing good information.

Cost Variations. While reading about the labor involved in a successful simulator project, the evaluator may raise for the first time the question of fixed and variable costs. Although you do not necessarily need to identify in your plan which costs are fixed and which are variable, understanding the difference between the two is integral to creating a realistic budget later in the process.

Fixed costs are costs that do not change based on the amount of output from your processes. A fixed cost remains the same whether you conduct one class or one hundred classes in a year. Examples of fixed costs as they pertain to a simulator center are the facility, the mannequin, the furniture, the computers, and salaried employees. As you can see in Figure 5, regardless of the number of attendees of your course the fixed costs do not change.

Variable costs (Fig. 6) change based on the number of simulator sessions that you conduct or the number of students that attend the sessions. Variable costs in a simulator center would probably include gloves, gases, hourly employees, paper, office supplies, programmer costs, marketing materials, and disposable supplies for the mannequin.

Depending on your desire to break down costs for budgetary purposes, you will notice that within both fixed and variable costs are levels of variation. Most notably, some variable costs will vary based on the number of students who use the simulator and some will vary based on the number of sessions offered with the simulator. Such a scenario lends to classifications of those expenses as either semifixed or semivariable costs.[13]

Salaried employees could be considered semifixed (Fig. 7) costs in certain circumstances. Suppose that demand for classes from the simulation center exceeds your expectations dramatically. While one salaried programmer may be able to facilitate a maximum of x number of visits, a second salaried programmer may be required if the volume approaches $2x$. In such a situation, programmer salary is no longer fixed; it is semifixed since it is constant over broad ranges of outputs. Like-

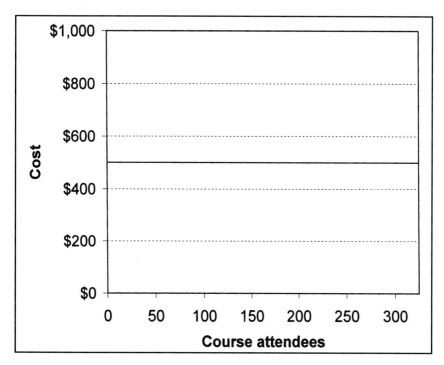

Figure 5. Fixed costs do not change as the output changes. Whether the simulator center hosts 20 or 300 attendees, this particular cost remains at five hundred dollars.

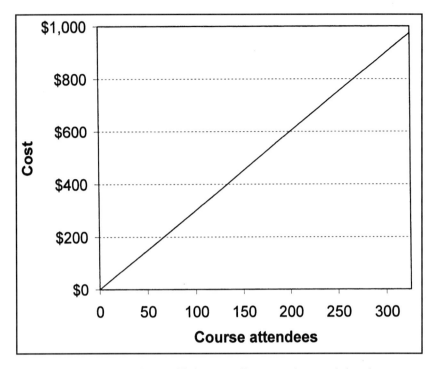

Figure 6. Variable costs change with the output. If no output is created, there is no cost.

wise, advertising may be considered semifixed because it will increase depending on how many sessions you need to advertise but will not be affected by the number of attendees at each session.

Semivariable costs (Fig. 8) will vary based on output, but not to the extent of a pure variable cost. Utilities are a prime example of a semivariable costs. Your disposable supplies for the mannequin are completely variable in that you will use them only when you are actually using the simulator, whereas electricity will be used to a lesser extent when the simulators are not in use and to a greater extent when they are.

Knowing the extent to which your costs are either fixed or variable provides you with vital information required to plan your budget, determine costs to allocate to internal customers for services, and arrive at a price to charge for sessions provided to external customers. Labor can fall into any of the cost categories depending on how the simulator project is staffed, and as long as you know who is being paid for what amount of work, you can determine whether the labor cost for that employee is fixed, variable, or somewhere between.

Environmental or Market Analysis. The purpose of the environmental or market analysis section is to provide the reader with essentially a SWOT analysis of both the internal and external factors that may impact the success of your simulator project. You should have discovered a great deal about both the external and internal environment during strategic planning. In the ongoing assessment section, you will learn why environmental analysis should not be frozen in time. All throughout the planning process you should be learning more about external and internal environments, making note of

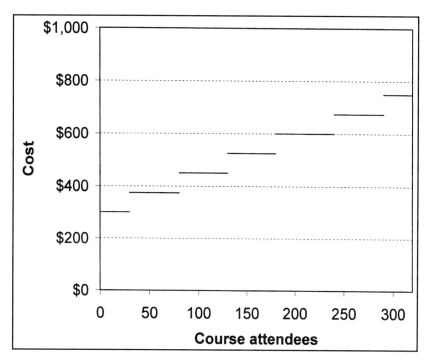

Figure 7. Semifixed costs behave like fixed costs over short intervals but vary over large ones.

any significant changes since the beginning of the process and discovering details that you did not know at the outset.

In the written business plan, the majority of the section should focus on external factors, but no environmental assessment is complete without looking into the internal environment. Within the internal environment, you will want to ask lots of questions to discern the skeleton of your internal environment SWOT analysis. Has the organization enjoyed success with similar projects? What is the support structure? What are the current alternatives within the organization to achieving a similar end? How do the costs of your proposed simulator project stack up against more traditional teaching methods? Are there differences in outcomes?

If you already have willing customers within the organization, describe them. Can parallels be drawn to other parts of the organization based on those who have already bought into the idea? Is the nature of simulator-provided coursework seasonal? Where are the current windows of opportunity to involve the simulators in the curriculum for the medical school, your department, the nursing school, and other internal customers? Within your organizational environment what are the policies and procedures for establishing a new project, center, institute or department. Can you move forward on a project and begin marketing it with the university's name displayed prominently without following the established chain of approval? Regardless of the beauty of your business plan and the success of gaining approval to do the project, the implementation may well be chaotic if during the planning stage you do not give consideration to the appropriate university procedures for establishing new projects.[14]

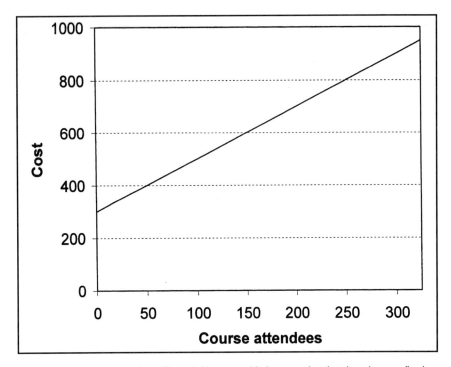

Figure 8. Semivariable costs behave like variable costs with the exception that there is some fixed component. Although long-distance phone charges are not costly unless you make long-distance calls, most telephone plans charge some level of base charge even if the phone is not used at all that month.

Is the infrastructure of the organization conducive to conducting research with your potential new simulators? If not, what might need to happen for you to get a research proposal written and approved by the institution, get funded by a sponsoring agency, and meet grant administration requirements within the organization? Are there currently investigators within the organization that have interests in simulator research?

What type of accounting does your organization use? Most likely the organization has some level of tax-exempt status, but is the organizational accounting based on an accrual or a cash basis? Accrual accounting is far more complicated than accounting on a cash basis but has many advantages and hence keeps droves of accountants employed. In the cash basis of accounting, cash is reported as revenue during the period it is received and costs are incurred as expenses when they are incurred.

Unfortunately, cash is often received in a different accounting period (month) than when the services are provided. If you are providing a class in the simulator center, perhaps the registration fees are received the month before the class, whereas the expenses of the class are not incurred until the subsequent month. From an extremely simplified view of that example, accounting on a cash basis would make the month preceding the class look extremely profitable, while the month of the actual class appears to lose money. Enter accrual accounting. Accrual accounting attempts to record all financial activity of an organization during the accounting period that the costs were incurred and the services were actually provided, regardless of when the cash was actually received or spent.

From the above example, the registration fees, although received in the month prior to the course, would still be credited to the course to the extent that the services provided during the course contributed to the total cost to provide the course. That is, if five percent of the budget was advertising costs incurred four months previously, five percent of the revenue is credited to the accounting period four months previously.

As you develop your budget, you will need organizational guidance as to what extent the organization utilizes various accounting tools such as accrual or cash-based accounting, depreciation, indirect cost allocations, and financial reporting. The earlier in the process that you know such details, the easier preparing the budget for the simulator effort will become.

Once you have completed a description of the internal market as it pertains to your simulator project, you want to address the external market. The analysis of the external market can be lengthy or somewhat short. At the very least you want to discuss who may be interested your services, how many of those potentially interested you can count on using the services, and how much those customers will be willing to pay for services.

Collecting external market data is not difficult, but it is time-consuming. Hopefully, since the very first time the idea of creating a simulator center crossed your mind, you have been collecting market data, at least informally. Perhaps you kept the brochure from a medical education conference, and you thought you could achieve the same, or even greater, educational objectives using a human patient simulator. Perhaps during the infancy of your simulator dream you attended a workshop at another simulator center and conveniently remembered the cost of the seminar. Probably you have already talked to other professionals and paramedical professionals about the types of continuing education and recertification that their specialties require and made note of whether or not such activities could be conducted in a simulator setting.

Before you begin your formal market analysis, you want to know what questions you need to answer about the market. Make a list of them, and begin the search for answers. You will certainly want to know the target market, the competition, a pricing strategy, your customers, advertisement opportunities, and vendors. This section of your business plan does not need to be presented in a question-answer format, nor will you need to describe all that you find. The reader already has a substantial document to digest. Hit the high points of what you find, and move on.

Do you already have sources for your market data? Do you have the time to search out resources? If not, you may need to outsource this function to a market research organization. If you are going to do it yourself, talk to representatives from each of the specialties, professionals, and paraprofessionals that might use your center. You may have done it already, but now you need to get specific. What do they need in way of training? How much does it cost them to do it in traditional ways? Are some training needs not being met in the immediate area? What have your peers done at other simulator centers by way of educating external medical and paramedical professionals? How do the members of your customer audience hear about continuing education opportunities?

Once you have probed into the sources for your market data, you need to refine the questions that the market analysis needs to answer. Instead of "Who are the competitors for my customers?," you will want to answer, "Where are the closest simulator training facilities?" and "How is my greatest competition reaching the nursing community?" You cannot get to the details without knowing the questions to ask, and you will not know the questions until you have answers to the basics. Knowing the questions is integral to knowing the answers. Once you know what it is that you need to know, you need to decide the best way of obtaining the information. Educational societies of the various specialties may have survey data regarding which universities have comparable simulator centers. Will you conduct your own survey? Will it be written or via phone? You do not need to describe your data-acquiring methodology in detail in your business plan, but you will report the results.

Once you have answers to your detailed questions, you need to organize and analyze the information. Group the data according to which of your global questions it answers. Use the answers to the detailed questions to answer each global question. Use your pricing data to set the prices for your services. By setting your price in the light of all that you know now, you will be making your best guess as to the equilibrium price based on what the market *demands* (market data) and what you can afford to *supply* (costs incurred for supplies, capital equipment, facilities, and salaries).

You should know now who your target customers are and how to effectively reach them. There may be better ways, but your research will have pointed out a proven way that works. Are the customers using booths at conferences, mass mailings, the media, telemarketing, or word of mouth most effectively?

Identify the suppliers of office and simulator supplies and discounts available for your specific situation. You should have determined what you need based on the alternative that stakeholders agreed to pursue and subsequent fleshing out of the proposal. During this phase, you need to find out who can provide the items, what the various alternatives are, and what they will cost so that you have the data when it is time to make the budget.

By now you will have identified your competition. One of the best ways to identify your competition is by asking your potential customers and your product suppliers. For instance, the Medical Education Technologies, Incorporated website[15] proudly displays who is using their simulation products and how many of each type of simulator each organization has as marketing for their own products. Your competition warrants special consideration in your business plan. You will want to list all of the major players in the area as well as any competitive advantages or disadvantages your simulator project may have. Compare your newly established prices to theirs in light of the aforementioned advantages and disadvantages. Is it possible that others could enter the marketplace, providing the same services as your simulator center? Is there room for growth among the types of education that you plan to offer the community to fund your simulator, or will the competition for a limited group of customers be bloody? If the competition will be fierce for a limited amount of resources, the depth of the analysis of both the organization and its competition will need to be much greater. As Sun Tzu says, "Know the enemy and know yourself, and you will never be defeated."[16]

By the time you have completed your environmental assessment, you should be able to communicate via the written business plan the following information: how the organizational infrastructure will affect the center, identities of potential customers (internal and external), what motivates the customers to use your services, a price for your services, how to best advertise to the customers, how your services will fit into the current marketplace, and perhaps even how fluctuations in the economy will affect your ability to conduct business in your simulator center.

Opportunities for Growth. Both opportunities for growth and potential threats can be provided within the market or environmental analysis section of your business plan, or you can break them out separately. The decision to include or provide separately should hinge on two factors: (1) the number of opportunities and threats you have discovered and (2) their potential impact on the future success of the project.

Unless both opportunities and threats are few in number and their potential impact on the future success of the simulator project somewhat minimal, you want to break the sections out separately. You do not want to be perceived as glossing over potentially important information. Upon completion, a good business plan should either suffuse you with confidence or convince you not to explore the project further. The business plan should not attempt to deceive or mislead the reader. The plan should provide enough facts, detail, and insight into the proposed venture so that the reader can make an informed business decision after reading it. If the opportunities are exaggerated and the threats are watered down, the plan stops being a business plan and becomes an attempt to convince people to buy something that they should not.

What are the opportunities for growth in the business of human patient simulators? Some factors that may lead to higher utilization of your simulator project may be obvious; others may not.

Are new hospitals or medical facilities opening in the region that will bring with it hundreds of medical and paramedical professionals to the area, who will then need continuing education classes? Instead of advertising to individuals, can you contract with other medical facilities to do group education? Some medical facilities might find such a situation attractive, especially if the alternatives to doing so involve paying travel expenses for all of the individuals at the medical facility to go elsewhere for training.

Is competition for the cream of the medical school applicant crop driving the need for quality human patient simulation? Can your school afford to keep up with the Joneses? Can it afford not to?

Is there a market for scenario development for simulators? If not a market, are there teaching grants for which you can apply? Can other specialties at your institution utilize the simulator center, even if they have been reluctant to do buy into the idea to date?

Potential Threats. You may have conducted an assessment of internal and external barriers to your proposed simulator venture during your market or environmental analysis; if so, you want to include them in this section of your business plan.

What are some of the barriers? Barriers are likely to exist in many formats both inside and outside the institution. A competitor for your customers with a dominating market share will be tough to overcome. If this is the case, do you have a plan to "steal" some of their customers? Are members of the medical school faculty resistant to changing the way medicine is taught? If you have faculty who still need assistance opening their e-mail, you can expect that they will not be the first in line to embrace the new teaching technology offered by a human patient simulator.

What about administrators unwilling to cope with economic risk? Simulators are expensive. One human patient simulator with very little optional equipment easily exceeds two hundred thousand dollars. Two hundred thousand dollars would buy a lot of smaller equipment for the school. Your business plan will be compared with all of the organization's other requests for institutional financial support. The case for a simulation center needs to be strong or have powerful advocates. Hopefully you built some of the latter in the early stages of the strategic planning process.

Will organizational politics be a factor? On whose toes might you step if your human patient simulator project becomes a huge success? Might the simulator center deprive any of the other departments of revenue-producing activities? Given the financial struggles of academic medicine in recent years, a negative economic effect experienced by one unit or department as the direct result of an action by a different department will certainly breed resentment and potential political undermining activities. Politics need not always be a reason not to do a project, nor do they necessarily need to be described in the business plan in detail, but the director-to-be of a simulator center should be intimately aware of the potential risks in order to steer clear of the pitfalls placed in the path by those who stand to lose by the simulator center's gain.

Productivity Goals. Before you begin to describe the productivity goals of the simulation center, you will need to address how productivity will be measured. Will productivity be measured by number of students, conference attendees, or visitors through the door? Will it be research dollars or academic papers? Is the organization interested in the local, regional, and national coverage by the media? Is revenue-producing productivity to be the measuring stick?

Depending on the number of productivity measurement instruments, this section of the business plan may quite short or comparable to others in length and scope. Tables are easy ways to convey the productivity goals if the measurement criteria are few. If the measurement criterion is simply the number of courses offered in a year internally and externally, list the ones that you plan to offer. If the bottom line of the simulator center is an issue early in the life cycle of the center, include for each set of courses the estimated revenue, cost, and contribution to the operational costs for each.

As the number of productivity goals for the simulator project increases, so should the length of this section of the business plan. Depending on where writing the business plan falls in the process for your specific situation (selling the idea or guide for implementation), your "goals" may include items such as "recruiting a world-class programmer to assist with scenario development" or "acquiring space." If you have not done something important yet, it is a goal, but remember that the more goals that you include in this section that are not productivity-related, the more it seems like a to-do list rather than measurements of productivity. While making a to-do list can certainly help the director stay focused and organized, productivity goals should stay positive in focus and not include a list of the important things that you have not done yet.

You should not list productivity goals in your business plan without discussing how the simulator center will reach them. For each goal, describe briefly how it will be reached. As you progress through each section of your business plan, you continue to draw on what has come before. Refer to, but do not repeat, your marketing strategy as it pertains to attracting 25 attendees to your intubation class. Refer to your class synopsis described in the Description of the Business as it relates to becoming part of the medical student curriculum.

Since you have not done so previously, one of the methods that you need to describe in some detail in this section is the extent of your marketing efforts. You know the market for your simulator project, thanks to the analysis conducted in the last section. You want to discuss the ways in which you plan to reach each segment of that market to achieve the goals outlined in this section.

Financial Estimates and Budget. All throughout the strategic and business planning process you have been accumulating data that will drive your budget. The budget may be the most time-consuming part of your plan, but it is also likely to be the most useful.

Budgets can take many formats, as shown by the many different formats used by various universities and sponsoring agencies for grant budget submission. There is no right or wrong way to do a budget so long as it meets your needs of providing a financial plan for the upcoming accounting periods.

Optimally, you want at least a skeleton of a budget for more than one year in the future. The budget for the upcoming year should include line-item detail, but subsequent years can consist of grouping budget categories together and attempting to account for potential variance in the subsequent years.

Start with a detailed budget for year one. Estimate any individual cost or revenue items as an individual line in the budget. Group similar small-ticket items together (such as office supplies), but separate any items that you know will vary based on revenue. Budgets should be dynamic—not frozen in time. Potentially, you may set up a spreadsheet or other accounting program to recalculate costs and revenues based on changing the number of simulator course attendees or courses offered. Since you know everything that you need by now, you can put it all in an organized format to paint a financial picture for the year to come. You need to calculate both estimated revenues and expenses. Do not clutter your budget page with the calculations used to arrive at revenue or cost figures. Keep each calculation as a separate table within your financial documents (Table 2).

You should use the calculated figures from each revenue or expense table to populate the budget (Table 3). The budget in your business plan can be as detailed or as simple as you wish. By now you should have a good feel for the stakeholders who will be passing judgment on what the plan contains. Do they need detail to make a decision? If so, include it. Regardless of whether or not you put a simple or detailed budget in the business plan, you should keep a detailed budget somewhere. To create a good simple budget, you *must* have created a good detailed one first!

Table 2.
Revenue Estimate*

State University Human Patient Simulator Budget Year One
External course revenue estimate

	Attendees	Revenue Per Visit	Semitotals
Course A	50	$500	$25,000
Course B	100	$400	$40,000
Course C	250	$300	$75,000
Course D	300	$200	$60,000
Course E	50	$500	$25,000
Course F	35	$750	$26,250
Course G	40	$600	$24,000
Course H	40	$550	$22,000
Total external course revenue			$297,250

* For each source of revenue, estimate the income based no market estimates and the price as determined from the attempt to price the product for an efficient market. Good detailed estimates will evolve into good categorized estimates for the simulator center annual budget.

Table 3.
Year One Budget*

REVENUE

External course revenue	$297,250
Endowment Income	$100,000
Director salary support–dean's office	$80,000
Director fringes support–dean's office	$20,000
Gift: Dr. Mrs. John Doe	$500,000
Loan	$350,000
Medical student tuition allocation	$15,000
Total revenues	$1,362,250

EXPENSES

Operational expenses

Director salary	($80,000)	
Director fringes	($20,000)	
Secretary salary	($25,000)	
Secretary fringes	($6,250)	
Computer technician salary	($60,000)	
Computer technician fringes	($15,000)	
Utilities	($3,000)	
Internet access	($500)	
Gases	($3,000)	
Office supplies	($1,500)	
Syringes, IV bags, hoses, moulage, soda lime	($2,000)	
Marketing	($2,000)	
Educational materials	($800)	
Insurance	($1,500)	
Entertainment	($1,000)	
Postage	($500)	
Office equipment	($2,000)	
Interest/loan payback	($35,000)	
Travel	($5,000)	
Total operational expenses	($264,050)	($264,050)
Renovation	($750,000)	
2 simulators	($400,000)	
Simulator warranties	($30,000)	
Simulator accessories	($82,000)	
Dean's tax on external revenue	($14,863)	
Rent/facilities cost	($100,000)	
Information systems infrastructure	($75,000)	
Computers	($25,000)	
Cameras	($10,000)	
Monitors	($8,000)	
Furniture	($150,000)	
Anesthesia machines	($45,000)	
Ventilators	($5,000)	
Intubation materials	($5,000)	
Training/site visits	($10,000)	
Projectors	($6,000)	
Total startup expenses	($965,863)	($965,863)
Total expenses		($1,229,913)
Revenue less expenses		$132,337.50
Contingency-10% of expenses		($122,991.25)
Projected balance for Year One		$9,346.25

* Compile specific revenue stream and expense budgets into a budget for the entire accounting period. Budgets can be created for any period. In an academic environment, where expenses and associated revenues often do not fall within the same month, creating monthly budgets becomes very cumbersome. A budget for the fiscal year should always be completed.

For subsequent years, you might want only the simple budget that has all of the line items from the Year One budget grouped together. For Year Two and beyond, probably the greatest expenses will be the human resources associated with the simulation center. Therefore, make sure to adjust salaries for estimated cost of living or merit increases. In planning for the budgets for subsequent years, remember fixed, variable, semifixed, and semivariable costs. Your categories of costs may change if you expect the number of courses offered to increase dramatically in the following years. Rent may not, but advertising and disposable supplies of all types most certainly will.

Remember to consider the accounting basis (cash or accrual), tax status, and reporting requirements of the organization in developing the financial statements for your simulator center. You may need to include income statement, balance sheets, or other accounting and financial documents if your organization uses them. You may need to account for depreciation, which is the decrease in value of your assets over time. You may need to account for taxes to local, state, or federal government. Any finance or accounting text can provide details on how to create those statements and how to include some of the more intricate finance and accounting methods within your business plan.

All throughout the strategic and business planning processes you questioned, researched, negotiated, and solicited. The budget for the project is the culmination of all of the answers that you received to every inquiry made throughout the entire process. Just as you will have asked questions and did not realize their impact on the budget at the time, you will undoubtedly find questions that you need to ask for other planning aspects of your simulator project as you complete the budget. A budget containing incorrect data is useless. As changes that impact the financial expectations of the simulator project occur, update the budget. Whether it is the budget or the simulator project as a whole, do not settle for "good enough."

Appendices. The appendices of your business plan should include all of the documents in their entirety referenced in the body of the business plan. Provide the items in the appendices in the order in which they were referenced in the body of the plan. Part of the appendices should detail the staffing, including a full organizational chart, curriculum vitae of the director and any other high-profile faculty or staff involved with the project, and any job descriptions yet to be filled. The budget, financial documents, and a layout of acquired space or the floor plan for the center-to-be should also be included in this section.

Ongoing Assessment

As of the time of this book, three of the most popular methods for measuring and managing effectiveness are Kaplan and Norton's Balanced Scorecard Collaborative,[17] Six Sigma,[18] and Total Quality Management.[19] Although the three systems are different in specific methodology and operational procedure, all three share the importance of identifying measurable outcomes, tracking them over time, and investigating the key business processes that contribute to fluctuations in them.

Numerous resources and publications exist on all three management systems and should be researched as you implement your project to determine which fits in with your organization's missions and strategies for continuous improvement. Do not complete the planning process without determining how you plan to maintain and improve quality in your new human patient simulator center.

Conclusion

Your business plan is now complete, and you are exploring alternatives for improving quality in the center. As difficult and time-consuming as the strategic planning and business planning processes are, the journey is far from over. Perhaps the scope of the original simulator dream has been altered, but the game plan is now set. Solicit final approval for the plan, toss the coin, and start implementation. Use the plan as a backbone for your tactics as you respond to your specific environment. You cannot take home the trophy yet—the game has just begun!

References

1. Warters RD, Katz J, Szmuk P, et al: Development criteria for academic leadership in anesthesiology: Have they changed? Anesth Analg 2002;95(4):1019–1023.
2. Academic Practice Management Compensation Survey: 2000 Report Based on 1999 Data. Englewood, CO, Medical Group Management Association, 2000.
3. Academic Practice Compensation and Production Survey for Faculty and Management: 2003 Report Based on 2002 Data. Englewood, CO, Medical Group Management Association, 2003.
4. Michaelson GA: Sun Tzu: The Art of War for Managers: 50 Strategic Rules. Avon, MA, Adams Media Corporation, 2001, p 3.
5. Michaelson GA: Sun Tzu: The Art of War for Managers: 50 Strategic Rules. Avon, MA, Adams Media Corporation, 2001, p 24.
6. Simyar F, Lloyd-Jones J, Caro J: Strategic management: A proposed framework for the health care industry. In Simyar F, Lloyd-Jones J (eds): Strategic Management in the Health Care Sector: Toward the Year 2000. Englewood Cliffs, NJ, Prentice-Hall, 1988, pp 6–17.
7. Slaton R, Bowers M: Strategic planning. In Bachrach DJ, Nicholas WR (eds): One Revolution: Managing the Academic Medical Practice in an Era of Rapid Change. Englewood, CO, Medical Group Management Association, 1997, pp 89–90.
8. Slaton R, Bowers M: Strategic planning. In Bachrach DJ, Nicholas WR (eds): One Revolution: Managing the Academic Medical Practice in an Era of Rapid Change. Englewood, CO, Medical Group Management Association, 1997, pp 98–99.
9. Drucker PF: Management: Tasks, Responsibilities, Practices. New York, Harper & Row, 1974, pp 86–102.
10. Hawley C: An environmental assessment is key. Provider 1988;14(4):14–20.
11. Slaton R, Bowers M: Strategic planning. In Bachrach DJ, Nicholas WR (eds): One Revolution: Managing the Academic Medical Practice in an Era of Rapid Change. Englewood, CO, Medical Group Management Association, 1997, p 101.
12. Mancuso JR: How to Write a Winning Business Plan. New York, Prentice Hall Press, 1985, pp 25–27.
13. Cleverly WO: Essentials of Health Care Finance, 4th ed. Gaithersburg, MD, Aspen Publishers, 1997, pp 223–225.
14. Rhodes NM, Purcell PM: The business plan for the academic clinical department. In Bachrach DJ, Nicholas WR (eds): One Revolution: Managing the Academic Medical Practice in an Era of Rapid Change. Englewood, CO, Medical Group Management Association, 1997, pp 131–132.
15. METI—New Installations. Sarasota, FL, Medical Education Technologies, Inc., 2003. (Accessed November 26, 2003, at *http://www.meti.com/installations1.html.*)
16. Michaelson GA: Sun Tzu: The Art of War for Managers: 50 Strategic Rules. Avon, MA, Adams Media Corporation, 2001, pp 100–101.
17. Balanced Scorecard Institute. Washington, DC: The Balanced Scorecard Institute, 2003. (Accessed November 26, 2003, at *http://www.balancedscorecard.org.*)
18. Samuels DI, Adomitis FL: Six Sigma can meet your revenue-cycle needs. Healthcare Finan Manage 2003;57(11):70–75.
19. Deming WE: The New Economics for Industry, Government, Education, 2nd ed. Cambridge, MA, Massachusetts Institute of Technology, Center for Advanced Engineering Study, 1994.

Section II

 SIMULATION:
PRACTICAL APPLICATIONS

Chapter 6

SIMULATION IN PHYSIOLOGY

Gary L. Anderson, PhD, and Michael S. Goodrow

Simulators are designed to teach students how to perform particular actions and to evaluate their ability to perform those actions. However, a well-designed and comprehensive simulator can also be used to teach basic concepts by reinforcing those concepts through demonstration.

This chapter describes an application that used patient simulators to teach physiologic concepts to medical school students. It also describes the existing physiology course and the logistics of incorporating the simulation sessions into the course structure. The response from the students and faculty is discussed. An overview of the simulator and the specific cases used for the course are also described. The teaching materials used during the sessions are included at the end of the chapter.

Working Within the Physiology Course Structure

The Medical Physiology Course is a 16-week course taught in the spring semester of the freshman year. About 150–160 first-year medical students take this course each year. The course consists of approximately 116 contact hours that include lectures (74 hours), quizzes with small group discussions (10 hours), problem-based learning case studies (12 hours), simulation exercises (8 hours), and examinations (12 hours). The course meets 6–10 hours per week, usually from 10:00 am to noon, Monday through Friday. Because the medical school curriculum is relatively rigid, we had to work within the 2-hour time block for Physiology in planning the simulation exercises. It was decided that four simulation exercises in the areas of cardiovascular and respiratory physiology would be done and that each exercise would be 1 hour in length. Each simulation exercise was written by a team of 3–4 faculty members, including both basic science and clinical faculty. The topics chosen are broadly described as (1) myocardial ischemia; (2) cardiac output and venous return; (3) pressure, flow, and resistance; and (4) pneumothorax. These simulation exercise case studies are provided at the end of this chapter.

Design and Logistics

The Simulation Center at the University of Louisville has a suite of 4 simulation rooms (simulated operating rooms with computerized mannequins) and 4 briefing (discussion) rooms. We randomly divided the class into two main groups (10:00 or 11:00 hour) and subdivided these two groups into two activity groups (simulation-first or briefing-first) for a total of four different logistical groups. Each simulation exercise or briefing discussion lasted 30 minutes. Then the simulation-first and briefing-first groups switched places. Half the class completed the simulation exercise (both simulation and briefing) from 10:00 AM to 11:00 AM, and the other half did the same from 11:00 AM to noon. Thus, there were a total of 16 groups of students (4 rooms × 2 hours × 2 activities) with 9–10 students per group for a total of 150–160 students.

The simulation exercise consisted of a clinical scenario conducted by one of the clinical faculty, and the briefing consisted of a discussion of the relevant physiology and was conducted by one of the physiology faculty. With this format, half the students had their briefing just before they went through the operating room portion of the simulation exercise, and the other half of the students had their briefing just after they had completed the operating room portion of the simulation exercise. In essence, half the students discussed what they were about to do and see in the operating room, and the other half of the students discussed what they had just done and seen in the operating room. It is not surprising but still interesting to note that both the clinical faculty and the physiology faculty commented that the second group of students (whether briefing-second or simulation-second) was better prepared to discuss and interact with each other and the faculty during the second session compared with the preceding group.

Each exercise contained several questions directed toward the students that were asked by the faculty member as the case unfolded (see the case scenarios in the appendices). These questions formed the basis for the discussion in the briefing room and for points of discussion in the operating room. The collective faculty had met earlier and agreed on answers to these questions in order to provide uniformity for the discussions among the different groups. However, each faculty member conducted his or her session according to what worked best for him- or herself. Based on a lack of student comments or concerns about whether they had briefing or simulation first, it was judged that there was no important difference between the two experiences. In fact, students in the two groups had the same average score later on exam questions related to the simulation exercises.

Student/Faculty Satisfaction

The simulation exercises were one of the most highly rated elements of the physiology course as judged by an end-of-course survey conducted by the Medical Curriculum Office. Among several items rated by students about the physiology course (e.g., organization, content, exams, overall quality) was a specific question about the simulation exercises. On a 1–5 point scale with 5 being best, the range of scores for all items was from 3.1 to 4.1 with an average score of 3.8. Physiology was among the most highly rated first-year courses in the medical school, and the simulation exercises were rated 4.0 in the physiology course.

Simulation Specifics

The simulations were implemented using the Human Patient Simulator (HPS) system, which is a product of Medical Education Technologies, Inc. (METI, Sarasota, FL). The HPS is a computer-controlled mannequin that incorporates a comprehensive physiologic model within the system. HPS cases have two sections: a "patient" and a "scenario." The patient contains the underlying, chronic status for the case. The scenario contains a sequence of changes that occur with that patient. These changes might represent the progression of an acute episode or the response to treatments.

As an example, the effects and treatment of an anaphylactic reaction can be demonstrated using the HPS system. A scenario can be designed to progress through the reaction, starting with mild symptoms (wheezing) and progressing through moderate (tachycardia and shortness of breath) to severe (hypoxia) symptoms. Additional steps include recovery after administration of the appropriate drugs. This scenario could then be used for a variety of HPS patients to show different levels of severity.

For the four physiology examples, scenarios were written to demonstrate the desired teaching objectives. The scenarios were also designed to facilitate the repeated execution of the scenarios, to fit within the time constraints of the sessions, and to simplify the operators' control and execution of the simulations.

The three cardiac simulations (ischemia, output, and circulation) were centered on simulated surgical cases. These cases started with the METI "Truck Driver" patient. Truck Driver is a 61-year-old man with a variety of health problems. Related to these cases, his specific conditions are hypertension, congestive heart failure, and chronic obstructive pulmonary disease. To facilitate the execution of the scenarios, these three cases started with the patient sedated, intubated, and ventilated. The fourth case was a respiratory physiology case based on a spontaneous tension pneumothorax. This case started with the METI "Standard Man" patient.

For the cardiac simulations, the physiology faculty members were specialists in cardiac or circulatory physiology, and the clinical faculty members were cardiac anesthesiologists. For the respiratory case, the physiology faculty members were respiratory physiologists or exercise physiologists, and the clinical faculty members were emergency medicine residents.

Cardiac Ischemia

The cardiac ischemia case is based on a patient presenting for a semi-emergent colectomy under general anesthesia. To demonstrate the effects of hypovolemia and peripheral vasodilation on blood pressure, the patient was given a bowel prep on the previous evening that caused hypovolemia; the anesthesia caused vasodilation, as evidenced by decreased systemic vascular resistance.

When the surgeon begins the procedure, the heart rate rises in response to the pain, and the blood pressure consequently decreases. The ECG begins to show ST-segment depression, indicating the possibility of ischemia. The initial treatment is fluid and sedatives, which somewhat resolve the problem, but the ST-segment depression increases. This problem is treated with a coronary vasodilator (nitroglycerin). The complete case is printed in Appendix A.

Cardiac Output

The cardiac output case is based on the same colectomy patient, 5 days postoperatively, returning to the operating room for an exploratory laparotomy. During the intervening days, the patient has also suffered a myocardial infarction. Before he enters the operating room, a pulmonary artery catheter is inserted in the patient.

The cardiac output (CO) is measured at several points during this procedure. The first reading is before the surgery begins. Then the following events occur during the surgery, and CO is measured after each event:

◆ Dobutamine infusion begun
◆ 500 ml blood loss (hemostasis clip comes loose, 2 hours into surgery)
◆ 1000 ml fluid infusion
◆ Additional 1000 ml fluid infusion
◆ Nitroglycerin infusion

The complete case is printed in Appendix B.

Peripheral Circulation

The peripheral circulation case is based on a patient presenting for the removal (resection) of an abdominal aortic aneurysm under general anesthesia. An intra-arterial catheter and a pulmonary artery catheter have been inserted prior to induction. The simulation starts with the patient sedated, intubated, ventilated, and on a monitor.

The surgeon begins the procedure by making an incision and mobilizing the intestines, which causes a marked decrease in blood pressure. This is resolved by administration of phenylephrine. Then, the aorta is clamped, which causes a very significant increase in proximal arterial blood pressure. This is then treated with nitroglycerin. At the end of the surgery, the aorta is unclamped, and the resulting hypotension is treated.

In addition to monitoring the alternations in the arterial and pulmonary blood pressures, the cardiac output was measured after each of the steps in the surgical procedure. The complete case is printed in Appendix C.

Tension Pneumothorax

The respiratory case is based on paramedics responding to an otherwise healthy patient complaining of sudden onset of shortness of air accompanied by severe chest pain. Initial condition is assessed, the patient is placed on four liters oxygen by nasal cannula, IV is inserted, and pulmonary artery catheter inserted.

The patient then exhibits increasing agitation and difficulty breathing. The patient's condition continues to deteriorate. Eventually, the students perform a needle decompression to relieve the spontaneous tension pneumothorax. The patient is then assessed, and follow-up treatment determined. The complete case is printed in Appendix D.

Simulation Exercise Case Studies

The students were provided copies of each exercise about 1 week prior to the date of the exercise and instructed to read and study the material and to be ready to discuss this among themselves and with the faculty leading the exercise. The general impression of the faculty was that many students did prepare, but certainly not all students read the material and were prepared for the discussions. The handouts provided to each student are listed below and provided in the following appendices: (A) Myocardial Ischemia, (B) Cardiac Output and Venous Return, (C) Pressure, Flow, and Resistance, and (D) Pneumothorax.

Appendix A: Patient Simulation Exercise 1:
ECG Alterations with Myocardial Ischemia
(Courtesy of John T. Fleming, Ph.D.)

The energy required to maintain the cardiac cycle is obtained via aerobic metabolism, which uses oxygen and glucose. Blood flow through the coronary arteries supplies these nutrients to the myocardial cells. If the blood supply becomes insufficient, causing an inadequate oxygen level, an energy deficiency occurs and the myocytes resort to anaerobic metabolism.

Specifically, oxygen delivery can become inadequate from either a decreased blood supply (e.g., atherosclerosis of the coronary arteries), or from an increased workload that outpaces supply. For patient care, we always try to maximize oxygen supply and minimize demand. Listed below are the factors affecting both myocardial oxygen supply and demand.

Supply

1. Coronary perfusion pressure: Hypotension reduces coronary blood flow.

2. Heart rate: Perfusion to the left ventricle occurs during diastole. Tachycardia is an undesired consequence because it reduces the time that the heart spends in diastole.

3. Oxygen content of the blood is affected by oxygen and hemoglobin levels within the blood. Anemia and hypoxia are a detrimental pair.

4. Coronary artery diameter: A patient with coronary artery disease has reduced blood flow secondary to the intraluminal obstruction.

Demand

1. Basal requirements of the myocytes.

2. Heart rate is the largest energy-consuming process for the heart (greater than preload or afterload). As such, tachycardia would be unfavorable.

3. Wall tension: Afterload > preload.

4. Contractility: Usually an increase in contractility causes an increase in myocardial oxygen consumption.

Normal cardiac function is dependent on adequate blood flow to cardiomyocytes and conductive tissues. An interruption of blood flow quickly leads to reduced oxygen delivery to these cells. The reduction of oxygen within the myocardium (known as ischemia) has profound effects on key biochemical events within the cells; these effects lead to altered physiologic function. Many of these oxygen-dependent cellular processes are involved in the distribution of ions (Na^+, K^+ and Ca^{++}) across the cell membrane. Thus, ischemia leads to significant changes in the transmembrane potential of the ischemic cells. The altered transmembrane potentials of the ischemic tissue alters the electrical currents produced by the heart. Since the electrocardiogram (ECG) "measures" the summated electrical activity of the heart, the ECG is altered during myocarial ischemia. Hence, the ECG is one of several important clinical tools used to diagnose myocardial ischemia.

Effects of Ischemia on Resting Membrane Potentials and ECG Segments

Under conditions of normal blood flow and oxygen delivery, cells of the heart generate adenosine triphosphate (ATP) via aerobic metabolism (oxidative phosphorylation). With a reduction in oxygen delivery, as occurs due to partial blockage of one or more coronary arteries, there is a shift to lesser efficient anaerobic metabolism. Intracellular levels of high-energy phosphate molecules (ATP and creatine phosphate) drop within minutes in the ischemic cells. Biochemical processes that depend on hydrolysis of ATP, such as the active transport of Na^+ and K^+ across the cell membrane by the ATPase pump, slow down. This pump plays a major role in maintaining the high extracellular Na^+ concentration and the high intracellular K^+ concentration of resting myocytes. A decrease in the activity of the pump alters the distribution of ions across the cell membrane and changes the resting membrane potential and the action potential.

In addition, the decline in intracellular ATP in ischemic cells causes ATP-regulated K^+ channels (I_{KATP}) to open, allowing more K^+ to diffuse out of the cell. Thus, the less active Na^+, K^+ pump and the increased efflux of K^+ through I_{KATP} channels raise the extracellular concentration of K^+. Because blood flow to the ischemic tissue is low, the high extracellular K^+ is not washed out but persists. The high extracellular K^+ reduces the concentration gradient of K^+ across the membrane and slows the rate of passive diffusion of K^+ out of the resting (unstimulated) cell.

Diastolic Current of Injury (Fig. 1). In resting cardiomyocytes, the slower rate of K^+ efflux from the resting cells causes a slight depolarization. Thus, during phase 4, the resting membrane potential of the ischemic myocyte is -70 mv rather than the normal intracellular resting potential of -90 mv. This differential between the electrical charge of the ischemic tissue and the normal tissue creates the flow of current across the surface of the heart when the heart is at rest. This abnormal current is referred to as the di-

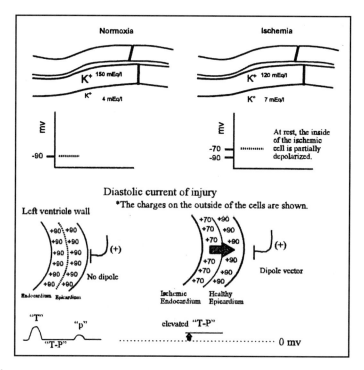

Figure 1.

astolic current of injury. Depending on the position of the ECG electrodes, the diastolic current of injury will produce an upward or downward displacement of the isoelectric line during the "T-P" segment relative to the true isoelectric line.

Systolic Current of Injury (Fig. 2). Ischemia also changes the permeability of cardiomyocytes during the plateau phase of the action potential. As discussed, ischemic endocardial cells have a less negative resting membrane potential compared to adjacent, healthy epicardial cells. When the hypoxic cells are presented with a sufficient depolarizing stimulus, the rate of depolarization (slope of phase 0) is less than normoxic cell. As a result, phase 2 of the action potential of hypoxic cells will be more negative, relative to normoxic epicardial tissue.

As shown in Figure 2 (upper right corner), the plateau phase of healthy epicardial cells reaches +10 mv (intracellular recording; −10 mv outside charge). By comparison, the hypoxic endocardial cells depolarize to only −20 mv during phase 2.) This charge differential at the interface of the hypoxic endocardial tissue and the normoxic epicardial tissue establishes an abnormal ventricular systolic current across the surface of the heart, known as the systolic current of injury. The "ST" segment of the ECG will be shifted above or below the normal isoelectric line depending on the position of the ECG electrodes.

Treatment of Myocardial Ischemia

Restoration of normal blood flow to the myocardium is the paramount concern of the clinician tending to a patient with evidence of myocardial ischemia. Various tools are available:

1. Agents that dilate coronary arteries are often used first to physiologically increase the diameter of the vessels. Nitroprusside and other nitrates are commonly used to treat

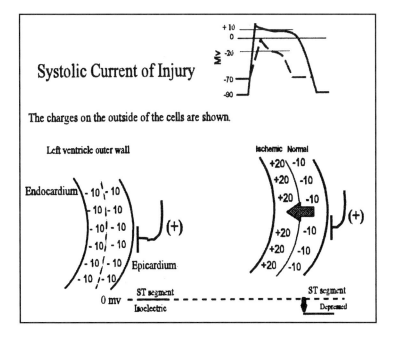

Figure 2.

angina (chest pain) symptoms because they act quickly and can be self-administered safely. Nitroprusside dilates coronary vessels by its conversion to nitric oxide (NO). NO stimulates the production of cyclic adenosine monophosphate (camp) inside the vascular smooth muscle cells in the walls of the coronary arteries. In turn, cAMP activates kinases, which dephosphorylate the myosin light chains that have been phosphorylated by the myosin light chain to promote the interaction of actin and myosin to initiate contraction.

2. Thrombolytic agents that lyse thrombi are often effective when the coronary artery is physically blocked.

3. Mechanical methods are also used to remove or compress the atherosclerotic material within the lumen of the artery.

4. Bypass surgery to circumvent coronary arteries that cannot be dilated, lysed, removed or compressed.

Clinical Scenario

(Courtesy of Dr. David Santamore)

The following will be used for the simulator session. It is a representative situation of the clinical diagnosis and management of myocardial ischemia. You will be divided into small groups of 8–9 students and will spend ½ hour in the Simulated OR (operating room) and ½ hour in the briefing room.

A 78 year-old male with a known history of coronary artery disease (stable angina, proven disease of the left anterior descending and circumflex coronary arteries on a previous cardiac catheterization — but he declined coronary artery bypass surgery) presents for a semi-emergent colectomy under general anesthesia (for colon cancer). He is given a bowel prep the night before surgery.

When you enter the simulator room, you will find that the patient is already under general anesthesia (intubated, on ventilator). Vital signs are stable (BP = 120/80, HR= 70, ECG = isoelectric, pulse oximetry = 100%)

Q1. What is a major determinant of myocardical oxygen demand?

Q2. What can compromise oxygen supply to the heart?

Then the surgeon begins the operation and makes the initial incision. The HR increases to 140, and BP decreases to 80/30. Discuss the fact that the patient is already hypovolemic from the bowel prep. The anesthesia, by causing vasodilation, has also decreased his systemic vascular resistance (SVR). There is sympathetic stress (pain) from the surgical incision. These factors all work to increase myocardial oxygen demand.

Q3. Why did our patient have an increase in heart rate when the surgeon began?

The ECG now begins to show ST-segment depression. Initial treatment includes a fluid bolus (500 cc of normal saline) and an agent to increase the depth of anesthesia (200 µg of fentanyl, a synthetic opioid). Discuss the possibility that myocardial ischemia is present.

Q4. Why does an ischemic area of the heart alter the ECG? (See Figs. 1 and 2.)

Q5. How do you treat pain and volume depletion?

Q6. How can you treat poor coronary perfusion?

The heart rate now slows down to 90 BPM, and the blood pressure comes back to 100/60, but there is still significant ST depression. Treatment with a potent coronary vasodilator is needed. We give a bolus of nitroglycerin, followed by a constant infusion.The ECG now shows a normal ST segment. The BP is now 110/60, with a pulse of 80 BPM. The surgery continues uneventfully. A postoperative 12-lead ECG shows no change from baseline, and serial cardiac isoenzymes are negative (no apparent permanent cardiac damage/infarction).

Instructions for Faculty Discussion Leaders

Four different groups of students will rotate through your briefing room (see assignments below) at half-hour intervals beginning at 8:00 AM and finishing at 10:00 AM. Attached is the handout that the students received. Please discuss this handout with each group of students. The main things to focus on are (1) Figures 1 and 2, which show why ischemic myocardium has an altered ECG, and (2) the various steps in the clinical scenario and why each treatment was given. An outline for this discussion is below. A list of students who will rotate through each briefing room is also attached.

All briefing rooms are in the Simulation Center B307

   Anderson: Briefing room 2   Wead: Briefing room 4

   Schuschke : Briefing room 1 Fleming: Briefing room 3

Questions and answers to discuss with the medical students:

Q1. What is a major determinant of myocardical oxygen demand?
- Work load of the heart, related to heart rate (high heart rate = high oxygen demand).

Q2. What can compromise oxygen supply to the heart?
- High heart rate (short filling time and short perfusion time for the heart—diastole).
- Poor coronary blood flow (low blood pressure or obstruction of coronary vessels).
- Poor lung function (low oxygen in blood).

Q3. Why did our patient have an increase in heart rate when the surgeon began?
- Pain from the surgical incision (inadequate anesthesia) and some volume depletion.

Q4. Why does an ischemic area of the heart alter the ECG? (See Figs. 1 and 2.)
- Loss of energy = K^+ loss by myocardial cells (lack of ATP for Na^+/K^+ pump).
- High concentrations of K^+ accumulate in the ischemic interstitium of the heart.
- Lack of perfusion = lack of potassium washout from the interstitium.
- High extracellular K^+ = reduced gradient for K^+ efflux and thus a less negative resting membrane potential (seen during phase 4).
- Current flows between ischemic and normal tissue during phase 4 because of the difference in resting membrane potential (see Fig. 1).
- The ST segment is not isoelectric (either elevated or depressed) because of changes in phase 2 of the sum of many cardiac action potentials (see Fig. 2).

Q5. How do you treat pain and volume depletion?
- Give an opiod drug (fentanyl) and 500 cc of normal saline IV.

Q6. How can you treat poor coronary perfusion?
- Dilate the coronary blood vessels with nitroglycerin.

Appendix B. Simulation Exercise 2:
Cardiac Output and Venous Return
(Courtesy of John T. Fleming, Ph.D.)

Study Heart Lecture Notes, pages 21–24

◆ Cardiac Output Regulation
◆ Frank-Starling Mechanism
◆ Inotropic State of the Heart

This simulation exercise is focused on understanding several factors that affect cardiac output (CO). We will demonstrate how to measure cardiac output in the operating room and then examine how the Frank-Starling mechanism, an inotropic agent, and a chronotropic agent affect cardiac output. It will be necessary to discuss central venous pressure (CVP) in this exercise. CVP is the blood pressure in the large veins immediately preceding the right atrium. The magnitude of this pressure (normally less than 10 mmHg) has a large impact on the amount of filling of the right ventricle during diastole.

Measuring Cardiac Output by Thermal Dilution

In the operating room, CO can be measured by a thermal dilution technique. This technique requires the use of a Swan-Ganz catheter. The catheter is inserted into the jugular (or subclavian) vein. The Swan-Ganz catheter has a balloon near its end that, when inflated, tends to float with the flow of blood and carry the catheter tip into the right atrium, right ventricle, and through the pulmonic valve into the right pulmonary artery and even to one of its major branches if desired. This catheter can be used to measure pressures in the above-mentioned segments of the circulation. When the catheter tip reaches the superior vena cava in the chest, venous pressure is seen to fluctuate with respirations. This is the central venous pressure (CVP). Advancing the catheter all the way to the pulmonary artery permits measurement of cardiac output by thermal dilution. The Swan-Ganz catheter has a thermister (temperature measuring probe) at its tip. Cold (usually room temperature, 22°C) saline (10 ml) is injected proximal to the thermister into the right atrium via one of several ports in the catheter. The cold saline dilutes the warmer blood (37°C) and lowers the temperature in proportion to the amount of blood flowing through the pulmonary artery, which equals the CO. The thermister is connected to a computer that (after careful calibration) converts the rate of temperature change into values for cardiac output.

Case Scenario

(Courtesy of Dr. David Santamore)

Mr. Smith is a 78 year-old male with a history of coronary artery disease (stable angina, proven 2-vessel disease on cardiac catheterization) who underwent a colectomy under general anesthesia. His intraoperative course was uneventful except for transient ischemia treated with nitroglycerin. Unfortunately, on the third day postoperatively Mr. Smith suffered a mild myocardial infarction. An echocardiogram (a noninvasive ultrasound device, which allows visualization of the heart walls) showed mild systolic dysfunction of the anterior apex of the left ventricle, with a mildly reduced ejection fraction of 45%. Cardiac isoenzymes had begun to improve by the fourth day, and his cardiology physician considered interventional treatment. However, on the fifth day the patient de-

veloped a small bowel obstruction requiring a return visit to the OR, and his further cardiac workup was put on hold. In preparation for the emergency bowel surgery (an exploratory laparotomy), a pulmonary artery (Swan-Ganz) catheter was inserted. Before
leaving for the operating room, Mr. Smith's initial cardiac output is 4.2 L/min.

When you enter the simulator room, you will find that the patient is already under
general anesthesia (intubated, on ventilator). The patient's vital signs are stable: BP =
110/70, HR = 70, ECG = isoelectric, pulse oximetry = 100%, and central venous pressure (CVP) = 9. Twenty minutes into the operation you perform a CO measurement,
which shows a value of 2.8 L/min.

Questions:
1. Why did we place a pulmonary artery catheter in this patient?
2. What information can you obtain from a pulmonary artery catheter?
3. What is the normal value for central venous pressure?
4. Is the patient's cardiac output normal?
5. How do you calculate stroke volume, and what are its normal values?
6. Explain why the CO was 4.2 L/min before surgery and is now 2.8 L/min during
surgery.

Dobutamine infusion: You decide to start an infusion of dobutamine at 4
μg/kg/min.

Questions:
7. What is the cellular mechanism of action of sympathomimetics (e.g., epinephrine,
dobutamine)?
8. What effect on CO do you expect to see with the addition of dobutamine?
9. What change in heart rate do you expect to see?

After the beginning the dobutamine infusion, you repeat the CO measurement.
The new value is 4.5 L/min, with a heart rate of 84. After altering your anesthetic regi-
men (using less myocardial depressant inhalational agents and more hemodynamically
stable opioids), you are successful in weaning the dobutamine off and keeping the patient's CO over 4.0 L/min.

Hemorrhage: Two hours into the surgery, a vascular hemostasis clip becomes loose and
there is an immediate blood loss of 500 cc. The vital signs are now BP = 88/60, HR = 110,
Pulse oximetry = 96%, ECG ST segment is isoelectric, CVP = 2, and CO = 2.4 L/min.

Questions:
10. What has caused this patient's hypotension (low arterial blood pressure)?
11. Should you restart the dobutamine?
12. Where on the Frank-Starling curve is this patient's cardiac function?
13. What treatment do you want to begin, and why?

Saline infusion: After administering a 1000-cc IV fluid bolus, the patient's vital
signs are now BP = 100/58, HR = 86, and CVP = 8. The CO has returned to 4.0 L/min.

Because of the slightly low blood pressure, you decide to repeat the fluid bolus with
another 1000 cc. Following the fluid administration, the BP falls to 86/40. The
CVP=18, and there is now 2.0 mm ST segment depression in the V5 ECG lead. The
CO is measured again, and is only 2.1 L/min.

Questions:
14. What do you think is occurring?
15. Why has the CO decreased to only 2.1 L/min?

16. Where did the second fluid bolus place the patient on the Frank-Starling curve?
17. Why did the central venous pressure (CVP) go up?
18. What medication should you administer?
19. What are the four determinants of myocardial O2 supply?

Nitroglycerin infusion: You start an infusion of nitroglycerin. Blood samples are sent to the lab, and the hemoglobin level is almost normal at 12.6. After a few minutes, BP = 120/80, HR = 70, CVP = 10, and pulseoximetry = 100%. The ECG returns to baseline, and the new CO is measured to be 4.0 L/min.

Questions:
20. Why did the CO increase after the use of nitroglycerin?
21. In this situation, why did the BP go up with the addition of a vasodilator?
22. What are the main factors that increase myocardial oxygen demand?

The surgeon removes several adhesions surrounding the bowel (remnants of the previous surgery), which explains the cause of the small bowel obstruction. Soon after, the operation is completed without incident. The patient spends an uneventful two days in the intensive care unit, where no elevations in cardiac isoenzymes are detected. He is then transferred to the cardiac wing for further management.

Faculty Guide for Answers to Questions (Simulation 2, 2003)
Initial Anesthesia
1. To measure CVP and also CO by thermal dilution.
2. Measure pressures from jugular through pulmonary wedge, and CO (see first page).
3. < 10 mmHg.
4. No. CO should be approaching 5 L/min in healthy adult (less in the elderly).
5. CO/HR = stroke volume (normal is 70–80 ml from a 50–66% ejection fraction).
6. Inhalation anesthetics depress cardiac function and performance (block Ca^{++} entry).
Dobutamine
7. Beta-1 agonist. A positive inotropic agent = increased contractility. Also a very mild positive chronotropic agent but with less effect to increase HR. Causes increased Ca^{++} flux into the myocardium via beta-1 receptors via G protein, adenylate cyclase, cAMP mechanism.
8. Increased CO by virtue of increased contractility.
9. A mild increase in HR (however, as CO improves, reflexes will decrease HR).
Hemorrhage
10. Low CO caused by hemorrhage (low blood volume, low CVP, low filling).
11. Yes, but that won't fix the blood volume problem.
12. On the low part of the upside of the curve (with too much overlap).
13. Give volume (normal saline) of 1000 ml.
Saline Infusion
14. Too much oxygen demand = ischemia (low hematocrit contributes to low oxygen of blood).
15. The heart is ischemic and cannot keep the work load.
16. Top of the curve (near end of functional maximum).
17. The heart is not effectively removing blood from the vena cava, and blood volume is too high. All this causes high CVP.

18. Give a positive inotrope and coronary vasodilator (nitroglycerin).

19. Lung performance (oxygen exchange), hematocrit (RBC content), blood pressure, and coronary vascular resistance.

Nitroglycerin

20. Improve cardiac perfusion and increase heart contractility.

21. Improved CO.

22. Heart rate, contractility, Frank-Starling effect.

Appendix C.
Clinical Simulation 3: Pressure, Flow, and Resistance

(Courtesy of Carol L. Lake, MD, MBA, MPH)

Goals of the Session
◆ To translate mechanical cardiovascular physiology into the clinical reality of cardiovascular anesthesiology.
◆ To apply Starling's law, preload, afterload, systemic and pulmonary vascular resistance, and myocardial compliance to clinical situations.

Student Preparation
To understand the mechanical cardiac physiology involved in this clinical correlation, you will need to understand some pathophysiology. Clinical practice requires integration of many subjects and does not follow the same pattern as your medical school curriculum. Additional information that you need for this clinical correlation is provided below. Use a medical dictionary for terms that are unfamiliar to you. Please be prepared in advance of this exercise so that you can get the most from it.

Coronary Anatomy, Physiology, and Pathophysiology. There are two coronary arteries that arise from the sinuses of Valsalva in the aortic valve. The right coronary artery serves the sinus node, AV node, right atrium and ventricle, interatrial septum, posterior fascicle of the left bundle branch, and posterior interventricular septum. The left coronary artery divides into the left anterior descending and circumflex coronary arteries. Atherosclerotic changes in these epicardial coronary arteries result in the formation of intimal lipoid plaques that cause both chronic stenosis and episodic thrombosis of the artery. When any of the coronary arteries becomes acutely occluded, the blood supply to the myocardium served by that artery is reduced. If this state persists for a prolonged period of time, a myocardial infarction (MI) or death of the myocardial tissue results. Following a MI, the patient may continue to have a myocardium at risk for ischemia or infarction. For 30 days after the MI, the patient has the highest risk if a surgery is performed during that time. After one month or following interventions such as thrombolytic therapy, coronary angioplasty, coronary bypass grafting, the risk of a prior MI places the patient at intermediate risk for additional problematic cardiac events. The use of specific monitors for ischemia such as the ECG or echocardiography may help in early identification of problems and thus also reduce this risk of ischemic/infarction.

Coronary blood flow is determined by perfusion pressure, myocardial extravascular compression, local myocardial metabolism, and neurohormonal influences. Stenosis or thrombosis of a coronary artery produces the changes of ischemia or infarction on the electrocardiogram. Acute ischemia causes elevation of the ST segment and inversion of the T wave while chronic ischemia or infarction produces Q waves and depression of the ST segment. Q waves or ST segment changes in leads V1 through V4 represent anterior ischemia/infarction (left anterior descending coronary artery, in I aVL, V5-V6 lateral ischemia/infarction (circumflex coronary artery), and in II, III, and avF inferior ischemia/infarction (right coronary artery). Intraoperatively, myocardial ischemia may result from an imbalance in myocardial oxygen supply/demand or from acute changes in coronary vascular tone (artery wall muscle tension). The factors involved in myocardial oxygen balance are listed below:

Oxygen Demand	Oxygen Supply
Wall tension	Coronary blood flow
Preload	Driving pressure (diastolic blood pressure–left ventricular end-diastolic pressure)
Afterload	Diastolic time
	Coronary resistance
	Coronary collaterals
Contractility	Arterial oxygen content (hemoglobin and oxygen)
Heart rate	Myocardial oxygen extraction

Abdominal Aorta and Aneurysm. The abdominal aorta has the following branches: superior mesenteric, inferior mesenteric, celiac, suprarenal, renal, spermatic or ovarian, and iliac. The abdominal aortic wall may weaken as a result of atherosclerotic disease in the media of the vessel. When this occurs, the wall of the aorta balloons outward, creating an aneurysm. When aneurysms grow larger than 6 cm in diameter, they are usually repaired to avoid rupture into the abdominal cavity, the retroperitoneum, the vena cava, or the duodenum. Repair of the aneurysm is a major surgical procedure in which the aorta must be clamped and a part of the aorta replaced by a woven Dacron, Teflon, or other prosthetic graft.

Monitoring During Abdominal Aortic Aneurysmectomy. During this operation, the patient is monitored with a catheter placed in the radial artery to measure the systemic blood pressure and with a pulmonary artery catheter placed in the right internal jugular vein to measure the pressure in the pulmonary vascular circulation. A multilead ECG (usually leads II and V5 which best detect ischemia) is continuously monitored through the perioperative period. The pulmonary artery catheter is placed percutaneously and passes through the right atrium, right ventricle, pulmonary artery, and finally into a wedged position in a small pulmonary artery. The typical waveforms seen during passage of this catheter through the heart are seen in the following diagram.

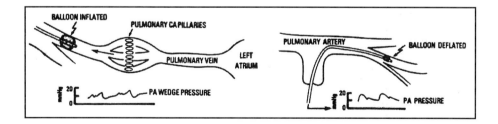

Because the pulmonary artery catheter has a thermistor, the thermodilution method (based on the dye dilution method) can be used to determine cardiac output intraoperatively. Once the cardiac output is known, the cardiac index, pulmonary vascular resistance, systemic vascular resistance, left/right ventricular stroke work can be calculated using the following formulas:

Variable	Calculation	Normal Values
Cardiac index (CI)	CO/body surface area (BSA)	2.5–4.0 L/min/M²
Stroke volume (SV)	CO/HR	60–90 ml/beat
Stroke index (SI)	SV/BSA	40–60 ml/beat/M²
Mean arterial pressure (MAP)	Diastolic pressure + 1/3 pulse pressure	80–120 mmHg
Systemic vascular resistance (SVR)	(MAP–CVP)/CO × 79.9	1200–1500 dyn-cm-sec⁻⁵
Pulmonary vascular resistance (PVR)	Mean (PAP–PWP)/CO × 79.9	100–300 dyn-cm-sec⁻⁵
Left ventricular stroke work index (LVSWI)	0.0136 (MAP–PWP) SI	45–60 g-m-beat⁻¹-M⁻²
Right ventricular stroke work index (RVSWI)	0.0136 (PAP–CVP) SI	5–9 g-m-beat-M⁻²

Direct monitoring of the blood pressure, heart rate, central venous, pulmonary artery pressures and thermodilution cardiac output allow the anesthesiologist, surgeon, and intensivist to precisely determine what physiologic changes are occurring to the patient during the operation. Typically there will be changes in preload, afterload, systemic and pulmonary vascular resistance, heart rate, and myocardial contractility during the various phases of the perioperative period.

Physiologic Principles Demonstrated by Abdominal Aortic Aneurysmectomy

Preload. Preload is defined as the end-diastolic stress on the ventricle (end-diastolic fiber length or end diastolic volume). The determinants of preload are:

◆ Blood volume
◆ Venous tone
◆ Ventricular afterload
◆ Myocardial contractility

The distribution of blood volume between intrathoracic and extrathoracic compartments also affects preload. Negative intrathoracic pressure during inspiration increases intrathoracic blood volume. Stroke volume is determined by the volume of blood in the heart at the beginning of systole (end-diastolic volume or EDV) and the amount of blood remaining in the ventricle at closure of the aortic valve at the end of systole (end-systolic volume or ESV). The degree of stretch of the left ventricular fibers, influenced by the amount of blood in the ventricle, helps determine the amount of work the ventricle can do. An increase in preload increases end-diastolic volume and wall tension. End-diastolic volume is *not* synonymous with end-diastolic pressure, nor are the two linearly related.

Afterload. Afterload is the wall stress or tension faced by the myocardium during ventricular ejection. It is the force opposing ventricular fiber shortening during ejection. Left ventricular afterload depends upon the shape, size, radius, and wall thickness of the ventricle; the principal factors are the radius (related to preload and chamber volume) and aortic impedance (controlled by arterial compliance and systemic vascular resistance). Other factors involved in afterload include arterial wall stiffness (aortic), blood viscosity, and the mass of blood in the aorta. Diastolic blood pressure (aortic) is a good index of afterload and is controlled by the above mentioned factors.

Clinically, systemic vascular resistance (one of the major factors controlling diastolic blood pressure) is frequently used as an estimate of afterload. However, systemic vascular resistance reflects only peripheral arteriolar tone rather than left ventricular systolic wall tension. A true measure of left ventricular afterload, such as left ventricular end-systolic wall stress, which incorporates left ventricular chamber pressure, ventricular dimensions, wall thickness, and peripheral loading conditions related to the diastolic blood pressure, should be used to accurately assess afterload.

When afterload is reduced, the ventricle shortens more quickly and completely. An increase in afterload decreases the extent and velocity of shortening, and increases active tension and the time to peak tension in cardiac muscle.

Contractility. The contractile or inotropic state of the heart is a measure of the functional state of the heart at any given preload and afterload condition. That is, at a set preload and afterload, an increase in the inotropic state of the heart will result in a greater increase in peak isovolumic pressure and a greater rate of pressure development by the heart. Conversely, a decrease in inotropic state results in a decrease in peak isovolumic pressure and decreased rate of pressure development at a given preload and afterload. The cellular basis for changes in the inotropic state is the concentration of free ionic calcium inside the myocytes. Norepinephrine (released from nerves) and various drugs have a positive inotropic effect on the heart. One common approach to assess the inotropic state of the intact heart is to measure the pressure within the left ventricle using a catheter. The slope of the pressure curve during isovolumic contraction is an index of contractility. The steeper the slope of the pressure curve, the greater the inotropic state.

Force of Contraction. An increase in the force of contraction by the heart in response to increases in end-diastolic volume (Frank-Starling principle) is achieved by a different mechanism. Stretching the myocytes beyond their resting length alters the three-dimensional spacing of the myofilaments and increases the sensitivity of the myofilaments to the existing intracellular levels of calcium. Therefore, the increase in force achieved by stretching occurs without any change in intracellular calcium concentration.

Pathophysiologic Changes during Abdominal Aneurysmectomy

Mesenteric Traction and Evisceration of the Small Intestines. There is a four-fold increase in 6-keto-prostaglandin F1α, a stable metabolite of prostacyclin in response to mobilization of the small intestine and mesentery during the transabdominal aneurysmectomy approach. This vasodilator causes decreased mean arterial pressure, decreased systemic vascular resistance, increased cardiac index, increased heart rate, and facial flushing. This response can be avoided by pretreatment with ibuprofen, an inhibitor of cyclooxygenase, a key enzyme needed for prostanoid synthesis.

Aortic Cross-clamping and Unclamping. The level at which the aorta is occluded affects the degree of hemodynamic response with thoracic clamping producing the most profound changes. Blood volume shifts from the lower to the upper half of the body during aortic crossclamping due to low splanchnic venous capacitance. Venous return is decreased by the exclusion of blood from the pelvis and lower extremities. Left ventricular end diastolic pressure and pulmonary wedge pressure may increase. Blood pressure increases and cardiac output may decrease particularly in patients with coronary artery disease. Systemic vascular resistance and afterload increase owing to increased impedance to ventricular ejection caused by the clamp. Ejection fraction may decrease. Myocardial ischemia and abnormal myocardial wall thickening may be present.

Before the aorta is unclamped, vasodilator drugs such as nitroprusside should be discontinued and intravascular volume restored with intravenous fluids or blood if the hemoglobin is low. Unclamping the aorta can result in severe hypotension because of acidosis in tissues distal to the occlusion, acute blood loss through the suture lines of the aorta, decreased venous return until the distal arterial circulation is refilled with blood, pre-existing hypovolemia, myocardial dysfunction, citrate toxicity, or inadvertent continued infusion of vasodilator drugs such as nitroprusside.

Clinical Scenario

A 68-year-old, 70-kg male with a body surface area of 2.2 M^2 and a history of a myocardial infarction (heart attack) one year ago is undergoing removal (resection) of an abdominal aortic aneurysm. An intra-arterial catheter and a pulmonary artery catheter have been placed for monitoring before the induction of anesthesia. Blood pressure (BP) = 130/90, heart rate = 70 beats per minute, central venous pressure (CVP) = 7, pulmonary wedge pressure (PWP) = 13, and cardiac index = 2.3 L/M^2/min.

1. What is the patient's systemic vascular resistance (SVR)?

The surgeon administers heparin to decrease clotting and prepares to clamp the aorta below the renal arteries. What are the abdominal branches of the aorta? Upon clamping of the aorta, the blood pressure increases to 200/110, CVP decreases to 3, PWP increases to 22, and heart rate decreases to 60.

2. What has happened to left ventricular afterload and preload?

The ECG shows decreased ST segments in leads II, III, avF, a pattern similar to that present at the time of the patient's prior MI.

3. Is the patient having another MI? If not, what is happening? Which coronary artery is likely to be stenotic to cause this ECG pattern?

The patient receives nitroglycerin to improve his coronary perfusion and other drugs to control his blood pressure. He becomes stable with BP = 160/90, HR = 84 bpm, PWP = 18, and CVP = 5.

4. Why is the PWP different from the CVP? Shouldn't they be the same?

The surgeon sews a bifurcated prosthetic graft from the abdominal aorta below the renal arteries to each iliac artery. He then releases the clamp on the aorta. What do you expect to happen to the cardiovascular variables (BP, HR, CVP, PWP, myocardial contractility, venous return) on unclamping the aorta? Two minutes after unclamping, BP = 90/70, HR = 90, CI = 1.9, CVP = 3, and PWP = 12.

5. Where is the patient now on the Starling curve? Should the patient be given intravenous fluid, blood, a drug to increase SVR, or a drug to increase ventricular contractility?

Reference

Lake CL: Cardiovascular Anatomy and Physiology. In Barash, Cullen, Stoelting (eds): Clinical Anesthesia. Philadelphia: Lippincott Williams & Wilkins, 2001, p 853.

Glossary of Terms

Anaphylactic/anaphylactoid reactions: an immediate reaction to injection of a molecule or antigen capable of stimulating antibody (immunoglobulin) production. When antigens bind to immunoglobulin E antibodies on the membranes of mast cells, histamine and other substances are released, causing bronchospasm, itching, vasodilatation, laryngeal edema, tachycardia, arrhythmias, urticaria, pulmonary hypertension, and systemic hypotension.

Bronchospasm: spasmodic stenosis of the bronchi, as in asthma.

Compliance: the relationship between ventricular volume and diastolic pressure; normally a curvilinear relationship.

Cyclooxygenase: the enzyme that converts arachidonic acid to prostaglandin intermediates.

Epinephrine (adrenalin): one of the catecholamines released by the adrenal medulla; also given as a drug to stimulate cardiac contractility.

Ibuprofen: a nonsteroidal anti-inflammatory drug whose pharmacologic action is probably related to prostaglandin synthase inhibition.

Impedance: resistance to flow; this term can be considered in light of electrical current as the sum of forces opposing electron movement in an alternating current circuit.

Isoproterenol: a sympathomimetic drug used to treat bronchospasm.

Nitroglycerin: a drug used to treat angina pectoris or chest pain resulting from inadequate blood supply to the heart. It relaxes the vascular smooth muscle to make the coronary arteries dilate or enlarge to supply more blood to the heart.

Prostaglandin: a naturally occurring substance found in semen and menstrual fluid that causes dilation of some vascular beds.

Vasoconstriction (vasoconstrictors): causing constriction of the blood vessels.

Clinical Scenario Answers

A 68-year-old, 70-kg man with a body surface area of 2.2 M^2 and a history of a myocardial infarction (heart attack) one year ago is undergoing removal (resection) of an abdominal aortic aneurysm. An intra-arterial catheter and a pulmonary artery catheter have been placed for monitoring before the induction of anesthesia. Blood pressure (BP) = 130/90, heart rate = 70 beats per minute, central venous pressure (CVP) = 7, pulmonary wedge pressure (PWP) = 13, cardiac index (CI) = 2.3 L/M^2/min.

Remember: SVR = (MAP–CVP)/CO $\times$ 79.9). Initial SVR (103–7)/5.1 $\times$ 79.9 = 1504.

1. What is the patient's systemic vascular resistance (SVR)?

SVR (103–7)/5.1 $\times$ 79.9 = 1504.

The surgeon administers heparin to decrease clotting and prepares to clamp the aorta below the renal arteries. What are the abdominal branches of the aorta? Upon clamping of the aorta, the BP increases to 200/110, CVP decreases to 3, PWP increases to 22, and HR decreases to 60.

◆ Increased afterload (decreased ejection time)
◆ Decreased venous return
◆ LV decreased preload (backed up)
◆ Baroreceptor reflex = decreased

2. What has happened to left ventricular afterload and preload?

Both are high.

The ECG shows decreased (depressed) ST segments in leads II, III, avF, a pattern similar to that present at the time of the patient's prior MI.

3. Is the patient having another MI? If not, what is happening? Which coronary artery is likely to be stenotic to cause this ECG pattern?

Ischemia is caused by increased heart work because of increased preload and increased afterload. Hypoperfusion is of the right coronary artery because it is best seen on leads II, III, and avF.

The patient receives nitroglycerin to improve his coronary perfusion and other drugs to control his blood pressure. He becomes stable with BP = 160/90, HR = 84 bpm, PWP = 18, and CVP = 5.

4. Why is the PWP so different from the CVP? Shouldn't they be closer?

PWP is the left side of the heart, and CVP is the right side of the heart. (Normal PWP = 9 mmHg). But the aorta clamp is still on, increasing pressure in the left heart (PWP).

The surgeon sews a bifurcated prosthetic graft from the abdominal aorta below the renal arteries to each iliac artery. He then releases the clamp on the aorta. What do you expect to happen to the cardiovascular variables (BP, HR, CVP, PWP, myocardial contractility, venous return) on unclamping the aorta? Two minutes after unclamping, BP = 90/70, HR = 90, CI = 1.9, CVP = 3, and PWP = 12.

5. Where is the patient now on the Starling curve? Should the patient be given intravenous fluid, blood, a drug to increase SVR, or a drug to increase ventricular contractility?

Decreased right and left ventricular filling are decreased (both PWP and CVP are decreased), so the patient is lower on the curve. Monitor the patient and give minimal fluids and possibly an inotropic drug to improve cardiac output.

Appendix D. Clinical Simulation 4: Pneumothorax: Pulmonary Mechanics, Gas Exchange, and Acid-Base Balance

(Courtesy of Richard W. Stremel, PhD, FACSM)

Goals of the Session
◆ To experience the clinical reality of the respiratory emergency of a pulmonary pneumothorax.
◆ To understand the mechanical, gas exchange and acid-base consequences of a pneumothorax.
◆ To understand the necessity and consequences for treatment of pneumothorax.

Student Preparation
A pneumothorax is an accumulation of air in the space between the visceral and parietal pleura. Air can enter the intrapleural space by a variety of mechanisms, the least common of which is the introduction of atmospheric air through the chest wall. In normal lungs, rupture of avleolar blebs (i.e., flaccid airspaces, often large in diameter) on the lung surface can occur spontaneously and through barotrauma (i.e., the use of a ventilator and positive pressure ventilation). Acute pneumothorax may occur also as a complication of other lung disease, such as emphysema, cystic lung disease, carcinoma, and pulmonary tuberculosis. Surgical (or "open") pneumothorax occurs when the chest wall is opened to atmospheric pressure.

Creation of a pneumothorax by "stabbing a classmate" (inflicting a penetrating chest wound) has been the example in class, but this is the least common cause of pneumothorax. Spontaneous pneumothorax is the most common form and is a consequence of rupture of a small bleb on the surface of the lung, typically near the apex. These blebs are usually no larger than small grapes. Spontaneous pneumothorax usually occurs in tall young males and may be related to the high mechanical stresses that occur in the upper zones of the upright lung (review pages 17–22 and 42–46). The presenting symptom is often sudden pain on one side accompanied by labored breathing (i.e., dyspnea). The chest pain is often worsened by body movement and attempts to take deep breaths. On auscultation, breath sounds are diminished on the effected side. An untreated pneumothorax gradually is reduced as the air is absorbed because the total gas pressure in the venous blood is much less than atmospheric air gas pressure.

In a small portion of spontaneous pneumothoraces, the site of leak between the lung and intrapleural space functions as a check valve. As a consequence, air enters the intrapleural space during inspiration, but cannot escape during expiration. The result is a large pneumothorax in which the intrapleural pressure may exceed atmospheric pressure and thus interfere with venous return to the thorax. This is a medical emergency and is recognized by increasing respiratory distress, tachycardia, and signs of mediastinal shift such as tracheal deviation and movement of PMI. Treatment consists of relieving the pressure by insertion of a chest tube. This tube is connected to an underwater seal that allows air to escape from the intrapleural space but not enter it.

A chest radiograph is usually diagnostic. Note in the radiograph below, the small collapsed right lung and radiolucency (dark area indicating absence of tissue to absorb x-ray energy), depression of the right hemidiaphragm, and overexpansion of the rib cage on the right. All are diagnostic signs of pneumothorax.

Clinical Scenario

Paramedics are called to a local soccer pitch where the World Cup is being held. They find a 22-year-old, physically fit male complaining of sudden onset of severe shortness of breath. The patient also reports pain in the left chest. No significant medical history is revealed and the patient denies medications or performance-enhancing drugs. The initial assessment reveals a blood pressure of 100/40, pulse rate of 96/min with sinus rhythm, respiratory rate of 36 that is shallow with diminished breath sounds on the left side. *Volunteer students should listen to the breath sounds.* The patient's skin is cool and clammy to the touch.

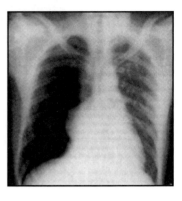

1. **What does the patient mean by the complaint of "shortness of breath," which is abbreviated on the chart as SOA (shortness of air)?**

Arterial blood gases (ABGs) are drawn and reported STAT. *Students must request data from attending physician.*

2. **How does his O_2 saturation compare to his P_aO_2? Why is there a difference?**

3. **How does the end-tidal PCO_2 compare to the P_aCO_2? Why is there a difference?**

The patient is given 4 L/min of O_2 by nasal cannula, IV lines are established (including pulmonary artery [PA] catheter), and a cardiac monitor is attached. He is immediately transported to the emergency department. Another ABG is drawn several minutes after the application of nasal cannula. *Students must request data.*

4. **Four L/min O_2 by nasal cannula provides a F_IO_2 of approximately 40%. What is the P_IO_2? Does this improve his O_2 Sat and P_aO_2?**

During transport, the patient shows signs of increasing agitation and difficulty breathing. Re-assessment reveals a blood pressure of 76/40, pulse rate of 124/min, respiration rate of 48 that is shallow and labored with an absence of breath sounds on the left side. Physical exam reveals hyperresonance to percussion on the left side. The patient is cyanotic with pronounced jugular venous distention (JVD) and tracheal and chest wall shift. Sample for ABGs is drawn. *Students must request data.*

5. **Why has the arterial blood pressure continued to decrease? Is there any effect upon PA pressure? Why?**

6. **Why has respiratory rate continued to increase?**

7. **Why is the skin cyanotic? What does this indicate?**

8. **Why is the left lung field hyperresonant to percussion?**

9. **What do you think has happened to D_LCO during this phase of the scenario compared to normal resting conditions?**

10. **What happens to arterial PO_2, PCO_2, pH, and $P_{ET}CO_2$ during this phase of the scenario?**

The patient's condition will deteriorate if treatment is inappropriate or not performed in a timely manner. Without proper decompression of the left pneumothorax the patient's cardiac rhythm will change to ventricular fibrillation. It will become necessary to intubate and ventilate the patient to avoid respiratory arrest.

Needle decompression of the left chest reveals positive pressure in the thorax, suggesting a tension pneumothorax. Following decompression, the patient's condition improves. Blood pressure is now 100/70, with a sinus rhythm and pulse rate of 120/min, respiratory rate is 28/min and diminished breath sounds are heard again on the left side. JVD is diminished and the trachea is more midline. Sample for ABGs is drawn. *Students must request data.*

11. Why is intrapleural pressure positive on the left side prior to decompression?

12. What has happened to the difference between P_aCO_2 and $P_{ET}CO_2$?

13. Has the patient completely recovered gas exchange function of the lung?

Glossary of Terms

P_a = arterial partial pressure of a gas (i.e., P_aO_2 = 100 mmHg, P_aCO_2 = 40 mmHg)
F_I = fraction of an inspired gas (i.e., F_IO_2 = 21%)
P_I = partial pressure of an inspired gas (i.e., P_IO_2 = 21% of 713 = 150 mmHg)
D_L = diffusion capacity of the lung for a gas (i.e., D_LCO = 25 ml/min/mmHg)
P_A = alveolar partial pressure of a gas (i.e., P_AO_2 = 100 mmHg)
P_{ET} = end-tidal partial pressure of an exhaled gas (i.e., $P_{ET}CO_2$ = 46 mmHg)

Teaching Notes for Mentor Sessions

The arterial blood gases provided in these notes are approximate for the scenario. They may change slightly when the students make their requests for results. The questions in the clinical scenario are answered serially in the section below.

General Comments for Discussion

Because the lungs have mass and we humans walk around in the upright position, the apices of the lungs experience mechanical stresses. In the upright posture, the lungs are effectively suspended from the trachea. When comparing apical vs. basal regions of the thorax, a consequence of this mechanical arrangement is a more negative intrapleural pressure, larger alveoli, reduced compliance, reduced alveolar ventilation, and reduced perfusion at the apices vs. the bases. This increase in mechanical stress in apical regions is also associated with disease processes (e.g., tuberculosis) and especially pneumothoraces. The mechanical stresses are accentuated in taller people.

The volume in the lungs at the end of a normal passive exhalation is referred to as functional residual capacity (FRC). At this lung volume, the recoil of the lungs inward and the recoil of the chest wall outward are equal and opposite in direction. It is this balance of recoil forces (both elastic and surface forces) that allows one to return to FRC simply by relaxing the respiratory muscles. It is also these recoil forces that produce some of the typical changes associated with pneumothorax. If the intrapleural pleural space is opened to the atmosphere, air will move from a region of relatively higher pressure to one of lower pressure and the intrapleural space will fill with air. The lung will recoil toward an airless state, which is depicted in the radiograph. The chest wall will also recoil outward towards its resting position. This only occurs on one side because humans have an intact mediastinum. This is an advantage in that only one lung will collapse and a disadvantage in that the negative intrapleural pressure on the right side will cause a shift of the mediastinum to the right, which will have a negative impact on right sided ventilation. Because the pressure on the side of the pneumothorax is atmospheric instead of sub-atmospheric, the diaphragm on that side will be flattened compared to the contralateral side. The negative intrapleural pressure helps hold the diaphragm in its normal dome shape at FRC.

Clinical Scenario Answers to Questions

1. What does the patient mean by the complaint of "shortness of breath," which is abbreviated on the chart as SOA (shortness of air)?

SOA is a complaint that can mean any number of things. It is not a specific complaint. Effectively, however, it means that the effort applied to the process of ventilation does not produce an adequate gas exchange match to the metabolic requirements of the situation.

2. How does his O_2 saturation compare to his P_aO_2? Why is there a difference?

At this first phase, before nasal cannula and supplemental O_2, the P_aCO_2 is 41.0 mmHg, the end-tidal PCO_2 is 14 mmHg, the P_aO_2 is 51 mmHg, the pH is 7.43, and the O_2 Sat is 82%. Because the relationship between PO_2 and hemoglobin saturation is sigmoidal in nature and fairly flat at high values of PO_2, the PO_2 can be reduced significantly before hemoglobin saturation begins to decrease. Thus, PO_2 will fall before O_2 Sat begins to fall.

3. How does the end-tidal PCO_2 compare to the P_aCO_2? Why is there a difference?

The patient is tachypneic. $P_{ET}CO_2$ is low because the right side is being hyperventilated and the left side (pneumothorax side) is being hypoventilated. Arterial PCO_2 is relatively normal because of some right-to-left shunting of blood is occurring and the right and left lungs are effectively balancing each other. The end result is an end-tidal CO_2 that is significantly less than the arterial value.

4. Four L/min O_2 by nasal cannula provides a F_IO_2 of approximately 40%. What is the P_IO_2? Does this improve his O_2 Sat. and P_aO_2?

Following 4 L/min of O_2 by nasal cannula, P_IO_2 increases to about 285 mmHg, the O_2 Sat increases to 89%, P_aO_2 increases to 61 mmHg, P_aCO_2 is 41.5, and $P_{ET}CO_2$ is 20 mmHg. The improvement in oxygenation is only slight because the pneumothorax is getting worse. The patient is developing severe ventilation/perfusion mismatch.

During the transport the pneumothorax worsens. The systemic arterial pressure continues to decrease throughout the scenario because the pressure in the pneumothorax side of the thorax increases to a pressure greater than atmospheric pressure. This is evidence of a tension pneumothorax. This positive pressure impedes venous return and therefore decreases arterial blood pressure. The ABGs at this point are as follows: P_aCO_2 of 47.4, $P_{ET}CO_2$ of 10, P_aO_2 of 42, and pH of 7.38.

5. Why has the arterial blood pressure continued to decrease? Is there any effect upon PA pressure? Why?

The pulmonary artery pressure rises throughout the scenario because the pulmonary vascular resistance on the pneumothorax side increases dramatically. The entire cardiac output must perfuse the normal right side and the collapsed left side—PVR is increased and PA pressure increases.

6. Why has respiratory rate continued to increase?

Respiratory rate increases (as does total ventilation) because of activation of pulmonary afferents (particularly irritant, stretch and C-fiber) that combine to stimulate ventilation and respiratory rate. In addition, the arterial PO_2 is perilously low and will stimulate breathing.

7. Why is the skin cyanotic? What does this finding indicate?

Cyanosis (blue or purplish color) is a sign in nail beds and mucous membranes that indicates deficient oxygenation. The patient is severely hypoxemic.

8. Why is the left lung field hyperresonant to percussion?

Hyperresonance indicates air filled regions on percussion. The space where the left lung should be is now occupied by atmospheric air and thus hyper-resonant. Hyporesonance would be associated with consolidation of lung tissue or fluid in the lung.

9. What do you think has happened to D_LCO during this phase of the scenario compared to normal resting conditions?

D_LCO is reduced because the left lung is now effectively a right-to-left shunt. If the left lung is completely collapsed, the D_LCO will be about one-half of the normal value (25 ml/min/mm Hg). If the students listen for breath sounds on the left side, they are now absent.

10. What happens to arterial PO_2, PCO_2, pH and $P_{ET}CO_2$ during this phase of the scenario?

ABGs cited above. If treatment is not initiated, the patient is likely to develop cardiac arrhythmias, ventricular fibrillation, and respiratory arrest.

Needle decompression of the left pneumothorax produces a significant improvement in the ABGs. P_aCO_2 is 39.9, $P_{ET}CO_2$ is 32, P_aO_2 is 76, and ph is 7.43. If the students listen carefully during the needle decompression, the sound of air rushing out of the thorax through the needle can be heard. This is confirmatory for a tension pneumothorax.

11. Why is intrapleural pressure positive on the left side prior to decompression?

The left side intrapleural pressure is positive with respect to atmospheric pressure because the patient has developed a tension pneumothorax. Air moves into the thorax during inspiration, but does not exit during expiration. The increase in pressure is a consequence of this continued movement of gases.

12. What has happened to the difference between P_aCO_2 and $P_{ET}CO_2$?

The a-ET difference in CO_2 is wider than normal, but improved from previous measurements. This is an indication of improved gas exchange since CO_2 is 20 times more diffusible than O_2.

13. Has the patient completely recovered gas exchange function of the lung?

The patient has not completely recovered and likely will not for several weeks. A collapsed lung has some long-term consequences to both mechanics and gas exchange. When pneumothorax was used as a treatment for tuberculosis (collapsing and "resting" the effected lung), patients would be maintained with the collapsed lung. When re-inflated patients exhibited fibrotic changes to the pleura that produced limitations to maximum breathing capacity and vital capacity. This acute scenario will not lead to such changes, but absorption of residual pleural air and re-inflation of atelectactic (collapsed) regions will occur.

Chapter 7

SIMULATION IN PHARMACOLOGY

Clinton Chichester, PhD, and Brian Felice, PhD, MBA

The use of medical simulators for training and instructing health care professionals has increased significantly in recent years. Universities and medical institutions around the world are realizing the benefits of highly realistic simulators. Of all medical personnel, anesthesiologists have undoubtedly made the greatest use of simulators, and as a result most of the advancements in this area can be attributed to them.

The simulators in current use provide instructors and trainees new, invaluable methods of teaching and learning that literally bring the classroom to life. The Human Patient Simulator (HPS), designed by Medical Education Technologies, Inc (METI) of Sarasota, Florida, physically resembles a real person, and contains all the physiologic parameters necessary to create a "real living-breathing" patient.[1] The full-scale mannequin has a complex respiratory system that monitors blood gases and allows proper airway management; a cardiovascular system that is sensitive to pressure changes throughout the vasculature; both heart and lung sounds; palpable pulses; eyes that respond to light; and several features related to trauma.

Describing all of the capabilities of the HPS is beyond the scope of this chapter. However, the variety of potential applications has generated interest from most health care disciplines. Most recently, the use of medical simulators has become an integral part of medical training. Health care disciplines now exploiting the use of these simulators as advanced training tools include nursing, emergency medicine technicians, surgical teams, radiology, and respiratory therapists. Groups that have evaluated the use of simulators in various fields of medicine have demonstrated a positive response from both trainees and trainers in terms of the simulator's effectiveness as a teaching aid.[2–7] Not to be forgotten in the excitement generated from these groups is the integration of high-fidelity simulators into academia. At both the undergraduate and graduate level, institutions have incorporated simulation into their curriculum to aid in teaching both basic physiology and physical diagnosis. The success of using simulators for these teaching purposes and the positive responses from educators and students alike have resulted in the development of simulator-based curricula in other related disciplines such as pharmacology.

Using simulation for pharmacology-based instruction is not a novel idea. For simplicity, pharmacology simulations can be divided into two major types: computer-based and full-scale patient mannequins. Computer-based simulation programs have been used to teach pharmacology since the mid 1980s and were designed to replace pharmacology and physiology laboratory experiments involving live animals.[8] In 1987 Robert D. Purves developed one such program, PharmaTutor, which simulates classic pharmacology laboratories, including the effect of catecholamines on blood pressure in whole animals and dose-response relationships using a tissue preparation suspended in an organ bath.[9] Although this program is now considered technologically outdated, at the time it introduced simulation as a novel teaching accompaniment to lecture material.

More recently pharmacologists have developed a library of software titles collectively called pharma-CAL-ogy, which is distributed by the British Pharmacological Society. This collection of software titles includes simulation programs encompassing various areas of pharmacology, such as clinical trial data, ligand-binding experiments, and an assortment of simulated animal experiments.[10] Titles include CardioLab (Biosoft), which allows the user to administer several agonists and antagonists to simulated anesthetized or pithed animals and to record heart rate and blood pressure.[11] In addition, simulations of isolated tissue preparations are also available. Simulated Vascular Rings is a program designed to illustrate the pharmacology of drugs affecting vascular smooth muscle and at the same time to demonstrate general pharmacologic principles. Other companies such as CoAcS, Ltd. also offer several computer-based simulation programs.[12] One such program, Cardiovascular System/Autonomic Nervous System Tutor (v.3.0) is an interactive simulation program showing the effects of autonomic nerves and transmitters on the cardiovascular system of an anesthetized animal. These and other computer-based simulation packages are advantageous because they are economically priced and remarkably user-friendly and require less expertise and personnel compared with full-scale simulators.

Whether they are called full-scale or high-fidelity models, the simulators deliver a feeling of realism. Life-sized simulators add a unique dimension to teaching pharmacology and other medically related topics because of the simulated human interface that they provide. As a group, health care-related instructors and teachers are just beginning to discover the possibilities of patient simulators in educating health professionals. This chapter explores the application of the HPS as a teaching tool for pharmacology and discusses whether simulation can play an essential role in pharmacy education now and in the future.

Modeling of Drugs Using the HPS

Dose-Response Relationships

A drug typically produces an effect by interacting with a specific target. The interactions of the drug and its target have been described mathematically by a number of investigators, most importantly Clark (1937), Ariens (1964), and Schild (1947).[13-15] These mathematical formulas suggest that the effect produced by a drug depends on the drug/receptor interaction. Thus, the effect produced by a drug is a function of the concentration of the drug at the effector site. This relationship can be illustrated graphically and is called a dose-response curve. Dose-response relationships are typically quantified using an in vitro system in which the amount of drug added to the system can be accurately measured. A typical dose response curve is illustrated in Figure 1. When the response to the drug is expressed in this manner, the shape of the curve is sigmoid. The concentration of the drug that produces 50% of the maximum effect is termed the EC_{50} (effective concentration for a 50% response). When all of the receptors are occupied by the drug, the curve reaches its maximal asymptote value.

When dose-response curves are created for humans or other whole animals, the adsorption and distribution of the drug become factors in the response. These variables modify the concentration of drug at the receptor site, and although the dose given to a

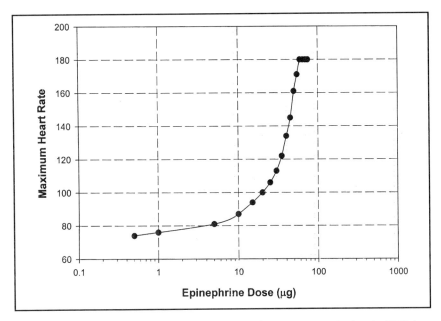

Figure 1. Epinephrine dose-response (maximum heart rate) curve generated using the HPS. Increasing doses of epinephrine were administered to the HPS and the maximum heart rate was recorded.

subject is known, the concentration at the effector site is not. Because of this variable the slope of the dose response curve may be altered in vivo.

Pharmacodynamic Model of the HPS

The HPS has a complex physiologic response that involves both a primary response and a series of secondary responses that result from reflexes elicited by the primary effect. Although physiologically relevant, the secondary effects complicate the development of physiologically relevant simulation of a drug effect(s). An example is the β-stimulation of the heart by isoproterenol. Initially one observes tachycardia, followed by a subsequent reflex that mutes this effect. In a typical experiment that quantifies a drug's effect in vitro or in situ, a drug is added to an isolated system and its primary effect is determined. In this way one can measure effects of the drugs using the EC_{50} and determine an affinity constant for the drug as in Kd. Computer simulation using affinity data is easy to do when simulating an in vitro effect of a drug. The concentration of drug added to the isolated system is directly determined, as is the response. Programs that simulate this in vitro effect are relatively easy to set up and provide students with situations that represent a close approximation of an actual experiment.

Simulation modeling of drug effects in vivo is more complicated. With the METI HPS, data are taken from direct observations of a drug's effects. Such data may be obtained from literature values or derived experimentally. These values are then programmed into the simulator. Values are adjusted so that the magnitude of effect closely mimics the real-life situation. Modifying the observed effect according to the dose administered creates a dose-effect relationship.

In the HPS, the effects of respiratory and cardiovascular drugs are modeled on direct effects on the respiratory and cardiovascular systems as well as indirect effects on physiologic control mechanisms. With the HPS, responses are produced in a direct linear relationship to the dose given. Most dose-response relationships have a logarithmic relationship between effect and dose of drug (i.e., the effect produced vs. the log of the dose of drug). A discussion of this relationship can be found in most pharmacology textbooks.[16] In the METI program, every drug that is modeled has a minimum dose below which it produces no effect. There is also a maximum dose, which, if exceeded, does not produce a direct effect. As an example, with the METI HPS, direct effects on the heart and respiratory system are given for parameters such as the following:

HR/D   Direct effect on the heart rate.
CONT/D   Direct effect on contractility
SART/D   Direct effect on systemic arteriolar resistance
PART/D   Direct effect on pulmonary arteriolar resistance
VUV/D   Direct effect on venous unstressed volume (venous capacitance)
VE/D   Direct effect on minute ventilation
VTRR/D   Direct effect on tidal volume over respiratory rate ratio

For effects on control mechanism:

PCV/D   Effect on the "potency" of the cardiovascular control mechanisms (baroreflex)
PRES/D   Effect on the potency of the respiratory control mechanisms (CO_2 and O_2 responses)

Thus the changes that the drug produces are in relation to the change from baseline response. For example, VE/D = 0.10 indicates that the drug produces a direct increase of the ventilation rate of 10% per mg/kg administered. All units are in inverse dose units.

Pharmacokinetic Model

The HPS uses a linear pharmacokinetics model. It assumes that the decrease in plasma concentration is of the second order. Third-order kinetics is not modeled because of the limited clinical relevance. All drugs are given intravenously. Both plasma and effector compartment concentrations are computed. However, the effector compartment concentration is normalized so that its maximum is linearly related to the dose of drug rather than the actual effector compartment concentration, which is difficult or impossible to measure. The advantage of this method is that the pharmacodynamics is based on the administered dose rather than compartment concentration.

Determination of Drug Parameters

For a drug to be modeled, dose-response data must be gathered for the appropriate parameters from the literature and then prepared as shown below. Effects are then quantified in terms of the dose administered. The resulting values are programmed into the HPS. The older version of the HPS software (version 5) has a user interface, called the drug recognition interface, that allows new drugs to be programmed into the software. In the newer version (version 6), this feature is still in the developmental phase. Once the parameters are determined for a drug and its kinetic rate constants are known, they

Table 1. Pharmacodynamic parameters used to determine a drug's effect on the cardiovascular system after a single bolus.							
Dose units	MAP (mmHg)	hr (bpm)	baroreflex sensitivity (bpm/mmHg)	SVR (dyne sec/cm^5)	PVR (dyne sec/cm^5)	LVSW or SV or EF	Change of VC (ml)

can be entered into the HPS drug recognition software and the drug effects can be modeled (Table 1). To obtain an accurate representation of a specific drug's effects, the parameters may require a certain amount of fine-tuning.

Simulation-based Pharmacology Instruction

The HPS teaching tool is highly adaptable to pharmacology instruction. This section explores the value of simulation-based teaching for both basic pharmacology laboratories and scenario-driven or more sophisticated role-playing exercises. In such classes, students evaluate drug action, determine the drug's physiologic effects, and are allowed to make critical decisions about the patient's condition. Drugs can be given to the HPS in a realistic manner, by loading liquid into a syringe and administering the drug through an IV port (Fig. 2). The liquid volume is measured by a flow meter, and the total dose is then calculated. Conversely, drugs can be administered using the computer interface, which allows quick

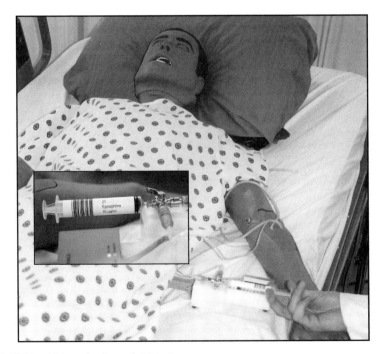

Figure 2. HPS and IV port for drug administration.

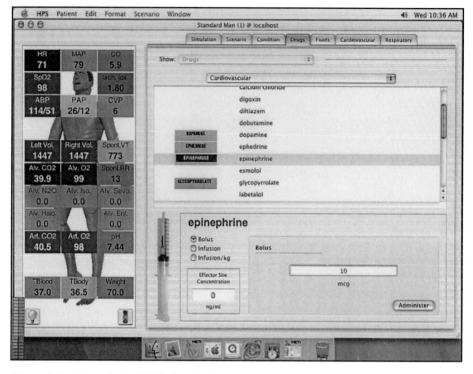

Figure 3. Heads-up display (HUD) showing the patient's physiologic parameters and drug administration utility.

and accurate dosing (Fig. 3). Once the drug is administered, pharmacokinetic and pharmacodynamic models programmed into the simulator determine the physiologic effects. These effects occur in real time, thus reinforcing the importance of accurate drug dosing.

The instructor has three options when multiple drugs are to be administered consecutively. The first option involves connecting to a new patient, which can be accomplished efficiently if the instructor preloads the patient into the virtual running mode. This method cancels out the possibility of residual drug responses and drug interactions and is highly recommended if the first drug is known to have a prolonged half-life. Alternatively, the second drug can be administered after metabolism and excretion of the first drug, which takes place in real time, or the metabolism can be fast-forwarded at a rate of 4-fold. This method is adequate for drugs that are metabolized quickly, such as epinephrine or succinylcholine. Finally, two drugs can be given simultaneously to investigate drug-drug responses and interactions.

The patient simulator is used in our curriculum at several different levels. In each year of the professional curriculum we have incorporated the simulator with an increasing degree of sophistication. Recently we have changed our curriculum to an all Pharm D program. Students enter the professional curriculum after two years of preprofessional preparation. They take autonomic pharmacology in the first semester. In the second semester students take a pharmacology lab that covers drug actions and reactions. In the past we have covered autonomic pharmacology using an in vivo experiment with rats. Now this lab has been converted to the patient simulator, and students are introduced to learning with a simulator.

In this laboratory, we introduce the students to our patient, a healthy 33-year-old male (70 kg), appropriately named "Stan D. Ardman." The HPS has over 30 preprogrammed patients, ranging from a 72-year-old with septic shock to a soldier with a snakebite injury. With a simple click of the mouse, the instructor can easily present new patients and investigate new topics. In this introductory laboratory, the objective is to familiarize students with vital signs (e.g., heart rate, blood pressure, oxygen saturation) and to use the simulator for a review of autonomic pharmacology. Students are encouraged to become comfortable with assessing the "patient's" condition, which includes listening to heart and breath auscultations and identifying the areas where pulses may be taken. This approach embellishes the realism of the laboratory and facilitates discussion. The HPS is pharmacologically programmed to display the effects of drugs interacting with alpha (α), beta (β), muscarinic, and nicotinic receptors. After drug administration the students can visually identify the physiologic changes by viewing either a patient monitor or, if the instructor chooses, the Heads-Up Display (HUD) found on the controller's monitor, which contains 25 selected physiologic parameters, including blood and lung gases (see Fig. 2).

To study autonomic pharmacology using the HPS, drugs were selected that are classified as either an agonist or antagonist to the previously mentioned receptors. Once the drugs were chosen, students were allowed to use online sources to calculate the correct IV doses. To demonstrate the physiologic response to α-receptor activation, norepinephrine and phenylephrine were chosen as agonists. When the drug was administered, the systemic vascular and cardiovascular effects of each drug were recorded for comparison and later discussion. After clearance of the agonist, a dose of phentolamine, a reversible, competitive, nonselective α-receptor antagonist, was administered, followed shortly afterward by the same dose of either norepinephrine or phenylephrine. The effect of the blocker on α-receptor activity was evaluated and compared with the results obtained with agonist alone. The students quickly recognized that phentolamine reduced the drug-induced hypertension associated with either norepinephrine or phenylephrine. With the HPS, students are able to associate a drug with a physiologic response—in this case, systemic vasoconstriction. If the class is somewhat confused, these types of experiments can be repeated as many times as necessary until the entire class is confident about explaining the results. Such experiments are straightforward and can be used to illustrate pharmacologic principles. However, the HPS is much more complex, and if one of the above experiments is repeated, it becomes obvious that the administration of an α-agonist causes reflex bradycardia driven by the increase in blood pressure. To investigate this phenomenon more closely, we designed an experiment that further explores the relationship between phenylephrine-induced hypertension and heart rate.

To further study the effects of phenylephrine and the capabilities of the HPS, dose-response curves were generated for both blood pressure and heart rate. At low doses of phenylephrine, the data clearly suggest a reflex bradycardia due to the increasing blood pressure. This response effectively demonstrates the capabilities and complexity of the HPS, but the response at higher doses of phenylephrine was quite unexpected. At doses higher than 250 μg (IV), the reflex bradycardia became less significant, and heart rate began to rise with increasing doses of phenylephrine, finally reaching a plateau of 63 beats/minute at doses higher than 500 μg (Fig. 4). Although the patient is still slightly

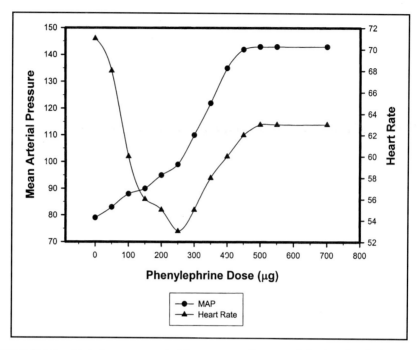

Figure 4. Relationship between mean arterial pressure and heart rate following phenylephrine administration.

bradycardic from the phenylephrine-induced hypertension, this effect does not fully explain the sudden physiologic change in heart rate. Through pharmacology class work and readings in the literature, students can learn that phenylephrine is classified as an α_1- selective agonist. Therefore, its administration should cause only hypertension and consequential reflex bradycardia. However, in addition to the α-receptor activation, phenylephrine also possesses β-adrenergic receptor activation at high doses. [17,18] This activation of β_1-receptors explains the sudden climb in heart rate after the administration of phenylephrine at doses greater than 250 μg. This simple experiment illustrates the complexity of the HPS's drug recognition system with respect to pharmacokinetic and pharmacodynamic models.

The next section of the lab focuses on drugs that activate or block β-adrenergic receptor activation. The HPS drug recognition system provides two β-agonists, epinephrine and isoproterenol, and four β-blocking agents, including esmolol, labetalol, metoprolol, and propranolol. For this experiment, epinephrine and metoprolol were chosen to demonstrate the effects of an agonist and antagonist to β-receptors, respectively. Much like the experiment with phenylephrine, students first administered a known dose of agonist, epinephrine, and recorded any changes that occurred. At this point the facilitator must make certain that all students can clearly explain the observed changes. Besides ensuring that everyone is comfortable with the material, this approach often stimulates instructor-student or peer-peer discussion.

Because epinephrine is rapidly metabolized, the altered physiologic parameters quickly return to normal values, and the β-blocking agent, metoprolol, can be administered. After metoprolol administration and allowance of time for sufficient uptake, the same dose of epinephrine is given. Physiologic changes are recorded, and the pharmacologic action of metoprolol can now be discussed. These results suggest that metoprolol blocked β_1-receptors in the heart, therefore decreasing the positive chronotropic effect of epinephrine. Additional experiments can be performed to compare the potencies of different β-blocking agents.

The exercises described above are simple in design, but they are effective teaching tools that support lecture-based material. With approximately 60 drugs to choose from and nearly 30 different patients that can be programmed into the HPS, countless pharmacologic exercises can be completed, each with a unique objective. This flexibility provides instructors the freedom to explore topics in pharmacology that may have been previously overlooked because of complexity or time requirements.

To further investigate the pharmacodynamic programming of the HPS, an experimental pharmacology study was designed to re-examine the interaction between metoprolol and epinephrine. Dose-response curves were generated for epinephrine in the presence of varying concentrations of metoprolol. Because the half-life of metoprolol is approximately 3 to 4 hours, a new patient was used for each dose level to increase the rapidity of the experiment and to eliminate any discrepancies due to metabolism or excretion. The response, which is maximum heart rate, is described as the maximum heart rate reached after each administration of epinephrine. A response curve was generated for epinephrine, followed by four additional dose-response curves of epinephrine in the presence of varying concentrations of metoprolol (2 mg, 5 mg, 10 mg, 100 mg). Time points for IV dosing of metoprolol and epinephrine were predetermined. Accuracy and reduced variability were achieved by administering epinephrine after a state of stabilized metoprolol-induced bradycardia was reached.

Receptor antagonists such as metoprolol are classified as reversible competitive antagonists. By definition, such compounds compete with the agonist for the active site. However, when the agonist reaches high enough concentrations, it effectively competes with the antagonist and produces the maximal response with an overall shifting of the dose-response curve to the right. True competitive antagonism was not achieved using the pharmacodynamic model programmed into the HPS (Fig. 5). Only a moderate shift of the dose-response curve was generated by increasing doses of metoprolol. Rather, the baseline heart rate was lowered with increasing doses of metoprolol, ultimately lowering the maximum response of individual epinephrine doses. Although the HPS may not be the perfect device to teach basic pharmacologic principles such as competitive or noncompetitive antagonism, it surely provides a visually powerful demonstration of drug responses and interactions.

Demonstrating the effects of atropine and succinylcholine concludes this series of experiments. A 3-mg dose of atropine produced a significant amount of cardiac stimulation because of vagal blockage. The lab is completed with the administration of a significant dose of succinylcholine to arrest breathing. Before the start of the lab we go over the relationships between alveolar carbon dioxide (CO_2) and oxygen (O_2) and arterial CO_2 and O_2. The succinylcholine effects allowed us to illustrate the relationships among alveolar O_2 and CO_2, arterial O_2 and CO_2 levels, and arterial pH. Finally, the patient was resuscitated by artificial respiration. Table 2 summarizes the drugs administered to the HPS and the observed effects.

In the fall semester of the second professional year, students have an integrated core curriculum that covers pulmonary diseases and infectious disease as well as appropri-

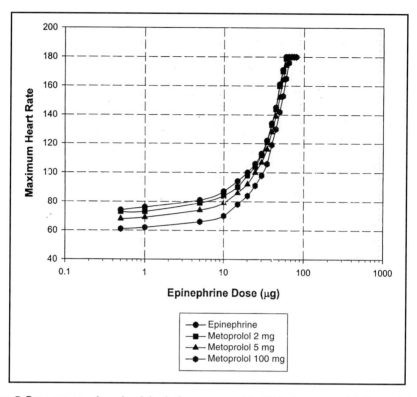

Figure 5. Dose-response for epinephrine in the presence of the β-blocker metoprolol. Metoprolol was administered to the HPS and the heart rate was allowed to stabilize, after which epinephrine was given and the maximum heart rate was recorded.

ate therapies. The biomedical science experiential course runs concurrently, allowing the use of the HPS along with the core lecture course. For example, it is important for the students to understand the sequence of events in an allergic drug reaction. In addition, students need to know that patients with penicillin allergies also may be allergic to the newer cephalosporins. A typical scenario presents a patient who has septicemia.

Table 2.
Effects of several drugs on the autonomic nervous system using the HPS.

Drug	Dose	BP	HR	Effect
None		114/52	71	—
Epinephrine	50 mcg	128/82	160	↑ HR
Epinephrine + metoprolol	50 mcg/50 mg	138/91	141	Lowered ↑ HR
Norepinephrine	100 mcg	150/84	80	↑ BP
Norepinephrine + Phentolamine	100 mcg/2 mg	128/65	83	Lowered ↑ BP
Atropine	3 mg	93/62	150	↑ HR
Succinylcholine	100 mg	112/59	94	Breathing Stops; ↑ PaCO2

Table 3.
HPS parameters that are modified throughout the anaphylaxis scenario.

Scenario Stage	Simulator Parameters changed During Stage	HR	SpO2	BP
Baseline		73	97	115/53
Begin Anaphylaxis	Start wheezing; increase shunt fraction; minus 400ml volume; decrease systemic vascular resistance; increase bronchial resistance	82	95	106/49
Mild Anaphylaxis	Increase shunt fraction; minus 600ml volume; decrease systemic vascular resistance	92	93	103/49
Worsening Anaphylaxis	Increase shunt fraction; minus 600ml volume; decrease systemic vascular resistance	105	91	99/50
Severe Anaphylaxis	Increase shunt fraction; minus 400ml volume; decrease systemic vascular resistance	119	89	81/43
Epinephrine Given/Recovery	Breath normal; decrease shunt fraction; increase systemic vascular resistance; decrease bronchial resistance	100	97	85/44

Various treatment options are discussed, and the "patient" is then administered an IV drip of imipenem (500 mg) and cilastatin (500 mg). An anaphylactic reaction soon ensues. Students must first diagnose this event and then initiate the proper treatment; in this scenario, a dose of epinephrine reverses the anaphylactic shock.

The simulator parameters that change during this scenario are shown in Table 3. The initial wheezing stage should be noticed by the students on examination of the "patient." In the initial stages, 400 ml of blood volume is taken out of the systemic circulation to simulate the redistribution of plasma to the peripheral tissues. During subsequent phases more volume is taken from the circulation, and the systemic vascular resistance parameter is decreased. The shunt fraction is altered so that less blood goes to the lungs to be oxygenated. In the severe anaphylactic stage, SpO_2 reaches 89% and hypotension is significant. A significant increase in heart rate occurs as a result of the hypotension. When the students recognize the situation, epinephrine is given. Epinephrine reverses the decreases in systemic vascular resistance, produces an increase in resistance, and increases blood flow to the lungs.

Advantages of the HPS

For teaching pharmacology, the HPS offers many obvious advantages as well as others that are less evident. With the growing concerns surrounding the use of animals for laboratory demonstrations, simulation presents a valid alternative for many standard pharmacology lessons. Animal demonstrations designed to show the physiologic effects (e.g., blood pressure changes) of cardiovascular or respiratory drugs can easily be demonstrated using the HPS. For example, the administration of a vasodilator such as nitroprusside results in a decrease in mean arterial blood pressure, followed by compensatory reflex tachycardia. The HPS shows these effects very well. With the pharmacokinetic and pharmacodynamic profiles of nearly 60 drugs, including narcotics, hypnotics, neuromuscular blockers, antagonists, cardiovascular drugs, and advanced cardiac life support (ACLS), the HPS provides a wide variety of responses for instructing pharmacologic demonstrations or scenarios for case studies.

The HPS also allows students to visualize the physiologic effects of drugs on humans. As other medical disciplines have shown, simulation facilitates the study of rare occurrences or side effects that cannot be shown in real patients because of ethical issues. Learning about the rare side effects of a particular drug or evaluating drug-drug interactions visually reinforces lecture-based material. If a major point of the lesson is missed or overlooked by the students, the simulator can be restarted and the lesson repeated—an option not easily accomplished with a real patient!

Besides the pharmacodynamic and pharmacokinetic characteristics that make simulators attractive teaching tools for pharmacology, the life-like physical presence and response capability of the HPS enhance the entire learning experience. Perhaps the greatest advantage of using a simulator for teaching pharmacology is the addition of realism, a factor that is often absent from lecture-based basic science courses. Whether the HPS is set up in an environment designed to represent a surgical theatre, a mock emergency room, or simply a nursing home, it forces students to become familiarized with critical care settings. The more props that are introduced, the more realistic the environment becomes, to the point that the instructor and students often believe that the patient is real. Once this stage is reached, the HPS becomes a powerful instrument to assess both individual and team performance.

Some may ask, "How does any of this relate to teaching pharmacology?" In our experience with undergraduate pharmacy students, we have noticed increased levels of student confidence in the ability to make decisions about drug therapy. The students can also be involved in role-play exercises with other health care providers such as nurses and doctors. This simulated atmosphere enhances both team-building and communication skills among the participants, thus preparing students for the professional interactions that they will encounter throughout their careers.

To optimize the simulator as an effective teaching tool, the class size should be smaller than lecture-based classes. We have found 8–10 students per session to be optimal. Although some may see small class size as a disadvantage of simulator-based teaching, we view it as an advantage because it promotes an open forum for questions and discussions. Initially students may feel apprehensive toward simulator training; therefore, an engaging facilitator is essential to encourage student participation. Once the students become comfortable with the simulator, they quickly appreciate the realism of the experience.

Limitations and Shortcomings of the HPS

Although the HPS is an effective teaching tool for pharmacology, it is not without limitations or shortcomings. Perhaps most formidable is the cost of the simulator, which can reach upward of $250,000 for a new full-scale mannequin. In addition, the simulators require a trained person for the day-to-day operations. Current simulators are complicated pieces of instrumentation and may require a significant amount of maintenance and troubleshooting. Depending on the realism of the simulator environment, props and other devices must also be included in the operating costs.

Another challenge that instructors must address is scheduling. Incorporating the HPS into an already intensive curriculum becomes extremely difficult, especially when a small class size is desired. We have found that simulation-based pharmacology classes are most effective with 10 or fewer students. Previously our pharmacology labs consisted of approximately 20 students; therefore, to run the HPS lab efficiently, we had to offer twice as many sections. Although this schedule was time-consuming and labor-intensive for the instructor, it was absolutely essential to achieve our teaching objectives. When our pharmacology lab classes are large, students have difficulty with following the material and do not feel part of the simulation experience; hence, the sense of realism is lost, the simulation environment no longer exists, and the transfer of knowledge is diminished.

Current simulators are far more advanced than their predecessors and provide instructors new opportunities of educating future health care providers. However, even the most advanced simulators lack some of the physical attributes of a real patient. For example, most simulators fall short of truly resembling a real person because they are often composed of rubber or plastic, which does not accurately reflect human skin. In addition, new advanced simulators are so physiologically complex that they cannot account for internal anatomic correctness; most simulators are completely filled with tubes and valves that allow the proper movements of gases and liquids. Although there is no replacement for the real thing, with the appropriate setting, medical props, and an enthusiastic facilitator, high-fidelity simulators create a dynamic learning experience that students will not quickly forget.

Future Directions

In the College of Pharmacy at the University of Rhode Island, we have just begun to explore the possibilities offered by simulation. To evaluate the success of the HPS as a teaching tool, we surveyed first-year professional students (n = 80). The survey included questions about educational self-assessment and provided students an opportunity to comment on the overall experience and advantages of using the HPS to teach pharmacology (Table 4). Our long-term goals include creating a simulation center that expands our teaching of pharmacology; forming relationships with other health care professionals at the university and at distant sites throughout the state; and implementing new simulation-based curricula to better prepare graduates for entering the health care arena. Short-term objectives are now focused on developing novel strategies to take advantage of the usefulness of the HPS in the curricula of both third- and fourth-year professional pharmacy students. New ideas include patient assessment and role-playing exercises designed to enhance team performance.

With the role of the pharmacist ever changing, increasing competencies in patient assessment are crucial. These competencies include familiarizing students with lung and heart sounds, pulses, blood pressures, blood gases, O_2 saturation, and arrhythmias. These sessions not only involve learning the normal values and recognizing heart and lung auscultations associated with a healthy patient; they also focus on identifying abnormalities, such as heart murmurs. The first encounter with a patient is sometimes overwhelming for many pharmacists; therefore, using the HPS to create a comfortable, yet realistic health care environment is invaluable to their education.

The College Of Pharmacy will include ACLS scenarios using the HPS as a part of

Table 4.
Survey of 1st professional year pharmacy students
to the University of Rhode Island.

Question:	% answering yes
Has the simulator increased your?	
Clinical knowledge	100
Basic Knowledge of Physiology	96
Awareness of Vital Signs	100
Basic Understanding of Pharmacological Principles	96
Did using the simulator enhance what you learned in lecture	97
	Most Common Answer
What did you enjoy most about using the HPS?	Being able to visualize previously learned topics
What is the greatest advantage of using the HPS for teaching pharmacology?	It produces a real life situation within a clinical environment

student training. In the foundations of human disease curriculum, taken during the third professional year, students learn about cardiovascular disorders, including pathophysiology, therapeutic interventions, and pharmacology associated with the disorders. There is a growing trend for hospital pharmacists to respond to emergency ACLS codes. As a result, ACLS certification is an important consideration for pharmacists.

Currently, pharmacists in health care facilities throughout the United States respond to codes. In addition, growing numbers of pharmacists are integral members of emergency health care teams. A major responsibility for these pharmacists is quick preparation of appropriate injectable medications. Because pharmacists are considered drug experts, they must be familiar with ACLS decision trees and dosing information and capable of anticipating which drugs are needed. They should be prepared to make recommendations or suggest interventions. Moreover, the pharmacy department in most hospitals is directly responsible for the crash cart. Pharmacists ensure standardized medication arrangements in the carts for ease of use in emergency situations as well as conduct regular inventory and expiration surveys. Therefore, it is beneficial for all parties involved that pharmacists are trained and become familiar with ACLS protocols.

Our pharmacy program focuses on the ventricular fibrillation/pulseless ventricular tachycardia algorithm, which is the most essential sequence to know for adult resuscitation. The treatment sequence is simple and includes defibrillation and ventilation. The recommended dose of epinephrine is 1 mg every 3–5 min, which is escalated if not effective. Typical medication sequence includes lidocaine, bretylium, magnesium sulfate, and procainamide (American Heart Association ACLS protocols). It is the intention of these training sessions to make students familiar with the process and the sequence of events involved with the treatments for arrhythmias and cardiac arrest.

In critical care situations teamwork is of utmost importance. Role-playing exercises designed to assess team performance can be practiced and evaluated.[19] The HPS is ideal for this situation. We also believe that pharmacists and pharmacy students who will be responding to codes must receive formal teamwork training in emergency medicine. The effectiveness of training and institutionalizing teamwork behaviors has been documented in emergency department staffs organized into caregiver teams.[20] Formal teamwork training with patient simulators improves team behaviors, reduces errors, and improves staff attitudes. Although pharmacists were not included in these teams, we believe that future inclusion of pharmacists will lead to a decrease in medication errors.

References

1. *http://www.meti.com* (last accessed May 30, 2003).
2. Tan GM, Ti LK, Suresh S, et al: Teaching first-year medical students physiology: Does the human patient simulator allow for more effective teaching? Singapore Med J 2002;43: 238–242.
3. Morgan PJ, Cleave-Hogg D: A Canadian simulation experience: Faculty and student opinions of a performance evaluation study. Br J Anaesth 2000;85:779–781.
4. Gordon JA, Wilkerson WM, Shaffer DW, Armstrong KG: "Practicing" medicine without risk: Students' and educators' responses to high-fidelity patient simulation. Acad Med 2001;76:469–472.
5. Chopra V, Gesink BJ, Delong J, et al: Does training on an anaesthesia simulator lead to improvement in performance? Br J Anaesth 1994;73:293–297.
6. Euliano TY: Small group teaching: Clinical correlation with a human patient simulator. Adv Physiol Educ 2001;25:36–43.
7. Holcomb JB, Russell DD, Crommett JW, et al: Evaluation of trauma team performance using an advanced human patient simulator for resuscitation training. J Trauma 2002;52: 1078–1086.
8. Hughes IE: The use of computers to simulate animal preparations in the teaching of practical pharmacology. Altern Lab Anim 1984;11:1078–1086.
9. Purves RD: Computer animations for teaching of introductory pharmacology. Trends Pharmacol Sci 1984;5:496–498.
10. Hughes IE: "Horses for courses"—categories of computed-based learning programs and their uses in pharmacology courses. Inform Serv Use 1998;18:35–44.
11. *http://www.biosoft.com* (last accessed May 30, 2003).
12. *http://www.coacs.com/software/published_titles/default.htm* (last accessed May 30, 2003).
13. Alberts et al: The Molecular Biology of the Cell, 2nd ed. New York, Garland Publishing, 1989.
14. Ariens EJ: Affinity and intrinsic activity in the theory of competitive inhibition. I: Problems and theory. Arch Int Pharmacodyn 1954;99:32–49.
15. Schild OH: Drug antagonism and pAx. Pharmacol Rev 1957;9:242–246.
16. Ross EM, Kenakin TP: Pharmacodynamics: Mechanism of drug action and the relationship between drug concentrations and effect. In Goodman and Gilman's The Pharmacological Basis of Therapeutics, 10th ed. New York, McGraw-Hill, 2001.
17. Simpson WW, McNeill JH: Blockade of the rate and force responses to phenylepinephrine on rate atria with labetalol. Res Commun Chem Pathol Pharmacol 1980;29:373–376.
18. Marquez MT, Mikulic LE, Aramendia P: Interactions between sympathomimetic agonists and blocking agents: Cardiac effects of phenylephrine and isoproterenol. Methods Find Exp Clin Pharmacol 1981;3:283–289.
19. Littlefield JH, Hahn HB, Meyer AS: Evaluation of a role-play learning exercise in an ambulatory clinic setting. Adv Health Sci Educ Theory Pract 1999;4:167–173.
20. Morey JC, Simon R, Jay GD, et al: Error reduction and performance improvement in the emergency department through formal teamwork training: Evaluation results of the MedTeam Project. Health Serv Res 2002;37:1553–1581.

Chapter 8

SIMULATION IN PHYSICAL DIAGNOSIS

Gary E. Loyd, MD, MMM

Simulation has been used to teach and evaluate the skills of physical diagnosis for decades. In 1975 Sajid et al. described the construction of a simulation laboratory for medical education at the University of Illinois College of Medicine. The goal of the center was to provide opportunities for students to improve their inpatient examination skills.[1] The importance of having such teaching equipment was well recognized and reported for at least 30 years. In 1973 Penta and Kofman reported that the use of simulation devices significantly improved students' ability to perform specific skills related to physical examination.[2] The evolution of the use of simulation to teach physical diagnosis has been significant. High-fidelity simulators, almost by definition, have an increased ability to provide this highly important function. Even though simulators have been used and described in the literature, they have not been universally accepted as the standard method of teaching health care providers the art and science of physical diagnosis. Anderson et al. identified several barriers to teaching current physical diagnosis at the University of Wisconsin. One of their suggestions for solving the problems was acquiring mid- or high-fidelity simulators.[3] The abilities of high-fidelity simulators have been described several times in this book. The intent of this chapter is to provide information about other simulation alternatives—some of them involving complex technology—used in the teaching and evaluation of physical diagnosis. This chapter is by no means an exhaustive collection of all of the products available, but rather a mere sampling; lists in catalogs are fairly substantial.

Value of Simulation

Assessing the actual value of simulation in teaching and evaluating the skills of physical diagnosis is difficult. For many, the value is almost intuitive and qualitatively evident. The quantifying of this assessment has been more problematic until recently. The assumption is that current methods of teaching and assessment are adequate and valid, as proved by decades of use and producing professionals who can provide a significant level of health care. Morgan et al. at the University of Toronto conducted a pilot study to evaluate the anesthesia simulator as an assessment tool for medical students. The interrater reliability was very high (0.87), but the correlation with written and clinical evaluations was low.[4] This finding begs the question of the validity of each evaluation tool in assessing whether we are producing a competent physician. Kahn et al. concluded that residency director evaluations of resident performances did not correlate with objective tests of either knowledge or clinical skills (using simulation). They suggested that more structured and objective evaluative tools might improve the validity and reliability of resident evaluations.[5]

Not only is the evaluation process questionable, but the traditional teaching methods are questionable as well. Morgan et al. found no correlation between students' clinical experiences and level of confidence and their ability to perform during standardized scenarios on a high-fidelity human simulator.[6] In a study evaluating physician reporting in medical records, Dresselhaus et al. found a high number of false positives in the physical examination in regard to history taking. Such a study may question the validity of assessment tools, such as portfolio checklists and chart-stimulated recall, in the assessment of residents.[7]

Other evidence also challenges our current system of teaching physical diagnosis. In 2000 Peitzman reported that both U.S. and non-U.S. international medical graduates performed lower than expected on specific tests included in the Clinical Skills Assessment of the Educational Commission for Foreign Medical Graduates certification.[8] Sayer et al. reported the results of a survey about the use of real patients for clinical skills education in the United Kingdom. They concluded that the great variation in the educational experiences of the learners raises many ethical and legal issues regarding the assessment of the learners' abilities.[9]

One of the current trends in simulation is to provide proof of the validity and reliability of simulators to create a superior educational experience. In 1982 Shain et al. compared students taught by plastic models and students taught by clinic patients at the University of Texas Health Science Center at San Antonio. There were few significant differences between the two groups.[10] Objective structured checklists were used to test interrater reliability in simulation and yielded good results.[11] Reznek et al. established the validity of using an intravenous catheter simulator for medical students, residents, and attending physicians.[12] Winckel et al. demonstrated the reliability and validity of a Structured Technical Skills Assessment (STSA) form in assessing the technical skills of surgery trainees.[13] In 2002 Glavin and Maran outlined a system for the development of a tool to assess clinical competence.[14]

Other advantages of using simulation to teach physical diagnosis have been appearing in the literature. A group of senior medical students who received seminar-based teaching were compared with a group of senior medical students who received simulator based-teaching in trauma management. There were no differences in knowledge acquired between the two groups when a surgery Objective Structured Clinical Examination (OSCE) was used as the evaluation tool. Yet students in simulator-based teaching felt more confident than their counterparts.[15] Marshall et al. demonstrated that using the human patient simulator not only augments the trauma management skills of interns but also improves teamwork and self-confidence compared with controls.[16] Karnath et al. suggest that one of the greatest benefits of using simulators during physical diagnosis is the possibility of introducing several abnormal physical findings during the examination without having to produce an unstable patient on which to do the examination. They also propose that simulated physical diagnosis allows completely valid standardization of a patient examination learning experience.[17] Issenberg et al. reported that using simulators in medical education engages learners in deliberate practice of clinical skills while producing large and significant improvements in their performance in a relatively short time. They also concluded that provision of simulator training requires little faculty involvement.[18]

Innovative uses of simulation in the teaching of physical diagnosis have been described in the literature. One example is its integration into existing teaching methods, such as problem-based learning. The University of Florida extended problem-based learning into the simulation laboratory.[19] Not all of the physical diagnosis simulators have been tangible replicators. At the University of Pittsburgh in 1995, White described the use of interactive video to demonstrate physical signs of a computer-based simulator for nurses instead of having the physical signs simply described. Twelve of the 16 first-time users reported that the simulations were similar or very similar to actual clinical encounters. The author concluded that the realism of interactive video-enhanced, computer-based simulations was a viable alternative to traditional approaches.[20] In 1999 Lyons and Milton described the integration of an innovative computer-based physical simulation and Laurillard's conversational framework in the effective teaching of midwifery in Australia.[21] The United States Army demonstrated the effectiveness of using a virtual reality simulator to improve complex decision making in the combat arena.[22]

From the natural evolution of simulation, as it relates to physical diagnosis, has come the development of clinical skills centers or laboratories. At the University of Dundee, OSCEs have been used since 1977. The university has used standard patients (SPs) and simulators in both teaching and learning and more recently performed assessments in a multistation area similar to a clinical skills laboratory.[23] Nicol and Freeth describe the development of the Bart Nursing OSCE, which also occurs in a clinical skills center.[24] Meharry Medical College has reported the use of simulations for teaching clinical skills breast examinations, examinations of male and female genitalia, pelvic examinations, venipuncture, lumbar puncture, intravenous catheter placement, and endobronchial intubations.[25] One of the newer and more comprehensive clinical skills laboratory exists at George Washington University's Clinical Learning and Simulation Skills (CLASS) Center.[26] Dent discusses in good detail the development of Clinical Skills Centers (for internet links see Table 1). He describes the variety of available patient simulators and simulated environments.[27]

System-Specific Simulators

Respiratory System

Respiratory system simulators are abundant. Perusal of teaching aids in catalogs demonstrates a variety of resuscitation mannequins and intubation heads. There have been many advances from the poorly mobile heads of 30 years ago to the articulated jaws and realistically distensible airways of modern simulators.[28] Both anatomy and physiology are replicated. The ability of simulators to replicate different respiratory physiologic states has been reported in critical care settings, emergency departments, and operating rooms.[29–32]

Virtual reality provides a new advancement in respiratory system simulation. Students can take a virtual tour of the airway using tools that clinicians use to evaluate airways.[33] Not all the advancements in respiratory system simulators have to be expensive. In 2000 Williams et al. described in a letter to the editor the inexpensive construction of an artificial throat to assist in the training of fiberoptic intubation.[34] The application of simulators has been reported for airway simulation in a variety of ways (see Table 2 for internet links). In teaching respiratory physiology to first-year medical students, the faculty at the University of Florida introduced the students to basic physical diagnosis with the simulator.[35] Skills in airway management have been introduced to first-year medical students as well.[36]

Table 1.
Internet Links to Clinical Skills Centers

1. The University of Minnesota Interprofessional Educational Resource Center {The University of Minnesota Interprofessional Educational Resource Center, 10-31-2003 #6679}
2. UW Medicine: Virtual Simulators Enhance Operating Skills {UW Medicine: Virtual Simulators Enhance Operating Skills, 10-31-2003 #6636}
3. University of Cincinnati: Clinical Skills Lab {University of Cincinnati Clinical Skills Lab, 10-31-2003 #6645}
4. PLAB {PLAB, 10-31-2003 #6662}
5. Harvard Medical School: Clinical Skills Lab {Harvard Medical School Clinical Skills Lab, 10-31-2003 #6663}
6. Southern Illinois University: Clinical Skills Lab {Southern Illinois University Clinical Skills Lab, 10-31-2003 #6664}
7. KU Wichita: Faculty Resources Clinical Skills Lab {KU Wichita Clinical Skills Lab, 10-31-2003 #6665}
8. University of Wales: The Clinical Skills Lab (CSL) {University of Wales Clinical Skills Lab (CSL), 10-31-2003 #6666}
9. LSU HSC Skills Lab {LSU HSC Skills Lab, 10-31-2003 #6667}
10. NHS UK: Clinical Skills Lab {NHS UK Clinical Skills Lab, 10-31-2003 #6668}
11. Indiana State University: School of Nursing {Indiana State University School of Nursing, 10-31-2003 #6669}
12. Clinical Skills Center: College of Medicine & Public Health: The Ohio State University {Ohio State University College of Medicine and Public Health, 10-31-2003 #6670}
13. University of Arkansas: Clinical Modules {University of Arkansas, 10-31-2003 #6671}
14. Huddinge University Hospital: Clinical Skills Center {Huddinge University Hospital Clinical Skills Center, 10-31-2003 #6672}
15. Huddinge University Hospital: Center for Advanced Medical Simulation {Huddinge University Hospital Center for Advanced Medical Simulation, 10-31-2003 #6673}
16. Program Coordinator (Curricular Affairs - Clinical Skills Center) - Staff Job Composite {Program Coordinator (Curricular Affairs–Clinical Skills Center)–Staff Job Composite, 10-31-2003 #6674}
17. What is the Clinical Skills Learning Center (CSLC)? {What is the Clinical Skills Learning Center (CSLC)?, 10-31-2003 #6675}
18. ACP Online–Clinical Skills Program {ACP Online Clinical Skills Program, 10-31-2003 #6676}
19. Student Assessment and Evaluation: Clinical Skills Testing and Assessment Center (University of KY) {University of Kentucky, last accessed 10-31-2003 #6677}
20. Basic Clinical Skills Harrell Center Activities {Basic Clinical Skills Harrell Center Activities, 10-31-2003 #6678}

 Table 2.
Internet links to Respiratory System Simulators

1. The R.A.L.E. Repository {The R.A.L.E. Repository, 10-31-2003 #6620}
2. Case One: The Choking Infant, age 0 to 1 year {The Choking Infant, 10-31-2003 #6656}

Cardiac System

One of the oldest simulators for the cardiac system is Harvey. In 1976, Harley suggested that a heart sound simulator improved students' ability to assess heart sounds accurately.[37] In 1976 Aloia and Jonas described how residents needed the appropriate educational environment to use a heart sound simulator to improve their skills.[38] Heart simulators have been used in several studies for both teaching and evaluation purposes (see Table 3 for internet links). In 2000 Gaskin et al. reported the use of a Harvey cardiology simulator to assess the clinical auscultation skills of pediatric residents at Duke

❖ Table 3.
Internet Links to Cardiac Simulators

1. Cardiac Auscultation Simulator {Cardiac Auscultation Simulator, 10-31-2003 #6615}
2. The Auscultation Assistant–Hear Heart Murmurs, Heart Sounds, and Breath Sounds {The Auscultation Assistant–Hear Heart Murmurs, 10-31-2003 #6616}
3. Heart Sounds {Heart Sounds, 10-31-2003 #6617}
4. ProLine Training, Inc.: Disclaimer {ProLine Training, 10-31-2003 #6618}
5. Auscultation Simulators {Auscultation Simulators, 10-31-2003 #6619}
6. Blaufuss Multimedia: Heart Sounds {Blaufuss Multimedia Heart Sounds, 10-31-2003 #6621}
7. MDchoice.com Advanced Cardiac Life Support (ACLS) Megacode Simulator {Mdchoice Advanced Cardiac Life Support Megacode Simulator, 10-31-2003 #6628}
8. Synapse Publishing Inc.–heart beats, heart sounds {Synapse Publishing Inc.–heart beats, 10-31-2003 #6629}
9. Basic EKG Rhythms {Basic EKG Rhythms, 10-31-2003 #6630}
10. CESLab - cardiac electrophysiological simulation package {CESLab - cardiac electrophysiological simulation package, 10-31-2003 #6631}
11. ACLS Electrical Therapy Quiz {ACLS Electrical Therapy Quiz, 10-31-2003 #6632}
12. Pediatric Advanced Cardiac life Support Simulator {Pediatric Advanced Cardiac life Support Simulator, 10-31-2003 #6633}
13. Pulmonary Arterial Catheterisation Simulator {Pulmonary Arterial Catheterisation Simulator, 10-31-2003 #6634}
14. Rhythm Master: test your rhythm recognition skill {Larson, 10-31-2003 #6635}

University Medical Center. They found that the residents' skills were suboptimal compared with practicing pediatric cardiologists.[39] St. Clair et al. describe how a Harvey cardiology simulator gave house staff difficulty when they tried to diagnose three valvular heart disorders.[40] Similarly, Jones et al. reported the difficulty of emergency medicine faculty and house staff in diagnosing three valvular abnormalities when assessed by the Harvey cardiology patient simulator.[41]

Newer developments in cardiac system simulators include internet, web-based systems. Kelsey et al. report the use of an online heart simulator to teach heart sounds.[42] The development of the multimedia computer-assisted instruction (MCAI) system by four institutions suggests a cost-effective alternative to expensive cardiac simulators.[43] Providing mass heart education to health care professionals could be very costly when considered in isolation;[44] providing the more expensive cardiac simulator as part of the total patient may be more prudent. Heart sound and other physiologic cardiovascular parameters are part of modern high-fidelity simulators. Studies are needed to elucidate this point.

Ophthalmology

The Center for Videoendoscopic Surgery at the University of Washington has refined a tissue-realistic physical simulator and virtual reality simulator to assess performance. It is assessing whether simulator training transfers to clinical practice.[45] Verma et al. described the development of a virtual reality simulator for vitreoretinal surgery.[46] In 1997 Kaufman and Bell described the benefits of using virtual reality simulation in the teaching and assessment of psychomotor, technical, and procedural skills. They also described the use of a virtual reality eye simulator at Dalhousie University Medical School[47] (see Table 4 for internet links).

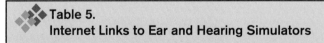

Table 4.
Internet Links to Ophthalmology Simulators

1 Eye Simulator Version 2.0 {Eye Simulator Version 2.0, 10-31-2003 #6639}
2. Neurological Eye Simulator {Neurological Eye Simulator, 10-31-2003 #6640}
3. Glaucoma Vision Simulators {Glaucoma Vision Simulators, 10-31-2003 #6641}
4. Insights From a Virtual Eye {Insights From a Virtual Eye, 10-31-2003 #6642}
5. Saint Louis University School of Medicine 2002's Class Material {Saint Louis University School of Medicine 2002's Class Material, 10-31-2003 #6643}
6. 3-D Eye Simulation Test {3-D Eye Simulation Test, 10-31-2003 #6644}
7. Eye Simulation Application {Eye Simulation Application, 10-31-2003 #6646}
8. Eye Reaction Simulator v1.11 {Eye Reaction Simulator v1.11, 10-31-2003 #6647}
9. IMTC Projects: Eye Surgery Simulator {Interactive Media Technology Center, last accessed 10-31-2003 #6648}

Ears and Hearing

Pichichero and Poole describe a system of testing technical competence in performing otoscopic examinations and tympanocentesis.[48] Such skills are reportedly necessary to distinguish between acute otitis media and otitis media with effusion and thus make appropriate antibiotic management decisions. Simulation of the different disease processes has demonstrated an improvement in this ability[49] (see Table 5 for internet links).

Genitourinary Simulation

At St. Mary's Hospital in London, Kneebone et al. integrated simulated urinary catheterization and wound suturing with a standardized patient to provide live feedback.[50] Matsumoto et al. validated the proposal that using hands-on simulation to teach urologic procedures enhanced the training of novices in ureteroscopic retrieval of a midureteral stone in the laboratory.[51] In 1985 Rakestraw et al. described the use of an anthropomorphic model, nicknamed Gynny, to teach the physical examination of the pelvis. Students who used the model performed significantly better than those who did not.[52] Pugh and Youngblood developed a pelvic simulator that provides raw numerical data to the learner. This simulator was demonstrated to be an objective, reliable, and valid assessment tool.[53] In 1984 Fang, et al. evaluated three groups of students at the University of Virginia School of Medicine. Students who were trained on plastic models were significantly more confident in their ability to perform a speculum exam than students who were taught either by lecture or standardized patients.[54] (see Table 6 for internet links).

Table 5.
Internet Links to Ear and Hearing Simulators

1. Artificial Ears and Ear Simulators {Artificial Ears and Ear Simulators, 10-31-2003 #6649}
2. AMS Acoustics: Ear and Mouth Simulators {AMS Acoustics Ear and Mouth Simulators, 10-31-2003 #6650}
3. Ear Examination Simulator {Ear Examination Simulator, 10-131-2003 #6651}

Decision Making

Floreck et al. reported the use of computer-based case simulations to examine students as part of the USMLE Step 3 examination.[55] The United States Army demonstrated the effectiveness of using a virtual reality simulator to improve complex decision making in the combat arena.[22] In 1989 Schwartz described how computer simulations were able to assess students' clinical reasoning skills at a cost of less than one dollar per student.[56] In 1998 Scheuneman et al. investigated the characteristics of computer-based case simulations that may be associated with case difficulty. The most interesting finding was that the difficulty of the case was related more to the length of the paragraph than to the structure of the simulation or the severity of the patient's condition.[57]

Miscellaneous Applications

This section includes a hodgepodge of interesting but isolated references to reported uses of simulation as it relates to specific physical diagnosis apparatuses or techniques (see Table 7 for internet links). Some of the items are popular, given the number of variations that are for sale in mail-order catalogs. Reznek, et al. established the validity of using an intravenous catheter simulator for medical students, residents, and attending physicians.[12] Hmelo and Day describe interjecting questions into computerized simulations and integrating them with problem-based learning. This approach was evaluated as having some value, but it was not superior to the traditional PBL.[58] In 1979 Schreiner et al. described the use of an independently produced abdominal mass simulator to teach pediatric physical diagnosis skills as related to ovarian cysts, neuroblastomas, and hepatic tumors. The device could also simulate a congenital hip dislocation or subluxation of the hip in a newborn.[59] In 1998 Chalabian et al. reported that primary care physicians who performed the poorest clinical breast examinations came from programs that did not have a dedicated breast curriculum.[60] Wiakakul et al. described a way to make an inexpensive simulated knee that can be used for the diagnosis of knee arthropathy and arthrocentesis and to simulate intra-articular injections.[61]

Conclusion

Physical diagnosis is one of the first areas in which simulation was used to teach health care professionals. Many devices have been created, and their uses have been reported in the literature. Modern high-fidelity simulators have integrated many individual organ simulators. Still there are many organ or system simulators on the market that provide teachers the flexibility to augment their instruction. As health care educators apply scientific scrutiny to the popular belief that simulation is a superior teaching and assessment instrument, they also are scrutinizing the current methods of instruction.

References

1. Sajid A, Lipson LF, Telder V: A simulation laboratory for medical education. J Med Educ 50:970–975, 1975.
2. Penta FB, Kofman S: The effectiveness of simulation devices in teaching selected skills of physical diagnosis. J Med Educ 48:442–445, 1973.
3. Anderson RC, Fagan MJ, Sebastian J: Teaching students the art and science of physical diagnosis. Am J Med 110(5):419–423, 2001.
4. Morgan PJ, Cleave-Hogg D: Evaluation of medical students' performances using the anesthesia simulator. Acad Med 74:202, 1999.
5. Kahn MJ, Merrill WW, Anderson DS, et al: Residency program director evaluations do not correlate with performance on a required 4th-year objective structured clinical examination. Teach Learn Med 13:9–12, 2001.
6. Morgan PJ, Cleave-Hogg D: Comparison between medical students' experience, confidence and competence. Med Educ 36:534–539, 2002.
7. Dresselhaus TR, Luck J, Peabody JW: The ethical problem of false positives: A prospective evaluation of physician reporting in the medical record. J Med Ethics 28(5):291–294, 2002.
8. Peitzman SJ: Clinical skills assessment using standardized patients: Perspectives from the Educational Commission for Foreign Medical Graduates. Am J Phys Med Rehabil 79:490–493, 2000.
9. Sayer M, Bowman D, Evans D, et al: Use of patients in professional medical examinations: Current UK practice and the ethicolegal implications for medical education. BMJ 324:404–407, 2002.
10. Shain RN, and et al: Evaluation of the gynecology teaching associate versus pelvic model approach to teaching pelvic examination. J Med Educ 57(8):646–648, 1982.
11. Bullock G, Kovacs G, Macdonald K, et al: Evaluating procedural skills competence: Interrater reliability of expert and non-expert observers. Acad Med 74:76–78, 1999.
12. Reznek MA, Rawn CL, Krummel TM: Evaluation of the educational effectiveness of a virtual reality intravenous insertion simulator. Acad Emerg Med 9:1319–1325, 2002.

13. Winckel CP, Reznick RK, Cohen R, et al: Reliability and construct validity of a structured technical skills assessment form. Am J Surg 167:423–427, 1994.
14. Glavin RJ, Maran NJ: Development and use of scoring systems for assessment of clinical competence. Br J Anaesth 88:329–330, 2002.
15. Gilbart MK, Hutchison CR, Cusimano MD, et al: A computer-based trauma simulator for teaching trauma management skills. Am J Surg 179:223–238, 2000.
16. Marshall RL, Smith JS, Gorman PJ, et al: Use of a human patient simulator in the development of resident trauma management skills. J Trauma 51:17–21, 2001.
17. Karnath B, Frye WA, Holden MD: Incorporating simulators in a standardized patient exam. Acad Med 77:754–755, 2002.
18. Issenberg SB, McGaghie WC, Gordon DL, et al: Effectiveness of a cardiology review course for internal medicine residents using simulation technology and deliberate practice. Teach Learn Med 14(4):223–228, 2002.
19. Euliano TY, Mahla ME: Problem-based learning in residency education: A novel implementation using a simulator. J Clin Monit Comput 15(3–4):227–232, 1999.
20. White JE: Using interactive video to add physical assessment data to computer-based patient simulations in nursing. Comput Nurs 13(5):233–235, 1995.
21. Lyons J, Milton J: Recognizing through feeling: A physical and computer simulation based on educational theory. Comput Nurs 17(3):114–119, 1999.
22. Pleban RJ, Matthews MD, Salter MS, et al: Training and assessing complex decision-making in a virtual environment. Percept Mot Skills 94(3 Pt 1): 871–882, 2002.
23. Davis MH: OSCE: The Dundee experience. Med Teach 25:255–261, 2003.
24. Nicol M, Freeth D: Assessment of clinical skills: A new approach to an old problem. Nurse Educ Today 18:601–609, 1998.
25. Hao J, Estrada J, Tropez-Sims S: The clinical skills laboratory: A cost-effective venue for teaching clinical skills to third-year medical students. Acad Med 77:152, 2002.
26. Blatt J: George Washington University has a Clinical Learning and Simulation Skills (CLASS) Center. Gary Loyf (ed), 2003.
27. Dent JA: Current trends and future implications in the developing role of clinical skills centres. Med Teach 23:483–489, 2001.
28. Agro F, Giuliano I, Montecchia F: A new human-dynamic simulator (Air Man) for airway training in emergency situations. Am J Emerg Med 20:495, 2002.
29. Arne R, Stale F, Ragna K, et al: PatSim—simulator for practising anaesthesia and intensive care. Development and observations. Int J Clin Monit Comput 13(3):147–152, 1996.
30. Berkenstadt H, A. Ziv A, D. Barsuk D, et al: The use of advanced simulation in the training of anesthesiologists to treat chemical warfare casualties. Anesth Analg 96:1739–1742, 2003.
31. Holcomb JB, Dumire RD, Crommett JW, et al: Evaluation of trauma team performance using an advanced human patient simulator for resuscitation training. J Trauma 52:1078–1085; discussion, 1085–1086, 2002.
32. Stringer KR, Bajenov S, Yentis SM: Training in airway management. Anaesthesia 57:967–983, 2002.
33. Rowe R, Cohen RA: An evaluation of a virtual reality airway simulator. Anesth Analg 95:62–66, 2002.
34. Williams KA, Harwood RJ, Woodall NM, et al: Training in fiberoptic intubation. Anaesthesia 55:99–100, 2000.
35. Euliano TY: Teaching respiratory physiology: Clinical correlation with a human patient simulator. J Clin Monit Comput 16(5–6):465–470, 2000.
36. Owen H, Plummer JL: Improving learning of a clinical skill: The first year's experience of teaching endotracheal intubation in a clinical simulation facility. Med Educ 36:635–642 2002.
37. Harley A: Evaluation of a heart sound simulator in teaching cardiac auscultation. J Med Educ 51:600–601, 1976.
38. Aloia JF, Jonas E: Skills in history-taking and physical examination. J Med Educ 51:410–415, 1976.
39. Gaskin PR, S.E. Owens, N.S. Talner NS, et al: Clinical auscultation skills in pediatric residents. Pediatrics 105:1184–1187, 2000.

40. St Clair EW, Oddone EZ, Waugh RA, et al: Assessing housestaff diagnostic skills using a cardiology patient simulator. Ann Intern Med 117:751–756, 1992.

41. Jones JS, Hunt SJ, Carlson SA, et al: Assessing bedside cardiologic examination skills using "Harvey," a cardiology patient simulator. Acad Emerg Med 4:980–985, 1997.

42. Kelsey R, Botello M, Millard B, et al: An online heart simulator for augmenting first-year medical and dental education. Proceedings of the AMIA Symposium, 2002, pp 370–374.

43. Waugh RA, Mayer JW, Ewy GA, et al: Multimedia computer-assisted instruction in cardiology. Arch Intern Med 155:197–203, 1995.

44. Karnath B, Thornton W, Frye AW: Teaching and testing physical examination skills without the use of patients. Acad Med 77:753, 2002.

45. Center for Videoscopic Surgery: http://depts.washington.edu/cves/edu.html. Last accessed 11-2-03.

46. Verma D, Wills D, Verma M: Virtual reality simulator for vitreoretinal surgery. Eye 17:71–73, 2003.

47. Kaufman DM, W. Bell W: Teaching and assessing clinical skills using virtual reality. Stud Health Technol Inform 39:467–472, 1997.

48. Pichichero ME, Poole MD: Assessing diagnostic accuracy and tympanocentesis skills in the management of otitis media. Arch Pediatr Adolesc Med 155:1137–1142, 2001.

49. Sorrento A, Pichichero ME: Assessing diagnostic accuracy and tympanocentesis skills by nurse practitioners in management of otitis media. J Am Acad Nurse Pract 13(11):524–529, 2001.

50. Kneebone R, Kidd J, Nestel D, et al: An innovative model for teaching and learning clinical procedures. Med Educ 36:628–634, 2002.

51. Matsumoto ED, Hamstra SJ, Radomski SB, et al: The effect of bench model fidelity on endourological skills: A randomized controlled study. J Urol 167:1243–1247, 2002.

52. Rakestraw PG, et al: Utilization of an anthropomorphic model in pelvic examination instruction. J Med Educ 60:343–345, 1985.

53. Pugh CM, Youngblood P: Development and validation of assessment measures for a newly developed physical examination simulator. J Am Med Inform Assoc 9:448–460, 2002.

54. Fang WL, et al: Evaluation of students' clinical and communication skills in performing a gynecologic examination. J Med Educ 59:758–760, 1984.

55. Floreck LM, Guernsey MJ, Clyman SG, et al: Examinee performance on computer-based case simulations as part of the USMLE step 3 examination: Are examinees ordering dangerous actions? Acad Med 77(10 Suppl):S77–S79, 2002.

56. Schwartz W: Documentation of students' clinical reasoning using a computer simulation. Am J Dis Child 143:575–579, 1989.

57. Scheuneman JD, Van Fan Y, Clyman SG: An investigation of the difficulty of computer-based case simulations. Med Educ 32:150–158, 1998.

58. Hmelo C, Day R: Contextualized questioning to scaffold learning from simulations. Comput Educ 32:151–164, 1999.

59. Schreiner RL, et al: Simulators to teach pediatric skills. J Med Educ 54:242–243, 1979.

60. Chalabian J, Formenti S, Russell C, et al: Comprehensive needs assessment of clinical breast evaluation skills of primary care residents. Ann Surg Oncol 5:166–172, 1998.

61. Waikakul S, Vanadurongwan B, Chumtup W, et al: A knee model for arthrocentesis simulation. J Med Assoc Thai 86:282–287, 2003.

Chapter 9

SIMULATION IN NURSING EDUCATION
Nursing in a Learning Resource Center

Lori Schumacher, RN, MS, CCRN

The use of simulation in nursing education provides exciting teaching and learning opportunities for everyone involved in the educational process and can be incorporated throughout the nursing curriculum. When using simulation in a nursing resource center, one needs to make sure that the content is realistic and current because simulation is an attempt to "replicate some or nearly all of the essential aspects of a clinical situation so that the situation may be more readily understood and managed when it occurs for real in clinical practice."[1] Through simulation, intellect can be developed, inductive thinking and reasoning take place, inquiry begins, and critical thinking and decision-making skills develop and become more refined.[2,3] Students are often anxious about the initial clinical experiences, and simulation provides them with a controlled environment that allows an opportunity to learn and practice without endangering a real patient.[4–7] This chapter explores the various uses of simulation in a nursing learning resource center. The list is far from exhaustive. Individual teaching methods and styles vary, and individual creativity in new situations may adapt aspects of the methods described below or create new methods.

According to Lupien and George-Gay (2001),[8] for simulation to be successful, a seven-step process should be used for developing and implementing simulation sessions:

1. Define educational objectives.
2. Construct a clinical scenario.
3. Define the underlying physiologic concepts.
4. Modify programmed patients and scenarios, as necessary.
5. Assemble the required equipment.
6. Run the program and collect feedback.
7. Repeat steps 2–6 until satisfied.

One may ask, "How can I use simulation in my current teaching practices?" or "Where do I even begin to incorporate simulation into the subjects I teach?" Nothing is impossible if you use creativity in developing new teaching strategies. The initial step in developing a simulation session is to determine the educational objectives and outcomes that you desire to achieve. The objectives may be as simple as having the participant select the appropriate equipment or perform the appropriate assessment for a specific clinical situation. Alternatively, the objective may be complex by combining numerous steps, such as initiation of the appropriate measures for an acutely ill patient and adjustment as indicated by patient condition, assessment findings, and response.

Once the educational objectives and outcomes have been determined, the next step is to construct the clinical scenario to be used in the session. The scenario may be basic in that the participants need to use basic assessment skills and management strategies, or the scenario may be complex in that participants need to use numerous skills and strategies, such as a mega code situation, in order to be successful.

During the development of the scenario, it is necessary to determine and define the underlying physiologic concepts that need to occur throughout the scenario according to patient condition and events presented. For example, if the learning objective of the session is to recognize symptoms of hemorrhage, the manifestations of decreased blood pressure and increased heart rate need to be exhibited. As the level of the learner changes and the session becomes more complex, then the scenario may need to be modified to achieve the objectives and outcomes of the session. One must learn to be flexible when using simulation because each learner or group will be different and the objectives and outcomes may switch or become revised as the session progresses. Some learners will progress through sessions successfully, and others will take time and require repeated attempts at skills and strategies to meet the objectives and outcomes.

Once the scenario is developed, all of the equipment necessary for the scenario must be collected and assembled. The more realistic a scenario can become, the better. Therefore, if the scenario takes places in an intensive care setting, the room or the set-up of the lab should resemble and contain the type of equipment and supplies found in the intensive care setting.

Next, the program and the scenario should be tested before they are used with students. Initially, testing assists in determining the flow of the scenario, whether the scenario has flaws, and/or whether additions or revisions need to be made. Once the session begins, the instructor needs to determine the degree of his or her involvement in the scenario. The instructor's involvement will vary from session to session and also with the learning level of the group. According to Lupien and George-Gay (2001), the instructor may be involved as "(1) a role model where critical thinking, decision making, and nursing interventions are modeled; (2) a coach who is available to assist students functioning in their nursing roles; or (3) a passive bystander who observes the scenario with minimal involvement."[8] Finally, the instructor must be able to actively debrief as the session is in progress. Active debriefing assists the participant in learning and also allows clarification of thoughts and actions, exploration of various skills and strategies, and improvement of performance.

Fundamental Skills

Simulation can provide a new and exciting way to introduce students to basic, fundamental skills such as taking blood pressure (BP) and obtaining pulse and respiratory rate. Students are usually nervous the first time that they need to perform these skills on a patient. By practicing these basic skills through various simulation scenarios, students should be more at ease when actually performing the skills. The student may encounter various scenarios:

1. A normal patient with normal vital signs
2. A patient with a weak, thready pulse
3. A patient who has an irregular heart rhythm, such as atrial fibrillation
4. A patient with a weak pulse for whom students need to obtain the BP through palpation or use of a Doppler device

Each scenario identified above certainly is realistic and increases in complexity; simulation should assist students in developing confidence in their skills. Not only does simulation assist in developing confidence, it is also the beginning of the student's development and lifelong performance of fundamental skills. Simulation provides students with feedback, and if the technique or performance is not adequate or appropriate, students may refine their techniques and practice until the performance is acceptable and meets the desired standards. In addition, the use of simulation at a simplistic level provides the foundation for the development of critical thinking and decision-making skills by taking each piece of patient data and each action performed and relating them to the management of the whole patient.[2,3,9]

Assessment Skills

Assessment skills, such as lung and heart sounds, may be produced, auscultated, taught, and reinforced by simulation. The student is able to listen actively to the mannequin's breath and heart sounds, which are more realistic than audiotapes of simulated lung and heart sounds. The realism of simulation in the learning of assessment skills can be quite challenging to the student. Most often students are unsure and have difficulty in auscultating and differentiating abnormal sounds and qualities. Simulation provides an excellent avenue to assist students in recognizing the various sounds and qualities that they may encounter in assessing real patients.

The location and quality of pulses can be used as an initial learning goal. Once students are comfortable with their assessment, the quality and even absence of pulses can be introduced, further challenging the student's assessment skills. Pupil size, pupillary reaction, and consensual light reflex can also be effectively assessed due to the realistic nature of the simulator's ability to change pupil sizes, types of reactions, and the consensual reflex.

Another assessment may include skin color. Even though the mannequin does not automatically change skin color, variation can be achieved by hanging a theater light above the simulator and changing the color of the film over the light bulb. For example, to produce a cyanotic, blue tint one may use a blue film over the bulb; if the appearance of a heat stroke or rash is desired, one may use a red film over the bulb; and if a jaundiced appearance is desired, one may use a yellow film over the bulb. If a theater light is not possible, moulage kits are available that allow the application of various types of make-up and tints that are also effective in producing the desired appearance.

Some simulators have the ability to produce a voice through a speaker in the mannequin. This feature requires that someone use a lapel microphone and speak as though he or she were the patient. The use of the microphone and speaker allows the student to ask the patient questions such as past history and pertinent items related to the findings of physical assessment.

To assess different types of wounds and stomas, various kits and overlays can be purchased or made by using cut-outs from pictures/scans or making the wound from felt or other supplies.

This list of ideas is not exhaustive. Instructors need to be creative and use imagination in creating the effect that they want to be assessed. As students become more comfortable and confident in their assessment abilities and recognition of the various sounds or assessment findings, another step in the development of critical thinking and decision-making can be made. Now the student may begin to place more of the pieces together, to infer patient problems and nursing diagnoses, and even to think about the types of actions that might be encountered in the particular situation.

Equipment Skills

Simulation also allows the development of technical and cognitive skills needed for initiating, using, and discontinuing various types of equipment encountered in the clinical arena. Simulation provides the student with a realistic situation or scenario to practice or even test certain skills and equipment. For example, a student may need to initiate an intravenous catheter and infuse fluids. Rather than performing this skill on an intravenous arm, the student has the opportunity to initiate the intravenous catheter and infuse the fluids on a simulator that resembles a realistic patient. Another skill that can be practiced is inserting, monitoring, and discontinuing a urinary catheter. Once again, simulation provides for a realistic opportunity to practice on a simulator that is breathing, with eyes blinking, and possibly talking (through microphone and speaker) as the student performs the skill.

Tracheostomy care and suctioning are two other equipment-related skills that can be performed through simulation. The simulator can be adapted so that a tracheostomy can be inserted. Then the student can be shown and taught the techniques, followed by practice sessions. The manipulation of the equipment and the steps to follow for each procedure are quite cumbersome to the student initially. But, after practicing the techniques, the student becomes more comfortable and is much more confident when performing the technique on a real patient. Models are available for students to practice tracheostomy care and suctioning; however, it is more realistic to allow the student to perform these skills on a simulator that is actually breathing. A disadvantage to using simulation for tracheostomy care and suctioning is that the simulator does not have the cough reflex like a normal patient. Therefore, to make the simulation more realistic, one may need to use the microphone and speaker capability.

Chest tube monitoring and care are challenges for any nursing student, but simulation should assist in making sense of the management of a patient with a chest tube. A chest tube can be inserted into the simulator, and the drainage product will drain into the attached drainage chamber. With a chest tube inserted and the simulator running, the student has the opportunity to perform chest tube care that is definitely more realistic than care performed on a chest model into which a chest tube has been inserted but does not produce drainage or simulate breathing. In addition, the simulator is able to produce various amounts of air leaks while the chest tube is connected to the drainage chamber and suction. This addition to teaching about chest tubes and drainage systems is invaluable since in most case air leaks are demonstrated and explained at the bedside.

As the student's skills and knowledge become more advanced, the scenarios for simulation can be made progressively more complex, requiring implementation of numerous assessments, skills, and actions. The continual progression and increasing complexity allow continual development of the student's critical thinking and decision-making skills.

Pathopharmacology Concepts

The pathopharmacologic effects of medications are another area that can be demonstrated with the simulator. The simulator can be used at a basic level to show the pharmacologic effects and length of actions of medications in a normal patient. For example, if epinephrine is administered, the instructor may ask the students what they would expect to see. Next, the medication can be administered so that the effects can be visualized and experienced. In this case, an increase in heart rate and blood pressure is seen when epinephrine is administered.

If a more complex learning objective is desired, the pathophysiology of various disease states may be introduced. Simulation provides a unique opportunity to program and experience the physiology of a disease state and then allow administration of various medications to observe their effects on the disease. For example, a patient who is hypotensive and possibly experiencing an acute myocardial infarction may present with a supraventricular tachycardia on the electrocardiograph. The learning objective might be to compare and contrast the pharmacologic mechanisms of a calcium channel blocker, such as diltiazem, and a beta blocker, such as metoprolol, when they are administered to this type of patient.

To meet the objective, the simulation scenario should be run twice: once to experience the effect of the administration of a calcium channel blocker, and again to experience the effect of the beta blocker. During the scenario, the students can experience and assess the pathophysiologic components of a hypotensive patient with myocardial infarction. The selection of a medication can be made. The pharmacologic effects of the medication can be discussed before or after administration. In either case, the student can experience the effects of the medication without compromising or putting a real patient in jeopardy. When metoprolol is administered in this scenario, the patient's heart rate begins to slow, but the patient also becomes more hypotensive or even suffers increased cardiovascular compromise or possible cardiopulmonary arrest. On the other hand, when diltiazem is administered, the patient's heart rate begins to slow, but the same degree of hypotension as with metoprolol does not occur.

For the more advanced student or the student rotating through the critical care units, the simulator provides an excellent way to experience the physiologic effects of continuous infusions of vasoactive medications. In the critical care setting, one has access to more assessment data from a patient's hemodynamic parameters obtained from a pulmonary artery catheter. When using simulation and administering vasoactive medications, one can observe the effects of the medication on cardiac output, cardiac index, systemic vascular resistance, blood pressure, pulmonary artery pressures, and pulmonary capillary wedge pressures. Next, the pathophysiology of a disease state can be created and introduced, and the student can see the physiologic effects of the medication on this type of patient.

Critical Care Monitoring Techniques

Teaching critical care concepts and principles is often challenging and difficult in nursing education because not every student experiences a clinical situation of what is being taught. The simulator is an excellent teaching tool and learning method to coincide with content.

Hemodynamic monitoring can be taught and observed on the simulator. In the past, educators have had to use posters or monitor simulators to produce the various waveforms. Fortunately, the simulator accomplishes the same goal and is able to simulate the waveforms, which students can visualize on a simulator that is breathing. Once the basics of hemodynamics have been taught, the complexities of pathophysiologic effects of various disease states and the pharmacologic effects on hemodynamics can be explored.

Ventilator management is another content area that can be taught and experienced on the simulator. The simulator can be intubated and placed on a ventilator. Next, the aspects, modes, and settings of the ventilator can be explained. Finally, once the student becomes comfortable with the simulated patient on the ventilator, different troubleshooting scenarios can be implemented to challenge the student's critical thinking and decision-making skills. Along with ventilatory management, neuromuscular blocking agents can be administered and a peripheral nerve stimulator can be used to assess the adequacy of the amount of medication that has been administered or is continuously infused.

Mock Codes and Advanced Cardiac Life Support

Simulation is an effective strategy and tool for teaching advanced cardiac life support (ACLS) and running mock cardiopulmonary resuscitations. Simulation for ACLS provides the participant with a scenario that appears very realistic and allows the team leader and the team to assess and intervene. The team members can administer appropriate medications, intubate, ventilate, perform chest compressions, and defibrillate with the appropriate joules as needed. Simulation is definitely an excellent realistic tool since a team can perform its various functions and the scenario can be developed to progress as needed to meet the learning objectives for ACLS.

Research has shown that with the passage of time, there is a deterioration of knowledge and skills of ACLS. Therefore, mock resuscitations should be performed routinely practice skills that might have been forgotten.

Developing a Virtual Hospital Experience

The basic purposes of developing the virtual hospital are to expose nursing students to a simulated clinical experience that allows them to exercise basic nursing skills, such as assessment and medication administration, and to challenge the students' critical thinking skills through a critical event that may occur to their patient at some point.

The virtual hospital should contain all of the necessary equipment and supplies that are normally found in the clinical setting. Besides the simulator, supplies should include such items as bar-coded syringes for medication administration, IV solution, and oxygen delivery devices.

Patient scenarios need to be developed according to the educational objectives that have been identified. For example, patients can be developed with the following medical diagnoses: exacerbation of chronic obstructive pulmonary disease with possible pneumonia; exertional angina and possible myocardial infarction; exacerbation of congestive heart failure; pelvic fracture and possible pulmonary embolus; thoracotomy exploration for chest stab wound; temporal contusion with loss of consciousness; sickle cell crisis; postoperative cholecystectomy patient with an allergy to a medication administered; and acute ischemic stroke patient after administration of recombinant tissue plasminogen activator (r-tPA). The patient scenarios should be based on clinical case studies that are relevant to subject matter to which the students have been or will be exposed throughout the semester. The length of time for the patient simulation can vary, but it is recommended that the scenario be for 2–4 hours in length. The reasoning is that the simulated experience should mimic a clinical experience the student can have in the hospital setting. The programming of the scenarios should be based on the patient's underlying disease and comorbidities, the time frame, and any other factors that may be included in the learning objectives, such as the occurrence of a critical event.

The virtual hospital should be created to be as realistic as possible, including forming and assembling a patient chart. Patient charts should contain categories of pertinent data such as orders, vital signs, medications, progress notes, nursing notes, and lab results. Flowsheets should be available so that the student can chart the relevant assessments, vital signs, nursing notes, and medication administration. Physician orders should be fashioned according to the patient's condition and should contain physician's order information such as patient diagnosis, allergies, vital sign frequency, intake and output, notification of physician of abnormal parameters, activity, diet, lab results or tests, and medications. Depending on the learning objectives, some of the physician orders may contain some erroneous medications as a vital check to see how observant and meticulous the student would be in the delivery of care to the patient. For example, in some simulations, students have actually administered a neuromuscular blocking agent because they misread the order and did not adequately look up the medication before administration.

Because human patient simulators are used primarily for a critical care environment, the bedside monitor that displays the hemodynamic readings should be adjusted to display the hemodynamic variables of the simulated patient. For the virtual hospital, all simulated patients have an arterial pressure tracing (which provides the student with a blood pressure reading) and a pulse oximeter value. An electrocardiograph tracing is provided for patients requiring telemetry. Simulated patients should also be given a hospital identification band and dressed in a hospital gown, just like actual patients in a hospital setting. Thus, throughout the preparation and creation of the simulated patient scenarios, the charts, and the environment, the student will receive a virtual hospital experience.

Prior to the actual clinical date for the virtual hospital experiences, students should receive an orientation packet, which contains such items as directions to the simulation lab, generic chart forms, and assignment information to be submitted after the experience. Depending on the learning objectives for this exercise, the student might be given the type of patient before coming to the virtual hospital experience. Sometimes the student receives no information about any of the patients or types of patients that they will encounter during their upcoming experience. The rationale for not giving the student information before the experience may be an attempt to duplicate a real-life experience of receiving a new patient in the acute care setting.

For the virtual hospital experience to be totally effective, the student should receive an orientation to the physical layout of the virtual nursing unit, basic functioning of the human patient simulator (location of best chest auscultation points, technique for medication administration), patient chart components, and an introduction to the key health care providers (physician, charge nurse). The roles of the physician and the charge nurse need to be assigned; depending on the level of the learner. These roles might need to be assigned to faculty or graduate students, if available. After the orientation to the virtual hospital setting, students should be given their patient assignments and proceed to work with the simulated patient. The students should review the patient charts, look up any information that they believe is needed, assess the patient to get a baseline status, acknowledge physician orders, and initiate charting.

If the learning objective for the virtual hospital is to challenge the students' critical thinking skills through a critical event, it is crucial that the developed scenario contain a critical event. The purpose of the critical event should be to observe the student's critical thinking abilities and response when they are put in a situation that became tenuous and possibly life-threatening if appropriate intervention does not ensue. One of the easiest critical events to develop is a respiratory event that may or may not lead to a compromise. Sometimes the critical event may be programmed into the scenario, whereas at other times the event might be caused by some action that the student performed. For example, when the student inadvertently administers a neuromuscular blocking agent, the simulator will stop breathing and respiratory compromise ensues. In some instances, the student may not have been previously exposed to any such event and will require coaching throughout. In the case of inadvertently administering a neuromuscular blocking agent, it is necessary for the student to make an astute assessment that the patient has stopped breathing and that the pulse oximeter reading is beginning to decrease. At that point, it is necessary to ventilate the simulator manually with an ambu bag. Sometimes the student performs this action automatically, but at other times the student needs to be told and coached on what appropriate actions need to take place. At the time of coaching and assisting in the management of the critical event, the student should perform an analysis of the situation and feedback should be given to the student. Hopefully, the student will realize the mistake that was made, and either a reversal agent can be administered or the patient can be intubated. The student will need to support the ventilations by manually ventilating the patient simulator with oxygen until the medication has been metabolized and the simulator begins to breathe spontaneously. In other cases, the outcome may be the least desirable, resulting in the expiration of the simulated patient.

Nurse Anesthesia Education

Alfred E. Lupien, PhD, CRNA

Approximately half of all anesthesia providers in the United States are certified registered nurse anesthetists (CRNAs). Nurse anesthetists practice both as members of anesthesia care teams and as sole providers of anesthesia care. The scope of practice for CRNAs includes preanesthetic assessment; administration of general, regional, and local anesthesia; insertion of invasive monitoring devices; and emergency resuscitation.[10]

To become a CRNA, a registered nurse must possess a minimum of a baccalaureate degree, have at least one year of acute- or critical-care nursing experience, complete a program of graduate study accredited by the Council on Accreditation of Nurse Anesthesia Education Programs (COA), and successfully complete a certifying examination administered by the Council on Certification of Nurse Anesthetists (CCNE).

Nurse anesthesia programs range in length between 24 and 36 months of full-time study. Specific content areas for didactic study and clinical experience are jointly defined by the COA and CCNE[11] (Table 1). Formats for nurse anesthesia programs are

Table 1.
Selected Minimum Requirements for Accredited Nurse Anesthesia Educational Programs

Coursework*	Requirement
Pharmacology	105 hours
Anatomy, physiology, and pathophysiology	135 hours
Anesthesia practice principles	105 hours

Clinical experiences†	Requirement
Geriatric patient	100 cases
Pediatric patient	35 cases
Obstetric patient	30 cases
Intracranial surgery	5 cases
Intrathoracic surgery	15 cases
Vascular procedure	10 cases
Subarachnoid anesthesia/analgesia	15 procedures
Epidural anesthesia/analgesia	15 procedures
Central venous catheter	5 procedures
Fiberoptic intubation	5 procedures

*Abridged from Standard III.C14.
†Abridged from Standard III.C17.

generally categorized either as "front loaded" with 6 to 12 months of classroom study followed by a clinical component or as "integrated" with didactic content and clinical experience intertwined throughout the program.

In 2001, Wren described three stages of learning for nurse anesthetists: (1) establishing a framework for practice based on principles of physiology, pathophysiology, and pharmacology; (2) the translation of principles into practice; and (3) the development of comfort, confidence, and finesse.[12] Applications of simulation in nurse anesthesia education can be divided into three types of activities (preclinical, transitional, and clinical) that generally parallel Wren's stages. Although the activities are presented sequentially in this chapter, as they might be introduced in a front-loaded curriculum, the same strategies can be implemented in an integrated curriculum.

Preclinical Experiences

Nurses entering graduate school to become nurse anesthetists are required to be experienced acute- and critical-care nurses. Clinical laboratory sessions using simulation focused on the respiratory and cardiovascular systems provide opportunities for the students to build on their knowledge of physiology and pharmacology and to gain additional insight that will be essential in their new roles as nurse anesthetists. Themes for laboratory sessions include respiratory dynamics with pressure/volume and flow/volume loops, modes of ventilation, and effects of vasoactive infusions. The precision with which patient variables can be manipulated is a particular benefit of using screen-based simulators (such as Anesthesia Simulator 2202, Anesoft Corporation, Issaquah, Washington) or mannequin-based high-fidelity simulators (such as the Human Patient

Simulator, Medical Education and Technologies, Inc., Sarasota, Florida) for these experiments in lieu of laboratory animals or lower-fidelity simulators. For example, individual respiratory resistances and compliances can be isolated to examine their influence on flow/volume or pressure/volume loops.

Simulation can also be used to explore specific aspects of anesthetic management of patients with cardiovascular disease, such as the effects of intravascular volume on patients with valvular lesions.[13] Following baseline measurements, a lesion (such as aortic stenosis) is introduced and hemodynamic parameters are observed as fluid volume is increased in 500-ml increments. Parameters to be measured include heart rate, arterial systolic and diastolic pressures, central venous pressure, pulmonary artery systolic and diastolic pressures, systemic vascular resistance, pulmonary vascular resistance, right and left ventricular stroke work, and cardiac output. Progressive changes in cardiac function are plotted as the relationship between left ventricular stroke work (or cardiac output) and pulmonary artery occlusion pressure (Frank-Starling curve). Once cardiac overload has been demonstrated, the simulated patient is returned to the baseline state and the experiment is repeated as fluid is withdrawn incrementally. To solidify the students' understanding of the relationship between fluid status and cardiac pathology, this same experiment can be conducted across the spectrum of stenotic and regurgitant lesions. The effect of administering various vasoactive medications can be demonstrated in a similar fashion. The combination of lecture plus mannequin-based high-fidelity simulation has been demonstrated to be more effective than instruction by lecture alone.[14]

Although identical experiments can be conducted using screen-based simulation, inclusion of the mannequin appears to keep students more engaged in the activity and has the additional benefits of requiring the students to mimic the activities that they would implement at the bedside (e.g., occlusion of the pulmonary artery balloon and administration of the thermodiluent) and reinforces the notion that these same techniques (such as the plotting of ventricular function curves) can be implemented with the standard monitoring equipment available in most clinical facilities.

Simulation can also be used to provide students with experience in monitoring techniques with which they are less familiar. Depending on each nurse's clinical background, capnography may be a monitoring modality that has never been used or used only with cursory understanding. The following exercise illustrates how mannequin-based simulation can be used to highlight the monitoring of respiratory function, with particular emphasis on end-tidal capnography.

Before the exercise students receive classroom instruction covering modalities for monitoring respiratory function. In a laboratory setting, students are provided the opportunity to manipulate the breathing circuit to observe the effects of variables such as incompetent one-way valves in the patient breathing circuit, carbon dioxide absorbent exhaustion, and rebreathing of respiratory gases on the capnographic waveform.

The exercise begins with a simulated patient with complete neuromuscular blockade and properly placed endotracheal tube. In the first phase of the exercise, students are asked to identify all available sources of information providing data about the patient's oxygenation and ventilation (such as chest excursion, breath sounds, in-line spirometer, inspiratory pressure manometer, pulse oximeter, capnographic waveform, end-tidal carbon dioxide, in-line oxygen monitor, and inspiratory pressure alarm on the ventilator). For the second phase of the exercise, the students are instructed to advance the tracheal tube into a mainstem bronchus and observe the patient for approximately five minutes while noting which patient and monitoring parameters change as well as the rate of change.

Changes to certain measures are predictable. For example, chest excursion and peak inspiratory pressure change immediately; changes in breath sounds depend on the site selected for auscultation; and hemoglobin saturation, as measured through pulse oximetry, may fall slowly, depending on the concentration of inspired oxygen used for the experiment. The inspired concentration of oxygen, as monitored in the inspiratory limb of the breathing circuit, will not change.

Drawing from their critical-care nursing experience and knowledge of physiology, students also anticipate hypercarbia. When experience with capnography has been limited, the fall in end-tidal carbon dioxide tension and attenuation of the capnographic waveform associated with endobronchial intubation are often unanticipated and appear paradoxical. The final phase of the exercise is a debriefing in which the characteristics of each monitoring modality are discussed. Capnographic waveform changes are an essential component of the debriefing session with particular attention to differences between arterial and end-tidal tensions of respiratory gases, factors that influence the relationship between arterial and end-tidal carbon dioxide measures, and the tenuous assumptions that must be valid before accepting the clinical "factoid" that end-tidal carbon dioxide tensions vary directly with arterial carbon dioxide levels.

Transition to Clinical Practice

Partial-task trainers, virtual reality devices, screen-based simulators, and mannequin-based simulators can be used to facilitate the transition from classroom to clinical practice. Partial-task trainers include upper torso mannequins to practice techniques for the placement of needles into the subarachnoid and epidural spaces. Virtual reality devices such as the AccuTouch Endoscopy Simulator (Immersion Medical, Gaithersburg, Maryland) enable the student to practice the psychomotor skills and identification of anatomic landmarks necessary for fiberoptic inspection of the trachea and fiberoptic intubation. Screen-based simulators provide opportunities to practice decision-making and management of emergent clinical situations. Mannequin-based high-fidelity simulators enable students to combine the technical elements learned through partial-task training with the dynamic interactive environment of screen-based simulators.

Perhaps one of the most comprehensive examples of using mannequin-based high-fidelity simulation is a compilation of exercises designed to introduce students to the steps for induction, maintenance, and emergence from general anesthesia. The expeditious and safe induction of general anesthesia requires the sequencing of psychomotor and cognitive tasks to include equipment preparation, the application of patient monitors, determination that physiologic and environmental conditions have been opitimized and are acceptable, preoxygenation, administration of induction agents, establishment of a patent airway, administration of paralytic agents, proper insertion of airway devices, evaluation of hemodynamic responses to induction, and a transition to the maintenance phase of the anesthetic. During the maintenance phase, anesthetic and paralytic agents are titrated in response to physiologic data, physical signs, and surgical considerations. Emergence activities include the sequencing of tasks associated with the determination of readiness for the return to consciousness; reversal, redistribution, or elim-

Table 2.
Simulation Themes Associated with Teaching the Administration of General Anesthesia

Topics	Simulator type
Basic airway management	Partial-task trainer
Introduction to ASA difficult airway algorithm	Mannequin-based
Operation of anesthesia machine and ventilator	Not applicable
Induction of general anesthesia	Screen-based simulator
	Mannequin-based
Uptake and distribution of anesthetic agents	Screen-based simulator
Maintenance of general anesthesia	Screen-based simulator
	Mannequin-based simulator
Management of common intraoperative problems	Screen-based simulator
	Mannequin-based simulator
Emergence from general anesthesia and tracheal extubation	Mannequin-based simulator

ination of anesthetic agents; removal of airway devices; assessing readiness for transfer from the operating room; and physical transfer of the patient to the postanesthetic care unit. Virtually all of these tasks and decisions can be practiced in the safety of the simulated environment. Example of the simulation modalities and exercises that are combined to teach basic management of general anesthesia are listed in Table 2. Given the range of simulation modalities and increasing availability of access to mannequin-based simulators, it is becoming increasingly difficult to justify a learner gaining initial experiences with common procedures using living patients rather than simulators.

During the transition from classroom learning to clinical practice, emphasis is placed on performance when anesthesia care progresses according to plan: concepts from reading or classroom lecture are clarified; sequences of activities are rehearsed; and readiness to progress from artificial to real clinical practice is confirmed. Outcomes of this phase should include increased confidence of both student and instructor and an ability to complete fundamental activities expediently. Successful completion of the transitional phase allows the student and preceptor to focus attention on the patient and the current clinical moment/situation rather than task achievement.

Building Clinical Experiences

In addition to the sequencing of skills and decisions associated with the management of "best-case" scenarios, simulation provides a safe environment for gaining experience in identifying and responding to critical events, both common (such as bronchospasm or myocardial ischemia) and uncommon (such as malignant hyperthermia or fire in the operating room). Textbooks, such as Crisis Management in Anesthesiology,[15] provide a reference point from which narrowly focused anesthetic management plans can be expanded to incorporate potential and unanticipated events. However, a comprehensive compendium of events, differential diagnoses, and management guidelines cannot place an event into the context of a specific clinical case. For example, even the relatively common event of hypovolemia caused by surgical blood loss generates a myriad of questions that are situation-dependent:

◆ What clinical signs or symptoms will prompt treatment: heart rate, blood pressure, EKG changes, decreasing hemoglobin, reduced SpO_2, or reaching the allowable blood loss?
◆ At what threshold would treatment be initiated: a heart rate greater than 120 beats/minute, blood pressure less than 20% of baseline, or a hemoglobin less than 8 gm/dl?
◆ What are the potential treatment options: crystalloids, plasma expanders, heterologous blood products, hemodilution, autologous transfusion, or vasopressors?
◆ What criteria will define successful resolution of the hypovolemia?
◆ How will it be determined whether the treatment should be continued or changed?

Through either screen- or mannequin-based simulation and guidance from faculty, the beginning practitioner can develop reasoning skills that can be integrated into clinical practice.

Simulation can also be used to create external events that all anesthesia providers should be prepared to manage. A contaminated oxygen source is an easy event to create by cross-splicing the oxygen and nitrous oxide hoses connecting the anesthesia workstation to its wall gas sources. The clinical scenario might begin with the anesthetist being called to the obstetric suite to provide general anesthesia for an emergent cesarean section (unaware that oxygen and nitrous oxide pipelines were inadvertently cross-connected during a recent renovation of the delivery room). Questions to be addressed with the learner during or after the simulation include:

◆ Could the contaminated oxygen source be detected during an equipment check?
◆ If the contaminated oxygen source is undetected before initiation of anesthesia care, what patient monitors should provide cautionary information once the case begins?
◆ How are manifestations of the problem affected by choices about the induction of general anesthesia (e.g., "routine" preoxygenation, preoxygenation with forced vital capacity breaths, skipped preoxygenation, maintenance with "pure" oxygen vs. oxygen with air or oxygen with nitrous oxide)?
◆ How would the problem manifest during regional anesthesia with the administration of supplemental oxygen through a high-flow mask vs. simple facemask or nasal prongs?

The second major goal of simulation in the clinical phase of instruction is to promote increased situational awareness, enhanced dynamic decision making, and effective resource management. Situational awareness is defined as the ability to maintain a comprehensive perspective of the clinical situation in its overall context, recognize developing problems, anticipate future developments, and focus team activities on optimal outcomes for the patient. Essential skills include the abilities to sustain vigilance, allocate attention, set priorities, utilize resources effectively, distribute workload, communicate effectively, and re-evaluate continuously the evolving situation.[15–18] Improved resource management and communication skills have been documented in first-year nurse anesthesia graduate students after only limited exposure to mannequin-based simulation and debriefing.[19]

The principles of situational awareness and resource management can be integrated into simulation experiences either through a formalized course, such as Anesthesia

Crisis Resource Management,[20] or reinforcement of Fletcher's ERR WATCH[17] principle during case-based simulation sessions. The ERR WATCH principles are as follows:

E = **E**nvironment
R = **R**esources
R = **R**e-evaluate
W= **W**orkload
A = **A**ttention
T = **T**eamwork
C = **C**ommunication
H = **H**elp

The following exercise in total electrical failure illustrates how the concept of resource management is incorporated into a simulation-based case study.[21] Although complete electrical failure in the operating room is an uncommon event, it is significant because it requires the anesthesia provider to assess the situation rapidly, understand his or her equipment, be aware of available resources, and manage the resources effectively. Because electrical failure is occasionally described in the literature, it is possible to draw from these experiences as part of the case study. Preparation for the simulation involves the following steps:

◆ Review the literature to identify circumstances and contributing factors that lead to power failure, problems that arose as a result of the failure, problem-solving and resource management techniques used during the failure, and lessons learned from the experience.
◆ Explore operating characteristics for all equipment to be used during the simulation to determine their reliance on electrical power (pneumatic power vs. electrical power, battery back-up for device operation vs. battery back-up for alarms only).
◆ Modify the environment to facilitate the scenario. Windows may be covered to create a "black-out" condition and temperature controls disabled at the moment of the electrical failure.
◆ Implement the scenario.
◆ Include in the debriefing session an examination of the participants' performance, integration of findings from the literature, and the development of a framework for how to respond in a comparable situation.

Well-constructed case studies can be videotaped and catalogued for repeated use.

Simulation and Evaluation

One of the most essential benefits of simulation is the opportunity to provide real-time and/or retrospective formative evaluation of student performance in a safe and controlled environment. Beyond its use as an educational tool, patient stimulators are used with increasing frequency to provide summative evaluation to be used for various purposes, including technical competency,[18,22] readiness to assume greater levels of responsibility (such as night call),[23] and readiness to re-enter clinical practice.[24] For the moment, the use of simulation to judge performance is somewhat controversial, although accumulating data suggest that mannequin-based simulation can differentiate provider abilities when measured with valid and reliable instruments.[25]

Practical Issues Associated With Simulation

The examples used in this chapter reflect two distinct approaches to simulation. Simulation involving clinical scenarios intended to mimic actual operating room conditions may require props and additional personnel to create a realistic environment. Participants are expected to suspend reality and enter into the new simulated reality. During the assimilation session, emphasis is placed on participant decisions and actions. The role of the faculty is to create the clinical context and then subtly control the scenario as it unfolds. The sessions are frequently recorded, and post-event debriefing is essential.

The second approach to simulation is more abstract and experimental. The suspension of reality is less important in this environment, which can be described as more like a laboratory than a clinical setting. Fewer personnel and supplies are needed to support the session under most circumstances. Faculty may become an integral part of the simulation by modeling skills and thought processes, directing actions, or focusing student thoughts. Debriefing may be simultaneous with the activity or may occur afterward.

The extent to which mannequin-based simulation can be integrated into the curriculum depends on a number of factors, including the availability of simulators and the number of students to be accommodated. Simulation experiences may be a one-time opportunity to practice an induction sequence in preparation for initial clinical experiences, occasional sessions focusing on specific learning objectives, intense multiday sessions focused on resource management, or frequent ongoing sessions. In a simulation-intense curriculum, each student may spend 75–100 hours in simulated environments before the first clinical day.

The number of students that can be accommodated simultaneously during a simulation varies depending on the intended outcomes of the session. For demonstrations of physiologic or pharmacologic principles, the number of learners may be limited only by the ability to keep the students intellectually involved in the exercise. Groups of four to six students, with some people taking on supporting roles, may be optimal for clinical scenarios involving resource management and communications. Critical thinking exercises can be implemented successfully with similarly sized groups. Groups of two to four students may be preferred when sessions are focused on learning technical skills and procedural sequences.

Faculty time commitment increases substantially as the number of learners increases and simulation become more integrated into the curriculum. A three-tier approach defines faculty involvement with simulation sessions:

1. *Directly precepted activities* require continuous faculty presence, usually with groups of four to six students and one faculty member, although the groups may be subdivided into pairs for practicing hands-on skills. Formative evaluation from faculty occurs in real time, and a student "buddy" may be included to monitor the learner's progress and provide correction as needed.

2. *Faculty-available sessions* typically involve discrete assignments, such as critical thinking exercises. A faculty member is designated to be available as needed but is not present throughout the session. The faculty member meets with the student group at the end of the session to validate findings and clarify remaining questions.

3. During *open laboratory sessions,* students working in groups of at least two can reserve simulator time to work unsupervised toward specified goals. Available simulator time can be increased by employing one or more graduate teaching assistants to keep

the laboratory open during extended hours. Debriefing and clarification of concepts after these more informal sessions is delayed and likely to be less extensive.

Conclusion

Simulation can be used to create a safe and effective learning environment for nurse anesthesia students. Activities may include clinical laboratory sessions, the rehearsal of technical skills, or exercises to refine decision-making and resource management skills. Faculty resources can be conserved by carefully matching faculty participation with the requirements for each specific session. For simulation to be used at peak benefit, the following adage can be applied to all simulated learning experiences: "Practice does not make perfect; *perfect* practice makes perfect."

High-Fidelity Simulation Across Clinical Settings and Educational Levels

Sheena Ferguson, Lorena Beeman, Mary Eichorn, Yolanda Jaramillo, and Mary Wright

Clinical educators are challenged with the need to identify and develop teaching modalities that facilitate the transition of the student/staff member from novice to expert, that are congruent with the learner's level of expertise, and that also foster critical thinking. The purpose of this section is to describe the use of high-fidelity simulation technology that can facilitate experiential learning and positively impact patient care in the clinical setting.

Background

Clinical care often requires rapid critical thinking in response to changing patient dynamics within an environment where the margin for error is limited. Creating educational opportunities that facilitate experiential learning is problematic. Limitations have included the inability to create realistic simulations that incorporate real-time critical thinking under pressure.

In the early 1980s, Patricia Benner conceptualized a skill acquisition model for critical care nurses founded on clinical experiences acquired over time in conjunction with the development of critical thinking in relation to the patient and clinical setting. It has been called Benner's Novice to Expert model of clinical development.[26-27]

At our facility, we have operationalized this model as a framework for tiering educational experiences provided to clinical care providers. Educational offerings are structured in a three-tiered program. Level one incorporates the Advanced Beginner to the Competent level. Course content for the Advanced Beginner is structured to achieve the following goals:

1. Development of a disease trajectory
2. Provision of a checklist of key assessment components for a patient population and/or disease process

3. Recognition of signs of patient deterioration or compromise within the disease trajectory or patient population

Course content for the Competent is predicated on the achievements of the Advanced Beginner with modifications in content and teaching methodology to achieve the following goals:

1. Initial development of critical thinking skills
2. Examples of how to present a case to a physician or other clinician
3. Individualization of the disease trajectory to a given patient
4. Recognition and reward of examples of successes to promote involvement in patient caring vs. technology (The objective is to prevent the nurse from becoming experienced but not expert.)
5. Provision of examples of best practices to prevent disillusionment

The second level of the program is predicated on the first level and involves clinical progression from Competent to Proficient. Course content and teaching methodologies are formulated to achieve the following goals:

1. Evidence-based practices
2. Ethical decision-making
3. Individualization of clinician application of the nursing process
4. Case studies facilitating the process of content plus context

The third level of the program involves clinical progression from Proficient to Expert. Once again, this level is predicated on the former levels but also recognizes the experiences that nurses at this level have acquired over time. Course content and teaching methodologies change to reflect acquisition of knowledge and skill. The educational opportunities within this level are designed to achieve the following goals:

1. Case studies involving multiple complexities
2. Case studies involving bioethical dilemmas and conflicts
3. Critical care challenges and puzzles
4. Demonstration of critical thinking skills through experiential learning

Within the second and third levels of skill and knowledge progression the use of the human simulator as a teaching and learning modality is best operationalized. At these levels, the nurse has a working understanding of anatomy and physiology, pathophysiology, and critical thinking, all of which are essential to optimize the effective utilization of this teaching modality.

Problem: Pulmonary Program

Needs assessment and clinical queries within the three critical care units at our facility revealed a knowledge and experiential deficit related to complex physiology and superimposed pathophysiology. One example is the pulmonary program (but the principles are easily applicable to any system): acute severe asthma, acute respiratory distress syndrome, and chronic obstructive pulmonary disease (COPD) with superimposed type II acute respiratory failure. The use of pulmonary calculations and ventilator graphics to optimize care of the patient on the ventilator were needed for our adult intensive care units.

In order to provide the content and experiential learning to address this problem, it was believed that the a full-body human simulator could be used to simulate the pathophysiology of each pulmonary state and, in so doing, interface with the attached ventilator to provide real-time conceptual reinforcement of didactic content (i.e., pulmonary calculations and ventilator graphics). In addition, patient compromise potentially associated with each of these states could be transitioned into the program. This approach allows the nurse to demonstrate critical thinking and interventions in action.

Description of Critical Care Program Development (Pulmonary Tier)

With interdisciplinary collaboration between critical care nursing and respiratory therapy, an interactive program was developed that consists of three phases. The first phase provides interactive didactic content and discussion related to pulmonary physiology and mechanical ventilation. This phase is provided by the critical care nurse educator. The second phase provides a detailed overview of pulmonary calculations and changes in ventilator graphics related to pulmonary pathophysiology and/or developing complications. The second phase is provided by an expert respiratory therapist. The third phase is experiential learning involving the participants and the full body human simulator. This last phase involves interaction with the simulator coordinator, the respiratory therapist, and the critical care nurse educator.

Application for approval to utilize the simulator in this capacity is approved by the Simulation Education Subcommittee, which is interdisciplinary and multispecialty in scope. This process facilitates and ensures the accuracy, validity, and representation of the simulations. It also prevents "reinvention of the wheel" since many departments see simulation exercises surrounding major categories of crises intervention. Table 1 outlines the programming changes made to simulate the pulmonary pathophysiology for acute severe asthma. Transitions are based on the nurses' assessment and interventions for the "patient." The complication built into this scenario is the need for rapid-sequence intubation. The case scenario on which the simulation is based was taken from an actual patient. The point in time at which the nurses are expected to begin interaction with the simulation program is identical to the actual case. Thus, the nurses have the detailed history and other information given in Table 2. Based on the nurses' interventions (appropriate or inappropriate), the simulation can be transitioned to simulate the actual patient response. Table 3 provides the assessment checklist that is used for this scenario.

Two additional scenarios are also given to the course participants. The second scenario involves a patient with COPD with superimposed acute respiratory failure type II and the development of tension pneumothorax. (The tension pneumothorax is preventable if the nurses recognize the changes in lung sounds, ventilator pressures, pulmonary calculations, and/or ventilator graphics). The final scenario involves a patient with septic trauma and developing acute respiratory distress syndrome (ARDS). In this case, the development of ARDS is the complication. The nurses are expected to recognize the causative condition of trauma and begin assessment for other findings involved with the identification of this condition (i.e., increasing pulmonary pressures, decreasing pulmonary compliance, development of hypoxemia, bilateral chest infiltrates, pulmonary artery wedge pressure $\leq$ 18 mmHg, and a PaO_2/FiO_2 ratio $<$ 200).[29,30]

To provide a comprehensive experience for the critical care nurse participants, the course is restricted to twelve participants. The group is then divided into four nurses per scenario. As would be expected in the actual critical care setting, the nurses may interact with and assist each other, although one is voluntarily assigned the role of primary nurse.

Table 1.
Simulator Program for Acute Severe Asthma: Advanced Ventilator Strategies

Progression of Simulation	Programming of Simulator
Baseline: Man awake	1. Heart rate factor to 1.8 2. Respiratory rate override to 32 bpm 3. Eyes: Blink control–both blinking 4. Resistance factor: systemic vasculature to 3.0 5. Breath sounds to wheezing 6. Shunt fraction to 0.2
Transition 1: Patient deterioration	1. Heart rate factor to 2.3 2. Respiratory rate override to 36 bpm 3. Resistance factor: systemic vasculature to 4.0 4. Shunt fraction to 0.5
Transition 2: Rapid-sequence intubation (RSI)	If sedation and neuromuscular blockade is initiated: 1. Heart rate factor to 2.0 2. Respiratory rate override to 10 bpm 3. Eyes: blink control–closed 4. Shunt fraction to 0.2 over 3 min
Transition option 3a: RSI failure	Simulator operator will superimpose patient deterioration if need for RSI is not recognized or is performed inadequately, resulting in failed airway. 1. Rhythm will change to VF 2. Respiratory arrest
Transition option 3b: Successful RSI mechanical ventilation with high peak pressure	1. Right bronchial resistance to 305 cmH$_2$O/lpm at 20 lpm 2. Left bronchial resistance as above 3. Resistance factor: systemic to 3.51 over 2 minutes
Transition 4: Moderate peak pressures (if successful at ventilator programming) End scenario	1. Right bronchial resistance to 200 cmH$_2$O/lpm at 20 lpm 2. Left bronchial resistance as above

bpm = breaths per minute, lpm = liters per minute, cmH$_2$O = centimeters of water pressure.
Programmers: David Wilks, MD; Lorena E. Beeman, RN, BSN, MS; Joe Morales, BS, RRT.

Nurses taking this course may range from competent to proficient to expert, and this mix has several advantages. First, it allows the expert to mentor the other nurses; secondly, it facilitates the achievement of the goals for each level. The nurses not involved in the scenario observe the others and are then part of the debriefing process, led by the clinical nurse educator. The debriefing process provides reinforcement of core content.

Debriefing

Before the start of the human simulation scenarios, the nurses are informed of the process for debriefing. Essential components include confidentiality, professional courtesy and respect, and constructive commentary. Debriefing permits reinforcement of key points in decision-making for each scenario based on patient presentation, correction of mislearning, and further discussion. The critical care nurse educator is the moderator and must also keep the debriefing focused in terms of content and time management.

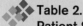

Table 2.
Patient Script Scenario for Acute Severe Asthma: Advanced Ventilator Strategies

Patient history
42-year-old Caucasian male
History of adult onset asthma 1994 following viral pneumonia
Has been intubated for acute severe asthma in the past
Nissen fundiplication 1997 for gastric esophageal reflux disease (GERD)
Hypertension (recent diagnosis)
Patient was seen in the asthma clinic for routine follow-up 4 days ago. No symptoms at that time, except nitric oxide (NO) level was increased.
Prednisone taper completed.
Patient developed viral symptoms (malaise, myalgia, low-grade temperature), decreasing peak flow, and wheezes the following day. Patient was again seen in the asthma clinic, where he received alternating albuterol and Atrovent nebulizer therapy to increase and maintain peak flow. The patient was sent home on every-4-hour treatment alternating albuterol and Atrovent nebulizer and was restarted on prednisone at 50 mg/day.
Patient developed fever spiking to 38.2°F two days ago, and was started on Bactrim DS twice daily. Peak flow dropped to under 150 approximately 1 hour ago (normally 300–350). Patient's wife called 911. Prior to paramedic arrival, the patient had completed 3 nebulizer treatments of 10 mg albuterol per treatment. (Treatments were back to back).

Paramedic report
Patient sitting upright, pale, diaphoretic.
Wheezes are audible, breath sounds decreased but present bilaterally.
Vital signs: blood pressure, 140/90; heart rate, 110; respiratory rate, 32 with use of accessory muscles with inhalation and exhalation.
IV started antecubitally, and 0.9% NS is infusing at 100 ml/hour.

Medications
Prednisone, 50 mg/day orally
Prilosec (omeprazole), 20 mg twice daily orally
Accolate (zafirlukast), 20 mg twice daily orally
Claritin (loratadine) 10 mg/day orally
Diovan (valsartan) 80 mg/day orally
Flovent (fluticasone proprionate,) 220 μg MDI 4 puffs 3 times/day
Serevent (salmeterol xinafoate) 21 μg MDI 2 puffs twice daily
Albuterol 2 puffs every 4–6 hours as needed

Direct admission to medical intensive care unit
Patient sitting upright on stretcher
Pale, diaphoretic
Patient anxious, oriented, unable to speak full sentences
Receiving albuterol 5 mg nebulizer treatment per mask
Using accessory muscles of breathing with inhalation and exhalation
Wheezes present with auscultation (not audible),and diminished breath sounds bilaterally.
Vital signs: blood pressure, 170/100; heart rate, 130; respiratory rate, 36–40 bpm, oxygen saturation, 78% on 10 L/mask.
Monitor shows sinus tachycardia with occasional PVCs
ABG results (Note: These are for high altitude): pH, 7.20; PaO_2, 45 mmHg; $PaCO_2$, 80 mmHg; HCO_3, 13 mEq/L; SaO_2 70%

Begin assessment and interventions
Patient assessments following above
Use of accessory muscles with inspiration and expiration; however, breath sounds are no longer audible with auscultation.

(continued)

Table 2.
   Patient Script Scenario for Acute Severe Asthma:
   Advanced Ventilator Strategies (*Continued*)

Patient assessments following above
   Patient is unable to speak.
   Less responsive to verbal commands.
   Vital signs: blood pressure, 180/100; heart rate, 140; respiratory rate, 10; oxygen saturation, 70%
Begin interventions
   Rapid-sequence intubation is expected at this point. Transition 3a or 3b, depending on interventions.
   Intubation successful and mechanical ventilation initiated. Nurses are expected to calculate pulmonary resistance,
      static compliance, and dynamic compliance and correlate with the pathophysiology.
   Ventilator mode, inspiratory time, expiratory time, flow rates, and adjuncts are to be programmed according to the
      pathophysiology.
   Changes in ventilator graphics correlating with the pathophysiology and response to ventilator programming are re-
      viewed.
End scenario and begin debriefing.
   PVCs = premature ventricular complexes, C = Centigrade, mmHg = millimeters of mercury.
   Developed by Lorena E. Beeman, RN, BSN, MS, CCVT.

Table 3.
   Performance Checklist for Acute Severe Asthma Scenario:
   Advanced Ventilator Strategies

Date: _____

Group: 1   2   3

Participants: _____
                _____
                _____
                _____

Performance Criteria	Acceptable	Remediation	Comments
Identification of key patient history information:			
a. Previous intubation	a. _____	a. _____	
b. Multiple triggers	b. _____	b. _____	
c. URI	c. _____	c. _____	
d. ↓ Peak flow	d. _____	d. _____	
e. Refractory to nebs	e. _____	e. _____	
Recognition of acute respiratory distress:			
a. Orthopneic	a. _____	a. _____	
b. Tachypneic	b. _____	b. _____	
c. ? O2 sat	c. _____	c. _____	
d. Use of accessory muscles	d. _____	d. _____	
e. Audible wheezes to inaudible with ↓ breath sounds	e. _____	e. _____	

(continued)

Table 3.
Performance Checklist for Acute Severe Asthma Scenario:
Advanced Ventilator Strategies (*Continued*)

Recognition of cardiovascular
compromise:
  a. Hypertension   a. _____   a. _____
  b. Tachycardia   b. _____   b. _____
  c. PVCs   c. _____   c. _____

Assessment of ABGs:
  a. Respiratory and metabolic acidosis   a. _____   a. _____
  b. Hypoxia   b. _____   b. _____

Interventions:
  a. Support oxygenation   a. _____   a. _____
  b. Solumedrol   b. _____   b. _____
  c. MgSO4   c. _____   c. _____
  d. Obtain K+   d. _____   d. _____
  e. Obtain lactate level   e. _____   e. _____
  f. Assess mentation   f. _____   f. _____

Recognize worsening respiratory
distress and need for intubation:
  a. Inaudible breath sounds   a. _____   a. _____
  b. ? Mentation   b. _____   b. _____
  c. Fall in RR   c. _____   c. _____

Rapid-sequence intubation:
  a. Prepare   a. _____   a. _____
  b. Preoxygenate   b. _____   b. _____
  c. Pretreat   c. _____   c. _____
  d. Paralysis with induction   d. _____   d. _____
  e. Protect   e. _____   e. _____
  f. Position   f. _____   f. _____
  g. Placement   g. _____   g. _____
  h. Proof of placement   h. _____   h. _____
  i. Secure tube   i. _____   i. _____

Postintubation management if
RSI recognized and successful
  a. Need for sedation/ analgesia   a. _____   a. _____
  b. Selection of mode   b. _____   b. _____
  c. Adjustment of I:E times   c. _____   c. _____
  d. Flow rates   d. _____   d. _____
  e. Assess lung sounds for tension
     pneumothorax   e. _____   e. _____
  f. ABGs   f. _____   f. _____
  g. Chest x-ray   g. _____   g. _____

Calculations and ventilator graphics:
  a. Resistance   a. _____   a. _____
  b. Compliance   b. _____   b. _____
  c. ID graphics showing ? resistance   c. _____   c. _____
  d. ID graphic showing development of auto-PEEP d. _____   d. _____

(continued)

Table 3.
Performance Checklist for Acute Severe Asthma Scenario:
Advanced Ventilator Strategies (*Continued*)

RSI not recognized or unsuccessful:

a. Ambu bag	a. _____	a. _____
b. Recognize failed airway (if RSI unsuccessful)	b. _____	b. _____
c. Appropriate ACLS	c. _____	c. _____
d. Reattempt intubation following difficult airway algorithm	d. _____	d. _____

URI = upper respiratory infection, nebs = nebulizer therapy, PVCs = premature ventricular complexes, ABGs = arterial blood gases, MgSO$_4$ = magnesium sulfate, K$^+$ = potassium, RR = respiratory rate, I:E = inspiratory-expiratory, PEEP = positive end-expiratory pressure, RSI = rapid sequence intubation, ACLS = advanced cardiac life support. Developed by Lorena E. Beeman, RN, BSN, MS, CCVT.

Description of Emergency Care Program Development (Advanced and Trauma Life Support)

Training of emergency care personnel has always been a problem due to logistic difficulties, access to teaching/training experts, and access to adequate facilities and various settings. In addition, freeing personnel to undergo training can be difficult. In order to mimic real life as closely as possible, a high-fidelity patient simulator can be used to train emergency care personnel. These full-body simulators can be used to teach students how to manage a wide variety of crises and provide practice of a wide variety of interventions. The authors maintain that the full impact of these experiences has yet to be achieved and that simulators are still underutilized. For the emergency department and prehospital crews, our facility has created simulations with ambulance and flight crews attending patients from the jump seats (bring the seats in from an old rig), in a night-time simulation (a darkened room with flashlight), and on a patient with copious emesis (simulated vomitus).

Our tiered curriculum has incorporated simulation into basic airway management courses and advanced rapid-sequence intubation and difficult airway management courses. Training is performed under a real-time constraint and is videotaped for later critique. The typical session takes approximately 20 minutes per scenario and another 30 minutes to debrief the participants about their actions and the results of those actions. Participants are encouraged to "think aloud" while in the scenario. During debriefing, the participants are asked to critique themselves, others in the team and the team as a whole. They are challenged to answer why they did (or did not do) what they did (or did not do) and to discuss their problem-solving aloud in a private room with the instructor and their team present. This process allows modeling and practice of critical thinking. Critical thinking can be defined as a process that challenges an individual to interpret and evaluate judgment: "self-consciously to monitor one's cognitive activities, the elements used in those activities, and the results educed, particularly by applying skills in analysis, and evaluation to one's own inferential judgments with a view toward questioning, confirming, validation, or correcting either one's reasoning or one's results." Appendix A outlines our simulation course for Advanced Cardiac Life Support.

Although this approach is an "expert" intensive method of training and does not allow large group participation, it provides direct evaluation of different skill levels and remediation of the emergency care provider. Typical passive lecture format does not take into account the different skill levels or evaluation of the individual and the team. Before the development of high-fidelity simulators, students would have learned these principles in a structured lecture, by animal experimentation in a physiology laboratory, or by observation in an intensive care unit. Implementation follows the basic-intermediate-advanced (novice-to-expert) tiered style of learning. The same scenario can be used to evaluate different abilities in various skill levels of personnel with different evaluations for each level of personnel. This approach fosters a sense of teamwork and diminishes participant anxiety about being held to unreasonably high performance criteria. The ultimate goal is clinical competence or the ability to use knowledge effectively and readily in order to perform a task and make decisions consistently and accurately, without direction. Used in this way, the full-body simulator provides an objective measurement of the student's ability to think critically and synthesize knowledge and skills for a particular critical health situation.

For example, a scenario can be designed to educate the basic level personnel in situations when trained paramedics are not available. The scene of the actual event (e.g., injury sustained following collapse of a building during an earthquake, injuries caused by fighting) can be transformed into a sequence involving evacuation and transfer to the level I facility, followed by subsequent stabilization and transfer to the critical care units. If the subsequent rehabilitation of the casualty is part of the training continuum, even a scenario of physical therapy and recovery can be included. Despite the questions that remain, it is certain that the ability to practice emergency skills with human patient simulators over and over in a safe environment will enable participants to achieve competency and confidence in practice. In addition, the opportunities presented for the objective measurement of knowledge, critical thinking abilities, and clinical skills guarantee the value of this technology for practitioners at all levels.

Description of Obstetric Program

Our facility uses both a full-body human simulator and simulators of mid-level fidelity that are obstetric-specific, depending on the objective to be simulated. Additional skills lab objectives (Appendix B) utilize specific task trainers, depending on the needs of the students. A particularly helpful aspect of simulation is the ability to include scenarios that are rarely and hopefully never witnessed. Our division of maternal/obstetric nursing uses the full-body simulator to demonstrate how to cope and comfort a distressed family as well as how to quantify blood loss in a postpartum hemorrhage scenario. The full-body simulator is converted to a female by use of a wig and a pregnant abdomen overlay to the stomach. The hemorrhaging uterus is a red fluid-soaked sponge in panty hose. Students are absolutely amazed to see the blood volume absorbed by "chux" or absorbent pads. Few can accurately assess blood loss, and this simulation identifies the inherent problems for the inexperienced clinician in doing so. Our series of simulations begins with the most routine cases and progresses to crisis management.

Obstetric Scenario

History. Jeanne, a 21-year-old G1P0 at 39 weeks' gestation, presented in the triage yesterday at 9:00 AM with spontaneous rupture of membranes (SROM) at 8:00 AM. Rupture of membranes was confirmed by sterile speculum exam (SSE) and positive ferning test. The cervix was closed per speculum exam. Jeanne reports feeling "menstrual-type cramping" and lower backache. The fetal monitor strip was reactive with baseline fetal heart rate (FHR) in the 140s. The prenatal course was normal except for slight anemia that was treated with iron supplementation. Prenatal labs: Blood type: O positive; rubella: immune; hepatitis B: negative; *Chlamydia* spp.: negative; group B streptococci: negative. Jeanne has an allergy to penicillin. Leopold's maneuvers confirmed a vertex presentation. All vital signs were in normal range.

Course of Labor. Jeanne ambulated the halls for several hours and was admitted to the birthing unit around 7:00 PM yesterday with regular uterine contractions of mild-to-moderate intensity at 3 minutes apart. At 11:30 PM, Jeanne was very uncomfortable and was 3–4 cm dilated on vaginal exam (VE). An epidural was performed, and vital signs remained stable. Uterine contractions were 4–5 minutes apart and of moderate-to-mild intensity after the epidural. At 3:00 AM today, Jeanne was 4 cm dilated, and an oxytocin infusion was started at 2 mU/min with orders to increase by 2 mU/min every 30 minutes until uterine contractions occurred every 2–3 minutes, lasted 50–60 seconds, and were of at least moderate intensity.

It is now 8:00 AM, and the oxytocin infusion is at 20 mU/min with uterine contractions every 3–4 minutes, lasting 40–50 seconds and of mild-to-moderate intensity. Jeanne is still very comfortable from the continuous epidural infusion. Vital signs are stable except for an increase in temperature to 37.8°C (100°F). Urinary output is steady at 50 ml/hr. Total IV rate of 125 ml/hr is maintained. An IUPC has now been placed; the Montevideo units are 150. Oxytocin was gradually increased over the next 2 hours to 25 mU/min, with rMontevideo units of 210.

At 11:00 AM today, Jeanne is dilated to 5 cm and 90% effaced, with vertex −1 station with molding palpable. Her temperature is now 38.3°C (101°F). Ampicillin, 2 gm IVPB, is now ordered, with 1gm IVPB to be given every 4 hours. Jeanne was also given acetaminophen, 650 mg. FHR baseline is in the 160s with early decelerations and average long-term variability (LTV).

At 1:00 PM Jeanne stated that she felt rectal pressure, and a VE confirmed that she was completely dilated with the vertex at +2 station. Jeanne's temperature was now 38.9°C (102°F), and she felt "chilled," although her skin felt hot and dry. FHR is in the 160s to 170s with minimal-to-average LTV. Oxygen is started at 10 L/min by facemask. Jeanne pushes for 2 hours with resulting descent of the fetal head to a +3/+4 station and then states, "I'm too tired." Pushing efforts become weaker despite several position changes. Vacuum extractor is applied, and with one contraction the fetal head is crowning. Jeanne gives birth to a 9-lb, 2-oz boy with Apgar scores of 6 and 9 at 3:15 PM.

Postpartum Hemorrhage Simulation

History. Monica is a 32-year-old G5P3, who gave birth to Jesse 72 hours ago. Jesse weighed 8lb 15 oz at birth. Monica was induced for postdates (41½ weeks) with dinoprostone (Cervidil) and oxytocin and was in labor for 36 hours. She had epidural anesthesia for 10 hours before delivery. Monica pushed for 2 hours and required forceps to rotate the baby from an OP to an OA position. Membranes were ruptured for 8 hours prior to birth. Group B streptococcal (GBS) status is negative. She has a secondary midline (ML) perineal laceration. She received an oxytocin infusion of 20 mU in 1000 ml over 4 hours after birth, and then her IV was discontinued. Placenta was expressed and delivered via the Duncan mechanism and was reported to be intact. Estimated blood loss (EBL) after birth was 350 ml. Vital signs have been stable. She is voiding without difficulty. At the last shift assessment, her fundus was at the umbilicus with a small amount of rubra lochia. Monica is bottlefeeding Jesse every 3 to 4 hours.

Scenario. Later Monica puts on her call light and asks if it is normal to pass a clot. Her nurse investigates, and Monica reports that she passed a clot about the size of a pancake in the toilet. She states that she feels like she is bleeding "a lot" right now. Her perineal pad is saturated with blood, and blood appears to be trickling out at a steady rate. Her fundus is at +1 and boggy. The nurse calls for help, and fundal massage is begun. Blood pressure, pulse, and respirations are within normal limits. An IV is established, 20 U of oxytocin is added to 1000 ml LR, and a bolus is started. Two more 5-cm clots are passed, but the fundus remains firm only with massage. Monica reports feelings of light-headedness and nausea. Her skin becomes clammy and pale in color. Her pulse is now 130, and respirations are in the 30s while blood pressure is slightly lower. Monica's physician arrives and does a manual inspection of the uterus. He removes more clots and a small piece of amniotic membrane with attached cotyledon of placental tissue. Methergine, 0.2 mg, is given IM per physician order. Bleeding is slowing, and the fundus is now 1 cm below the umbilicus and firm but relaxes without massage. Pulse is still 130. Blood pressure is dropping. A Foley catheter is inserted, and a second IV is started. Physician orders a D&C and Monica is sent straight to the operating room via stretcher. One smaller piece of amniotic membrane is removed during the D&C, and bleeding returns to normal. Blood pressure slowly rises over the next 30 minutes with continued IV bolusing. After 30 minutes, her pulse rate is 100 and her respiration rate is 22 with blood pressure slightly low but in normal range. Recovery continues, and Monica is returned to the postpartum floor.

Outcomes

To determine whether the use of simulation for experiential learning is effective, nurses attending the courses are asked to provide examples of the application of these strategies via narrative understanding at 3-month and 9-month intervals following the course. Narratives were used by Benner et al. to differentiate the levels from advanced beginner to expert as participants developed critical thinking skills (thinking in action) and clinical experiences.[31] Since the facilities educational tiered system is founded on Benner's model, it was decided to incorporate this evaluation process as a measure of course outcomes. Narratives also serve to demonstrate the urgency, temporality, and practical understanding of content in the actual clinical setting. The narratives have thus far consistently demonstrated successful and ongoing incorporation of the desired core concepts into patient care.

Summary and Recommendations

Within the spectrum of hospital-based nursing education, the use of human simulation technology can serve to provide experienced nurses with an alternative learning modality that provides realistic patient pathophysiology and responses within a safe environment. The evaluator is given the opportunity to see the nurse's ability to apply the nursing process and to demonstrate real-time critical thinking under pressure. The educator, however, must have a clear understanding of the population for which this learning modality is intended and be able to determine whether other forms of simulation may meet the needs of the intended audience. The population must be considered not only in terms of the three-tiered educational system as utilized in this example, but also in terms of the age or generation of the participants. We have noted that nurses familiar with low-fidelity simulators and instructor-guided cases have a longer learning curve in terms of effectively interfacing with the high-fidelity human simulator that does not require instructor responses to questions. Finally, faculty/educators must be aware of the ramifications of the debriefing process that is necessary after use of high-fidelity simulation. The participants involved in high-fidelity human simulation are a potentially vulnerable group. It is recommended that faculty/educators involved in the debriefing process formally state the ground rules for how their debriefing process will be structured to prevent the consequences of destructive criticism and mislearning.

Discussion

The previous section highlights three examples of our tiered approach to critical thinking and the benefits of high-fidelity simulation. The reader may have noted that each specialty has adapted flowsheets and critique forms to its specific needs. It was our goal to illustrate three methods of the simulation-based education program currently used in the clinical education department. In addition to the pulmonary program, our facility has developed tiered programs with regard to sedation, airway management, trauma, cardiac, bioterrorism, obstetrics, and advanced life support. In addition, simulation for nurses has been incorporated into our medical-surgical floors, subacute care, intensive care, emergency department, life-guard air ambulance, and surgery. Additional programs that have incorporated simulation into their undergraduate education are the schools of respiratory therapy and physical therapy. For additional information about these or any other simulation experiences, readers are encouraged to contact the authors, who will refer them to faculty who are willing to share programs, scenarios, flowsheets, and other materials they have stumbled across during this adventure.

Faculty initiating simulation as a teaching modality should expect that staff participants need time to acquaint themselves with the simulator as well as some introduction to the goals of the program. Our facility introduced the staff participants to the benefits of simulation practice and debriefing for the patient, and understanding the need for teamwork and team development smoothed the introduction of the program throughout our facility.

As these programs are integrated into our college of nursing (undergraduate and graduate), the percentage of staff who have "grown up" with simulation also increases. In fact, simulation has been incorporated into annual clinical competencies for nursing throughout our organization. Trends, new procedures, medications, variances, accreditation standards, and a variety of methods help to determine which scenarios are used during annual competencies. To reiterate, staff participants find the observation of their perfomrnace and the performance of others as educational as the performance aspect itself. Our department has been able to use the human simulator for videotaping scenarios for teaching "best practices" and team communication.

APPENDIX A. Human Patient Simulation: Course Development Request Form

Date Submitted:_____ Date Approved:_____

Instructor:	Mary L. Eichorn, MSN, RN, CEN
Organization:	University of New Mexico Hospitals
Department:	Community Training Center
Date of Class:	Ongoing
Learners:	Experienced ACLS providers
Number of Students:	Eight
Course Title:	Advanced Cardiac Life Support Fast Track
Description:	Case-based simulations, which require the experienced ACLS provider to demonstrate critical thinking , make decisions based on the clinical assessment on the Human Patient Simulation (HPS).

Providers will receive one of three scenarios involving cardiac and respiratory emergencies (see attachment) and will work in a team situation to treat the HPS.

The ALS cases/skills include respiratory arrest with a pulse, pulseless ventricular tachycardia, pulseless electrical activity, acute ischemic stroke, bradycardia, stable tachycardia, PSVT, acute coronary syndrome, asystole, airway mamagement with ET tubes, combitubes, LMA, IV access, defibrillation, cardioversion, and appropriate drug dosing.

Objectives:

1. Identifies a variety of cardiac arrhythmias, correlates rhythms with the clinical assessment, and chooses clinical interventions for treatment of the arrhythmia, as indicated.
2. Demonstrates the ability to successfully pass an endotracheal tube, combitube, and laryngeal mask airway, via the oral route, with appropriate evaluation of placement.
3. Correctly defibrillates patient, observing safety precautions each time.
4. Evaluates common complications related to code management and treats HPS appropriately in accordance with the etiology and clinical manifestations.

Schedule

11:50–12:05 Registration
12:05–1325 BLS Video
13:30–1430 BLS skills check off
14:30–1545 Group I takes tests (ACLS, Arrhythmias, BLS)
            Group II performs scenarios
15:45–17:00 Group II takes tests (ACLS, Arrhythmias, BLS) videotape debriefing
            Group I performs scenarios, then videotape debriefing

ACLS Simulations: Case I   **Patient options: Baseline Man**
Scenario options: ACLSFT1
Rate 1.50
A 55-year-old man with IDDM and ESRF; dialysis-dependent; weight = 100 kg.
Presents with weakness, nausea, vomiting, dyspnea, malaise.
Vital signs: HR = 140 bpm, BP = hypotensive via automatic cuff, RR = 26/min,
temp = 35°C, oximetry = 92% on 100% O_2 via NRBM mask.

History:
Depressed, taking TCAs
Missed last 2 dialysis treatments

Physical assessment:
Rales over lower half of chest
Gasping, using accessory and abdominal muscles to breathe
S_3 heart sounds
Abdomen benign
Weak pulses, diaphoretic skin
Eyes blink; Glasgow score of 12; moans
SVT on monitor with ECG changes: peaked T waves, ST ischemia, hypotensive
Respiratory arrest with a pulse-〉 patient becomes unresponsive.
Respiratory rate drops to 4 breaths/min and shallow, then apneic.
Participant shakes victim, calls his name, calls for help.
Opens airway with head tilt, chin lift. Looks, listens, and feels; patient not breathing
Gives two slow breaths using bag-valve-mask with 100% O_2.
Check for a pulse at the carotid artery-> weak, thready pulse
Participant should begin ventilations using BVM, 1 breath every 5 seconds.

Airway:
Place airway device as soon as possible; takes no more than 30 seconds to place
    device.
If airway is placed and assessed afterward (checking for placement at five points),
    participant will find that airway is not in place.
Stomach has gurgling sounds with each breath delivered; no breath sounds.
If participant or group fails to check placement, abdomen will distend, patient will
    vomit, victim will not improve.
Participant must remove the airway device, bag the patient with 100% O_2 for
    approximately 30 seconds, and repeat placement of airway device.
This time, there will be equal breath sounds over both lung fields and no sounds over
    the stomach.
Confirm proper placement by second method: end-tidal CO_2 and/or esophageal
    detector devices. (If participant inserts LMA, esophageal detector is ineffective and
    inaccurate—use CO_2 detector). Inflates airway devise with the appropriate amount
    of air.
Prevent airway device dislodgment. Use purpose-made tube holder or proven tape-
    and-tie or other technique

Participant monitors oxygenation and ventilation for effectiveness via O_2 saturations on pulse oximetry; BVM used to raise chest with equal rise and fall of chest.

Rhythm change: torsades
Defibrillation as soon as available.

IV access:
Participant simultaneously attempts IV access, with success, and hangs 0.9 % NS via IV, blood for labs (electrolytes, cardiac enzymes, bedside glucose). Results: potassium = 7.2, glucose = 345, BUN = 50, creatinine = 4.2.
Participant orders ABGs.

Drugs:
Drugs if using LMA. Participant does not consider using LMA for drug administration. Considers ETT route if using ETT and IV access not available
Participant gives either epinephrine (1 mg of 1:10,000 IVP, repeat every 3–5 minutes) or vasopressin (40 U IV, 1 time only).

Differential diagnosis:
Participant should look for most likely cause = hyperglycemia, TCA overdose (associated with torsades)

Drugs:
Consider antiarrhythmics.
Aminodarone, 300 mg IVP; consider repeating at 150 mg in 3–5 minutes (maximum cumulative dose of 2.2 gm/24 hours); if given, will widen QRS more. OR gives:
Lidocaine, 1 mg/kg IVP (100 mg with Stan)
May give magnesium, 1–2 gm, diluted in 10 ml, by IVP. No change in rhythm, pattern, or physical assessment.
Defibrillate at 360 J within 30–60 seconds of medication; call all clear, wait for others to clear.

Rhythm change: sinus bradycardia, rate of 45 on monitor; ECG changes: peaked T waves, oximetry 100% on 100% O_2 via BVM.
Participant gives epinephrine, 1 mg , 1;10,000 concentration, IVP; repeats every 3–5 minutes.

End Scenario:
Here the participants can discuss other drugs/treatments.

ACLS Fast Track Check Sheet I	Satisfactory	Needs Remediation/Comments
Respiratory arrest with a pulse		
Assesses responsiveness		
Calls for help/defibrillator		

ACLS Fast Track Check Sheet I	Satisfactory	Needs Remediation/Comments

Opens airway
Determines breathing
Provides first rescue breaths with ambu bag
Checks pulse (present)
Prepares to achieve advanced airway control
Achieves within 30 seconds–knows if it takes too long
Confirms tube placement through:
   Visualizes tube passing through vocal cords
   Uses end tidal CO_2 device
   Performs 5-point auscultation
   Looks for chest expansion/rising O_2 levels/vapor in tube
   Uses EDD
Secures tube in place

Pulseless VT
Monitor shows VT; checks pulse–no pulse
Defibrillator attached
Stacked shocks: 200-300-360
Calls "all clear" with each shock
Pulse check/rhythm check
Starts chest compressions
Establishes IV/sends labs
Gives vasopressin (40 IU)/epinephrine (1:10,000; 1 mg
   IV or 2 mg) ETT (not per LMA/combi)
Gives fluid bolus/raises extremity/circulates
   meds for 60 seconds
Shocks at 360
Calls "all clear" with each shock
Pulse check/rhythm check
Starts chest compressions
Gives antiarrhythmics:
   Aminodarone, 300 mg IVP; consider repeating
     at 150 mg in 3–5 minutes
   Lidocaine, 1 mg/kg IVP (100 mg with Stan)
Considers that procanamide and amniodarone may
   widen QRS more
     Magnesium, 1–2 gm, diluted in 10 ml, IVP.
Defibrillate at 360 J within 30–60 seconds
   of medication
Calls "all clear" with each shock
Pulse check/rhythm check

Pulseless Electrical Activity
Sinus bradycardia on monitor
Pulse check/rhythm check
Starts chest compressions
Epinephrine, 1mg , 1;10,000 concentration, IVP;
   repeat every 3–5 min
Atropine, 1 mg IV push, to a total of 0.04 mg/kg
Assesses for occult blood flow with Doppler
Differential diagnosis: 5 Hs/5 Ts
Looks for specific cause

ACLS Fast Track: Debriefing Tool

Case I: Team Leader:_____

Airway:
Breathing:
Circulation:
Defib/drugs/disability/differential diagnosis: What was done well?
What would you do differently?

Case 2: Team Leader:_____ _____

Airway:
Breathing:
Circulation:
Defib/drugs/disability/differential diagnosis: What was done well?
What would you do differently?

Case 3: Team Leader: _____

Airway:
Breathing:
Circulation:
Defib/drugs/disability/differential diagnosis: What was done well?
What would you do differently?

APPENDIX B. Skill Station 2: Deep Tendon Reflexes, Clonus, and Homans' Sign

Deep Tendon Reflexes

1. Demonstrate ability to elicit bilaterally
   a. Patellar reflex
   b. Biceps reflex
   c. Triceps reflex
   d. Brachioradialis
2. Grade reflexes
   - 0= No response
   - 1= Diminished response
   - 2= Average response
   - 3= Brisker than average
   - 4= Hyperactive with clonus

Clonus Assessment

3. Demonstrate ability to assess for clonus bilaterally
   a. Knee flex and leg supported
   b. Firmly dorsiflex the foot
   c. Maintain dorsiflexion momentarily
   d. Release
4. Report findings
   a. Normal: Foot returns to its normal position of plantarflexion
   b. Clonus present if the foot jerks or taps against examiner's hand
   c. Number of taps or beats is recorded
   d. Record differences between right and left

Deep vein thrombosis assessment

5. Identify risk factors for DVT
   a. Pregnancy
   b. Past history of DVT
   c. History of DVT in current pregnancy
   d. Surgery during pregnancy
   e. Cesarean birth
   f. Pregnancy-induced hypertension
6. Describe signs and symptoms of DVT
   a. Edema of the ankle and leg on the affected side
   b. Initial low-grade fever followed by high temperature and chills
   c. Complaints of pain
      1. Politeal and lateral tibial areas (politeal veins)
      2. Entire lower leg and foot (anterior and posterior tibial veins
      3. Inguinal tenderness (femoral vein)
      4. Lower abdomen (iliofemoral vein)
   d. Affected limb sometimes cool to touch
   e. Peripheral pulses may be decreased on affected limb
   f. Tender and or reddened, warm area on affected limb
7. Demonstrate Homans' sign

   a. Knee slightly flexed (decreases risk of embolization)
   b. Dorsiflex client's foot
   c. Describe findings
      1. Pain in foot is positive Homans' sign
8. Client teaching
   Prevention
   a. Dorsiflexion of feet on hourly basis while on bedrest (or passive range of motion)
   b. Early and frequent ambulation
   c. Avoiding pressure behind knees
   d. Avoiding use of knee-gatch on the bed
   e. Avoiding crossing legs

Instructor _____ Instructor's initials _____

References

1. Morton PG: Creating a laboratory that simulates the critical care environment. Crit Care Nurse 1996:16(6):76–81.
1. Rauen CA: Using simulation to teach critical thinking skills. Crit Care Nurs Clin North Am YEAR;13(1):93–103.
2. Aronson BS, Rosa JM, Anfinson J, Light N: Teaching tools: A simulated clinical problem-solving experience. Nurse Educ 1997;22(6):17–19.
3. Joyce JH, Zerwic JJ, Theis SL: Clinical simulation laboratory: An adjunct to clinical teaching. Nurse Educ 1999:24(5):37–41.
4. Whitis G: Simulation in teaching clinical nursing. J Nurs Educ 1985:24(4):161–163.
5. Satish U, Streufert S: Value of a cognitive simulation in medicine: Towards optimizing decision making performance of healthcare personnel. Qual Safe Health Care 2002;11(2):163.
6. Issenberg SB, McGaghie WC, Hart IR, et al: Simulation technology for health care professional training skills training and assessment. JAMA 1999;282:861–866.
7. Lupien AE, George-Gay B: Fuszard's Innovative Teaching Strategies in Nursing, 3rd ed. Gaithersburg, MD, Aspen Publishers, 2001, pp 134–148.
9. Weis P, Guyton-Simmons J: A computer simulation for teaching critical thinking skills. Nurse Educ 1998:23(2):30–33.
10. Http://www.aana.com/crna/of/scope.asp [accessed June 12, 2003].
11. Council on Accreditation of Nurse Anesthesia Educational Programs: Trial Standards for Accreditation of Nurse Anesthesia Educational Programs [adopted trial standards for 2003]. Park Ridge, IL, Council on Accreditation of Nurse Anesthesia Educational Programs, 2003.
12. Wren KR: Learning from a nurse anesthetist perspective: A qualitative study. AANA J 2001;69:273–278.
13. Exercise designed by Richard Haas, Med, MS, CRNA. Medical College of Georgia Nursing Anesthesia Program, Augusta, GA.
14. Tan GM, Ti LK, Suresh D, et al: Teaching first-year medical students physiology: Does the human patient simulator allow for more effective teaching? Singapore Med J 2002;43(5):238–242.
15. Gaba DM, Fish KJ, Howard SK: Crisis Management in Anesthesiology. New York, Churchill Livingstone, 1994.
16. Craig PA: Situational Awareness. New York, McGraw-Hill, 2001.
17. Fletcher JL: ERR WATCH: Anesthesia crisis resource management from the nurse anesthetist's perspective. AANA J 1998;66:595–602.
18. Gaba DM, Howard SK, Flanagan B, et al: Assessment of clinical performance during simulated crises using both technical and behavioral ratings. Anesthesiology 1998;89:8–18.
19. Henrichs BH, Rule A, Grady M, Ellis W: Nurse anesthesia students' perceptions of the anesthesia patient simulator: A qualitative study. AANA J 2002;70:219–225.
20. O'Donnell J, Fletcher J, Dixon B, Palmer L: Planning and implementing an anesthesia crisis

resource management course for student nurse anesthetics. CRNA Clin Forum Nurse Anesthet 1998;9(2):50–58.

21. Exercise designed by Donna Michele Bork while enrolled as a graduate student in nurse anesthesia. Medical College of Georgia Nursing Anesthesia Program, Augusta, GA.

22. Monti EJ, Wren K, Haas R, Lupien AE: The use of an anesthesia simulator in graduate and undergraduate education. CRNA Clin Forum Nurse Anesthet 1998;9(2):59–66.

23. Henson LC, Richardson MG, Stern DH, Shekhter I: Using the Human Patient Simulator to credential first-year anesthesiology residents for taking overnight call [abstract]. In Proceedings of the 2001 International Meeting on Medical Simulation, Scottsdale, AZ.

24. Rosenblatt MA, Abrams KJ: The use of a human patient simulator in the evaluation of and development of a remedial prescription for an anesthesologist with lapsed medical skills. Anesth Analg 2002;94:786–787.

25. Byrne AJ, Greaves JD: Assessment instruments used during anaesthetic simulation: Review of published studies. Br J Anaesth 2001;86:445–450.

26. Benner P, Tanner C, Chesla C: From beginner to expert: Gaining a differentiated clinical world in critical care nursing. Adv Nurs Sci 1992;14(3):13–28.

27. Benner P, Wrubel J: Skilled clinical knowledge. The value of perceptual awareness: Part I. J Nurs Administr 1982;May:1–14.

28. Benner P, Wrubel J: Skilled clinical knowledge. The value of perceptual awareness: Part II. J Nurs Administr 1982;June:28–33.

29. Bernard GR, Artigas A, Brigham KL, et al: Report of the American-European consensus conference on acute respiratory distress syndrome: Definitions, mechanisms, relevant outcomes, and clinical trial coordination. J Crit Care 1994;9:72–81.

30. van Soeren MH, Diehl-Jones WL, Maykut RJ, et al: Pathophysiology and implications for treatment of acute respiratory distress syndrome. AACN Clin Issues 2000;11:179–197.

31. Benner P, Hooper-Kryiakidis P, Stannard D: Clinical Wisdom and Interventions in Critical Care: A Thinking-in-Action Approach. Philadelphia, W.B. Saunders, 1999.

Chapter 10

SIMULATION IN CRISIS MANAGEMENT

Crisis management has been an evolving topic in medicine for the past dozen years as reports of medical errors have increased and performances of health care providers have become more frequently based on patient outcomes. Given that crisis management is a relatively new topic in health care, this chapter is divided into three sections: an introduction by Alicia Vogt, application of current knowledge by Michelle Lewis, and finally targeted instruction in crisis management by Gary Loyd. With this information, the reader should be able to provide effective teaching of crisis management by using patient simulation.

Introduction to Crisis Management

Alicia C. Vogt

Every health care professional with even the slightest experience knows whom she or he would select to handle emergency care in a crisis. As David Gaba writes in *Crisis Management in Anesthesiology,* "when a crisis does present itself . . . it is obvious to everyone who works in an operating room that some anesthetists cope better than others. These anesthetists take more steps to prevent a crisis, and they are better prepared when crises occur."[1] Applying Gaba's words to all health care professionals immediately poses a question: Why are some health care professionals better crisis managers than others? Why are there certain people whom Gaba describes as those "most of us would choose to administer our anesthetic if we needed it?"[1] The most efficient crisis managers are chosen because they possess certain conspicuous abilities: to categorize crises, to practice flexible responses, to develop behavior-monitoring mechanisms that prevent errors, to train groups to recognize individual errors, to understand objectives, and to coordinate responses to manage the crisis and its consequences.

Once these qualities are identified, they can be taught to others. It is true that some are inherent personality traits, whereas others are acquired skills, but the origin of these characteristics is inconsequential. What is important and constitutes the foundation of this chapter is that these qualities are teachable—and, perhaps more significantly, they are learnable. Therefore, although some health care professionals are by nature efficient crisis managers, those who are not can attain an equivalent level of efficiency through training. It is absolutely vital that they do so, for crises in medicine are inescapable and often affect the patient's quality of life and survival.

As W. Timothy Coombs asserts in *Ongoing Crisis Communication,* "no organization is immune to crises."[2] From this inevitability arises the need to manage efficiently both the crises themselves and their consequences. To accomplish this goal, an organization needs to train its workforce proficiently in crisis management. Having recognized this need, several organizations have introduced crisis management plans to prepare for the unavoidable. For example, the federal government's CONPLAN specifically coordinates federal, state, and local emergency responses to acts of terrorism, and the aviation industry's Crew Resource Management instructs personnel aboard an airplane how to manage in-air crises. Instruction in the medical sciences, however, offers neither comparable training nor an analogous crisis management plan to health care professionals. Since the gravity of the crises encountered in medicine approximates that of terrorism and aviation, such training should exist to contribute to the prevention of mismanaged crises. To put it another way, as Ian Mitroff states in *Managing Crises Before They Happen,* "While not all crises can be foreseen, let alone prevented, all of them can be managed far more effectively if we understand and practice the best of what is humanly possible."[3] This section explains how certain components of and approaches to crisis management training achieve "the best of what is humanly possible" by exploring existing crisis management plans in fields other than medicine, by targeting training to the particular psychology of the trainees, by investigating the way in which individuals learn, and by analyzing the dynamics and psychology of individuals and teams.

Discussing crisis management first requires defining a crisis, and because definitions are as varied as crises themselves, each definition must be assessed to discover a unifying theme. This theme leads to the definition of a crisis as an "event that affects or has the potential to affect the whole of an organization."[3] Based on this definition, it is apparent that health care providers encounter crises on a daily basis, for numerous patient cases and outcomes "affect or have the potential to affect" the whole of the hospital or all of health care. The dynamic and uncertain nature of the risks of medically intervening in a patient's life means that crises are inherent to health care; therefore, training in crisis management ought to be equally intrinsic to medical education. For this training to have optimal effect, according to the Institute for Crisis Management, the innumerable types and forms that crises may assume must be categorized; otherwise one risks futile instruction in crisis management by overwhelming trainees with a random presentation of countless crises.

The Institute for Crisis Management defines four causes or categories of crises[4]: acts of God, mechanical problems, human errors, and management decision/indecision. Research into crisis management demonstrates that the most successful organizations — with success defined as the minimization of the duration and damage of a crisis — generate a list of specific crises, fit them into a category, and practice and prepare for at least one particular crisis within each category[3] (Fig. 1). During health care providers' preparation and training for the chosen crisis, research finds that instructors who suggest alternative paths for a given crisis during training may produce more flexible crisis managers who are better able to anticipate how to respond to crises of varying forms and who are more prepared for a broad array of crises. This flexibility in crisis management is precisely the reason that these organizations are so successful. They avoid facing the impracticality of training for every possible crisis and concurrently ensure that time and resources are used efficiently. Training with flexibility permits the preparation of re-

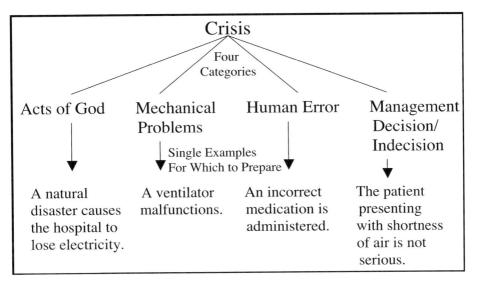

Figure 1. Flow chart depicting four categories of crises and a sample crisis under each category title. Crisis management training specifically prepares health care providers for one crisis in each category but does so in a flexible manner. This flexibility allows trainees to recognize and, in fact, prepare for other crises that fall under the same category while technically training for just one.

sponses to an encompassing spectrum of crises while planning for just one. This preparation is a key feature of efficient crisis management.

Another aspect of efficient crisis management involves the minimization of errors during the actual management of the crisis, and although preparing for one crisis within each of the four categories curtails the number of errors in and of itself, only complete crisis management training addresses and truly minimizes errors. Minimization of errors requires an understanding of their nature. The most notable errors are of two types: slips and fixation errors. Slips occur "when a person does an action that is not intended,"[5] whereas fixation errors involve maintaining an incorrect course of action when emerging data indicate a different course. Crisis management training functions to restrict these types of errors by instructing trainees to monitor and coordinate their actions. Monitoring eliminates slips while coordinating eradicates fixation errors. Each is discussed in turn. Slips are inevitable in medicine, for health care providers directly execute their orders and actions without any intervening party. Thus, they are more prone to slips because any error in a field whose members execute their own actions is by definition a slip. Research suggests that slips are a result of competing and, in fact, conflicting actions or thoughts, such as all of the options for treatment an anesthesiologist weighs when a patient's blood pressure drops.

It is clear that health care professionals are susceptible to slips. What is paramount, however, is not the susceptibility to slips but rather the ability to detect them. Herein lies the ability to control and manage the outcome of errors. The effect of this ability on instruction in crisis management is considerable; as Norman writes, "many slips are caught at the time they are made. . .(so) there must exist some monitoring mechanism of behavior."[5] Furthermore, "for a slip to be detected, the monitoring mechanism must be made aware of the discrepancy between intention and act."[5] Instructors of crisis management who understand and cultivate this monitoring mechanism in trainees produce health care providers whose consideration or monitoring of their own actions catches slips. To recognize the incongruity between intention act, Norman suggests training people in two ways: (1) by positively reinforcing actions that efficiently manage the crisis during training and (2) by promoting active use of the behavior-monitoring mechanism. Thus, during training instructors permit health care providers to anticipate the types of maneuvers that they may expect to perform during a crisis and to practice these actions in an atmosphere in which the behavior-monitoring mechanism has been instilled and nurtured. Again, such instruction minimizes errors of execution or slips by training health care professionals to heighten their level of behavior monitoring. What about minimizing fixation errors? An indispensable part of any instruction in crisis management is a delineation of the roles of the numerous people and entities responding to the crisis as well as a description of the coordination among their responses. The risks of ignoring training in coordination are outlined in the federal government's CONPLAN, a crisis management plan to coordinate emergency responses to terrorism (see below). Training in this type of coordination minimizes fixation errors. Instruction has now progressed beyond teaching crisis management to individuals into the realm of training in group decision making, which involves a unique psychology. R. Scott Tindale concludes in his essay in *Individual and Group Decision Making* that "groups make less errors on problem-solving tasks."[6] Through research in decision making, he discovers that the particular quality that makes groups superior problem solvers relative to individuals involves the group's ability to "check errors."[6] Crisis management, then, benefits from the coordinated effort of an entire health care team as individual errors are checked by the group, whose role cannot be underestimated. The group prevents a decision in error from progressing into a fixation error by checking it through a re-evaluation of the current germane data. Instruction in crisis management, therefore, includes developing the behavior-monitoring mechanism of individuals to minimize slips, but it must also incorporate training groups of people to recognize slips that conflict with prevailing data and to act on these data to manage the crisis.

The dynamic and unpredictable nature of health care dictates that both slips and fixation errors occur. Because crisis management training allows health care professionals to prepare and practice their actions with instructors who encourage evaluation of those actions, it fosters development of a behavior- monitoring mechanism. Instruction also specifies how to coordinate the group's response to emerging information, thereby minimizing the number of errors committed and managing the crisis efficiently. Because there is no definitive training in crisis management for the field of medicine, instructors of health care providers must turn to the federal government's CONPLAN, in which emphasis on coordination creates a consummate paradigm for educating health care providers about the significance of working as a team.

CONPLAN, the United States Government Interagency Domestic Terrorism Concept of Operations Plan, is a crisis management plan designed to coordinate the response to a crisis, such as terrorists' use of weapons of mass destruction, to ensure efficient management. Because CONPLAN provides "overall guidance to Federal, State, and local agencies,"[7] coordination is its primary theme, and its application to medicine is immediate. A medical crisis mandates a bedside (local), departmental (state), and hospital-wide (federal) response, and coordination of the three is the crux of CONPLAN. To achieve the requisite coordination to manage crises efficiently, CONPLAN emphasizes three goals[7]: (1) it establishes a structure for a systematic, coordinated, and effective national response to threats or acts of terrorism; (2) it defines procedures for the use of federal resources to augment and support local and state governments; and (3) it encompasses both crisis and consequence management responsibilities and articulates the coordination relationships between these missions.

For a corresponding health care crisis management plan, known as HEALTHPLAN, the preceding three objectives might read as follows: HEALTHPLAN (1) institutes a framework for a methodic, coordinated, and effective hospital-wide response to events that may become crises or are currently crises; (2) outlines protocol for the use of hospital-wide resources to supplement and support bedside and departmental responses; and (3) encompasses both crisis and consequence management responsibilities and articulates the coordination relationships between these missions. The third objective reads the same as CONPLAN, for consequence management and coordination of responses are vital to the management of any crisis, regardless of the size of the organization.

To accomplish these three goals, CONPLAN defines the role of various agencies; for example, it designates the Federal Bureau of Investigation as the lead agency for crisis management and the Federal Emergency Management Agency as the lead agency for consequence management. Additionally, it explicates how to integrate the responses of these and other agencies to achieve a coordinated response and thus manage the crisis efficiently. CONPLAN also describes the consequences of crisis management instructors' neglecting education about the importance of coordination.

The risks of disregarding coordination as an integral theme of instruction in crisis management include a failure to manage the consequences of the crisis and a wasteful duplication of training and responses that may be tragic during a real crisis. First, a crisis can never be considered managed if its consequences themselves constitute crises. For example, a postoperative patient with a pulmonary embolism constitutes a crisis, and the management of this crisis includes administration of tissue plasminogen activator to dissolve the clot. Shortly thereafter, the patient's blood pressure falls significantly because of profuse bleeding from wounds received in the initial trauma responsible for the patient's surgery. In this case, a consequence of the original crisis (pulmonary embolism) is itself a crisis (drop in blood pressure), and one cannot consider this course of action to be efficient crisis management. Because CONPLAN is a "coordinating plan between crisis and consequence management,"[7] it ensures an efficient resolution to the existing crisis and precludes the emergence of another crisis from consequence mismanagement. Instruction to health care providers must likewise illustrate how primary responses manage the crisis and coordinated secondary responses manage the consequences.

Secondly, a crisis is not managed efficiently if numerous entities train several personnel for a task that a single person can accomplish with ease, and one goal of CONPLAN is to eliminate futile duplication of training. The solution is that "each agency should coordinate its training programs with other response agencies to avoid duplication,"[7] for then no two people interfere with one another during the management of an actual crisis. Instructors of health care providers learn from this section of CONPLAN that proficient allocation of training to bedside, departmental, and hospital- wide responders is crucial. For instance, if a technician from elsewhere arrives at the bedside to initiate operation of a ventilator that was, in fact, begun earlier by someone else, then the presence of two identically trained technicians in one place does not constitute efficient crisis management. One of the trained technicians may be needed to manage a crisis somewhere else, and their simultaneous attendance at the same bedside is a direct consequence of a lack of training and communication. Instructors must competently allocate training to bedside, departmental, and hospital-wide personnel to coordinate responses and avert duplication and inefficient crisis management. This type of coordination benefits from interpersonal communication, which is a theme of the aviation industry's Crew Resource Management, a second training program to which health care providers must turn since medicine possesses no systematic training of its own in crisis management.

In 1979 NASA held a workshop to discuss the causes of airline accidents and concluded that "the human error aspects of the majority of air crashes [are] failures of interpersonal communications, decision making, and leadership."[8] Attendees at this conference decided on a training program that focused on the utilization of all human resources on the airline to reduce pilot errors. They labeled this program Cockpit Resource Management (CRM). United Airlines undertook the first comprehensive CRM program in 1981, and the training included two novel notions for the time: (1) simulator training in interpersonal skills must accompany traditional classroom instruction, and (2) CRM training is not a single incident in a crew's career but rather occurs periodically as new technology or safety standards emerge. Because medicine is as dynamic and technologically dependent as aviation, instruction to health care providers must incorporate the same guidelines. Instruction must include patient simulators that realistically portray events leading to or constituting a crisis; then health care providers are able to practice managing the crisis using the techniques and concepts that they learned in a classroom. In addition, as biomedical engineers present physicians with new devices that improve the standard of care, efficient crisis management is redefined by the use of new technology, and training must occur periodically to ensure that crisis management is not outdated.

Later CRM training programs instituted other concepts from which crisis management training in medicine may benefit. For example, in 1986 Cockpit Resource Management was renamed Crew Resource Management to reflect that the training was now more team-oriented rather than pilot-centered. The change was also an acknowledgment that it truly takes an entire crew to manage a crisis efficiently. Therefore, training was extended to include flight attendants, dispatchers, and maintenance personnel. Instruction to health care providers must similarly be concerned with training all responders individually and as a group. It must not be solely physician-centered, for the team of health care professionals who resolve a crisis includes nurses, technicians, and physicians alike.

In addition, in the early 1990s airlines integrated CRM with pilots' technical training. Previously pilots learned to fly through one school of instruction and attended another for CRM training, but because being a pilot involves both flying an airplane and managing a plane whose wing is on fire, divorcing CRM training from technical training made little sense. By incorporating CRM into technical training, aviation has admitted that simply instructing a pilot in how to fly a plane does not guarantee that the pilot knows how to manage a crisis. This admission is precisely what medicine resists. Medical school and residency training produce physicians, not crisis managers; however, if instruction in crisis management were integrated into the medical training that all physicians must complete (as CRM training is for pilots), physicians could indeed be efficient crisis managers on completion of their residency. As it is now, there is no systematic crisis management training whatsoever, and implementation of a CRM-like program in medicine should occur as an integrated aspect of physicians' technical training during medical school and residency. As more airlines began adopting CRM programs, they determined individually the teaching of which concepts yielded the best results and refined their CRM programs to focus on that instruction. CRM training, therefore, continues to evolve.

Helmreich and colleagues refer to the most recent updates to CRM training in an article in *The International Journal of Aviation Psychology,* in which they equate present CRM with error management. The premises underlying this latest CRM training are that "human error is ubiquitous and inevitable"[8] and that training must confront the commitment of errors through three lines of defense. The first line is to avoid the error altogether by preparing and training thoroughly for the tasks that one is expected to perform. The second line involves trapping incipient errors and is accomplished by reviewing and re-evaluating one's own actions as well as the actions of the crew. The third and final line of defense is to allay the consequences of errors that are neither avoided nor trapped by monitoring the outcomes of actions. Instruction in crisis management to health care providers must feature these same three lines of defense (Fig. 2) because human error is one of the four categories of crises in medicine for which instruction prepares health care providers. This instruction affects trainees the most when

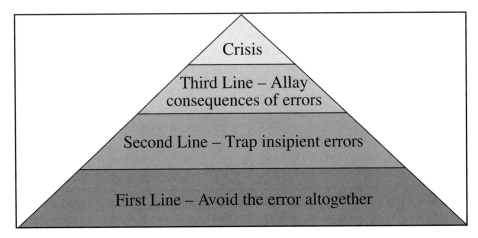

Figure 2. The three lines of defense to confront the commitment of human error. The area of each of the four levels of this pyramid represents the relative number of errors to be confronted by that line of defense. The pyramidal shape of the figure, therefore, is instructive, for only errors that make it through the first line of defense are available for confrontation with the second line, which is a smaller level of the pyramid to represent a reduced number of errors. Likewise, confrontation with the third line is a smaller area still, and errors penetrating this level reach the peak—a crisis. An error may be confronted and a crisis managed at any level as one ascends the pyramid.

it is carried out with a "non-punitive approach."[8] Once a hospital is able to identify the nature and source of the human errors that preclude efficient crisis management, it can attempt training along the three lines of defense, but if that training occurs in a punitive manner, trainees do not "gain acceptance of the error management approach."[8] Instruction, therefore, must indicate to healthcare providers that the three lines of defense to confront human errors exist because error is unavoidable and patients are best served by this training. This approach removes any threatening chastisement when instructors in crisis management commence this portion of training, which, if approached punitively, may appear like health care providers are being blamed for the occurrence of crises. CRM describes precisely how this instruction must proceed.

Because the goal of the three lines of defense involves error management, the basis of training should be "formal instruction in the limitations of human performance."[8] A large part of this instruction in aviation involves illustrating how stressors such as fatigue, work overload, and emergencies promote human errors aboard airlines. The same stressors permeate the field of medicine. Furthermore, research demonstrates that pilots believe that they are not susceptible to allowing occurrences within their personal lives to influence decision making in the airplane, but in fact, pilots "hold unrealistic attitudes about the effects of stressors on their performance."[8] Again, there are parallels with medicine, for "this attitude of personal invulnerability is a negative component of the professional culture of pilots and physicians."[8] The aim of instruction is first to explain that everyone experiences certain stressors, which undoubtedly have a negative effect on decisions and actions, in order to correlate those stressors with poor job performance. Second, instruction must clearly relate the minimization of errors during an actual crisis to participation in crisis management training. Thirdly, instruction must connect crisis management training to optimum job performance. Figure 3 depicts these interrelationships, whose presentation to health care providers during training as a measure to confront poor performance increases the likelihood that they will embrace all other aspects of training.

A second measure designed to increase the probability that health care providers will welcome their entire training also originates in CRM. This measure involves the use of observation both to measure the health care team's performance and to provide feedback and reinforcement. The idea is to offer trainees evidence through the use of checklists that they are, in fact, managing crises efficiently; such proof validates their training and encourages their acceptance of additional sessions. Helmreich's research proves that "observers could readily identify errors, their sources, and management strategies"[8] aboard a U.S. airline. Thus, instruction in crisis management training that includes teaching someone to respond to the crisis solely as an observer allows the entire team of health care providers to gain feedback and reinforcement concerning its actions. Certainly this observer is expected to find examples of errors avoided, errors trapped, and errors mitigated along the three lines of defense under which the health care providers are trained. The reinforcement offered by a primary source at the actual crisis improves acceptance of the training by illustrating its direct impact on patient outcomes. Ultimately CRM offers the field of medicine an admission that no training can ever entirely eliminate error or guarantee safety in high-risk professions such as aviation and health care, for "error is an inevitable result of the natural limitations of human performance and the function of complex systems."[8] However, CRM and other training programs al-

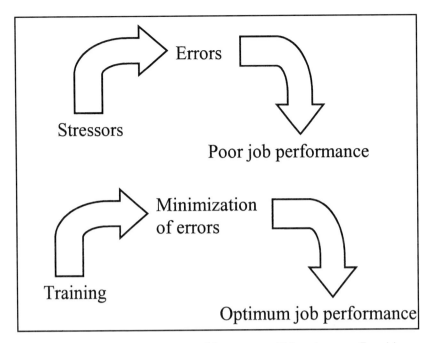

Figure 3. The interrelationship among stress, training, errors, and job performance. For crisis management training to have optimal effect, these relationships must be communicated clearly to health care providers. If they are not, trainees view instruction on minimizing human error in a negative and punitive manner as if they are being blamed for the occurrence of crises. Such an atmosphere precludes acceptance of all the remaining components of crisis management training.

low error to be managed, and because human error is a category or cause of medical crises, where errors are managed, crises are managed as well.

Thus far, this chapter has described the informational content that instructors must present to produce efficient crisis managers, but there is another aspect of instruction in addition to content: the method of instruction or how one teaches the content. Anderson calls these two aspects of teaching the intentional and the reasoned. The intentional aspect of teaching "concerns how teachers help students achieve the teacher's objectives,"[9] and the reasoned aspect involves what objectives teachers choose for their students. Instruction in crisis management is an intentional and reasoned act. The goal of efficient crisis management requires (1) being aware of content, (2) categorizing crises, (3) practicing flexible responses, (4) developing behavior-monitoring mechanisms, (5) training groups to recognize individual errors, and (6) coordinating responses to manage consequences. Once instructors determine the elements of content, the question remains: how do they teach these elements? Answering this question is vital, for the distinct personalities of health care providers determine how they best learn. Knowing how they learn translates into knowing how to teach (the intentional aspect). What is a plan worth without the ability to teach it in a manner that promotes effective learning? If an instructor is aware of precisely what to say but knows not how to say it, that instructor is no less deficient than if she or he ignored aspects of content altogether. Efficient crisis management results only when instructors are conscious of both the content and the method of instruction. The method arises from information about how people learn.

Nelson and others discuss in *Metacognition* various theories of learning and intelligence and cite a classic study conducted by Dweck and colleagues as "some of the strongest evidence"[10] that learners can be divided into two types: entity theorists and incremental theorists. Entity theorists believe that one simply possesses or lacks the capacity for certain intellectual tasks, whereas incremental theorists hold that it is possible to improve one's intellectual capacity ultimately to accomplish a task. It is essential that instructors of crisis management recognize these two types of learners when they encounter them, for teaching crisis management to the varying personalities that compose a team of health care professionals as if they all learned in the same manner alienates and neglects those who learn differently. For instance, entity theorists are perpetually anxious about performance results and scores, and temporary disappointments engender in them feelings of failure, helplessness, and self-contempt. On the other hand, incremental theorists respond comparatively well to transient setbacks since they are oriented toward ultimate goals and improvement through learning from mistakes. Recognizing these two types of learners, an instructor can target tailor-made training in crisis management to the particular style of learning the members of the health care team exhibit. This directed training is as simple as encouraging an entity theorist to persevere when he or she commits an error or focusing an incremental theorist on the detailed features of a task when he or she is considering only the ultimate goals. By adapting the style of training to the psychology of the learner and, as outlined below, by understanding how the learner comes to know the objectives of the training, instructors acknowledge the intentional aspect of teaching and offer the opportunity for utmost acquisition of knowledge, which ultimately culminates in optimally efficient crisis management.

How do learners come to understand the objectives an instructor chooses? The answer is that they categorize the objectives within a framework of which they have existing knowledge. Consider the phylogenetic framework, as Anderson does. A phylogenetic framework contains categories such as mammals and arthropods, organized according to criteria such as type of birth or type of body skeleton. If an instructor selects as an objective that the student will learn to differentiate a beetle from a hyrax, the student turns to the phylogenetic framework to satisfy that objective. Such a framework enhances the ability to understand this objective by allowing one to learn the characteristics of each category within the framework and subsequently to infer information about a particular organism by virtue of its placement in a known category. For example, mammals are defined by nursing of their young and breathing of air. As Anderson and Krathwohl discuss in *A Taxonomy for Learning, Teaching, and Assessing,* if a hyrax is a mammal, immediately one appreciates particular qualities of a hyrax due to the phylogenetic framework.[9] The framework, therefore, enhances understanding. Likewise, since a beetle is an arthropod and belongs in a distinct category from a hyrax, a student who employs this framework satisfies the objective from existing knowledge of the categories within the framework.

A special type of framework, known as a taxonomy, is simply a framework whose "categories lie along a continuum."[9] In terms of crisis management training, a taxonomy of objectives, in which objectives are defined as "explicit formulations of the ways in which students are expected to be changed by the educative process,"[9] is of utmost importance. Objectives contain a reference to a cognitive process followed by a statement of the knowledge students are expected to acquire. Take, for example, the objective that the student will learn to differentiate a beetle from a hyrax. The cognitive process includes the expectation that "the student will learn to differentiate," and the knowledge consists of differentiating "a beetle from a hyrax." Just as a hyrax is associated with a category of mammals and a beetle with arthropods inside a phylogenetic framework, so, too, are the cognitive process and knowledge components of an objective associated with categories within a taxonomy of objectives. The six cognitive process categories are remember, understand, apply, analyze, evaluate, and create. The four knowledge categories are factual, conceptual, procedural, and metacognitive. These categories are no different from the categories of mammals and arthropods, for they allow students to draw conclusions about objectives from previous knowledge of the categories into which they fall in the same manner that they arrive at conclusions about a hyrax from information about the category to which it is assigned.

Categorizing the two components of objectives enhances students' understanding of the objective. Likewise, a clearer understanding of the objective results in more efficient satisfaction. If the objective is to teach health care professionals to manage crises, instructors and patients alike desire efficient satisfaction. Here is how this categorization works. The interrelationship between the two components cognitive process and knowledge is referred to as the "Taxonomy Table"[9] (Table 1). Return again to the previous example that the student will learn to differentiate a beetle from a hyrax, but now place the cognitive process and knowledge into proper categories in the table. "Differentiate" corresponds to the category "analyze," and beetles and hyraxes are types of organisms. Types of things are concepts and, therefore, are associated with the category conceptual knowledge. The "X" in the table indicates that this objective requests that students analyze conceptual knowledge, but how does this process increase their understanding and facilitate satisfaction of the objective?

Once students understand the meaning of the categories analyze and conceptual

Table 1.
The Taxonomy Table*

	Cognitive Process Component					
Knowledge Component	Remember	Understand	Apply	Analyze	Evaluate	Create
Factual	0					
Conceptual				X		
Procedural		Z				
Metacognitive						

*The six cognitive process categories are listed horizontally across the top of the table, and the four knowledge categories are arranged vertically along the left side. Any single unit on the table indicates both a cognitive process and a knowledge category. The Z, for example, denotes an objective that requires trainees to understand procedural knowledge. The Taxonomy Table's categorization of objectives provides immense utility to crisis management training by allowing instructors to teach more exactly and trainees to learn more efficiently. See text for discussion.

knowledge, they are able to understand the objective completely, just as knowing the meaning of the categories "mamma" and "arthropod" allowed them to comprehend a beetle and a hyrax. Instructors must also understand the categories within the Taxonomy Table if they are to help students satisfy objectives. Because "different types of objectives require different instructional approaches,"[9] instructors must adjust how they teach, the intentional aspect of teaching, depending on the particular objective. For example, satisfaction of objectives that require students to analyze conceptual knowledge is assisted by the extensive use of examples that allow students to form proper classification systems, which are really concepts of different types of things like organisms. If during crisis management training an instructor's objective is to teach a health care professional to differentiate between hyperventilation and tachypnea in order to manage an actual crisis efficiently, the instructor is well served by using numerous examples of each type of breathing so that the student can formulate a classification system of the concepts of distinct types of breathing. If the instructor does not know that this objective belongs in the "analyze conceptual knowledge" categories, the instructor disregards the use of examples, which is the foundation of instructing students to satisfy objectives requiring an analysis of conceptual knowledge.

Objectives that correspond to other categories benefit less, if at all, from examples; instead, their satisfaction is enhanced by instruction particular to the categories under which they fall. For instance, imagine an instructor whose objective for a health care provider is simply to learn the names and pager numbers of all the surgeons in the cardiothoracic specialists group so that the proper person can be notified during a crisis. In the Taxonomy Table, the cognitive process "learn" belongs in the category "remember," and knowledge of names and pager numbers belongs in the category "factual." Factual knowledge is the categorization of this objective ("O" in the table), and instruction in satisfying it includes strategies and techniques to aid the process of memorization. Anderson suggests that instructors encourage rehearsal and repetition as strategies and the use of mnemonic devices or word associations as examples of techniques, all of which promote memorization.[9] Copious examples are futile, for memorization satisfies this objective, which does not require construction of classification systems as the previous sample objective does. Instructors and students, therefore, benefit from knowledge of the categories in the Taxonomy Table. Instructors are able to teach their objectives more clearly, and students are able to understand those objectives more precisely. Again, the ultimate result is efficient crisis management.

All health care providers can be trained to be efficient crisis managers if the instruction that they receive includes the content described throughout this section and if the manner by which they receive it corresponds to the recommendations within this text. The content includes training individual health care providers to recognize a crisis and categorize it appropriately, to practice flexible responses during the preparation for a sample crisis within each category, to confront human errors through three lines of defense, and to develop within themselves behavior-monitoring mechanisms. The content further includes training groups to recognize individual errors and to coordinate bedside responses with those of the department and the hospital at large in order to manage the crisis and its consequences. Many of these principles are derived from systematic crisis management plans in other fields, such as antiterrorism (CONPLAN) and aviation

(CRM). A point that this section attempted to emphasize was that presentation of this content is equally as important as the content itself. Instructors must understand the Taxonomy Table to know how to categorize the objectives that they intend to teach as well as how trainees categorize those same objectives in order to comprehend them. Such recognition and understanding lead to targeted training that is directed at the particular psychology of the learner. By teaching the content in the manner described above, instructors create through training health care providers who are truly efficient crisis managers. Previous attempts at training crisis managers in medicine utilized algorithms and a provider's own past experiences and common sense. The components of instruction lacking in this training include aspects of dynamic decision-making skills, organization and leadership skills, and skills that allow providers to anticipate a crisis. It is to these components that this chapter now turns.

Applying the Prinicples of Crisis Management

Michelle T. Lewis

Health care professionals rely primarily on the use of algorithms, work-related experiences, and common sense for training in all genres of medicine, including crises. Algorithms are undoubtedly an essential element for training in the health care professions. They format a logical, stepwise method of describing the decision-making process and are an asset to the planning of patient care on a daily basis.[11] These systematic decision-tree approaches, although helpful, lend themselves to deleterious dilemmas. What do you do when the scenario does not fit into any currently recognized algorithm, or the necessary algorithm has been unintentionally forgotten? In such a predicament, one turns to prior experiences, general knowledge relating to the situation, and common sense for an effective solution. In episodes such as this, problems are most likely to arise and mistakes are most likely to be made. Because of the low occurrence of many rare crises, an individual may never have received exposure to a similar event or may be unable to reason an acceptable explanation and satisfactory treatment that resolves the predicament. Clearly, this approach to training has inevitable flaws that can result in dire consequences for the patient and the medical professional alike. The incorporation of effective crisis management training into the educational programs of health care professionals is the additional element needed to reduce the likelihood of such an outcome and to assure patients that those to whom they have entrusted their care have the critical skills essential for coping with a crisis.

Education in effective management of crises is not a recent notion. In fact, simulations have been used for years to teach crisis management skills to a variety of professionals, such as pilots, military personnel, firefighters, and nuclear power plant workers.[12] The medical field, however, has only recently initiated the exploration of this training option. The specialties of anesthesia and radiology have pioneered the idea by instituting programs and engaging in several studies involving the use of realistic and computer-based simulators for training in crisis management. This chapter now explores the basis for these models and methods.

The majority of current medical training models for crisis management reflect similar models used for years in the aviation industry. Cockpit resource management training (CRM), considered previously, has been used by the aviation industry since 1979. At that time a National Aeronautics and Space Administration (NASA)/ Industry workshop addressed the concepts of crew coordination and effective utilization of all available resources in flight operations.[13] Since then there has always been the question, "Is cockpit resource management effective?" If one looks at the proliferation of CRM training programs, and the enormous investment of time and money that they entail, it appears that the question has been answered in the affirmative, but empirical evidence is just beginning to accumulate.[14] As for analogous training in medicine, studies have shown that this approach has considerable merit, but undisputed, nonsubjective data have not yet been realized.

Methods of evaluation currently used to examine the outcome and potential benefits of crisis management training in anesthesia and radiology include participant self-evaluation and testing and observer responses and ratings. These are highly subjective investigative methods, but as Weller, Wilson, and Robinson recognize in *Survey of Change in Practice Following Simulation-based Training in Crisis Management,* "It would be desirable to demonstrate improved management of crises in the operating theater, but problems with scheduling a standardized, repeatable crisis, and the ethical issues of observation limit the reliability and feasibility of this option."[15] Thus, several different criteria measuring the effectiveness of simulation-based crisis management training programs have been employed. In a 1998 study conducted at the Department of Radiology at the Brigham and Women's Hospital, Harvard Medical School, the mode of analysis utilized two reviewers' evaluations of videotapes that captured elements of the clinical scenarios conducted. Participants were rated by performance based on a range of behavioral responses both in the entire group of trainees and using a standard ordinal rating scale.[12] A similar study in anesthesia conducted at the Wellington Simulation Centre in 2001 used anesthesiologists' own perceptions of changes in their clinical practice as a measure of the efficacy of the program.[15]

Results of these studies and others like them have been exceedingly encouraging. Most participants express enjoyment of the courses and acknowledge that they are indeed a helpful and worthwhile educational experience. Those who conducted studies focusing on improved management of crisis simulations found marked advancement in the performance of both residents and attending physicians following a crisis management training course. Practicing physicians also thought that the training was a valuable resource and noted significant improvement in their problem-solving and communication skills in routine practice. Information relating to the need for and benefits associated with crisis management and knowledge of research and methods supporting its application are essential for developing a genuine appreciation of the concept. The fundamental ideas inherent in crisis management must be taught in order to manage crises effectively, and it is to these basic principles the chapter turns (Table 2).

Educating health care personnel in the elements of crisis management is a fairly complex process but can begin with the simple concept of anticipating problems and planning ahead. Whether the person is a unit secretary on the floor or a surgeon in the operating room, this concept is of primary importance. A patient whose condition has slowly deteriorated is a simple example of a case in which preparedness and anticipation should come into play. Physician's phone or beeper numbers should be easily accessible, a code

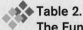

Table 2.
The Fundamental Elements of Crisis Mangement Training*

1. Anticipation of problems and planning ahead.
2. Problem-solving and decision-making skills
    • Observations and recognition
    • Data verification
    • Assessment of the situation
    • Systematic and nonsystematic responses
    • Re-evaluation
3. Teamwork
    • Verbalizing and sharing the problem with colleagues
4. Organization and leadership
    • Need for a leader
    • Delegation and prioritization of tasks
5. Calling for help

*These basic concepts are the key components that one must learn to manage crises effectively. Team members must learn and rehearse these ideas through discussion, simulation, and debriefing in order to refine and perfect the required skills.

cart should be positioned close by, family should be alerted to the impending problems, and other staff members should be notified of the precautionary measures taken in case a crisis ensues. All of these measures help avoid panic and permit a more organized crisis management response.

Another illustration of this idea involves a surgical team in the operating room. Before surgery the team receives knowledge that the patient has well-controlled asthma and moderately controlled high blood pressure. With this information the team must make preliminary decisions about which medications will be given, taking care not to exacerbate any of the patient's preexisting conditions, and prepare for crises which they foresee may arise in light of the patient's current situation. These preparatory actions enable the case to run smoothly with a low occurrence of problems, and, if a crisis should occur, the likelihood of a rapid and accurate resolution, with no unfavorable consequence to the patient, is extremely high.

The next element necessary for effective crisis management training is problem-solving and decision-making skills. Gaba established two key objectives that an instructor must address when conducting crisis management training. The first is to familiarize participants with the underlying processes of dynamic decision making—in particular, to enhance their acquisition of precompiled responses to common events. The second is to instruct participants in the coordinated integration of all available resources to maximize safe patient outcomes.[16] These objectives help taper the scope of the discussion to the individual level of crisis management training. To constitute an efficacious training program, the instructor must educate health care professionals about the fundamentals of key components in areas of dynamic decision making, leadership, and communication.

In conjunction with Gaba's first objective, it is crucial that the elements of dynamic decision making be further investigated. To accomplish this goal, let us focus on the perspectives of Orasanu and Connolly in *Decision Making in Action: Models and Methods,* which considers a model slightly different from the structured, systematic classical decision-making model. Known as naturalistic decision-making, or the act of making decisions in natural settings, this revised approach addresses seven factors, traditionally ignored in the classical model.[17]

The first factor involves "ill-structured problems." It is uncommon for the problems faced by medical professionals to conform to only one algorithm or construct. It thus becomes essential for an individual to evaluate all of the given variables and to decide which are of vital importance. The most effective method for acquiring and enhancing this faculty is through multiple exposures to a variety of different scenarios. This type of training can be achieved most expediently through the use of simulations. Exposure to thousands of trials, it has been argued, allows experts to build up a set of patterns for organizing information in their domain. These patterns facilitate rapid action and reduce workload.[18] Previously this chapter discussed four different categories from which a particular crisis may originate, acts of God, mechanical problems, human error, and management decision/indecision. Experiencing many simulations aids in the discovery of common patterns within each of these general classifications and ultimately leads to proficient decision-making and more effective crisis management.

Within the medical profession the work environment is rapidly changing. This change brings us to the second characteristic of naturalistic decision settings, "uncertain dynamic environments." The problems that one must confront in this field possess qualities capable of changing from moment to moment. An immediate diagnosis of the situation is often elusive, and observations can at times be deceiving. Here again, the use of simulators is of profound importance. Multiple trials can help to resolve problems associated with discerning key components of a developing or ongoing crisis and also promote pattern recognition, enabling timely evaluation and regulation of the situation.

A third factor to be considered is "shifting, ill-defined, or competing goals." This concept addresses the uncertain, rapidly changing, and often unclear nature of the objectives, which medical professionals must define and interpret in crises and on a daily basis. It is rare for a decision to be dominated by a single, well-understood goal or value.[17] Conflicts that revolve around the interests and well-being of patients can be exacerbated by the dynamic nature of a situation. Through simulated training exercises conducted with multiple players performing specific roles, individuals learn to address and resolve problems together, attend to disagreements, and deal with shifting intentions without compromising patient outcome.

Arenas in which natural decision making is prevalent employ the use of "action/ feedback loops" to cope with a series of events or actions intended to resolve a single problem. A physician, for example, may prescribe the antibiotic Biaxin to a patient who presents with symptoms that she believes are indicative of sinusitis. Two weeks latter the patient returns to the office with intensified symptoms. On talking to the patient, the physician discovers that she has been under tremendous stress while dealing with a messy divorce and that the pain, which had been originally associated with sinusitis, may instead be a manifestation of migraine headaches. A prescription is written for Naproxin, and on the next follow-up visit the patient's symptoms have resolved. This simplistic illustration represents the basic ideas pertinent to adequate comprehension. Situations that involve actions, evaluation of the effects of those actions, and then further actions to alleviate a particular problem arise each day in every aspect of the medical field. In a crisis situation it is imperative that actions are taken quickly and that components of the action are orchestrated in a smooth and coordinated fashion. To accomplish this goal, training cannot be taught in such a manner as to isolate the decision-making component alone. Decision-making processes must be taught within the context of a reasonable situation so that an individual can learn to combine these skills with other components required in the execution of a complex task.

"Time stress" and "high stakes" are two more vital qualities of natural decision- making that can significantly affect one's ability to cope with and manage situations. Especially within the context of crisis management, these two elements are at the forefront of almost every event. In a crisis event, time is of the essence, and this sentiment is particularly valid within the medical profession. A patient's condition in a crisis may change in minutes or even seconds, and if these variations are not accounted for and dealt with in an acceptable and timely manner, severe consequences may ensue. Indeed, the result of a mismanaged crisis in medicine may compromise the health and well-being of the patient or even result in loss of life—high stakes indeed. Such enormous responsibility can also create personal stress that, on reaching extreme levels, may impede effective decision-making processes. Zakay and Wooler discovered that practice without time pressure did not enhance decision-making under time constraints. This finding suggests that if decision-making is likely to be required under time pressure or other stressful conditions, practice should include task performance under those conditions (or their simulation).[18] Therefore, to prepare for these two elements effectively, simulated events must be realistic in terms of the pace at which incidents occur and the expected severity and consequences of actions taken.

The final characteristic of naturalistic decision settings that differs from that of classical decision- making is the involvement of "multiple players." It is seldom the case that medical professionals confronted with crisis situations will manage the emergency entirely alone. Thus, cooperation among all of the team members is paramount. Everyone must be kept aware of situational goals, the ongoing status of events as they unfold, and any other information that might be pertinent to the decision- making goals of each member of the team. The many theories that address ideas about training for team performance are discussed in more detail later.

Now that the essential parts that make up decision-making in natural settings have been discussed, along with training for each characteristic component, it is time to elaborate on the cognitive attributes that problem solving and dynamic decision making entail: observations and recognition, data verification, assessment of the situation, systematic and nonsystematic responses, and re-evaluation (Fig. 4).

Observations and recognition include being attentive to all of the surrounding variables influencing a given situation and recognizing when any one or many attributes are incongruent with the overall data. The knowledge of such deviations, whether from clinical observances, laboratory tests, or monitored variables, may be the only premonition to an impending crisis situation. Once these variances are identified one must assess whether they represent a problem, and if so, what actions are appropriate to manage the situation.

Once observations have been made and specific data are available, one must be able to evaluate properly whether the information collected is valid and reliable. Gaba as-

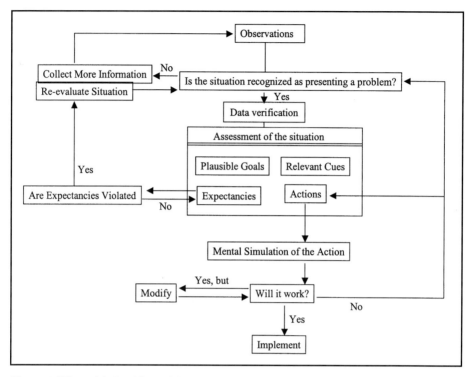

Figure 4. This model of problem-solving and dynamic decision-making in complex environments illustrates the thought processes that occur when an individual is confronted with a complex decision-making task. Understanding these components helps to organize the decision-making process and, as an individual becomes more experienced, facilitates faster and more efficient decision-making strategies. This model is based in part on Gary A. Klein's Recognition-Primed Decision Model.[10]

serts that data are not always reliable and must often be verified before acting upon them. He notes that even direct clinical observation can be misleading and outlines seven different methods for verifying data[16]:

1. Repeating the observation or observing the short-term trend
2. Observing an existing redundant channel
3. Correlating multiple related variables
4. Activating a new observation modality
5. Calibrating or testing an instrument's function
6. Replacing and instrument with a backup
7. Asking for a second opinion

Often the magnitude of the crisis or the time frame in which actions must be taken limits the type of data verification that can be effectively employed. It is essential, however, when circumstances permit that data be properly scrutinized, to limit the number of errors made through the acquisition of erroneous or misleading information.

Once it is clear that the data attained are correct representations of the current situation, it is possible to proceed in assessing the situation. In discussing his Recognition-primed Decision Model of Rapid Decision Making, Klein asserts that people use situation assessment to generate a plausible course of action and mental simulation to evaluate that course of action. He elaborates by outlining four important aspects of situation assessment: (1) understanding the types of goals that can be reasonably accomplished in the situation, (2) increasing the salience of cues that are important within the context of the situation, (3) forming expectations that can serve as a check on the accuracy of the situation assessment (i.e., violation of the expectations suggests that the situation has been misunderstood), and (4) identifying the typical actions to take.[19]

Once a suitable action has been identified, Klein found that most people, if time permits, run through a mental simulation of the event to identify any problems. If this mental exercise uncovers no flaws, then the action is implemented; if problems are foreseen, the action is modified. It is easier to understand these constituents of assessment in the context of an example. For instance, an anesthesiologist in the operating room realizes that the patient is not receiving an adequate amount of oxygen through the ventilation system. The ultimate goal is to restore proper breathing to the patient, but the first step in doing so is to locate the source of the problem. Initial expectations may lead one to check the endotracheal tube for obstructions, the oxygen monitoring device to ensure its correct functioning, and the ventilation unit to ensure that it is adjusted to the correct settings. If all of these elements appear to be operating accurately, the expectancies originally constructed are violated. At this point it is imperative that the ultimate goal be achieved or the patient is going to suffer adverse consequences. The initial ultimate goal now becomes the immediate goal, and new expectations and actions are considered. The ventilator is subsequently disconnected, and the patient is manually given oxygen via an ambulatory bag. The patient's oxygen level returns to normal, and the patient suffers no negative consequences from the experience.

Many first responses to crisis situations are systematic responses based on specific algorithms that fit well with the observed variables. In situations that do not fit a specific set of rules or a precompiled procedure, one must develop a logical plan that will determine and treat the given problem. In such instances and in situations in which the planned procedure does not produce the desired effect, medical professionals experience dilemmas. Slips and fixation errors, as discussed previously, can further facilitate such incidents. Although these errors are two of the most commonly made, they are also exceedingly preventable. One must learn to recognize these tendencies and work diligently to avoid them.

Norman describes various slips that may occur during execution of a necessary action[5]:

1. Capture error: a common action takes over from the one intended (e.g., force of habit).

2. Description error: performing a correct action on the wrong thing (e.g., flipping the wrong switch).

3. Memory error: forgetting an item in a sequence.

4. Sequence error: performing an action out of sequence with other actions.

5. Mode error: actions appropriate for one mode of operation are incorrect in another mode.

In a dynamic field such as the medical profession, particularly in crisis situations, one must constantly reassess the patient and adapt the treatment accordingly. Re-evaluation is a key feature in the complicated process by which complex decisions are made. Frequently the initial assessment of a patient's condition is incorrect or incomplete, and further measures may need to be taken to ensure a positive outcome. Likewise, some treatments may have adverse or unexpected effects, and failure to reevaluate the situation can have devastating consequences. As a crisis progresses, a patient's status changes, and faulty adaptation to these changes may result in a fixation error. Despite this possibility, errors can be prevented by developing a good behavior- monitoring mechanism or by having a member of the team check and assess the data to catch any errors that may be made.

This problem brings us to another fundamental aspect of crisis management training—teamwork. The ability to function optimally as a team is essential for the proper regulation of any medical emergency. To begin, it is important first to establish what team means. Orasanu et al. developed a list of specific characteristics that define a team: a set of two or more individuals, more than one information source, interdependence and coordination among members, adaptive management of internal resources, common valued goals, defined roles and responsibilities, and task-relevant knowledge.[20] These characteristics allow us to distinguish between a team and a group, and for our purposes the above definition applies. The central attribute in team performance is communication. Individual skills and knowledge are not sufficient for successful team performance. An individual must be able to utilize appropriate resources through interaction processes.[20] An effective way to procure successful communication skills is through simulation and encouragement by the instructor to verbalize data to the entire team and make all problems immediately known. Practicing this process prevents miscommunication of pertinent information and misunderstanding of the severity of an event. Because this vocal response adds yet another task to an already demanding workload, it is recommended that such strategies be incorporated in a safe and controlled environment, such as a patient simulation.

Within a team it is important to establish leadership in order to maintain integrity and proper organization. A charge nurse and physician are two examples of people who often are in charge of an emergent event. A proficient leader can divide his or her attention among many tasks and possibly many different problems. Allocation of attention is a critical aspect of leadership. It determines which data streams are observed and how frequently and the priority given to different routine actions and to handling different potential problems.[16] A leader assumes the responsibility of prioritizing and delegating tasks among members of the team and seeing that those tasks are correctly executed. Without a prominent leader it is difficult to coordinate team members. Lack of leadership can lead to confusion, uncertainty, and a chaotic environment, which may foster inappropriate and misinformed decisions and is not conducive to effective crisis management.

The final and possibly most disregarded factor involved in managing crises is calling for help. This factor may seem simple, but when time is short and stakes are high, it is often perceived that there is no time to call for support. Such a belief often leads to tragic consequences for both patients and medical professionals. Thus, it is necessary to educate individuals about their duty to call for help and therefore ensure that proper steps are taken to generate the most positive outcome achievable under the particular circumstances.

Now that all of the primary elements used to establish crisis management training have been discussed, it is necessary to review the instructional components of a course that can be practiced and perfected. The method of action centers on the use of simulations to exercise the methods and skills that at this point trainees should understand and possess. In the following section, two scenarios mentioned in previous chapters are revisited. Each is discussed briefly, leading to a crisis situation that elicits the behaviors and cognitions that have been the principal focus of this chapter.

The first of these scenarios comes from the chapter on pharmacology. A situation is manufactured for the purpose of teaching the sequence of events that occur in an allergic drug reaction. It is not difficult, however, to modify the scope of this incident so that the new objective is to practice the skills required for proficient management of a crisis. This particular crisis falls into the category of human error (an incorrect or improper medication is administered) and plays out as follows. A patient has arrived in the emergency department and after thorough examination is diagnosed with septicemia. This systemic disease, formerly known as "blood poisoning," is caused by the multiplication of microorganisms in the circulating blood.[21] Treatment options are discussed, and it is decided to administer an IV drip of imipenem (500 mg) and cilastatin (500 mg). No one thinks to review whether the patient acknowledged any drug allergies, although they are indicated in the chart. Indeed, the patient is allergic to penicillin and the newer class of cephalosporin drugs, one of which has just been administered. The patient soon goes into anaphylactic shock, and thus a crisis has develeloped. The trainees involved in this simulation must now adhere to the fundamental concepts for crisis management, which have been discussed throughout this chapter, to identify the problem, take appropriate actions, and yield a positive outcome for the patient.

A second category to which a crisis may be assigned is that of mechanical problems. The chapter on obstetrics and gynecology presents a case with the potential to fit perfectly into this genre. The scenario, introduced as Case No.2: Molar Pregnancy and Thyroid Storm, can be briefly summarized as follows: An 18-year-old girl presents in the emergency department with severe vaginal bleeding. The fetus is at a gestational age of 12 weeks, and this is the girl's first pregnancy. After the physical examination and extensive laboratory tests have been performed, it is determined that the patient has a molar pregnancy and needs to undergo urgent dilation and curettage (D&C). The crisis management trainees in this simulation begin in the operating room with the patient. During the evacuation procedure the patient suddenly goes into atrial fibrillation, her body temperature elevates to 38.6°C, and her blood pressure rises to 200/120 mmHg. These are all signs of a thyroid storm and should be treated by the trainees who are performing the anesthesia. In the midst of this turmoil, the Berkeley suction machine that the surgeons are using to evacuate the uterus breaks down. The trainee surgeons must now decide what actions to take in order to complete the procedure successfully. To accomplish this goal, they must advance through all the elements previously discussed as fundamental to effective crisis management (see Table 2).

After each simulation has been completed, participants must be required take part in a debriefing session. The team members are allowed to observe a videotape of their performance and then discuss the concepts from their training that they observed and those that were forgotten. This segment of instruction is critical to the comprehension, encoding, and analysis of the concepts and procedures performed in the simulation and to the understanding and incorporation of avenues not pursued.

Teaching Crisis Management

Gary E. Loyd, MD, MMM

The cases explained above are examples of how just about any simulation scenario can be converted into crisis management (CM) education. In contrast, the remainder of this chapter focuses on teaching CM directly as the main learning objective. Arguments can be made that life experiences can teach CM, but the literature shows that this argument may not be true. Morgan found no correlation between students' clinical experiences and level of confidence and their ability to perform on standardized scenarios on a high-fidelity human simulator.[22] Therefore, formal CM training courses seem to be indicated. Several people have taken the lead in developing CM courses and teaching initiatives. CM has been taught to medical students and surgery interns learning trauma management.[23, 24] The CM courses have used various methods to achieve successful teaching. At the University of Toronto, an integrated approach to crisis resource management was attempted successfully, using seminars, computer-based programs, and an anesthesia simulator.[25] Schwid and O'Donnell described the successful use of a screen-based program for teaching CM.[26] Nyssen et al. compared learning on a screen-based CM program and a patient simulator learning session and found no difference in acquired knowledge but a significant improvement in teamwork and performance with the patient simulator. Reznek et al. demonstrated the successful portability of an ACRM type of course in emergency medicine using patient simulators.[27]

The impact on crisis management is difficult to assess because crises do not occur with sufficient frequency. Prospective studies may have to be conducted over extended periods or among multiple institutions. Retrospective analysis of crises may yield some evidence, but in the author's opinion the variables will be too great to produce iron-clad results. Studies so far are primarily limited to the benefit perceived by the learners in CM courses. In the study by Holzman et al., for example, senior attending physicians and residents who finished training in an ACRM thought that the benefit was significant enough to warrant yearly training and retraining.[28] Another study by Kurreck et al. found that anesthesiologists who had never even seen a simulator before the ACRM training workshop reported benefit and indicated that such training should be taken every 18 months.[29] Participants in a CM course in New Zealand recommended that the course to be repeated every two years.[30]

Emerging studies are using simulation to test the impact of CM training courses. The successful teaching of crisis management in radiology using simulation demonstrated higher scores than courses with lectures only.[12] In a follow-up survey of participants in a CM course, respondents reported that the CM course had changed their practices and that the principles learned in the CM course had been applied to crises similar to, but not the same as, those experienced in the CM course.[15]

Government and military agencies laid some of the basic groundwork for the study of crisis management, and their results have spilled over into the medical arenas. When Berkenstadt et al. found that using full protective gear against bioterrorism increased the intubation time of experienced anesthesiologists and decreased communication ability during crisis management, important information emerged about limitations or hindrances can manifest during crisis management.[31] The value of simulation in crisis management goes beyond its educational value; simulation also provides insights into how we approach crises. The United States Army demonstrated the effectiveness of using a virtual reality simulator to improve complex decision making in the combat arena.[32]

At the University of Louisville, teaching crisis management has been an evolving process. The class has been taught to varying audiences more than 40 times, with the approach changing to better initiate a change in the long-term behaviors of the learners. The pioneers in this field as it applies to medicine, such as Drs. Gaba, Howard, and Schwid, have taken a systematic approach to translating how CM has been taught in health care. The workshop presentations at the American Society of Anesthesiologist have been based on hands-on, interactive learning sessions, advocating four principles of crisis management, as set forth by the pioneers. When this method is taught to medical students and anesthesia residents, the behaviors outlined under each principle are readily accepted and short-term improvement in crisis management skills is noticed. Yet, when retested a few months later, the student and resident learners exhibited no change in crisis management behaviors. The methodology is being refined in preparation for a research study. Therefore, the methodology presented here is anecdotal.

The current approach, which is a hybrid of work done by Wong[33] and Reznek,[27] concentrates on seven essential behaviors. Students and residents prepare for the crisis management session by reading the Wong and Reznek article—not for their conclusions, but for the way the authors taught crisis management. The CM session begins with the students listing all kinds of crises. Usually the learners list medical crises and need challenging to think of other examples. They then quickly list the common characteristics of the example crises. The instructor usually must provide the last common characteristic: effectively managed in a similar manner. The next part of the session begins with the presentation of an acronym, **LIPCRUD,** which summarizes the seven essential behaviors mentioned earlier: **l**eadership, **i**nformation management, **p**ractice/**p**lanning, **c**ommunication, **r**e-evaluation, **u**tilization of resources, and **d**istribution of workload.

The students describe their perceptions of what leadership is, which range from the tyrannical dictator to the docile facilitator. This information is quite helpful to the instructor as he or she works on realigning the student's perceptions with the principles of CM. One of the most popular perceptions is that the leader dictates the distribution of workload to personnel as they line up awaiting their instructions. When asked to diagram leadership, the most common sketch places the leader at the top of a pyramid, with instructions streaming down to the bottom and information streaming up to the top (Fig. 5). Although many health care institutions and departments are set up in this traditional manner, it is not the most effective model in CM. Yet the most common reason for ineffective CM is the lack of effective leadership.

All of the medical students and residents at the University of Louisville taking CM training are ACLS-certified. Yet when asked how they would perform in adhering to the guidelines of ACLS in resuscitating the instructor, they unanimously reply "poorly." They usually agree that they would have a better chance of resuscitating the instructor collectively rather than individually. From this example, the concept of group thinking develops, and the new leadership diagram begins to look like Figure 6, with a web of communication in place. Not all communication needs to be between team members and the leader, but most of it is. Leadership does not take place in a vacuum; it is the pivot

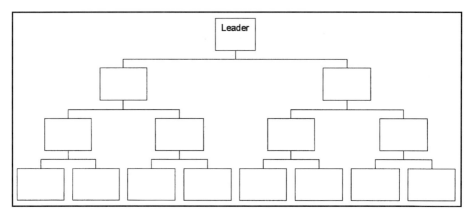

Figure 5. The leader is designed as the top box. Each box represents a person involved in the CM situation and each lines represents a line of communication.

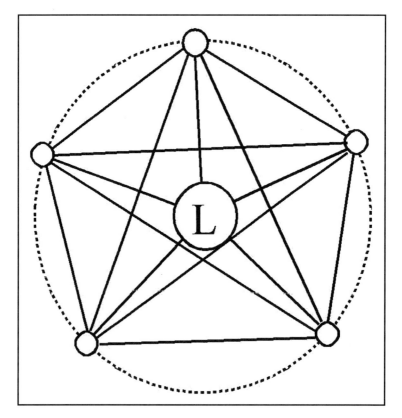

Figure 6. Each circle is a person in the CM situation and the circle with the "L" is the leader and each black line is a line of communication, producing a web of communication.

for the other behaviors to align themselves. When asked who should be the leader in a crisis, the learners routinely reply that it should be the one with the most experience with the crisis or the one who is most senior.

At this point an example is presented of a situation at University of Louisville Hospital. A sewage pipe in the ceiling of an unoccupied operating room burst, spilling large amounts of sewage into the room. The housekeeper, who had finished a course in contamination containment 2 weeks earlier, was able to get the doctors, nurses, and technicians to mobilize quickly and produce appropriate barriers for containment. The housekeeper performed all of the necessary functions of effective leadership .The instructor advocates to the learners that the job of the leader is to perform/facilitate the other six behaviors. From this point the other behaviors are addressed.

Since each line in the diagram (Fig. 6) represents communication, communication is the next logical behavior to address. When the learners are asked to describe how effectively or ineffectively their special orders are handled during lunch hour at a popular fast-food hamburger chain, they can almost always break it down to effective and ineffective communication. Effective communication is two-way so that the sender gets a reply confirming the information sent, resulting in correct production and delivery of the special order. The other part of communication addresses the group thinking perspective. If a team member sees a flat-line and declares that the patient is in asystole and another team member calls the first team member a dunce because he or she has identified a lead off the patient, the likelihood that the first team member will speak up again or that other team members will speak up for fear of being ridiculed becomes greatly reduced. The learners usually can develop some strategies for the leader to re-establish the group communication and facilitate the communication of ideas.

Communication is the second most common reason for ineffective CM. Two main items are communicated: instructions and information. Delegation of tasks or distribution of workload appears straightforward. The learners appear quick to accept the logic of the concept and how it can originate from the leader. The instructor then gives examples of the situation providing a distribution of workload, such as the organized chaos of the trauma operating room at University of Louisville Hospital, or team members asking for help in doing their tasks and others volunteering without the intervention of the leader. Information in a crisis can be quite large and daunting. The learners are asked to reflect on the days when they received their learner's permit for driving and the amount of information that they had to manage at one time to accomplish the task of driving. They can readily relate to this analogy and, after some pondering, come up with what mental gymnastics are required.

Then the instructor presents the concept of fixations as the mental information management ability that we develop through practice. As presented earlier in this chapter, fixations are normal mental functions that allow us to perform complex tasks efficiently so that we become unconsciously competent in those tasks. When we perform a fixation in error, accidents occur, and when we allow the fixation error to bias our actions, poor patient outcomes occur.

When fixation errors occur, the re-evaluation behavior is the mechanism whereby we catch such errors and attempt to correct for them. Students seem to have the most difficulty in describing what re-evaluation behavior, as a concept, should look like—perhaps because it is a mental skill in which they are only consciously incompetent. The instructor should take care to put this behavior in context, such as an ACLS code situation or even a local crisis with which the learners are familiar either directly or via extensive news coverage. The behavior can be described as several team members (which usually include the leader) physically and mentally stepping back from the action and reviewing the physical actions of the team, the mental conclusions drawn from the data, and the resulting responses. During the review, the validity of the action or conclusion drawn must be challenged. The optimal members of this review team should be those with expertise in the situation, but not in the critical tasks that they are still performing. Having a housekeeper with no medical training or a surgeon struggling to re-anastomose a lacerated artery in the re-evaluation group would probably not be optimal during a medical crisis.

Utilization of resources also appears to be an easy concept for the learners to understand. Calling for help during a code is acceptable behavior. The learners can usually give examples of observing a health professional not calling for help—either as a perceived preservation of ego or because the person was unaware of what resources were available. Another aspect of the utilization of resources is "thinking outside the box." When asked to describe what this term means, usually only one or two learners in a group are able to do so. A decent definition is to utilize items or other resources for functions for which they were not intended. Examples cited include using syringes for oxygen hose connectors or ballpoint pens for emergent surgical airways.

The last of the behaviors is practice/planning. Algorithms for common crises such as an ACLS code or a fire are accepted as good skills to possess for training. Yet without proper feedback and reinforcement of skills, the short-term memory storage does not make it to the long-term memory. It is impossible to produce an algorithm for every conceivable crisis. It would be rare for a hospital in Kentucky to have a hurricane disaster plan or for a hospital in Hawaii to have a blizzard plan. Some crises are simply not anticipated until they happen. Consider the September 11 disaster of the twin towers in New York City as an example. We can fill whole libraries with algorithms and still not include them all, not to mention the time required to practice and prepare.

After an interactive small-group session on CM, the students or residents go to an adjacent human patient simulation laboratory to practice a scenario such as a standard anesthetic induction or placement of a pulmonary artery catheter. The learners are warned that sometime during one of the scenarios, there will be a surprise crisis that they will have to manage as a team. Even though the team is warned that a crisis will occur, they are usually surprised when it does.

When the CM scenario is finished, the students are allowed to watch themselves perform on videotape. They are asked to identify the leader, identify the fixation errors, and grade themselves as a team on the seven essential behaviors on a four-point scale. Then they are asked to develop strategies to address or improve their most poorly performed behaviors. During a didactic session for CM, one student said he had crisis management training in his former life as a businessman and that the material was just repackaging. To his surprise, he was challenged when the repackaged material focused on changing his behavior. After watching his inadequate CM behavior on the videotape, he announced that it was apparent to him that simply knowing the principles of CM was not enough. Practicing the behavior changes was the key to producing effective CM.

The purpose of this educational unit is to change behavior in an effort to improve outcome. The data, so far, are inconclusive that crisis management training will improve patient outcomes, but given the impact on airlines, emergency response teams, and the military, it seems intuitive that it should. The University of Louisville experience is just one method of teaching CM. and its effectiveness has not yet been proven.

Examples used at the University of Louisville program are divided into individual tasks in case there are separate teachers, simulator operators, hands-on learners, and observers. The detail provided should be sufficient to program a high-fidelity simulator but also easily adaptable to a lower-fidelity simulator. Three cases have three distinct audiences, although with some modifications each can be adapted to other audiences, such as nursing or allied health professionals. The following descriptions are not given in great detail because of the detail provided in the boxes in the Appendix.

Anaphylaxis and Pneumothorax Case. Box 1 contains the instructions to the simulator operator for students learning a standard anesthetic induction on an anesthesia rotation. The instructor gets the page of instructions in Box 2 in case he or she is filling in for the person who wrote the scenario. The learners receive the third handout (Box 3). Even though they have only one learning objective about standard induction, they focus on Box 3 because they know that it is the immediate task to perform. The instructor reviews and demonstrates the induction protocol and then leaves the room to allow students to perform the tasks as a team, with the instructions that everyone on the team must perform the induction at least once in the role as an anesthesiologist. After one or two runs at induction and intubation, the students become somewhat comfortable with the protocol and their confidence rises. Thus the third or fourth learner usually gets the CM scenario added onto the induction scenario. If there are any observers, they receive at least Box 4. Some observers are interested in how to teach with the simulator and receive all four of the boxes.

No Oxygen Cholecystectomy Case. The no-oxygen example is usually too advanced for medical students and frequently trips up junior residents. As in the previous example, there is a handout for the simulator operator (Box 5), the instructor (Box 6), students (Box 7), and observers (Box 8). However, the learner's handout has a misguiding learning objective, leading the learners to think that the CM will be about latex allergy. The instructor must not get so involved in whether or not the learners pick up on the lack of oxygen supply that he or she forgets the other 80% of learning objectives: to learn about and perfect the essential behaviors for effective CM. This scenario can be easily adapted to a critical care setting.

Pediatric Seizure Case. The third example (Boxes 9–12) is situated in a critical care setting. The intended audience is stated as graduates of an anesthesiology program, but it may include any physician or nurse providing care to critical care patients. Experienced health care providers usually catch the simple problems like those presented in the first two examples; they must be challenged with multiple problems simultaneously to create a truly chaotic environment. The purpose of the more challenging situation is to force the participants into CM behaviors to the point that they can identify which behaviors need strategies for improvement.

Conclusion

The conversion of aviation CM to medical CM has been facilitated by several medical pioneers. They have adapted the basic principles to medical situations and have begun to validate the effectiveness of teaching CM principles to students. The best method to produce the desired behavior changes that positively affect patient outcomes remains to be proven. As the area of medical CM becomes part of medical school curricula and becomes entrenched in postgraduate training for all specialties, our knowledge of how to be effective crisis managers will increase.

References

1. Gaba D: Theory of dynamic decision making and crisis management. In Gaba D, Fish K, Howard S (eds): Crisis Management in Anesthesiology. New York, Churchill Livingstone, 1994, pp 1–29.
2. Coombs WT: A need for more crisis management information. In Health RL, Vasquez GM (eds): Ongoing Crisis Communication Planning, Managing, and Responding. Thousand Oaks, CA, Sage Publications, 1999, pp 1–7.
3. Mitroff II, Anagnos G: Why crises are an inevitable and permanent feature of modern society. In Mitroff II (ed): Managing Crises Before They Happen: What Every Executive Needs to Know about Crisis Management. New York, Amacon Books, 2001, pp 5–34.
4. Institute for Crisis Management: http://www.crisisexperts.com/crisisdef_main.htm. Last accessed 11-2-2003.
5. Norman DA: Categorization of action slips. Psychol Rev 88:1–14, 1981.
6. Tindale R: Decision errors made by individuals and groups. In Individual and Group Decision Making : Current Issues. Hillsdale, NJ, Lawrence Erlbaum Associates, 1993, pp 109–123.
7. United States Government Interagency Domestic Terrorism Concept of Operations Plan: www.fbi.gov/publications/conplan/conplan.pdf. Last accessed 11-2-2003.
8. Helmreich RL, Merritt AC, Wilhelm JA: The evolution of Crew Resource Management training in commercial aviation. Int J Aviat Psychol 9(1):19–32, 1999.
9. Anderson LW, Krathwohl DR, Bloom BS: A Taxonomy for Learning, Teaching, and Assessing : A Revision of Bloom's Taxonomy of Educational Objectives. New York, Longman, 2001.
10. Nelson TO: Knowing thyself and others: Progress in metacognitive social psychology. In Yzerbyt V, Lories G, Dardenne B (eds): Metacognition: Cognitive and Social Dimensions. London, Sage Publications, 1998, pp 69–89.
11. Bready LL: Decision Making in Anesthesiology: An Algorithmic Approach, 3rd ed. St. Louis, Mosby, 2000.
12. Sica GT, et al: Computerized realistic simulation: A teaching module for crisis management in radiology. Am J Roentgenol:301–304, 1999.
13. Cooper G: Resource management on the flight deck. In Proceedings of a NASA/Industry Workshop, 1980. Moffet Field, CA, US: NASA-Ames Research Center.
14. Helmreich RL, et al: How effective is cockpit resource management training? Exploring issues in evaluating the impact of programs to enhance crew coordination. Flight Saf Dig 9(5):1–17, 1990.
15. Weller J, Wilson L, Robinson B: Survey of change in practice following simulation-based training in crisis management. Anaesthesia 58.471–473, 2003.
16. Gaba D: Dynamic decision making in anesthesiology: Cognitive models and training approaches. In Evans D, Patel V (eds): Advanced Models of Cognition for Medical Training and Practice. New York, Springer-Verlag, 1992, pp 123–147.
17. Orasanu J, Connolly T: The reinvention of decision making. In Klein GA (ed) Decision Making in Action : Models and Methods. Norwood, NJ, Ablex Publications, 1993, pp 3–20.
18. Means B, et al: Training decision makers for the real world. In Klein GA (ed): Decision Making in Action: Models and Methods. Norwood, NJ, Ablex Publications, 1993, pp 306- 326.
19. Klein GA: A recognition-primed decision (RPD) model of rapid decision making. In Klein GA (ed): Decision Making in Action: Models and Methods. Norwood, NJ, Ablex Publications, 1993, pp 138–147.
20. Orasanu J, Salas E: Team decision making in complex environments. In Klein GA (ed): Decision Making in Action: Models and Methods. Norwood, NJ, Ablex Publications, 1993, pp 327–345.

21. Stedman TL, Dirckx JH: Stedman's Concise Medical Dictionary for the Health Professions, 4th ed. Philadelphia, Lippincott Williams & Wilkins, 2001, p 897.
22. Morgan PJ, Cleave-Hogg D: Comparison between medical students' experience, confidence and competence. Med Educ 36:534–539, 2002.
23. Gilbart MK, et al: A computer-based trauma simulator for teaching trauma management skills. Am J Surg 179:223–238, 2000.
24. Marshall RL, et al: Use of a human patient simulator in the development of resident trauma management skills. J Trauma 51:17–21, 2001.
25. Byrick R, Cleave-Hogg D, McKnight D: A crisis management program for residents in anesthesia. Acad Med 73:592, 1998.
26. Schwid HA, O'Donnell D: The Anesthesia Simulator-Recorder: A device to train and evaluate anesthesiologists' responses to critical incidents. Anesthesiology 72:191–197, 1990.
27. Reznek M, et al: Emergency medicine crisis resource management (EMCRM): Pilot study of a simulation-based crisis management course for emergency medicine. Acad Emerg Med 10:386–389, 2003.
28. Holzman RS, et al: Anesthesia crisis resource management: Real-life simulation training in operating room crises. J Clin Anesth 7:675–687, 1995.
29. Kurrek MM, Fish KJ: Anaesthesia crisis resource management training: An intimidating concept, a rewarding experience. Can J Anaesth 43(5 Pt 1):430–434, 1996.
30. Garden A, et al: Education to address medical error—a role for high fidelity patient simulation. N Z Med J 115(1150):133–134, 2002.
31. Berkenstadt H, et al: The use of advanced simulation in the training of anesthesiologists to treat chemical warfare casualties. Anesth Analg 96:1739–1742, 2003
32. Pleban RJ, et al: Training and assessing complex decision-making in a virtual environment. Percept Mot Skills 94(3 Pt 1):871–82, 2002.
33. Wong SH, Ng KG, Chen PP: The application of clinical simulation in crisis management training. Hong Kong Med J 8:131–135, 2002.

APPENDIX

 Box 1.
Instructions for Simulator Operator
Anaphylaxis and Pneumothorax Case (Standard Induction)

The adult male mannequin is intubated with a #8.0 oral ETT and is on the OR table ready for induction. The EKG, pulse oximeter, arterial pressure wave, central venous pressure, intracranial pressure waveform, ETCO2 and NIBP are the monitors attached.

Connect:
- Art line, but do not turn on
- PA catheter, but do not turn on
- CVP catheter, but do not turn on
- ICP, turned off
- All standard monitors except temp are on the manikin

Other:
- Mannequin on back awake
- Anesthesia machine fully working
- Anesthesia cart fully stocked
- Induction drugs laid out

Run:
- Start Standard Man awake
- Eyes to automatic
- Set weight to 70 kg

States/Interventions:
- The first two or three students will be allowed to perform a standard induction uneventfully.
- The next student will have the scenario play out
- Administer all drugs according to verbalized desire if they are not in a syringe
- Follow all the fluid instructions.

Scenario events:
- As soon as the induction agent is given start the anaphylaxis scenario.
- As soon as the student gives the first breath through the endotracheal tube successfully placed, then start the left tension pneumothorax scenario

- Anaphylaxis Scenario
  Begin
    set breathing to wheezing
    set shunt fraction to 0.15 over 1 min
    remove 800 ml of fluid
    set SVR to 0.9 over 1 min
    set both bronch resistances to 40 cm
  Mild
    set shunt fraction to 0.2over 1 min
    remove 800 ml of fluid
    set SVR to 0.8 over 1 min
  Worsening
    set shunt fraction to 0.25 over 1 min
    remove 800 ml of fluid
    set SVR to 0.7 over 1 min
  Severe
    set shunt fraction to 0.3 over 1 min
    remove 800 ml of fluid
    set SVR to 0.6 over 1 min
    set ischemic index to .8 over 5 min
- If epinephrine given, then restore all to normal

- Tension Pneumothorax Scenario
    set chest wall compliance to 0.1 over 1 min
    set left lung compliance to 0.1 over 1 min
    set left intrapleural volume to 1000 ml over 1 min
    set chest wall capacity to 2300 over 1 min
    set shunt fraction to 0.5 over 15 sec
    set left bronchial occlusion to total occlusion over 1 min
- If left chest is needled, then restore all to normal

Box 2.
Briefing Instructions (FOR the instructor)
Anaphylaxis and Pneumothorax Case (Standard Induction)

Intended audience is third- and fourth-year medical students.

This is based on a REAL case.
+ Let them READ their case. Explain what each step of the standard induction requires and why it is performed.
+ Demonstrate the standard induction for them and tell them they each will be required to be the anesthesiologist and do an induction and intubation. You, the instructor, will be out of the room and your classmates will help you as need be.

Only if asked:
+ Any other lab or x-ray values are "drawn and pending"
+ The monitors visible (EKG, NIBP, pulse oximeter) are what you have.
+ If they call for an attending anesthesiologist, they are doing a code in another room.
+ If they call for a surgeon, they are still in their car in the parking garage.

- -

Problems to be encountered in addition to the Case (do **NOT** reveal to the participants):
+ *The patient will have an anaphylaxis to the induction agent.*
+ *The patient will have a left tension pneumothorax from the first breath after successful intubation.*
+ *They will review their performances on videotape and score themselves.*

❖ Box 3.
Learner's Handout (Standard Induction)

Learning Objectives: After this session the learner should be able to:
   1) understand the components a standard induction and intubation for an elective surgical procedure
   2) understand their ability to manage a crisis
   3) improve their teamwork skills
   4) improve their communication
   5) understand the essential behaviors for effective crisis management

An 18-year-old man is scheduled for an elective hernia repair under general anesthesia.

PMHx: None
Allergy: NKMA
Medications: None
Review of Systems: All systems are negative except for PMHx.
Preoperative Physical Examination:
   BP = 120/65, HR = 65, RR = 15, SpO2 = 98% on room air
   Airway = Malampati class II, teeth in good repair
      Neuro = Awake, Alert, Oriented times three
   Skin = Normal
   Pulmonary = Clear to auscultation, no wheezing
   Cardiac = Regular rate and rhythm without any murmurs
   Weight is 70 Kg
      Height of 5' 11"
Laboratory:
Hemoglobin = 15.0, Hematocrit = 45.0, Platelets are 250,000 and WBC = 6.8
Access:
One 18g IV right forearm
IV fluid going at 130 ml per hour

Standard Induction Protocol:
1) Prepartion of tools and drugs
2) Preparation of patient, monitors, and positioning
3) Preoxygenation
4) Induction
5) Ventilate patient
6) Paralyzation
7) Intubation
8) Check endotracheal tube placement

Box 4.
OBSERVERS' DEBRIEFING WORKSHEET
Anaphylaxis and Pneumothorax Case (Standard Induction):
Specific debriefing points

Standard Induction . . . . . Did they?
+ prepare tools and drugs?
+ prepare the patient with monitors and positioning?
+ preoxygenate the patient?
+ induction the patient appropriately?
+ ventilate the patient?
+ paralyze the patient?
+ intubate the patient successfully and appropriately?
+ check endotracheal tube placement?

Crew (Crisis) Resource Management . . . . . Did they?
+ Have leadership?
+ Manage their information?
+ Show evidence of systematically dealing with an unknown crisis?
+ Have good communication skills?
+ Re-evaluate for fixation errors?
+ Utilize all their resources?
+ Delegate responsibilities?

Box 5.
Instructions for Simulator Operator
No Oxygen (Cholecystectomy)

The adult female mannequin is not intubated on the OR table ready for general anesthesia.

Connect:
• Art line, turn on
• PA catheter, but do not turn on
• CVP catheter, but do not turn on
• ICP, turned off
• All standard monitors except temp

Other:
• Mannequin on back awake
• Anesthesia machine fully working
• Anesthesia cart fully stocked
• Induction drugs laid out
• Put in a faulty oxygen analyzer

Run:
• Start Standard Woman awake
• Eyes to automatic
• Set weight to 90 kg
• Set age to 45 yr

States/Interventions:
• The resident will do a standard induction on this patient.

Scenario events:
• As soon as the resident has put down the mask to intubate, switch the oxygen supply line to nitrogen and start videotaping.
• Increase the oxygen consumption to 2000 ml/min
• Increase the shunt fraction to 0.5
• Set the ischemic index to 0.8
• If the residents identifies the problem and starts to ventilate with room air, then put the patient into severe bronchospasm and reduce the oxygen consumption to 400 ml/min.

Box 6.
Briefing Instructions (FOR the instructor)
No Oxygen (Cholecystectomy)

Intended audience is residents of any experience.

This is based on a REAL case.
+ Let them READ their case. No need for verbal explanation.
+ They have completed their preoperative evaluation and have the patient on the OR table ready for induction

Only if asked:
+ Any other lab or x-ray values are "drawn and pending"
+ The monitors visible (EKG, NIBP, Pulse Oximeter) are what you have
+ If they call for the other anesthesiologist, they are doing a code in another room.
+ If they call for a surgeon, they are still in their car in the parking garage.

- -

Problems to be encountered in addition to the Case (do **NOT** reveal to the participants):
+ *The oxygen supply line will be switched to nitrogen as soon as the resident puts down the mask so he/she can intubate.*
+ *If the resident correctly diagnoses the problem, then the patient will have severe bronchospasm as well.*
+ *They will review their performances on videotape and score themselves.*

❖ Box 7.
Learner's Handout (Cholecystectomy)

Learning Objectives: After the session, the learner will be able to:
  1) manage the anesthesia equipment on a patient with a latex allergy
  2) resuscitate a patient in crisis
  3) improve their teamwork skills
  4) improve their communication
  5) understand the essential behaviors for effective crisis management

A 44-year-old-woman, scheduled for an elective cholecystectomy, is on the table and ready for induction.

PMHx:
  Cholecystitis with gall stones
  Good exercise tolerance
  History of mitral valve prolapse, palpitations controlled with medication
Allergy:
  Eggs and latex (anaphylaxis)
Medications:
  Metoprolol
Review of Systems:
  All systems are negative except for PMHx.
Preoperative Physical Examination:
  BP = 110/65, HR = 65, RR = 25, SpO2 = 941% on 2 L nasal cannula
  Airway = Malampati class II, teeth in good repair
  Neuro = Awake, alert and oriented time three
  Skin = Normal
  Pulmonary = Clear to auscultation, no wheezing
  Cardiac = Regular rate and rhythm without any murmurs
  Weight is 100 Kg
    Height of 5′ 6″
Laboratory:
  Hemoglobin = 11.0, Hematocrit = 33.0, Platelets are 224,000 and WBC = 10.8
  ABG = pH = 7.4, PCO2 = 39 mmHg, PO2 = 141 mmHg
    Basic electrolyte/metabolic panel is WNL
    Chest x-ray demonstrates no acute disease.
Access:
  Intravenous line in the left arm
  IV fluid going at 140 ml per hour total

◆◆◆ **Box 8.**
OBSERVERS' DEBRIEFING WORKSHEET
No Oxygen (Cholecystectomy): Specific debriefing points

Standard Induction . . . . . Did they?
+ prepare tools and drugs (include de-latexing)?
+ prepare patient with monitors and positioning?
+ preoxygenate the patient?
+ induction the patient appropriately?
+ ventilate the patient?
+ paralyze the patient?
+ intubate the patient successfully and appropriately?
+ check endotracheal tube placement?

No oxygen supply . . . . . Did they?
+ check the oxygen analyzer?
+ check the side-stream gas analyzer?
+ ventilate the patient with room air?
+ attempt to get another oxygen source?

Optional Bronchospasm . . . . . Did they?
+ recognize and diagnose the bronchospasm?
+ treat the bronchospasm appropriately?
+ rule out anaphylaxis from latex?

Crew (Crisis) Resource Management . . . . . Did they?
+ have leadership?
+ manage their information?
+ show evidence of systematically dealing with an unknown crisis?
+ have good communication skills?
+ re-evaluate for fixation errors?
+ utilize all their resources?
+ delegate responsiblities?

Box 9.
Instructions for Simulator Operator
Pediatric Seizure Case

The Pediatric Sim is intubated and being weaned from the ventilator. The ICU specialist is making rounds and checking the blood gases on the patient before extubating him. The EKG, pulse oximeter and NIBP are the only monitors attached. The defibrillator needs to be away from the patient in the farthest corner.

Connect:
- Art line, but do not turn on talking
- PA catheter, but do not turn on
- CVP, but do not turn on
- All standard monitors
- Left ankle saphenous IV

Other:
- Intubate the child with ETT barely in the trachea taped in place
- Ventilator settings to CPAP
- Laryngoscope blade missing from code box
- Drugs, IVs and other equipment in code box

Run:
- Start Standard Child
- Set weight to 27 kg
- Between baseline and set patient, zero all catheters (baseline sets all catheters to atmosphere)
- Remove colloid 350ml
- Add crystalloid 700 ml
- Increased venous capacity to 1.4
- Change extrathoracic elastance of arteries to 1.1
- Change respiratory rate factor to 1.1
- Change shunt fraction to 0.2
- Change heart rate factor to 1.1
- Eyes blink control: both closed
- Spontaneously breathing

States/Interventions:
- Start videotaping as soon as the instructor finished

  (before the mock seizure)
- Administer all drugs according to verbalized desire
- Follow all the fluid instructions until IV comes out

Scenario events:
- Patients seizes (*Instructor shakes patient*), IV comes out, ETT dislodges during seizure.
- Make a complete bilateral bronchospasm (completely occluded)
- Change O2 consumption to 800 ml/min
- After the patient is extubated, and masking is attempted, you may take the laryngoscope into the room
- When patient becomes reintubated, he is in bronchospasm with oxygen saturations continuing to drop
- When instructor signals, relieve the bronchospasm and reset the O2 to normal

Box 10.
Briefing Instructions (FOR the instructor)
Pediatric Seizure Case

Intended audience is graduates of anesthesiology training programs.

This is based on a REAL case.
- ✦ Let them READ their Case. No need for verbal explanation.
- ✦ There is NO time to delay in treating the crisis. The scenario plays out in real time.

Only if asked:
- ✦ Any other lab or x-ray values are "drawn and pending"
- ✦ The monitors visible (EKG, NIBP, Pulse Oximeter, ETCO2) are what you have
- ✦ Laryngoscope broke on last intubation and went to be fixed.

Problems to be encountered in addition to the Case (do **NOT** reveal to the participants):
- ✦ *The patient will simulate a seizure.*
- ✦ *The IV will come out when the seizure occurs.*
- ✦ *The ETT will become dislodged during the seizure.*
- ✦ *The laryngoscope blade will be missing for cleaning.*
- ✦ *The situation is videotaped and they will watch it to score themselves*

⬧⬧⬧ Box 11.
Learner's Handout (Pediatric ICU Case)

Learning Objectives: After this session, the learner will be able to:
1) understand their ability to manage a crisis
2) improve their teamwork skills
3) improve their communication
4) understand the essential behaviors for effective crisis management

A 7-year-old-boy is intubated and in the pediatric ICU secondary to a severe closed head injury he suffered one week ago. He has made terrific progress and is in the process of being weaned from the ventilator. The ICU specialist is making rounds and checking the blood gases on the patient before extubating him. The EKG, pulse oximeter and NIBP are the only monitors attached.

PMHx:
  Seizure disorder
Allergy:
  NKMA
Medications:
  Tegretol
Review of Systems:
  All systems are negative except for PMHx.
Physical Examination:
  BP = 100/65, HR = 90, RR = 18, SpO2 = 91% on 50% oxygen/air mixture
  Airway = Malampati class II, teeth in good repair, patient intubated and ETT taped in place
  Neuro = Asleep sedated for fighting the ventilator
  Skin = Normal
  Pulmonary = Clear to auscultation, no wheezing
  Cardiac = Regular, tachycardic rhythm without any murmurs
  Weight is 27 Kg
    Height of 4′ 2″
Laboratory:
  Hematocrit = 29
Access:
  One 20g Intravenous lines in left saphenous vein
  IV fluid going at 67 ml per hour total

Box 12.
OBSERVERS' DEBRIEFING WORKSHEET
Pediatric Seizure Case: Specific debriefing points

ACUTE SEIZURE SCENARIO.......Did they:
 ✦ Recognize the seizure?
 ✦ Recognize the extubation?
 ✦ Recognize the disconnected IV?
 ✦ Attempt to treat the seizure?
 ✦ Attempt to restart the IV?

REINTUBATION . . . . . .Did they:
 ✦ Mask the patient?
 ✦ Discover the laryngoscope blade is not in the code box?

Crew (Crisis) Resource Management . . . . . Did they?
 ✦ Have leadership?
 ✦ Manage their information?
 ✦ Show evidence of systematically dealing with an unknown crisis?
 ✦ Have good communication skills?
 ✦ Re-evaluate for fixation errors?
 ✦ Utilize all their resources?
 ✦ Delegate responsiblities?

Chapter 11

SIMULATION IN ANESTHESIOLOGY

Gary E. Loyd, MD, MMM

Technologic simulation in anesthesiology can take many forms and be implemented in a variety of ways. Simulations can be as basic as a computer screen-based system or as advanced as a high-fidelity human patient simulator used to facilitate education and research in anesthesia.[1] Beneken et al. described in detail different types of simulation models. He expounded on the process involved in developing a simulation model and which models had proved themselves useful.[2] Early in simulation, Byrne et al. described the design and initial testing of a computer screen-based anesthesia simulator, simulating emergency situations. This simulator, called ACCESS (anesthetic computer-controlled emergency situation and simulator) was rated by learners as a realistic and easy-to-use tool of educational value.[3] Other popular screen-based systems include the Anesthesia Simulator Consultant,[4] Gasman,[5] SIMA,[6] Body Simulation,[7] and Virtual Anesthesia Machine.[8]

The Anesthesia Simulation Consultant is a computer screen-based program that allows one to prepare the patient, induce the patient graphically, intubate the patient, and manage the patient intraoperatively. The system is designed for decision-making skills. Gasman demonstrates, in a visual format, uptake and distribution of anesthetic gases in the different body compartments under varying conditions. The Virtual Anesthesia Machine is an internet-based program, free for use, for the visualization of how a typical anesthesia machine operates. Nobs and switches are movable, and appropriate changes take place in the graphical representation. Examples of high-fidelity simulators include the Laerdal SimMan,[9] METI (Medical Education Technologies, Inc) HPS,[10] MedTec PatSim,[11] MedSim,[12] and Leiden Anesthesia Simulator.[1] These simulators simulate breathing and cardiovascular functionality.

Not only can the type of simulator vary, but the methods in which they are implemented vary considerably too. Some systems are totally departmentally based and used only to instruct anesthesiologists or emergency medicine personnel. Other simulators are organized to fulfill the needs of a health sciences campus, such as the center at the University of Louisville.[13] Still others are organized into simulation services to address the needs of multiple medical training institutions, like the simulator-based medical education service developed at Harvard for medical teaching institutions in the Boston area.[14] Staffing for these facilities varies also. People trained to run high-fidelity simulators are few and usually are trained within the institution in which they work. Frequently the physician using the simulator is also running the simulator, which ultimately is not a cost-effective approach if you are doing a sufficient number of simulations.

It is difficult to discuss simulation in anesthesiology without acknowledging the role that standardized patients play. Earlier articles about standardized patients referred to them as simulated patients. Over the past few decades, the label "simulated patient" evolved into "standardized patient" to reflect the training that gave these valuable teaching tools validity and reliability. There is no intention in this chapter to downplay or negate the value of standardized patients in teaching medical students or residents. The focus of this chapter is on the technologic simulation of patients and medical situations to enhance the education of the medical learner. In 1992, David Gaba wrote an editorial about improving performance by simulating reality to address this very point.[15]

From the standpoint of an anesthesiologist, The history of simulation in anesthesia practically can be considered the history of simulation itself. Yet a review of 3,700 articles and manuscripts about medical simulation revealed that only 6% were by anesthesiologists or about anesthesia. These 6%, however, were primarily about high-fidelity simulation and its use in medical education or patient safety training. In 2002, Morgan et al. published a survey of simulation institutions, of which 77% were involved in undergraduate education and 85% in postgraduate education. Very few were using their simulators for any sort of assessment. She concluded that simulators tend to be underutilized for a variety of reasons and that more training and research are needed to develop this modality of education.[16] Supporting her findings, Heard et al. reported in 2002 the results of a survey of program directors, which indicated that they needed assistance in regard to developing and implementing a successful simulation program.[17]

One of the greatest hurdles has been the expense of a simulation center and the lack of adequate studies demonstrating a superior teaching and learning outcome, which would justify the added expense. In 1997, Kurrek et al. described the building of a simulation center at the University of Toronto, which cost $665,000 (Canadian) and had a projected operating cost of $165,000 (Canadian).[18] The four METI (Medical Education Technology, Inc) HPSs and three METI ECSs (Emergency Care Simulators) in a four-simulation laboratory, four-classroom facility at the University of Louisville cost a total of approximately $2,000,000 to build and furnish. The operating costs are a little more than those of the University of Toronto.

Malignant Hyperthermia

Malignant hyperthermia (MH) is well suited for study in simulation, because its rarity negates most anesthesiologists' personal experiences with the disease process, making changes in behavior more attributable to the training received. Clearly defined protocols for dealing with MH assist with standardization. There are two main types of MH simulations. The first is the computer screen-based type,[19] which has been used successfully to self-teach and self-assess management of MH. Hotchkiss et al. describe how this type of simulation has been used to teach nurse anesthetists.[20] The other type is the full-scale, hands-on model, which most recent studies have used.

One of the values of simulation is the ability to assess what behaviors actually occur. Gaba et al. used simulated exercises in malignant hyperthermia and cardiac arrest to establish the value of technical and behavioral assessments via videotaping in the simulation laboratory. Interrater variability for this study ranged from 0.62 to 0.65, which is good.[21] Chopra et al. demonstrated that simulation improved performance in the recognition and management of malignant hyperthermia when the learners were tested 4 months after the training compared with controls.[22] In one study, only 44% of 32 teams hyperventilated the patient with MH, even though 100% had indicated that they needed to hyperventilate.[23]

Airway

When most nonanesthesiologists assess the value of an anesthesiologist, they usually emphasize airway management. Airway management was the early catalyst for the advancement of simulation in anesthesiology. In an editorial in 1998, Mason describes the use of simulation and standardizing anesthesia resident training and airway management as a substitute for the traditional haphazard training.[24] Does Mason's call for standardization in airway training for residents make sense? In 1999 Thwaites et al. reported the results of a survey of anesthesiologists in the United Kingdom. Their findings suggest considerable variation in the application of rapid-sequence induction.[25] Yet in 2002 Forrest et al. used a human patient simulator to track the improvement of novice anesthetists with rapid-sequence induction.[26] Given that such variability exists and can be tracked, standardization seems appropriate.

Stringer reviewed basic training in airway management and covered multiple simulation modalities.[27] Airway simulators are usually a manikin head with a replaceable larynx. Some of the airways on high-fidelity simulators have movable larynxes, which can be obstructed, put into laryngospasm or bronchospasm, have the tongue swollen, and have gastric contents fill the mouth via the simulated stomach and esophagus. The difficulty with high-fidelity simulators is poor portability, which makes field training difficult. A common portable airway management simulator model available is the Laerdal AirMan,[28] which is used to train emergency medical personnel in management of the difficult airway.[29] This model is also used by airway device suppliers to demonstrate their products.[30]

Airway simulators have been used for years, and the benefit of simulator practice has been intuitive. Scientific evidence indicates that simulation does improve performance in airway management. In 1997 Roberts et al. demonstrated that training in the use of laryngeal mask airway was just as effectively done on mannequin as on living patients.[31] In 2001 Naik et al. described the results of a transference study, which demonstrated that fiberoptic orotracheal intubation skills learned in simulation transferred to clinical practice better than didactic training.[32] In 2002, Rowe and Cohen reported how a virtual-reality flexible bronchoscopy simulator improved resident skills at fiberoptic intubation of pediatric patients.[33]

How does one get maximum value from using an airway model? A teaching exercise may not provide the results desired. In 2003 Olympio et al. discovered a failure of anesthesia residents to change their behavior in the management of esophageal intubation when exposed to a simulation scenario on esophageal intubation.[34] Personal experiences with teaching residents in the simulation center support Dr. Olympio's report. An anecdotally successful response has been to request that residents repeat the procedure until they get it correct. They also need to demonstrate the correct way to do the procedure, whether in real time or on video. Then they need to have their performances videotaped so they can watch and compare as they progress. Just as in the teaching and assessment of malignant hyperthermia, videotapes of simulations of airway management can be used to identify flaws in performance.[35]

So how many attempts does it take? Hosking evaluated how the practice of intubation on a manikin improved medical students' skills. Although not published in a peer-reviewed publication, his paper indicates that at least 30 intubations by each individual in their study would have been necessary to demonstrate some transference of the laboratory skill to the clinical setting.[36] In a letter to the editor in 2000, Cross raised the question of whether 20 intubations a week is impractical to maintain clinical competence, because it would require approximately 1040 intubations per year—more than anesthetists perform, given the widespread use of LMAs and regional anesthesia.[37]

Advancements in airway management simulation will continue. Berkenstadt et al. reported that airway management is complicated by the protective gear worn during a simulated bioterrorism attack.[38] There have been reports of using people instead of simulated patients for practice in airway management. In 2002, Patil et al. reported the results of using learning subjects as the simulated patient, locally anesthetizing the airway, and practicing fiberoptic intubation. Reported complications include paresthesias, nasal bleeding, coughing, and sore throat.[39] In 2003 Frerk raised the ethical problems with using learners as simulated patients.[40] Simulating a difficult airway demonstrated that providers, otherwise skilled in airway management, could produce several complications, including esophageal intubations and ischemia.[41] The author has no wish to participate in such a workshop when acceptable simulation is available.

Resuscitation

Patient resuscitation has always been a part of an anesthesiologist's practice because patients lose bodily fluids during surgery. Given the stresses of surgery, cardiac events are not uncommon, requiring cardiac resuscitation like that taught in Advance Cardiopulmonary Life Support (ACLS). Simulation improves the performance of ACLS providers. The ACLS course is even taught with a degree of simulation. In 1998 Kurrek et al. reported that when residents were assessed for adherence to the ACLS guidelines, residents with previous training in ACLS performed better than those who had not received the training. The startling finding was that both groups did poorly.[42] Compared with students who received only lectures, students trained with computer screen-based simulation performed better.[43]

Long-term retention of resuscitation algorithms, since certification can last up to several years, is a major concern for effective use of the ACLS protocol to save lives. Simulation can facilitate this process. Ten to 11 months after taking an ACLS course, students who used a computer screen-based method not only retained their information 19% better than those who used the traditional approach but also passed the algorithms section 56% better.[44] Now a computer screen-based program allows one to practice the resuscitation of a patient for European Advanced Life Support (ALS).[45]

Crisis Resource Management in Anesthesiology

Anesthesiology has helped lead the way in the development of crisis resource management (CRM) in health care. Chapter 10 deals with the history and suggests an approach in teaching CRM, but the richness of the studies deserves some mention here. Simulation has helped establish the need for CRM in health care. In 1990 DeAnda and Gaba reported that 87% of the critical incidents during anesthesia simulations were found to be due to human error and only 3% to equipment failure.[46] There is also no evidence that anesthesia training or regular private practice experience prepares one for dealing with crises. In 1989 Gaba and DeAnda found that experience by anesthesia residents did not correlate with their ability to detect the simulated critical incidents. There was a correlation in experienced residents to respond appropriately to the critical incident once it had been detected.[47] In 1991 DeAnda and Gaba reported that during simulated critical incidents, the more rapid response by experienced anesthesiologists over residents was not statistically significant due to the high variability within each group.[48] Such evidence suggests the need for regular training in crisis management.

In another study, Schwid and O'Donnell compared ten anesthesia residents, ten faculty anesthesiologists, and ten anesthesiologists in private practice in their management of simulated emergency situations. They discovered many errors in the management of emergency situations, even among anesthesiologists with years of experience. The results were startling: misdiagnosis of a simulated anaphylactic reaction (60%); inadequate treatment of simulated myocardial ischemia (63%); and mismanagement of a simulated cardiac arrest according to ACLS guidelines (70%). The root of many of the problems was fixation errors (63%).[49] In a similar study involving residents, none of the 21 teams of anesthesia providers diagnosed and treated anaphylaxis within 10 minutes in the simulation laboratory.[50] Anesthesiology may have six sigma quality, but the evidence seems compelling that we can do better.

The effectiveness of crisis management courses for anesthesiologists is becoming evident. In 2003 Weller et al. surveyed anesthetists who had taken a crisis management course the year before to evaluate any change in their professional behaviors during crisis management. They found that 70% of those who had a critical incident in the past year felt that their crisis management skills had improved, and they credited the improvement to the crisis management course. In addition, 88% of the respondents indicated that they would return for future crisis management training.[51] Even though continuing education courses are lecture-based, the evidence suggests that simulation should be the preferred method of providing CRM training. Schwid et al. demonstrated that computer screen-based training for emergent critical incidents during an anesthetic was better than training with a handout.[52]

CRM training can occur with computer screen-based programs, such as the Anesthesia Simulator Consultant, which simulates the operating room environment graphically while an automated record-keeping system produces a detailed summary of the case. An additional expert system provides interpretations of patient information, differential diagnosis, and treatment for abnormal patient conditions. The combination of the simulator, recorder, and expert system allows a self-study and assessment tool.[53] How to create a course is addressed in an article by O'Donnell et al., who describe implementation of an ACRM using a high-fidelity human simulator, including the key supportive and logistic resources necessary. The authors also provide feedback from students and faculty as well as lessons that they learned.[54] Since 2002, high-fidelity simulators have been used at the annual meeting of the American Society of Anesthesiologists to teach CRM and have been well received by the participants. Further advancements may follow the lead of the U.S. military. The United States Army demonstrated the effectiveness of using a virtual reality simulator to improve complex decision making in the combat arena.[55]

Patient Safety

Patient safety is a paramount concern in health care today. All of the sections of this chapter relate directly or indirectly to patient safety, yet some research addresses patient safety directly. As consumers become more aware of the health care product that they are buying, they are demanding more information about the quality of the product. Simulation is providing some answers as well as an avenue for safe testing of new procedures and systems in an ethical environment.[56,57] Byrne and Jones described the charting habits of 11 anesthetists during several simulated incidents. They found that the anesthetists recorded typical rather than actual events. This study opens scrutiny of why this would occur and to what degree it does occur in actual practice or training.[58]

Fatigue is a large enough concern that legislation governs the work hours of truck drivers, airplane pilots, and residents. Howard et al. state that the quandary of whether fatigue and sleep deprivation significantly affect the performance of anesthesia providers will not have a comfortable solution until psychomotor testing and vigilance testing can be performed realistically and safely in simulated conditions.[59] In 2003 Murray and Dodds evaluated the effect of sleep deprivation on the performance of anesthetists. One finding was that a good night of undisturbed sleep provided an improvement in the anesthetists' vigilance scores. Disturbing the anesthetists' sleep during the first third of the night interfered with vigilance most significantly.[60] In 2000 Gander et al. surveyed anesthetists in New Zealand and found that 71% of residents and 58% of practicing anesthetists exceeded their own self-defined safety limits with regard to work hours. These same anesthetists reported a greater incidence of medical errors in their practice.[61] It is intuitive that alcohol impairs ability to work, but simulation has provided evidence. Dorafshar et al. demonstrated that alcohol ingestion impaired performance on a MIST virtual reality surgical simulator.[62] Simulation is also now used to identify the components of medical tasks both in complexity and workload requirements so that more effective management schemes can be created.[63] Such information will guide the ability to set reasonable working conditions and provide optimal safety for patients.

Testing new products in a simulator is an ethical alternative to live testing. Berkenstadt et al. found that using full protective gear against bioterrorism increased intubation time among experienced anesthesiologists and decreased communication ability during crisis management.[38] Such a study may have endangered real patients, especially given the outcomes of the study. A simulator was used to evaluate the efficacy of a graphical object display during shock states. This allowed a safe evaluation in case the graphical display became a hindrance to the anesthesiologist during a crisis situation.[64] Another example is a study in which an anesthesia machine was contaminated with bacteria as it anesthetized a human patient simulator. This experiment would be totally unethical in real patients, yet it provided important information about the safety of the devices that we use every day.[65]

Simulation has been specifically directed at training for patient safety. Ashish Jha et al. described the use of simulation in the training for patient safety.[66] Garden et al. reported the results of a participant evaluation of a course designed to address medical errors. He found that 80% of the participants would recommend the course to a colleague and approximately one-third thought the course should be repeated every two years.[67] Murray et al. used the simulator to instruct anesthesiologists in the use of a new drug, remifentanil. The participants thought that the use of the simulator facilitated their understanding of the drug.[68] In another study, Syroid et al. were able to improve the performance of anesthesiologists in computer-based simulation by giving them simulated graphical displays of plasma levels of different drugs. This is an example of bringing simulation into the operating theater to augment current practice.[69] Such use of simulation as it relates therapeutic interventions to improve quality is advocated by Haux.[70]

Anesthesia-Related Medical Education

So far this chapter has presented specific task- or topic-oriented areas relevant to medical education. In this section, the emphasis is on medical education, especially in anesthesiology. Even though the anecdotal evidence is compelling medical education facilities to invest in health simulation technology, absolute scientific evidence of the modality as the superior education tool has not been shown. This section presents some of the literature on health care simulation as it relates to anesthesia-related education.

Advantages of simulation in the literature are numerous. As far back as the 1960s, Abrahamson et al. reported the advantages of computer-based simulations.[71-73] Anesthesiologists at the University of Florida use the simulator to teach basic physiology to first-year medical students.[74] In another report, first-year medical students rated physiology as taught by anesthesiologists via the human patient simulator superior to the traditional lecture method.[75] Zvara et al. also describe the use of the human patient simulator in teaching cardiovascular physiology to first-year medical students.[76] Cleave-Hogg and Morgan reported that the experience of fourth-year medical students in the human patient simulation center was overwhelmingly positive.[77]

Simulation allows flexibility in teaching. The University of Florida extended problem-based learning into the simulation laboratory.[78] The use of small group learning in the human patient simulation laboratory is effective and well received by first-year medical students.[79] Simulation allows instructors to break down a difficult topic or scenario and students to explore different options available to them. In so doing, the students also learn how the physiologic parameters interact to produce the hemodynamic responses encountered.[80]

Ethical dilemmas are avoided when simulation is used for training instead of human subjects. In 1997 Roberts et al. demonstrated that training in the use of laryngeal mask airway was just as effectively done on mannequins as on live patients without traumatizing people in the process.[31] Simulation is also expanding to allow training in regional anesthesia.[81] One does not have to be a physician to learn; simulation is appropriate for anyone who deals with patients. The simulator is used successfully to teach conscious sedation to nonphysicians. Participants rated the experience highly.[82] In 1995 van Stralen et al. reported that emergency medical service personnel could be trained in retrograde intubation via the use of mannequins.[83]

Growing evidence indicates that education in simulation is superior to traditional approaches in some areas, although the studies have not reached a critical mass of conclusiveness. In 1999 Anastakis et al. reported how six basic procedures were taught equally as well on the bench model as on a cadaver. They also demonstrated that both simulation and cadaver training are superior to training from a prepared text. The gold standard for this study was performance of the procedure on cadavers.[84] In 2001 Naik et al. described the results of transference in a study demonstrating that fiberoptic orotracheal intubation skills learned in simulation transferred to clinical practice better than the same skills learned from didactic training.[32] Ten to eleven months after taking an ACLS course, students who used a computer screen-based method retained their information 19% better than those who used the traditional approach and also passed the algorithms section 56% better.[44]

The literature also has reported some pitfalls with simulation. Olympio et al. discovered a failure of anesthesia residents to change their behavior in the management of esophageal intubation after exposure to a simulation scenario on esophageal intubation.[34] Building on the Olympio article, Glavin and Greaves discuss some problems of simulator-based instruction and make some recommendations, including the belief that simulation lessons should be appropriate to the learner's situation.[85] In 2002 Byrne et al. were not able to demonstrate a significant improvement between learning subjects who observed their own performance on videotapes compared with those who did not.[86] This finding should make everyone aware that just walking into a simulation center does not guarantee automatic success at teaching. How one teaches is more important than the teaching environment. When using problem-based learning, general surgery residents believed that the thought-provoking tutor was more important than the case chosen.[87]

Since it is becoming obvious that we must pay attention to how we teach in the simulation laboratory to be effective, we must pay detailed attention to the methodologies used by those who create success in their simulation laboratories. First, when using the human patient simulator for the first time, it is the preference of the learner to have an introductory session to the simulator first so that he or she can acclimate to the environment.[88] Hartland et al. describe the use of simulation to produce instructional videos for teaching.[89] Such an approach, plus allowing practice until success was achieved. may have been the answers to Olympio's findings, but we will not know until further study is done. Videotaping is an important part of many simulation studies.[85,86] Simulation templates developed for anesthesiologists can be used in other disciplines, such as emergency medicine.[90] Libraries of simulation scenarios and templates are being built to be shared. One such library, sponsored by Duke University, is called SimDot .[91] In a related area are texts on such topics as anesthesia OSCEs.[92]

The type of simulation device used for the instruction really depends on the intended goal. In 2002 Nyssen et al. compared the training of screen-based simulation and mannequin-based simulation. They found little difference between computer screen-based and mannequin-based simulations for managing light shock. They also demonstrated again that simulators can significantly improve the performance of anesthesia residents.[93] Computer screen-based programs have been shown to be quite successful in teaching uptake and distribution of inhaled anesthetics, ACLS instructions, and critical event management.[42,52,94-96] These programs are also being developed for full anesthesia training.[97]

Just as important as the methodology is the assessment scheme. Simulation allows for evaluation of all three domains of Bloom's taxonomy, which is an expansion from the confinements of the previous knowledge-based only assessments. Due to the abstract concept and lack of a standard model, critical thinking is difficult to teach. Weis and Guyton-Simmons present a methodology that meshes with simulation education.[98] Morgan et al. demonstrated that experiential learning in a human patient simulation laboratory was equal but not superior to videotape presentation in getting students to learn knowledge-based material.[99] Marshall et al. demonstrated that using the human patient simulator not only augmented the trauma management skills of interns but also improved teamwork and self-confidence over the controls.[100] One group of senior medical students who had seminar-based teaching was compared to another group who had sim-ulator-based teaching for trauma management. There was no performance difference, but students in simulator-based teaching felt more confident and more prepared for the real event.[101] Morgan et al. found no correlation between students' clinical experiences and level of confidence and their ability to perform on standardized scenarios on a high-fidelity human simulator.[102] These studies raise the question of whether or not our current instruction and evaluation modes are adequate. In 2001 Brailovsky et al. argued that they proved the construct validity of a script concordance (SC) test. This test was pitted against short-answer management problems (SAMPs), simulated office orals (SOOs), and objective structured clinical examinations (OSCEs).[103] Even though the script concordance test was not designed specifically for low- and high-fidelity simulation laboratories, the author sees the potential for their possible introduction.

The various uses for simulation as an educational tool are increasing as well. In 2002 Rosenblatt and Abrams described the use of the patient simulator to evaluate and develop a remedial program for an anesthesiologist who had allowed his medical skills to lapse. They described two phases of the evaluation process. Phase one included a personal history, extensive psychological assessment, and assessment of general medical knowledge, for which objective structured clinical evaluations (OSCEs) were used. Phase two included an anesthesiology-specific evaluation, which identified deficient areas and suitability for retraining.[104] Kofke et al. introduce the idea of using simulation of acute crises to educate juries during legal proceedings.[105] Tooley et al. discussed the planning and implementation of telemedicine as it related to simulation training for learners who could not personally attend the simulation environment.[106] Yet Xiao et al. caution that evaluation of behaviors by students via remote telemedicine connections may be a real challenge because these remote activities are multidisciplinary and rapidly changing.[107] The use of simulations in large meeting formats has also been addressed successfully.[108]

As the scientific study of medical education with simulation evolves, our understanding of how to provide a better education for students and residents will increase. Prystowsky and Bordage studied three years' worth of medical education literature and found that the preponderance of the articles used the assessment of trainee performance as the outcome, whereas patient outcomes represented less than 1%.[109] Such a study suggests that better performance is always associated with better outcomes. Since our ability to educate beyond the paradigms of the past is exploding with possibilities, so should our ability to think "outside the box." Wong et al. best summarize this section: "Although there is evidence demonstrating the popularity, reliability, and validity of simulator training, its superiority over conventional training has not yet been proven, and research in this area is required."[110]

Assessment and Certification

Assessment is an important part of education. It is the mechanism by which we find out whether the learner learned and whether our strategy to optimize learning was successful. Assessment in the literature so far focuses on two main areas: diagnostics and competency assessments. Diagnostics are not always so flattering to the work that we think we are doing. Devitt et al. demonstrated that in simulation 63% of charting of critical events and simulated anesthetics was not complete, regardless of level of training or experience.[111] When just under 50% of trainees and graduates of anesthesia programs cannot correctly diagnose anaphylactic shock or correctly treat myocardial ischemia in simulation, major warning flags should appear.[49] This finding does not appear to be a fluke, although more studies of such searching depth are indicated.[112] Not only does it appear that anesthesiologists cannot perform optimally, but when events occur, they tend to document a significant number of the values in error of the real value by more than 25%.[113] There may be reasonable explanations for these variations, but until more simulation studies are completed, it will not be known how much they have to improve as a specialty to acquire perfection. Rosenblatt and Abrams described how the simulation laboratory was used to diagnose insufficient skills of an anesthesiologist who had let those skills lapse. They were able to use the data to tailor a remedial program for that individual.[104] Morgan et al. used the simulation center to identify gaps in senior medical students' performances as they related to achieving the goals and objectives of the anesthesia rotation that they had just completed. They were able to demonstrate areas where teaching had not been successful on a program level rather than on an individual basis.[114]

Increasing reports of how simulation detects inappropriate decision-making skills or patient management skills are providing momentum for simulation to be used in an evaluative role. Schwid et al. reported the results of a multi-institutional study that identified numerous management errors by anesthesia residents from 10 institutions. They concluded that such evidence may benefit a program by catching these errors since they occurred at all levels of training. Yet they conceded that improvements were necessary in the development and implementation of standardized simulation scenarios and in assessment criteria before mannequin-based simulation should be used for certification.[115]

In 2001 McGaghie et al. outlined an eight-step procedure in developing reliable and valid evaluation tools.[116] In 2002 Glavin and Maran outlined a system for the development of a tool for the assessment of clinical competence.[117] Specific tools have been described and used. One of the most popular is videotaping. In 2003 Weller et al. reported the use of videotapes in the assessment of performance of anesthetists in simulated crises. Their findings suggest that two judges of performance should be adequate.[118] One of the evaluation tools uses videotaping so that performances can be evaluated by competent judges when the judges become available. Devitt et al. showed excellent interrater agreement between evaluators when videotape was used.[119] Videotaping can also be used to demonstrate directly to learners how their performance is improving over time. In 1994 Weinger et al. described an objective method for analyzing the vigilance and efficiency of anesthesiologists in training.[120] Objective structured checklists were used by Bullock et al. to test interrater reliability in simulation with good results.[121] Morgan et al. evaluated the reliability and validity of using global assessment vs. checklists for assessing a student's performance in an artificially small testing window of 15 minutes.[122] Although not designed specifically for simulation, the anesthesia OSCE book could be of great benefit.[92] Though used to assess the technical skills of surgery trainees and not anesthesia trainees, Winckel et al. demonstrated the reliability and validity of a structured technical skills assessment (STSA) form.[123]

Growing evidence supports simulation assessment of competency as the evaluation tools are developed. King et al. reported how evaluation of performance in the simulation laboratory was able to differentiate between residents of different training levels. The authors proposed that simulation can be a valid and useful tool to evaluate the safe practice of anesthesia providers.[124] In 1998 Devitt et al. demonstrated that a patient simulator-based evaluation tool can be used with acceptable reliability to differentiate between residents and staff anesthesiologists.[125] Devitt et al. were also able to use the simulator to distinguish between residents-in-training and practicing anesthesiologists. All of the participants rated the simulation environment highly realistic.[126]

Once tools are established, one has to assess whether or not they evaluate what they were intended to evaluate. An article in the *British Journal of Anesthesiology* analyzed 13 reports dealing with the assessment of anesthesia performance with an anesthesia simulator. Of these, only four were designed to address validation or reliability.[127] In 2000 Morgan and Cleave-Hogg reported that a simulator can be a reliable assessment tool for evaluating the performance of medical students on an anesthesiology rotation.[128] Weller et al. described how the validity and reliability of a performance assessment tool were established. The implication is that simulators can potentially be used to make evaluations of anesthesia providers for establishing competency and/or certification.[118] At the University of Toronto Morgan et al. did a pilot study to evaluate the anesthesia simulator as an assessment tool for medical students. The interrater reliability was very high (0.87), yet the correlation to written and clinical evaluations was low.[129] This finding begged the question of the validity of each evaluation tool in assessing whether or not we are producing a competent physician. The authors produced a full study assessing the performance of medical students in the simulation laboratory and again found a poor correlation between subjective clinical scores and objective checklist scoring from videotapes.[130] Subjective clinical scores have been the foundation of establishing competency in medicine. However, if the objective checklist scoring is more accurate, the entire paradigm of how medical students and residents are assessed has to change. Schupfer et al. presented his rationale of why simulators and simulation are not ready to begin assessing trainees for certification because of a lack of adequate training in decision-making skills and other behavioral skills to which the simulations allow access.[131] Nothing seems to have stressed residents at the University of Louisville more than telling them that they will be graded on a simulation scenario. They prefer to have their performances graded on real patients, in whom critical incidents seldom occur, whereas almost every simulated scenario contains one such incident. Their attitudes changed when they discovered that the assessments were self-evaluations meant to show improvement over time. Still the debate over when and under what circumstances simulation can be reliably used to assess competency and ultimately certification will be ongoing.[132-134]

Veterinary Medicine

Delivery of veterinary anesthesia is now also taught via simulation. Some institutions rely on interactive videodisc systems.[135] Others have taken the novel approach of using human patient simulators to teach skills that transfer directly to animals, such as providing anesthesia. The students induce and maintain anesthesia on their patients while they monitor vital signs. They are provided several critical events that they must diagnose and treat as they occur. In a randomly controlled study, the students who received simulation scored significantly higher on their clerkship examination, which dealt with concepts reviewed by simulation, than students who engaged in self-study instead of the simulation exercise (p < 0.001). The authors concluded that the human patient simulator was a valuable educational venue for students to learn veterinary medicine. The reality of the scenarios permitted the students to learn without subjecting live patients to their mistakes. Being able to make mistakes and determine why their therapies were unsuccessful allowed critical decision making and facilitated correlation of basic science knowledge with clinical data. This learning model was very exciting for the students.[136]

Innovations

As anesthesiologists and other physicians embrace simulation for its current worth and potential profits in teaching, learning, and assessment, their innovative minds create advances for the field of medical simulation. Some of the advances related to the cardiovascular system are recent. In 2002 Schwarz et al. demonstrated how to successfully make arteries pulsate in a cadaver with a pneumatically driven pulse generator.[137] Eason et al. reported the development of a simulated internal jugular device that can be incorporated into a METI HPS. This device allows the percutaneous Selinger technique and placement of a central venous catheter or cordis.[138] Euliano modeled obstetric cardiovascular physiology on a full-scale patient simulator.[139]

There have been several advances in neurophysiology simulation. Thoman et al. were able to demonstrate a brain physiology simulation program that remained within 9% of literature data for related physiologic states.[140] In 2001 de Beer et al. described the development of an EEG simulator to educate anesthesiologists in EEG monitoring during the anesthetics that they provide.[141] Because of the safe environment that simulations provide, many different devices and techniques can be evaluated, and their efficacy and safety can be demonstrated before they are introduced into a patient environment. One such piece of equipment is a specialized anesthesia-providing device useful in low oxygen reserve situations. Testing such equipment may be hazardous for real patients as anesthesia providers learn to use them.[142] The simulator was used to evaluate the efficacy of a graphical object display during shock states. This approach allowed a safe evaluation to be conducted.[64] The U.S. Army used simulators and a simulated environment to test a compact patient monitoring system.[143] Syroid et al. were able to improve the performance of anesthesiologists in computer-based simulation by giving them simulated graphical displays of plasma levels of different drugs. This is an example of bringing simulation into the operating theater to augment current practice.[69] Not all new simulation ideas need to be costly devices. In 2000 Williams et al. described in a letter to the editor the inexpensive construct of an artificial throat to assist in the training of fiberoptic intubation.[144] Peg boards and tortuous piping were used successfully to familiarize learners with how to manipulate a fiberoptic bronchoscope.

Virtual reality and haptics are exciting innovations that may prove to revolutionize current simulation modalities. Virtual reality has been discussed in the anesthesia literature for at least eight years.[145,146] Surgery has been the leader in this area because laparoscopic instruments are easily adapted to current virtual reality technology.[147-149] Introduction into critical care is one of anesthesiology's virtual reality venues. Rowe and Cohen reported the results of using a flexible bronchoscope in a virtual reality trainer to teach fiberoptic intubation to residents learning to intubate children fiberoptically. They reported that after an average of 17 cases, the time to completion of successful intubation with a fiberoptic bronchoscope decreased from 5.15 to 0.88 minutes. The number of times that the tip of the bronchoscope hit the mucosa decreased from 21.4 to 3.0.[33] Also in critical care, Arne et al. described a PC-controlled mannequin designed for use in the intensive care unit. The simulator, named "PatSim," was capable of laryngospasm, lung compliance variability, scalable airway resistance, pneumothorax, leakage of the intubation tube cuff, blocking of the breathing sounds from one lung, secretion, gastric regurgitation, and diuresis in addition to standard hemodynamics, which could be monitored via any standard critical care monitor.[150]

How the Author Writes an Educational Simulation Session

The author's first steps are to decide the topic or title of the educational session and to acknowledge the intended audience. The audience is extremely important. The next step is to choose learning objectives. If the audience is a mixture of residents and medical students or junior and senior residents, separate learning objectives may be created for each group. The learning objectives are crucial and should not be done as an afterthought. You may return to them after creating the educational session and update or revise them. The author's learning objectives are structured to Bloom's taxonomy and attempt to include at least one learning objective in each domain. The rest of the simulation is then molded to fit the learning objectives. *Yao and Artusio's Anesthesiology: Problem-oriented Patient Management*[151] and Reed's *Clinical Cases in Anesthesia*[152] were great helps early in the author's simulation career to guide thinking in putting simulations together. Seropian outlines a system similar to the author's.[153]

Next the author works to create the simulation. The preoperative evaluation and intraoperative course of an actual patient may be recreated from the medical records, or the likely medical course may be recreated from case reports. The next step is to browse the simulation library for previously prepared patients and scenarios that may need only minor adjustments to fit. More than 160 scenarios are in the University of Louisville simulation library. After the patient and the scenario are recreated at the simulator, real-time parameters are adjusted to fit into the allotted time for the didactic. Any remaining time is used to create handouts or short mini-lectures of about 12–15 minutes. The total time for creating the first few of these simulations was about an hour longer than the time required to create an hour of lecture. Now creation of a simulation takes about the same amount of time and is a lot more fun.

Examples

The following pages include three examples of cases used at the University of Louisville. All of the cases are intended for the instruction of residents. Cases intended more for medical students and graduates of anesthesiology training can be found in Chapter 10. The attached figures are similar to what one would find in the simulation library at the University of Louisville. Each case is accompanied by a brief description and explanation. Four separate pieces are written specifically for each case to accommodate the variations in available assistance and size of audience. At the University of Louisville, we classify instructors into three categories. The class A instructors can sit at the simulation computer and program the simulator with all the variables seen in Figure 1 to produce the desired responses and to make the four pieces for the simulation. Class B instructors make the instructor, learner, and observer handouts but must use the simulation specialists to

Background: The adult male manikin is intubated with a #8.0 oral ETT and is on the OR table ready for induction. The EKG, Pulse Oximeter, arterial pressure wave, central venous pressure, intracranial pressure waveform, ETCO$_2$ and NIBP are the monitors attached.

Connect:
- ☺ Art line, turn on
- ☺ PA catheter, but do not turn on
- ☺ Left subclavian triple lumen catheter
- ☺ CVP attached to 3lumen cath, turn on
- ☺ ICP, turn on
- ☺ All standard monitors except temp
- ☺ Attached ETT to anesthesia breathing circuit
- ☺ Set the ventilator to a rate of 12 and a tidal volume of 700

Other:
- ☺ Manikin on back, not awake
- ☺ Eyes are closed
- ☺ 8.0 oral ETT in trachea, secured at 25 cm at the teeth
- ☺ Anesthesia machine fully working
- ☺ Anesthesia cart fully stocked
- ☺ Induction Drugs laid out
- ☺ Body warmer/cooler in room
- ☺ Fluid warmer in the room

Run:
- ☺ Start Standard Man
- ☺ Set weight to 70kg
- ☺ Patient's ICP should be 25
- ☺ Add 1000ml of fluid
- ☺ Increase SVR factor to 1.4
- ☺ Increase heart rate factor to 1.8
- ☺ Decrease the venous capacitance to 0.9

States/Interventions:
- ☺ If the learner checks placement of the ETT and readjusts, clear the right mainstem occlusion and if ICP not treated, raise ICP to 35 mmHg
- ☺ If the learner increases the venitlation, reduce the ICP by 3 mmHg
- ☺ If the learner gives mannitol, reduce the ICP by 3 mmHG

- ☺ If learner positions patient's head up 30 degrees reduce ICP by 3 mmHg
- ☺ If learner opens the IVC drain reduce the ICP by 5 mmHg
- ☺ If learner loosens the trach tape, reduce the ICP by 3 cm mmHg

NOTE: the ICP low limit will be 15 mmHg
- ☺ When induction pentothal or propofol is given, reduce the ICP by 3 mmHg
- ☺ If places esophageal temp probe raise ICP to 30 mmHG if untreated
- ☺ If ETT suctioned without ICP treatment, raise ICP to 45 mmHG
- ☺ If intubation occurs, raise the ICP to 30 mmHg if previously treated, 45 mmHG if not previously treated
- ☺ Administer all drugs according to verbalized desire if they are not in a syringe
- ☺ Follow all the fluid instructions
- ☺ If the learner cools the patient, drop the body temperature to 34 degrees C°

Scenario events:
- ☺ The patient has an increased ICP, right mainstem intubation, and no temperature probe, no warming/cooling blanket
- ☺ After induction, the ETT will become partially clogged with secretions.
- ☺ Any time before the cranium is open, the INSTRUCTOR may choose for the brain to herniate, set periperal baros= 8, SVR= 8 and Venous capacitance= 0.8, and Extrathoracic art elast= 0.5, HRF=1
- ☺ The surgeon is ready to clip the aneurysm and wants the blood pressure low
- ☺ The INSTRUCTOR may choose to let the aneurysm burst, then take out 2000 ml of colloid, Venous Capacitance=3

Figure 1. Instructions for simulator operator: cerebral aneurysm case (management of intracranial pressure [ICP]). ETT = endotracheal tube, OR = operating room, EKG = electrocardiogram, ETCO$_2$ = end-tidal carbon dioxide, NIBP = noninvasive blood pressure monitoring, PA = pulmonary artery, CVP = central venous pressure, SVR = systemic vascular resistance, IVC = inferior vena cava.

make the operator instructions. The class C instructors take the four pieces, which class A and B instructors have prepared, and teach an educational session. In the following examples, the simulation operator instructions are specific to METI's version 6 of HPS software. From the experience of having four of these HPS simulators, one can expect similar but not exactly identical results from running the scenario on different simulators. Even though the simulators are supposedly identical, each has its own individual characteristics and reactions. The cases are also written so that the instructor can perform a demonstration and teach in an interactive small-group environment or a large-group environment via live audio and video link. The author rarely does demonstrations because of a firm belief in active learning. Each case is also designed to be taught in one- or two-hour blocks.

Before the class session begins, it is important that a rehearsal takes place. This rehearsal begins with preparation of the room in which you are doing the simulation. Once preparations are made, the author frequently takes a digital picture of the set-up for future reference. Even though the instructions to the operator are detailed, significant details, such as positioning of the OR table, anesthesia machine, IV poles, and cameras, may influence the session. Rehearsing with the simulation operator allows the operator to understand how you want the session to play out and gives practice for interaction. Even though the states, interventions, and scenario events seem very concrete, there will be considerable variability between each session in which this case is done. Not every case needs a simulation operator separate from the instructor, but rehearsal is recommended. In addition to the instructor and operator rehearsal, learners need an introduction to patient simulation if they have had no previous experience. Learners have difficulty trying to learn simulator capabilities and limitations at the same time that they are learning the educational material planned for them.

Cerebral Aneurysm Case

The instructions to the operator for the cerebral aneurysm (management of intracranial pressure [ICP]) case are shown in Figure 1. The specifying of a male mannequin is necessary, because gender sometimes is overlooked as everyone attempts to concentrate on the case at hand. Even though everyone gets a chuckle when the gender is wrong, it breaks the realism that everyone is creating in his or her mind as the scenario unfolds. Any pressure lines that may be needed during the case should be connected and prepared before the learners arrive. Intrusion of the simulation operator into the educational theater is not fatal, but it does tend to interrupt—at least temporarily—the suspension of disbelief. In this cerebral aneurysm case, the learner is presented with a patient for whom he did not get to prepare. Arterial and central venous pressures already have been transduced. The anesthesia cart or supplies have not been sabotaged. The patient appropriate for this simulation is stipulated as any kind of patient that can be programmed into the software. Several ready-for-use simulated patients come with the software program. In this case it is a regular healthy patient called "standard man." At this point you can make alterations to his physiology to simulate the conditions to be encountered by the learner.

The state and intervention sections are separate from the scenario section because the interventions by the learner or instructor tend to be quick and require the immediate attention of the operator. When written into a file in the HPS program, frequently the interventions follow in a logical sequence between the planned scenario events. There are multiple ways to treat an increased ICP, and specific values are given. Experienced simulation operators with some physiology background easily adapt and can improvise, but the operators who are more technically oriented need the detailed values. The scenario events are those which the instructor plans for the course of the simulated patient. The ICP management case begins with an increase in ICP and a right mainstem intubation, neither of which is declared by the instructor. The instructor may or may not be in the room while the scenario unfolds, depending on how he or she wants the educational experience to take place.

The instructor's page (Fig. 2) is important to have, even if you programmed the scenario. At the bottom of the page is a quick review of where the simulation is going. The instructor's page also serves as a quick reminder of any script that the instructor needs to know or cite during the scenario. If other actors are involved in the case, they too can have either the instructor's page or a separate page prepared specifically for them with their individual scripts. In Figure 3, the learner is not told in the title that the case is about ICP management, even though it is listed in the learning objectives. The details in the learning objectives can be changed, depending on how much notice the instructor wants to give the resident about unexpected events during the case. If the simulation were be-

---

Intended audience is first- and second-year anesthesiology residents.

This is based on a REAL case.
- ✦ Let them READ their case. No need for verbal explanation.
- ✦ The preoperative evaluation was completed for them and they have the patient on the OR table ready for induction

Only if asked:
- ✦ Any other lab or x-ray values are "drawn and pending"
- ✦ The monitors visible (EKG, NIBP, Pulse Oximeter, $ETCO_2$, A-line, CVP) are what you have
- ✦ No transesophageal echo is available
- ✦ The anesthesia tech dropped and broke the only precordial doppler you have on the way to the room

- -

Problems to be encountered in addition to the case (do **NOT** reveal to the participants):
- ✦ *The patient will have an increased ICP at the start of the case.*
- ✦ *The patient has a right mainsteam endobronchial intubation.*
- ✦ *The patient does not have a warming/cooling blanket on, nor a temperature probe in place.*
- ✦ *If the learner must perform several of the ICP reducing mechanisms to get an acceptable ICP measurement.*
- ✦ *The ETT will become partially clogged with secretions for which suctioning will stimulate the rise in ICP if no treatment given.*
- ✦ *At any time the INSTRUCTOR may signal for the patient to herniate or for the aneurysm to burst.*

Figure 2. Briefing instructions for the instructor: cerebral aneurysm case (management of intracranial pressure [ICP]). OR = operating room, EKG = electrocardiogram, NIBP = noninvasive blood pressure monitoring, $ETCO_2$ = end-tidal carbon dioxide, CVP = central venous pressure, ETT = endotracheal tube.

ing done for an evaluation of performance, the learning objectives would not be included. One can use a complete preoperative evaluation form instead of the learner's handout. Finally, the observer's debriefing worksheet (Fig. 4) is available for either real-time observers via a direct or audio-video link or for audiovisual playback for the learner to view. The author always includes a section for crisis management at the bottom of

---

Learning Objectives: After this session the learner should be able to:
1) understand the components intracranial pressure (ICP)
2) choose the appropriate actions to manage the ICP
3) remain vigilant of what each action takes on the patient's ICP
4) choose appropriate measures to maintain cerebral perfusion pressure (CPP)
5) choose appropriate measures to provide cerebral protection

A 48 year-old man is intubated and just arrives in the OR via transport of a CRNA, who is now leaving because her shift is finished. You have arrived to take over the case. The patient has a right MCA aneurysm, which the surgeon is going to attempt to clip. The patient has already been moved to the OR table, monitors placed and is ready for your induction.

PMHx:
Heavy 70 pack year smoker who fell down yesterday
Allergy:
NKMA
Medications:
None
Review of Systems:
All systems are negative except for PMHx.
Preoperative Physical Examination:
BP = 120/65, HR = 105, RR = 25, SpO_2 = 98% on 50% oxygen/air mixture
Airway = Malampati class II, teeth in good repair, patient intubated and #8.0 oral ETT secured with trach tape
Neuro = Patient responds to painful stimuli with movement
Skin = Normal
Pulmonary = Clear to auscultation, no wheezing
Cardiac = Regular, tachycardic rhythm without any murmurs
Weight is 70 Kg
Height of 5' 11"
Laboratory:
Hemoglobin = 15.0, Hematocrit = 45.0, Platelets are 350,000 and WBC = 10.8
ABG = pH = 7.48, PCO_2 = 31 mmHg, PO_2 = 134 mmHg
Basic electrolyte/metabolic panel is WNL
Chest x-ray demonstrates no acute disease with an ETT 2 cm above the carina.
Access:
One left subclavian central venous triple lumen catheter
IV fluid going at 130 ml per hour

Figure 3. Learner's handout: cerebral aneurysm case. OR = operating room, CRNA = certified registered nurse anesthetist, MCA = major coronary artery, PMHx = past medical history, BP = blood pressure, HR = heart rate, SpO_2 = pulse oximetry, ETT = endotracheal tube, WBC = white blood cells, ABG = arterial blood gases, PCO_2 = partial pressure of carbon dioxide, PO_2 = partial pressure of oxygen, WNL = within normal limits, IV = intravenous.

Increased ICP . . . . . Did they:
- ✦ Recognize the increased ICP?
- ✦ Treat the increased ICP with multiple modalities?

Cerebral perfusion and protection . . . . . Did they:
- ✦ Choose appropriate anesthetic agents?
- ✦ Provide moderate cerebral hypothermia?

Right mainstem intubation . . . . . Did they:
- ✦ Recognize the right mainstem intubation?
- ✦ Provide ICP protection before the manipulated the ETT?
- ✦ Readjust the ETT to an appropriate level?

Induction . . . . . Did they:
- ✦ Choose appropriate induction agents?

Obstructed ETT . . . . . Did they:
- ✦ Recognize the obstructed ETT?
- ✦ Treat the ICP before suctioning?
- ✦ Suction the ETT quickly?

Aneurysm clipping . . . . . Did they:
- ✦ Choose the appropriate drugs to drop the pressure?
- ✦ Choose the appropriate drugs to restore the pressure?

Optional herniation or aneurysm burst . . . . . Did they:
- ✦ Recognize the event?
- ✦ Choose appropriate management?

Crew (Crisis) Resource Management . . . . . Did they:
- ✦ Have Leadership?
- ✦ Manage their information?
- ✦ Show evidence of systematically dealing with an unknown crisis?
- ✦ Have good communication skills?
- ✦ Re-evaluate for fixation errors?
- ✦ Utilize all their resources?
- ✦ Delegate responsibilities?

Figure 4. Observers' debriefing worksheet: cerebral aneurysm case (management of intracranial pressure [ICP]). Specific debriefing points. ETT = endotracheal tube.

the debriefing worksheet. From experience with many simulations, the learner creates a crisis or allows a crisis to happen and must manage the crisis, even though he may not have planned it to happen. Human error is the number-one cause of crises.

Repair of Abdominal Aortic Aneurysm

The operator instructions for the Abdominal Aortic Aneurysm Repair Case (Fig. 5) are significantly more involved than those for ICP management (see Fig. 1). This intricacy did not evolve in one simulation planning meeting. From repeating the educational session many times and constantly improving the scenario, handouts, and teaching method, something like Figure 5 evolves. Note that compared with the ICP management case, we are using a different patient called "Grandma." She is the "standard man" who has aged and changed gender, with the appropriate changes in vascular and pulmonary anatomy and physiology for a 65-year-old woman. This simulated patient is now the starting point for our scenarios. We add modifications to Grandma to achieve our desired patient, such as increasing the weight to 100 kg. The instructor's page (Fig. 6) is fairly simple, since no extraordinary events are planned. The case is difficult enough, and the learning objectives are targeted to the management of this case only. The latex allergy mentioned on the learner's page (Fig. 7) is intended to raise awareness but not meant to be a complicating event. If the resident misses this point, another scenario called "anaphylaxis" (see Chapter 10) can be overlaid on the AAA repair scenario and allowed to act simultaneously. The observer's page (Fig. 8) follows the major events of the case and has the crisis management evaluation ready if appropriate.

Thoracotomy Case

The thoracotomy case has fewer portions to the scenario on the operator's page (Fig. 9) than the AAA repair case (see Fig. 5), but the set-up is more elaborate with the need for double-lumen tubes, fiberoptic intubation, and continuous positive airway pressure (CPAP) devices. Also note that the interventions include steps that rely on the instructor to give verbal cues. Rehearsal is required to get them correct, because the operator, if not anticipating the instructor's speech, will miss the step. The instructor and operator may also set up a visual cue. For any of the cases, the ability to run the program from a wireless laptop computer exists. Even though this may seem convenient for the instructor to run, it distracts the instructor from paying total attention to the behaviors of the learners. Less complicated scenarios lend themselves quite well to the instructor's role as wireless operator. There is also an option for the instructor to communicate with the operator via a headset. Almost all instructors, including the author, who start using a headset will opt not to use it by the third or fourth time they teach a session.

The instructor's page (Fig. 10) for the thoracotomy case outlines multiple options that can take place at the discretion of the instructor. The learner's page (Fig. 11) has multiple other pieces of valuable preoperative information, such as the patient's poor respiratory status and poor IV access. These issues, if not addressed, will become important later in the scenario. Unlike the observer's page on the AAA repair case, the observer's page (Fig. 12) for the thoracotomy case outlines the events to take place and finishes with any crisis management that was required.

Figure 13 is a copy of a self-assessment form, which serves several functions. First, it serves as evidence that the learner was present and an active participant in the learning experience. Second, it provides a trail of self-assessment so that learners can demonstrate progress throughout their training. Third, it provides feedback to the simulation session in both the comments and the learning objectives that they must fill in. Experience has demonstrated that learners usually do not complete the learning objectives section until last, and what they write does not necessarily match the learning objectives provided before the simulation. The self-assessment form has provided the author with valuable information for refinement of future educational sessions.

From the author's experience at getting residents and medical students to change

Background: The adult female manikin is awake and alert on OR table ready for induction for general anesthesia. The EKG, Pulse Oximeter, and NIBP are the only monitors attached. The defibrillator needs to be away from the patient in the farthest corner.

Connect:
- ☺ Art line, off
- ☺ PA catheter, off
- ☺ CVP catheter, off
- ☺ All standard monitors

Other:
- ☺ Manikin on back, awake
- ☺ Anes machine working
- ☺ Anesthesia cart stocked
- ☺ Induction Drugs laid out
- ☺ Fluid warmer in room

Run:
- ☺ Start Grandma
- ☺ Eyes to automatic
- ☺ Set weight to 100kg
- ☺ Set Heart rate factor (HRF)= 1
- ☺ Set Syst Vasc Resist (SVR)= 1.5
- ☺ Set Pulm Vasc Resist (PVR)= 1.5

States/Interventions:
- ☺ Administer all drugs according to verbalized desire if they are not in a syringe
- ☺ Follow all the fluid instructions.
- ☺ If intestinal mobilization treated with phenylephrine, then:
  Add 500ml of volume over 30 sec
  HRF=0.85
  venous return (VR)= 1.8
  venous capacit (VC)= 1.4
  SVR= 1.2

- ☺ If ischemia on aortic clamping treated with nitroglycerin, then:
  Ischemic Sensitiv (IS)= 0.9
  barorecep min (BMn)= 80
  barorecep max (BMx)= 160
  R vent contract (RVC)= 0.75
  L vent contract (LVC)= 0.75
  extrathoracic arterial elastance (EETA)= 2
  intrathoracic arterial elastance (EITA)= 3
  HRF= 1

- ☺ If hypotension from unclamping is treated with fluid and vasopressors, then:
  Add 500ml volume
  VC= 1.5
  PVR= 1
  EPA= 0.23
  HRF=0.85

Scenario events:
- ☺ Resident will perform standard induction. Do not make any changes at this time.

- ☺ Intestinal Mobilization
  HRF=1
  SVR= 1.5
  Overall barorecep (OB)= 0.1
  EITA= 1.5
  VR= 2.5
  VC= 1.8

- ☺ Aortic Cross Clamping
  O₂ consumpt (O2C)= 150

IS= 0.5
ischemic averag (IA)= 0.9
right femoral pulse off
left femoral pulse off
right pedal pulse off
left pedal pulse off
BMn= 120
BMx= 220
Barorecep periph gain= 0.5
RVC= 0.9
LVC= 0.9
VR= 1
SVR= 7
VC= 1.5
pulm vasc resist (PVR)= 7
pulm art elast (EPA)= 1
EETA= 3
EITA= 5
HRF= 0.7

- ☺ Unclamping Aorta
  O2C= 200
  BMx= 120
  SVR= 1
  VC= 2
  PVR= 2.2
  EPA= 0.5
  EETA= 1.1
  EITA= 2
  HRF= .92
  right femoral pulse on
  left femoral pulse on
  right pedal pulse on
  left pedal pulse on

Figure 5. Instructions for simulator operator: abdominal aortic aneurysm (AAA) repair case. OR = operating room, EKG = electrocardiogram, NIBP = noninvasive blood pressure monitoring.

their behavior in the long term, simply playing in the simulation laboratory or watching themselves on video does not usually provide the intended result. The author's experience is consistent with that reported by Olympio et al.[34] Success requires the setting of a standard of performance for the resident to see and experience, followed by repeated attempts until success is achieved. Learner review of videotaped performances has been an important tool for their self-improvement. Even though the literature is growing to support the author's experiences, not enough study has been done to validate it.

Intended audience is for anesthesiology residents of any level. This case is meant to be an instruction step-by-step recreation of a AAA repair.

This is based on a REAL case.
+   Let them READ their case. No need for verbal explanation.
+   They have completed their preoperative evaluation and have the patient on the OR table ready for induction

Only if asked:
+   Any other lab or x-ray values are "drawn and pending"
+   The monitors visible (EKG, NIBP, Pulse Oximeter, $ETCO_2$, temperature) are what you have
+   No transesophageal echo is available

- -

Problems to be encountered in addition to the case (do **NOT** reveal to the participants):
+   *The case should be straight forward without additional hidden scenarios*

Figure 6. Briefing instructions for the instructor: abdominal aortic aneurysm (AAA) repair case.

Resident Orientation

The first few weeks during which a new resident tries to learn and function can be extremely stressful and challenging for both residents and faculty.[118] No new resident can receive a majority of a faculty member's teaching time because of multiple room assignments and patient care procedures allowed under the Medicare rules. Evaluation of a new resident's performance has been difficult because residents received so much help from the senior residents with whom they were initially paired. In addition, the teaching ability of the senior residents and the degree of difficulty of cases to which the new residents were assigned result in a haphazard clinical experience on which their education has been primarily based. The amount of time, in weeks, required to bring new residents up to a competency level where they can be left alone in an operating room for a few minutes after induction and intubation kept the total number of personnel available to provide anesthesia, breaks, and patient work-ups at a suboptimal level compared with the demand for surgical procedures. Despite the efforts of faculty to teach, residents were not ripening and deemed ready for solo work at the same rate; their skills were not consistent due to the haphazard clinical exposure.

Murray et al. described a three-day introductory course to familiarize new residents with the basics of the operating room and anesthetic theater.[154] At the University of Louisville in 2001, a three-day pilot study was conducted to orient new anesthesiology residents to the anesthesia machine, basic equipment, and a standard induction in addition to the traditional method of initial training using the new HPS systems from METI. The goal was to see if this course could replace the traditional system of daily lectures and haphazard clinical exposure. The results of the pilot study were quite amazing. Both senior residents and clinical faculty assessing the new residents' performances thought the new course to be consistent and superior to the traditional method for the knowledge

Learning Objectives: After the session, the learner will be able to:
1) understand the succession of events which typically occur in a AAA repair
2) prepare for the events as they occur
3) choose the appropriate drugs and maneuvers for management of events

A 58 year-old-woman is on the table and ready for induction with only standard monitors on.

PMHx:
Came to ER with back pain, found to have slowly leaking AAA
Good exercise tolerance
Allergy:
Eggs and latex (anaphylaxis)
Medications:
Metoprolol
Review of Systems:
All systems are negative except for PMHx
Preoperative Physical Examination:
BP = 110/65, HR = 65, RR = 25, SpO$_2$ = 941% on 2 L nasal cannula
Airway = Malampati class II, teeth in good repair
Neuro = Awake, alert and oriented times three
Skin = Normal
Pulmonary = Clear to auscultation, no wheezing
Cardiac = Regular rate and rhythm without any murmurs
Weight is 100 Kg
Height of 5' 6"
Laboratory:
Hemoglobin = 11.0, Hematocrit = 33.0, Platelets are 224,000 and WBC = 10.8
ABG = pH = 7.4, PCO$_2$ = 39 mmHg, PO$_2$ = 141 mmHg
Basic electrolyte/metabolic panel is WNL
Chest x-ray demonstrates no acute disease
Access:
One 20g Intravenous line in the left arm
IV fluid going at 100 ml per hour total

Figure 7. Learner's handout: abdominal aortic aneurysm (AAA) repair case. ER = emergency room, PMHx = past medical history, BP = blood pressure, HR = heart rate, RR = respiratory rate, SpO$_2$ = pulse oximetry, WBC = white blood cells, ABG = arterial blood gases, PCO$_2$ = partial pressure of carbon dioxide, PO$_2$ = partial pressure of oxygen, WNL = within normal limits, IV = intravenous.

areas taught. Therefore, an eight-day, total curriculum based in the simulation laboratory was designed to replace the mentor and basic lecture series. In the new curriculum each day, without any human patients, a faculty member presented the lecture material in short, interactive learning modules. To ensure adequate faculty availability, faculty members were not allowed to be on vacation during the first two weeks of July. Each day the session was taught by a different faculty member so that one faculty member could concentrate on the goals and objectives for that day. The modules were followed with the new resident practicing the skills in simulation until he or she was deemed proficient by the teaching faculty member. Each day built on what was taught the day before, and new residents rehearsed the skills that they had learned on previous days, again

IV access . . . . . Did they:
- ✦ Place a central line like a PA catheter?
- ✦ Place an arterial catheter?

Latex allergy . . . . . Did they:
- ✦ Remove the latex objects which may come in contact with the patient?

Induction and intubation . . . . . Did they:
- ✦ choose appropriate drugs to minimize hemodynamic responses?
- ✦ complete the intubation in less than 15 seconds?

Bowel manipulation . . . . . Did they:
- ✦ anticipate the fluid third spacing?
- ✦ treat the problem with fluid?

Aorta cross clamp . . . . . Did they:
- ✦ anticipate the clamping with preparation of drugs?
- ✦ treat the hemodynamic changes appropriately?

Aortic clamp release . . . . . Did they:
- ✦ anticipate the unclamping of aorta?
- ✦ treat the hemodynamic changes which accompany the unclamping?

Crew (Crisis) Resource Management . . . . . Did they:
- ✦ Have Leadership?
- ✦ Manage their information?
- ✦ Show evidence of systematically dealing with an unknown crisis?
- ✦ Have good communication skills?
- ✦ Re-evaluate for fixation errors?
- ✦ Utilize all their resources?
- ✦ Delegate responsiblities?

Figure 8. Observers' debriefing worksheet: abdominal aortic aneurysm (AAA) repair case. Specific debriefing points. PA = pulmonary artery.

proving proficiency to a different faculty member. On a daily basis the teaching faculty completed an objective evaluation form for the residents, documenting their competency in basic skills in the simulation laboratory.

The simulation curriculum was then followed with clinical performance in the operating room with a resident mentor in case skills were not transferred from the simulation laboratory. This segment lasted for as many days as necessary until the new resident was deemed ready for solo work with a supervising faculty member. The advantages to this new system were several. The instruction of the new residents was now standardized compared with the traditional method and verified consistently to the satisfaction of eight different faculty members. The time paired with a senior resident decreased from weeks to only one or two days. Faculty stress levels decreased too. The most recent group of residents took a national Anesthesia Knowledge Test (Metrics Associates, Inc.), improving from the 38th percentile on the first day test (before simulation) to the 48th percentile on

Background: The adult male manikin is supine on an OR table ready for induction with the standard monitors placed.

Connect:
- Art catheter, but do not turn on
- PA catheter, but do not turn on
- CVP catheter, but do not turn on
- All standard monitors except temp

Other:
- Manikin on back
- Anesthesia machine fully working
- Anesthesia cart fully stocked
- Induction Drugs laid out
- Body warmer/cooler in room
- Fluid warmer in the room
- Axillary support in room
- A #39 and #41 left and right double lumen endotracheal tubes on the anesthesia cart
- A fiberoptic intubating bronchoscope with light source in room
- Additonal oxygen tank available to attach to the CPAP device for the double lumen tube
- 20g IV right forearm

Run:
- Start Standard Man
- Eyes to automatic
- Set weight to 90kg

States/Interventions:
- The patient has a right lower lobe empyema. Breath sounds are diminished on the right.
- Set heart rate factor to 1.4
- Set functional residual capacity to 1530 ml
- Set shunt fraction to 0.2
- Set oxygen consumption to 300 ml/min
- Set ischemic index sensitivity to 0.2
- Administer all drugs according to verbalized desire if they are not in a syringe
- Follow all the fluid instructions
- If PEEP is applied to the left lung, do nothing
- If CPAP is applied to the right lung, then reset shunt fraction to 0.2
- If the instructor says the learner's management should help, then set the venous return resistance to 10
- If the instructor says the learner's management should fix the patient's hemodynamics, then set the venous return resistance to 1

Scenario events:
- The learner will first induce the patient and place a double lumen endotracheal tube
- After the non-dependent lung is deflated, set shunt fraction to 0.4 over 1 minute
- After the CPAP is applied, then set the venous return resistance to 50 over 1 minute
- Upon cue from the instructor (can happen at any time), either put on bronchospasm bilaterally 40cm H_2O pressure or a left pneumothroax (intrapleural volume =500ml) as instructor signals

Figure 9. Instructions for simulator operator: thoracotomy case. OR = operating room, PA = pulmonary artery, CVP = central venous pressure, CPAP = continuous positive airway pressure, PEEP = positive end-expiratory pressure.

the 30th day test (after simulation). Even though a large amount of information and numerous skills are packed into two weeks, this system was used successfully with three different sets of new residents between July of 2002 and July of 2003. The anesthesiology faculty overwhelmingly approves of disallowing faculty vacations during the first two weeks of July to provide this much-needed education for new residents.

The schedule for the first two weeks is reproduced in a generic form in Figure 14. Some of the details of daily activity follow almost an OSCE format and look like those

This is based on a REAL case.
+ Let them READ their case. No need for verbal explanation.
+ They have completed their preoperative evaluation and have the patient on the OR table ready for induction

Only if asked:
+ Any other lab or x-ray values are "drawn and pending"
+ The monitors visible (EKG, NIBP, Pulse Oximeter, ETCO₂, temperature, arterial catheter, PA catheter) are what you have
+ Transesophageal echo is broken and unavailable

Problems to be encountered in addition to the case (do **NOT** reveal to the participants):
+ *The learner must induce and place a double lumen tube correctly or the patient will either have bronchospasm or pneumothorax on the unoperable side will occur.*
+ *The learner must position the patient on his side for the thoracotomy correctly or the patient's saturation will fall or the patient will have postoperative neurologic deficits.*
+ *The learner must recheck his double lumen tube for correct placement or the patient will either have bronchospasm or pneumothorax on the unoperated-on side.*
+ *The patient's saturation will decrease on one-lung ventilation which only responds to 10cm of H₂O of CPAP.*
+ *The patient will have a decrease in the venous return to the heart after the CPAP is applied.*

Figure 10. Briefing instructions for the instructor: thoracotomy case. EKG = electrocardiogram, NIBP =- noninvasive blood pressure monitoring, ETCO₂ = end-tidal carbon dioxide, PA = pulmonary artery, CPAP = continuous positive airway pressure.

found in *Anaesthesia OSCE.*[92] Below are brief overviews of each day except the orientation day. When July 1 does not fall on a didactic afternoon, that didactic time is replaced in the schedule to do baseline videotaping. The videotaping was started as part of an ongoing study, which has some interesting results yet to be reported and published.

On the first day the new residents get a tour of the simulation center with a hands-on introduction to the high-fidelity simulators. If the first day is not a didactic day, the afternoon is used to obtain baseline video of the new residents' performances. Their homework assignment is to read about preoperative evaluations. On the second day, the new resident gets a demonstration of how to take a history and do a physical exam oriented toward anesthesiology and how to appropriately document the encounter. New residents are allowed to practice with a standardized patient until they feel comfortable. Next, they are shown how to use the basic equipment, including the anesthesia machine and monitors, and how to start intravenous lines. They must complete a full FDA check-out of the equipment to complete the day. Their homework is to study induction agents and general anesthetics.

On the third day in the simulation center, they again must prove they can successfully perform an FDA check-out of the equipment and do a preoperative evaluation of the instructor acting as a healthy 18-year-old male scheduled for a right inguinal hernia repair. The new residents are given a short lecture on the induction agents, general anesthetics,

Learning Objectives: After this session, the learner will be able to:
1) place a double lumen endotracheal tube appropriately
2) manage one-lung ventilation
3) appropriately position a patient in the decubitus position
4) diagnose and manage the hemodynamic changes that can occur on one lung ventilation in the right lateral decubitus position

A 38 year-old-man, scheduled for an open thoracotomy to remove a right lower lobe secondary an empyema unresponsive to antibiotic therapy, is on the OR table ready for induction.

PMHx:
    Known IV drug abuser
Allergy:
    NKMA
Medications:
    Cefazolin IV
Review of Systems:
    All systems are negative except for PMHx
Preoperative Physical Examination:
    BP = 130/75, HR = 105, RR = 20, SpO$_2$ = 93% on 50% oxygen/air mixture
    Airway = Malampati class III, teeth in poor repair
    Neuro = Awake, alert
    Skin = Normal
    Pulmonary = No breath sounds in right lower lobe, congestion heard throughout all other lung fields
    Cardiac = Regular, tachycardic rhythm without any murmurs
    Weight is 90 Kg
    Height of 6' 6"
Laboratory:
    Hemoglobin = 10.2, Hematocrit = 31.0, Platelets are 650,000 and WBC = 18.4
    ABG = pH = 7.43, PCO$_2$ = 36 mmHg, PO$_2$ = 75 mmHg
    Basic electrolyte/metabolic panel is WNL
    Chest x-ray demonstrates a normal sized heart and a right lower lobe opacity
Access:
    One 20g Intravenous line in left forearm (obtained via ultrasound)

Figure 11. Learner's handout: thoracotomy case. OR = operating room, IV = intravenous, PMHx = past medical history, BP = blood pressure, HR = heart rate, RR = respiratory rate, SpO$_2$ = pulse oximetry, WBC = white blood cells, ABG = arterial blood gases, PCO$_2$ = partial pressure of carbon dioxide, PO$_2$ = partial pressure of oxygen, WNL = within normal limits.

and paralytic agents. They receive a detailed demonstration of the proper way to prepare, induce, maintain, and emerge the patient from an anesthetic as well as the proper way to document the anesthetic course. Each new resident must perform the short anesthetic in simulation to complete the day successfully. During the day residents are also given a short lecture and demonstration on the internal workings of the anesthesia machine. Their homework assignment is to read about fluid management and prepare for the list of crises that they will encounter on the next day.

IV access . . . . . Did they:
+ start a central IV access?
+ start an arterial catheter?

Induction and double lumen intubation . . . . . Did they:
+ induce appropriately for the reduced FRC of the patient?
+ place the double lumen endotracheal tube corrrectly?
+ check the placement with auscultation and fiberoptic confirmation

Right lateral decubitus position . . . . . Did they:
+ guard the airway during patient movement?
+ check for pressure point problems?
+ check for proper placement of axillary support?
+ check placement of double lumen endotracheal tube?

One lung ventilation . . . . . Did they:
+ open the correct lumens to deflate the lung?
+ correct the ventilatory settings for one-lung ventilation?

One lung hypoxia . . . . . Did they:
+ optimize ventilatory settings for one-lung ventilation?
+ apply CPAP appropriately to the deflated lung?

Hemodynamic changes . . . . . Did they:
+ recognize the hemodynamic changes?
+ diagnose the reason for the change?
+ treat the problem appropriately?

Crew (Crisis) Resource Management . . . . . Did they:
+ Have Leadership?
+ Manage their information?
+ Show evidence of systematically dealing with an unknown crisis?
+ Have good communication skills?
+ Re-evaluate for fixation errors?
+ Utilize all their resources?
+ Delegate responsiblities?

Figure 12. Observers' debriefing worksheet: thoracotomy case. Specific debriefing points. IV = intravenous, FRC = forced residual capacity, CPAP = continuous positive airway pressure.

The fourth day is devoted to crises that may happen in the perioperative period. Before they start, the new residents must again demonstrate an adequate FDA check-out of the anesthesia equipment. Then they are given short talks about each of the listed crisis topics, including how to recognize, diagnose, and treat each. To complete the day successfully, each resident must anesthetize the patient again while recognizing, diagnosing, and treating whatever three or four crises may occur. Fluid management is included in the anesthetic management for this day. The residents' anesthetic records are more carefully scrutinized for completeness. Their homework is to study the difficult airway algorithm of the American Society of Anesthesiologists (ASA) and to read about obesity.

Date: _____   Resident Name: _____

Faculty Presenting/Facilitating: _____   Simulation Title: _____

What was/were the Goal(s) of this simulation:

Faculty Comments:

Competency	Required Skill	Circle those which apply	Faculty concurrence with your assessment *(Faculty fills out)*
Patient Care	Develop & carry out-patient Management plans	N/A 1 2 3 4	☐ YES ☐ NO
	Performance of procedures a) Routine physical exam	N/A 1 2 3 4	☐ YES ☐ NO
	Work with in a team	N/A 1 2 3 4	☐ YES ☐ NO
Medical Knowledge	Investigatory & analytic thinking	N/A 1 2 3 4	☐ YES ☐ NO
	Knowledge & application of basic sciences	N/A 1 2 3 4	☐ YES ☐ NO
Practice-Based Learning & Improvement	Analyze own practice for needed improvements	N/A 1 2 3 4	☐ YES ☐ NO
Professionalism	Ethically sound practice	N/A 1 2 3 4	☐ YES ☐ NO
	Other Objective:	N/A 1 2 3 4	☐ YES ☐ NO
	Other Objective:	N/A 1 2 3 4	☐ YES ☐ NO
	Other Objective:	N/A 1 2 3 4	☐ YES ☐ NO

N/A = not applicable, 1 = Very Unsatisfactory, 2 = Borderline Failing, 3 = Average, 4 = Excellent

Comments from Resident:

Faculty Signature _____

Figure 13. Simulation evaluation tool. N/A = not applicable.

Tuesday, July 1, 2003		Wednesday, July 2, 2003	

Tuesday, July 1, 2003	Wednesday, July 2, 2003
8:00 a.m. Orientation - Chair of Department	Faculty #1
Welcome	7:00 a.m. Simulation Lab - Basic Equipment
Process of Board Certification	Anesthesia Machine Checkout
Expectations of residents	Anesthesia Monitoring orientation
Expectations of faculty	Anesthesia cart orientation
Expectations of staff	Preoperative Evaluation
8:30 a.m. Resident Coordinator	Proper Documentation
Lab Coats	IV starting
General Paperwork	All day Baseline Videotaped Evaluations
Vacation Requests	
ABA Paperwork	**Thursday, July 3, 2003**
Pyxis numbers	Faculty #2 / Faculty #3
Resident Lounge/ mailboxes	7:00 a.m. Simulation Lab
8:50 a.m. Business and Billing Mangers	General anesthesia for right inguinal
Pagers	hernia repair on healthy 18 y/o male
Messages	Preinduction/standard monitoring
Library Materials	Induction
Copier and Supplies	Inhaled Anesthetics
Palm Pilots	Induction Agents
Billing Paperwork	Paralytics
Compliance	Intubation
Obtaining Books	Positioning
Reimbursements	Maintenance
ASA & SEA memberships	Emergence
9:30 a.m. ULH HIM staff	Postoperative care
ULH Health Info. Management	Proper Documentation
10:00 a.m. Vice Chair for Education	Anesthesia Machine Function
Didactic Curriculum	Uptake and Distribution
Rotations	
Competency Curriculum	**Friday, July 4, 2003**
In-training exams	Holiday
Mock Orals	
Journal Clubs & Social Events	**Monday, July 7, 2003**
Computers/ Blackboard	Faculty #4
Research	7:00 a.m. Conference
11:00 a.m. Chief Residents	8:00 a.m. Simulation Lab - Crisis Management
Call requests and call schedules	General anesthesia for right inguinal
Tour of ULH facilities	hernia repair on healthy 18 y/o male
12:00 p.m. Lunch on own	Can't Intubate!
1:00 p.m. Billing Company	Hypotension
Billing	Hypertension
2:00 p.m. Assistant Dean for Ed./ Pt. Simulation	Hypoxia
Tour of Paris Sim Center	EKG changes
2:30 p.m. Didactics (see schedule)	ACLS protocols
4:30 p.m. AKT-1 Pretest	Hypothermia

Figure 14. New resident education schedule, July 2003. (*continued*)

On the fifth day the new residents watch demonstrations of fiberoptic intubations as well as other airway interventions found in the ASA algorithm on difficult airways. They are allowed to practice and, after successfully completing an FDA check-out of the anesthesia equipment, use their new airway techniques to intubate the simulated patient and provide an anesthetic. At least one of the crises from the day before will appear during the anesthetic. There are also mini-lectures about the anesthetic management considera-

Hypercarbia
Laryngospasm
Bronchospasm
Hemorrhage
Crystalloid Management
Oliguria
Malignant Hyperthermia
Proper Documentation
(*Anything from previous days can be thrown in unexpectedly during the practices*)

Tuesday, July 8, 2003
Faculty #5
8:00 a.m. Simulation Lab - with crisis General anesthesia for right inguinal hernia repair on 40 y/o male with Pickwickian Syndrome
Preinduction/standard monitoring
Induction
Intubation
Maintenance
Emergence
Postoperative care
Proper Documentation
I-Stat/GEM/ACT training
Practice all of above on HPS
2:30 p.m. Didactics (see schedule)

Wednesday, July 9, 2003
Faculty #6
8:00 a.m. Simulation Lab - with crisis General anesthesia for right inguinal hernia repair on healthy 78 y/o male with coronary and carotid artery disease
Preinduction/standard monitoring
Arterial Line Placement
Appropriate Induction
Intubation
Appropriate Maintenance
Emergence
Postoperative care
Proper Documentation
(*Anything from previous days can be thrown in unexpectedly during the practices*)

Thursday, July 10, 2003
Faculty #7
8:00 a.m. Simulation Lab - with crisis General anesthesia for total pelvic exenteration on 48 y/o female with sickle cell anemia disease
Blood product administration
Preinduction/standard monitoring
Practice Induction
Practice Intubation
Practice Intraop Maintenance
Practice Emergence
Provide Postoperative care
Practice Proper Documentation
(*Anything from previous days will be thrown in unexpectedly during the practices*)

Friday, July 11, 2003
Faculty #8
8:00 a.m. Simulation Lab-Regional anesthesia for ORIF right ankle fracture on healthy 18 y/o female
Preinduction/standard monitoring
Local Anesthetics
Indications & Contraindications
Techniques
Maintenance and adjuncts
Emergence and Complications
Postoperative care
Proper Documentation
(Fresh Tissue lab for spinals and epidurals)
1:00 p.m. Final videotaped performances

Saturday, July 12, 2003
8:00 a.m. In-training exam - **DON'T MISS IT!!!**

Thursday, July 31, 2003
Vice Chair for Education
3:00 p.m. Classroom
Orientation Reinforcements
Research (Vice Dean for Research)
Computers
Questions & Answers
4:00 p.m. AKT-1 Post Test

Figure 14. *(continued)*

tions of obesity. While some residents are practicing, others are receiving training and competency assessments in portable blood analysis machines. The homework assignment is to study how to manage a patient with coronary artery disease for noncardiac surgery. On either the fifth or sixth day, the schedule of events is adjusted to account for the Tuesday afternoon didactics, which the new resident must still attend.

The sixth and seventh days contain more review and practice than introduction of new material. The sixth-day material revolves around how to manage a patient with coronary artery disease. The new residents practice placing central venous access catheters in simulation and learn how to interpret pulmonary artery catheter readings as well as obtain cardiac outputs and calculate systemic vascular resistances. On both days they still have to do the FDA checklist, anesthetize their patients, and deal with any crisis. The twist on these two days is that the anesthetic equipment has been sabotaged, and residents must discover the problems via the checklists. The subject of the seventh day is a large fluid-shifting case in a patient with sickle cell disease. The mini-lecture is about maintaining vigilance, tight fluid control, and temperature management. The new residents must also demonstrate accurate documentation of their anesthetic. The homework assignment is to study for spinal and epidural anesthetics.

On the eighth and final day of the simulation course, the morning is devoted to teaching spinal and epidural anesthesia. There are short presentations about local anesthetics and techniques for providing regional anesthesia. The demonstration and practice take place in the fresh tissue laboratory at the University of Louisville. In the afternoon, the new residents do follow-up videotaping of their performances at anesthetizing a patient and managing a crisis. The videotapes are viewed by the residents for self-evaluation and later by faculty to ascertain the amount of improvement in each resident since the beginning tapes. While new residents are waiting their turn in front of the camera, they will go and see the real patients to whom they have been assigned. The next clinical day is a Monday, and residents provide anesthesia to real patients.

Conclusion

Anesthesiology has played a leading role in medical simulation. Many advances over the past 10 years allow more accurate anatomic and physiologic modeling. With these great tools, medical educators are unleashing the potential to teach and evaluate objectively as medicine has not been able to do before. Much work still lies ahead in finding appropriate teaching methods and in establishing valid and reliable evaluation tools. The examples provided in this chapter are based on anecdotal experiences. The author looks forward to the time when they are replaced with tested and scrutinized material. The future of patient simulation, with the integration of virtual reality and the development of human-cyborg type interactions, seems unlimited. Standardized patients were the first simulated patients and will probably continue to play an important role in medical education. Technical simulations can standardize a teaching experience, but only humans can provide the rich variety of experiences. Anesthesiology is known to be the only specialty to achieve six sigma quality, and now it is poised to achieve even greater quality.

References
1. Chopra V, et al: The Leiden anaesthesia simulator. Br J Anaesth 1994;73:287–292.
2. Beneken JE, van Oostrom JH: Modeling in anesthesia. J Clin Monit Comput 1998;14: 57–67.
3. Byrne AJ, Hilton PJ, Lunn JN: Basic simulations for anaesthetists: A pilot study of the AC-CESS system. Anaesthesia 1994;49:376–381.
4. Anesoft Corporation: Anesthesia Simulator 2002. Available at *http://www.anesoft.com/Products/as.asp*. Accessed 11–26-2003.
5. Med Man Simulations, Inc., GasMan. Available at http://www.gasmanweb.com/. Accessed 11–26-2003.
6. Math-Tech: SIMA. Available at *http://www.math-tech.dk/sima/*. Accessed 11-26-2003.
7. Advanced Simulation Corporation: Body Simulation. Available at *http://www.bodysim.com/BodySim/Index.htm*. Accessed 11–26-2003.

8. University of Florida: The Virtual Anesthesia Machine. Available at *http://vam.anest.ufl.edu/*. Accessed 11-26-2003.
9. Laerdal: SimMan—Universal Patient Simulator. Available at *http://www.laerdal.com/document.asp?nodeID*=1855430. Accessed 11-26-2003.
10. METI: HPS. Available at *http://www.meti.com/hps.html*. Accessed 11-26-2003.
11. MedTek: PatSim-1. Available at <http://www.ux.his.no/tn/medtek/patsim.htm> Accessed 11-26-2003.
12. MedSim: Advanced Medical Simulations, L., Med-Sim Eagle. Available at *http://www.medsim.com/*. Accessed 11-26-2003.
13. University of Louisville: University of Louisville Paris Simulation Center. Available at *http://www.louisville.edu/medschool/psc/psc.htm*. Accessed 11-26-2003.
14. Gordon JA,. Pawlowski J: Education on-demand: The development of a simulator-based medical education service. Acad Med 2002;77:751–752.
15. Gaba DM: Improving anesthesiologists' performance by simulating reality. Anesthesiology 1992;76:491–494.
16. Morgan PJ, Cleave-Hogg D: A worldwide survey of the use of simulation in anesthesia. Can J Anaesth 2002;49:659–662.
17. Heard JK, Allen RM, Clardy J: Assessing the needs of residency program directors to meet the ACGME general competencies. Acad Med 2002;7:750.
18. Kurrek MM, Devitt JH: The cost for construction and operation of a simulation centre. Can J Anaesth 1997;44:1191–1195.
19. Schwid HA, O'Donnell D: Educational computer simulation of malignant hyperthermia. J Clin Monit 1992;8:201–208.
20. Hotchkiss MA, Mendoza SN: Update for nurse anesthetists. Part 6: Full-body patient simulation technology: gaining experience using a malignant hyperthermia model. AANA J 2001;69:59–65.
21. Gaba DM, et al: Assessment of clinical performance during simulated crises using both technical and behavioral ratings. Anesthesiology 1998;89:8–18.
22. Chopra V, et al: Does training on an anaesthesia simulator lead to improvement in performance? Br J Anaesth 1994;73:293–297.
23. Gardi T, et al: How do anaesthesiologists treat malignant hyperthermia in a full-scale anesthesia simulator? Acta Anaesthesiol Scand 2001;45:1032–1035.
24. Mason RA: Education and training in airway management. Br J Anaesth 1998;81:305–307.
25. Thwaites AJ,Rice CP, Smith I: Rapid sequence induction: A questionnaire survey of its routine conduct and continued management during a failed intubation. Anaesthesia 1999;54:376–381.
26. Forrest FC, et al: Use of a high-fidelity simulator to develop testing of the technical performance of novice anaesthetists. Br J Anaesth 2002;88:338–344.
27. Stringer KR, Bajenov S, Yentis SM: Training in airway management. Anaesthesia 2002;57:967–983.
28. Laerdal, Deluxe Difficult Airway Head. Available at *http://www.laerdal.com/document.asp?nodeID*=3805268. Accessed 11-26-2003.
29. Agro F, Giuliano I, Montecchia F: A new human-dynamic simulator (Air Man) for airway training in emergency situations. Am J Emerg Med, 2002;20:495.
30. Loyd GE (ed): Dan Sirota C. Inc: Models Used in Airway Device Demonstrations. Louisville, KY, 2003.
31. Roberts I, et al: Airway management training using the laryngeal mask airway: A comparison of two different training programmes. Resuscitation 1997;33:211–214.
32. Naik VN, et al: Fiberoptic orotracheal intubation on anesthetized patients: Do manipulation skills learned on a simple model transfer into the operating room? Anesthesiology 2001;95:343–348.
33. Rowe R, Cohen RA: An evaluation of a virtual reality airway simulator. Anesth Analg 2002;95:62–66, table of contents.
34. Olympio MA, et al: Failure of simulation training to change residents' management of oesophageal intubation. Br J Anaesth 2003;91:312–328.
35. Mackenzie CF, et al: Comparison of self-reporting of deficiencies in airway management

with video analyses of actual performance. LOTAS Group. Level One Trauma Anesthesia Simulation. Hum Factors 1996;38:623–635.

36. Hosking EJ: Does practising intubation on a manikin improve both understanding and clinical performance of the task by medical students? Anaesth Points West 2003;31(2):25–28.

37. Cross J: Airway management—a current training problem? Anaesthesia 2000;55:515–516.

38. Berkenstadt H., et al: The use of advanced simulation in the training of anesthesiologists to treat chemical warfare casualties. Anesth Analg 2003;96(6):1739–1742, table of contents.

39. Patil V, et al: Training course in local anaesthesia of the airway and fibreoptic intubation using course delegates as subjects. Br J Anaesth 2002;89:586–593.

40. Frerk C: Training course in local anaesthesia of the airway and fibreoptic intubation using course delegates as subjects. Br J Anaesth 2003;90:258; author's reply, 258–259.

41. Goldberg JS, et al: Simulation technique for difficult intubation: teaching tool or new hazard? J Clin Anesth 1990;2:21–26.

42. Kurrek MM, Devitt JH, Cohen M: Cardiac arrest in the OR: How are our ACLS skills? Can J Anaesth 1998;45:130–132.

43. Attia RR, Miller EV, Kitz RJ: Teaching effectiveness: Evaluation of computer-assisted instruction for cardiopulmonary resuscitation. Anesth Analg 1975;54:308–311.

44. Schwid HA, et al: Use of a computerized advanced cardiac life support simulator improves retention of advanced cardiac life support guidelines better than a textbook review. Crit Care Med 1999;27:821–824.

45. Christensen UJ, et al: ResusSim 98—a PC advanced life support trainer. Resuscitation 1998;39(1–2): 81–84.

46. DeAnda A, Gaba DM: Unplanned incidents during comprehensive anesthesia simulation. Anesth Analg 1990;71:77–82.

47. Gaba DM,. DeAnda A: The response of anesthesia trainees to simulated critical incidents. Anesth Analg 1989;68:444–451.

48. DeAnda A, Gaba DM: Role of experience in the response to simulated critical incidents. Anesth Analg 1991;72:308–315.

49. Schwid HA, O'Donnell D: Anesthesiologists' management of simulated critical incidents. Anesthesiology 1992;76:495–501.

50. Jacobsen J, et al: Management of anaphylactic shock evaluated using a full-scale anaesthesia simulator. Acta Anaesthesiol Scand 2001;45:315–319.

51. Weller J, Wilson L, Robinson B: Survey of change in practice following simulation-based training in crisis management. Anaesthesia 2003;58:471–473.

52. Schwid HA, et al: Screen-based anesthesia simulation with debriefing improves performance in a mannequin-based anesthesia simulator. Teach Learn Med 200;13(2):92–96.

53. Schwid HA, O'Donnell D: The Anesthesia Simulator Consultant: Simulation plus expert system. Anesthesiol Rev 1993;20(5):185–189.

54. O'Donnell J, et al: Planning and implementing an anesthesia crisis resource management course for student nurse anesthetists. CRNA 1998;9(2):50–58.

55. Pleban RH, et al: Training and assessing complex decision-making in a virtual environment. Percept Mot Skills, 2002;94(3 Pt 1):871–882.

56. Ziv AS, Wolpe SD, Root P: Patient safety and simulation-based medical education. Med Teach 2000;489.

57. Grube C, et al: [Changing culture—simulator-training as a method to improve patient safety. Report on an international meeting on medical simulation. Scottsdale: January 12–14, 2001]. Anaesthesist 200;50(5):358–362.

58. Byrne AJ, Jones JG: Inaccurate reporting of simulated critical anaesthetic incidents. Br J Anaesth 1997;78:637–641.

59. Howard SK, et al: Simulation study of rested versus sleep-deprived anesthesiologists. Anesthesiology 2003;98:1345–1355; discussion, 5A.

60. Murray D, Dodds C: The effect of sleep disruption on performance of anaesthetists—a pilot study. Anaesthesia 2003;58:520–525.

61. Gander PH, et al: Hours of work and fatigue-related error: a survey of New Zealand anaesthetists. Anaesth Intens Care 200;28:178–183.

62. Dorafshar AH, O'Boyle DJ, McCloy RF: Effects of a moderate dose of alcohol on simulated laparoscopic surgical performance. Surg Endosc 2002;16:1753–1758.
63. Xiao Y, et al: Task complexity in emergency medical care and its implications for team coordination. LOTAS Group. Level One Trauma Anesthesia Simulation. Hum Factors 1996; 38: 636–645.
64. Blike GT, Surgenor SD, Whalen K: A graphical object display improves anesthesiologists' performance on a simulated diagnostic task. J Clin Monit Comput 1999;15:37–44.
65. Leijten DT, Rejger VS, Mouton RP: Bacterial contamination and the effect of filters in anaesthetic circuits in a simulated patient model. J Hosp Infect 1992;21:51–60.
66. Jha AK, Duncan BW, Bates DW: Simulator-based training and patient safety. In Markowitz AJ, et al (eds): Evidence Report/Technology Assessment, No. 43, pp 511–518.
67. Garden A, et al: Education to address medical error—a role for high fidelity patient simulation. N Z Med J 200;115(1150):133–134.
68. Murray WB, et al: Learning about new anesthetics using a model driven, full human simulator. J Clin Monit Comput 2002;17(5):293–300.
69. Syroid ND, et al: Development and evaluation of a graphical anesthesia drug display. Anesthesiology 2002;96:565–575.
70. Haux R: Aims and tasks of medical informatics. Int J Med Inf 1997;44:9–20; discussion, 39–44, 45–52, 61–66.
71. Abrahamson S, and et al: A computer-based patient simulator for training anesthesiologists. Educ Technol 1969;9(10):55–59, 69.
72. Abrahamson S, et al: Effectiveness of a simulator in training anesthesiology residents. J Med Educ 1969;44: 515–519.
73. Abrahamson S, Denson JS, for the University of Southern California Los Angeles. School of Medicine: A Developmental Study of Medical Training Simulators for Anesthesiologists. Final Report. Los Angeles, 1968, p 216.
74. Euliano TY: Teaching respiratory physiology: Clinical correlation with a human patient simulator. J Clin Monit Comput 2000;16(5–6):465–470.
75. Tan GM, et al: Teaching first-year medical students physiology: Does the human patient simulator allow for more effective teaching? Singapore Med J 2002;43(5):238–242.
76. Zvara DA,. Olympio MA, MacGregor DA: Teaching cardiovascular physiology using patient simulation. Acad Med 2001;76:534.
77. Cleave-Hogg D, Morgan PJ: Experiential learning in an anaesthesia simulation centre: Analysis of students' comments. Med Teach 2002;24:23–26.
78. Euliano TY, Mahla ME: Problem-based learning in residency education: A novel implementation using a simulator. J Clin Monit Comput 1999;15(3–4):227–232.
79. Euliano TY: Small group teaching: clinical correlation with a human patient simulator. Adv Physiol Educ 2001;25(1–4): 36–43.
80. Register M, Graham-Garcia J, Haas R: The use of simulation to demonstrate hemodynamic response to varying degrees of intrapulmonary shunt. AANA J 2003;71(4):277–284.
81. Hiemenz L, Stredney D, Schmalbrock P: Development of the force-feedback model for an epidural needle insertion simulator. Stud Health Technol Inform 1998;50:272–277.
82. Farnsworth ST, et al: Teaching sedation and analgesia with simulation. J Clin Monit Comput 2000;16(4):273–285.
83. van Stralen DW, et al: Retrograde intubation training using a mannequin. Am J Emerg Med 1995;13:50–52.
84. Anastakis DJ, et al: Assessment of technical skills transfer from the bench training model to the human model. Am J Surg 1999;177:167–170.
85. Glavin R, Greaves D: The problem of coordinating simulator-based instruction with experience in the real workplace. Br J Anaesth 2003;91:309–311.
86. Byrne AJ, et al: Effect of videotape feedback on anaesthetists' performance while managing simulated anaesthetic crises: a multicentre study. Anaesthesia 2002;57:176–179.
87. Schwartz RW, et al: Residents' evaluation of a problem-based learning curriculum in a general surgery residency program. Am J Surg 1997;173:338–341.

88. Morgan PJ, Cleave-Hogg D: A Canadian simulation experience: Faculty and student opinions of a performance evaluation study. Br J Anaesth 2000;85:779–781.
89. Hartland W, Biddle C, Fallacaro M: Accessing the living laboratory: Trigger films as an aid to developing, enabling, and assessing anesthesia clinical instructors. AANA J 2003;71(4): 287–291.
90. Reznek M, et al: Emergency medicine crisis resource management (EMCRM): Pilot study of a simulation-based crisis management course for emergency medicine. Acad Emerg Med 2003;10:386–389.
91. Duke University: SimDot. Available at *http://www.simdot.com*. Accessed 11–26-2003.
92. Arthurs G, Elfituri KM: Anaesthesia OSCE, 2nd ed. London, Greenwich Medical Media, 2002, p 453.
93. Nyssen AS, et al: A comparison of the training value of two types of anesthesia simulators: computer screen-based and mannequin-based simulators. Anesth Analg 2002;94:1560–1565, table of contents.
94. Garfield JM,. Paskin S, Philip JH: An evaluation of the effectiveness of a computer simulation of anaesthetic uptake and distribution as a teaching tool. Med Educ 1989;23:457–462.
95. Philip JH: Gas Man—an example of goal oriented computer-assisted teaching which results in learning. Int J Clin Monit Comput, 1986;3(3):165–173.
96. Heffernan PB, Gibbs JM, McKinnon AE: Teaching the uptake and distribution of halothane. A computer simulation program. Anaesthesia 1982;37:9–17.
97. Christensen UJ, et al: The Sophus anaesthesia simulator v. 2.0. A Windows 95 control-center of a full-scale simulator. Int J Clin Monit Comput 1997;4:11–16.
98. Weis PA, Guyton-Simmons J: A computer simulation for teaching critical thinking skills. Nurse Educ 1998;23(2):30–33.
99. Morgan, PJ, et al: Simulation technology: A comparison of experiential and visual learning for undergraduate medical students. Anesthesiology 200;96:10–16.
100. Marshall RL, et al: Use of a human patient simulator in the development of resident trauma management skills. J Trauma 200;51:17–21.
101. Gilbart MK, et al: A computer-based trauma simulator for teaching trauma management skills. Am J Surg 2000;179:223–238.
102. Morgan PJ, Cleave-Hogg D: Comparison between medical students' experience, confidence and competence. Med Educ 2002;36:534–539.
103. Brailovsky C, et al: Measurement of clinical reflective capacity early in training as a predictor of clinical reasoning performance at the end of residency: An experimental study on the script concordance test. Med Educ 2001;35:430–436.
104. Rosenblatt MA, Abrams KJ: The use of a human patient simulator in the evaluation of and development of a remedial prescription for an anesthesiologist with lapsed medical skills. Anesth Analg 2002;94:149–153, table of contents.
105. Kofke WA,. Rie MA, Rosen K: Acute care crisis simulation for jury education. Med Law 200;20:79–83.
106. Tooley MA, Forrest FC, Mantripp DR: MultiMed—remote interactive medical simulation. J Telemed Telecare 1999;5(Suppl 1):S119–S121.
107. Xiao Y, et al: Information acquisition from audio-video-data sources: An experimental study on remote diagnosis. The LOTAS Group. Telemed J 1995;5(2):139–155.
108. Lampotang S, et al: Logistics of conducting a large number of individual sessions with a full-scale patient simulator at a scientific meeting. J Clin Monit 1997;13(6):399–407.
109. Prystowsky JB, Bordage G: An outcomes research perspective on medical education: The predominance of trainee assessment and satisfaction. Med Educ 2001;35:331–336.
110. Wong SH, Ng KF, Chen PP: The application of clinical simulation in crisis management training. Hong Kong Med J 2002;8(2):131–135.
111. Devitt JH, et al: The anesthetic record: accuracy and completeness. Can J Anaesth 1999; 46:122–128.
112. Byrne AJ, Jones JG: Responses to simulated anaesthetic emergencies by anaesthetists with different durations of clinical experience. Br J Anaesth 1997;78:553–556.

113. Byrne AJ, Sellen AJ, Jones JG: Errors on anaesthetic record charts as a measure of anaes-thetic performance during simulated critical incidents. Br J Anaesth 1998;80:58–62.
114. Morgan PJ, et al: Identification of gaps in the achievement of undergraduate a 2003;97:1691–1694.
115. Schwid HA, et al: Evaluation of anesthesia residents using mannequin-based simulation: A multiinstitutional study. Anesthesiology 2002;97:1434–1444.
116. McGaghie WC, et al: Assessment instruments used during anaesthetic simulation. Br J Anaesth 2001;87:647–648.
117. Glavin RJ,. Maran NJ: Development and use of scoring systems for assessment of clinical competence. Br J Anaesth 2002;88:329–330.
118. Weller JM, et al: Evaluation of high fidelity patient simulator in assessment of performance of anaesthetists. Br J Anaesth 2003;90:43–47.
119. Devitt JH, et al: Testing the raters: Inter-rater reliability of standardized anaesthesia simu-lator performance. Can J Anaesth 1997;44:924–928.
120. Weinger MB, et al: An objective methodology for task analysis and workload assessment in anesthesia providers. Anesthesiology 1994;80:77–92.
121. Bullock G, et al: Evaluating procedural skills competence: Inter-rater reliability of expert and non-expert observers. Acad Med 1999;74:76–78.
122. Morgan PJ, Cleave-Hogg D, Guest CB: A comparison of global ratings and checklist scores from an undergraduate assessment using an anesthesia simulator. Acad Med 2001;76: 1053–1055.
123. Winckel CP, et al: Reliability and construct validity of a structured technical skills assess-ment form. Am J Surg 1994;167:423–427.
124. King PH, et al: A proposed method for the measurement of anesthetist care variability. J Clin Monit Comput 2000;16:121–125.
125. Devitt JH, et al: Testing internal consistency and construct validity during evaluation of per-formance in a patient simulator. Anesth Analg 1998;86:1160–1164.
126. Devitt JH, et al: The validity of performance assessments using simulation. Anesthesiology 2001;95:36–42.
127. Byrne AJ, Greaves JD: Assessment instruments used during anaesthetic simulation: review of published studies. Br J Anaesth 2001;86:445–450.
128. Morgan PJ, Cleave-Hogg D: Evaluation of medical students' performance using the anaes-thesia simulator. Med Educ 2000;34:42–45.
129. Morgan PJ, Cleave-Hogg D: Evaluation of medical students' performances using the anes-thesia simulator. Acad Med 1999;74:202.
130. Morgan PJ, et al: Validity and reliability of undergraduate performance assessments in an anesthesia simulator. Can J Anaesth 2001;48:225–233.
131. Schupfer GK,. Konrad C, Poelaert JI: [Manual skills in anaesthesiology]. Anaesthesist 2003;52:527–534.
132. Wantman A: Can simulators be used to assess clinical competence? Hosp Med 2003;64(4): 251.
133. Kapur PA, Steadman RH: Patient simulator competency testing: Ready for takeoff? Anesth Analg 1998;86:1157–1159.
134. Gouvitsos F, Vallet B, Scherpereel P: [Anesthesia simulators: benefits and limits of experi-ence gained at several European university hospitals]. Ann Fr Anesth Reanim 1999;18: 787–795.
135. Swanson CR: Teaching clinical veterinary anesthesia with an interactive videodisc simula-tion: Perceptual and academic results. J Vet Med Educ1991;18:17.
136. Modell JH, et al: Using the human patient simulator to educate students of veterinary med-icine. J Vet Med Educ 2002;29:111–116.
137. Schwarz G, et al: Pneumatic pulse simulation for teaching peripheral plexus blocks in ca-davers. Anesth Analg 2002;95:1822–1823.
138. Eason MP, Goodrow MS, Gillespie JE: A device to stimulate central venous cannulation in the human patient simulator. Anesthesiology 2003;99:1245–1246.

139. Euliano TY, et al: Modeling obstetric cardiovascular physiology on a full-scale patient simulator. J Clin Monit 1997;13(5):293–297.
140. Thoman WJ, et al: Autoregulation in a simulator-based educational model of intracranial physiology. J Clin Monit Comput 1999;15(7–8):481–491.
141. de Beer NA, et al: Educational simulation of the electroencephalogram (EEG). Technol Health Care 2001;9:237–256.
142. Fritz LA,. Kay JA, Garrett N: Description of the oxygen concentration delivered using different combinations of oxygen reservoir volumes and supplemental oxygen flow rates with the Ohmeda Universal Portable Anesthesia Complete draw-over vaporizer system. Mil Med, 2003;168:304–311.
143. Johnson K, et al: Clinical evaluation of the Life Support for Trauma and Transport (LSTAT) platform. Crit Care 2002;6:439–446.
144. Williams KA, et al: Training in fiberoptic intubation. Anaesthesia 2000;55:99–100.
145. Burt DE: Virtual reality in anaesthesia. Br J Anaesth 1995;75:472–480.
146. Doyle DJ, Arellano R: The Virtual Anesthesiology Training Simulation System. Can J Anaesth 1995;42(4):267–273.
147. Johnston R, et al: Assessing a virtual reality surgical skills simulator. Stud Health Technol Inform 1996;29:608–617.
148. Ziegler R, et al: Virtual reality arthroscopy training simulator. Comput Biol Med 1995;25:193–203.
149. Sung WH, et al: The assessment of stability and reliability of a virtual reality-based laparoscopic gynecology simulation system. Eur J Gynaecol Oncol 2003;24:143–146.
150. Arne R, et al: PatSim—simulator for practising anaesthesia and intensive care. Development and observations. Int J Clin Monit Comput 1996;13(3):147–152.
151. Yao F-SF: Yao and Artusio's Anesthesiology: Problem-oriented Patient Management, 5th ed. Philadelphia: Lippincott Williams & Wilkins, 2003, p 1231.
152. Reed AP: Clinical Cases in Anesthesia, 2nd ed. New York, Churchill Livingstone, 1995, p 437.
153. Seropian MA: General concepts in full scale simulation: Getting started. Anesth Analg 2003;97:1695–1705.
154. Murray WB, Schneider AJ, Robbins R: The first three days of residency: An efficient introduction to clinical medicine. Acad Med 1998;73(5):59.

SIMULATION IN CRITICAL CARE

Elizabeth H. Sinz, MD

The practice of critical care medicine is highly complex and technical. By definition, critically ill patients are at risk for rapid deterioration, and they are not resilient when delays or errors in management occur. These characteristics make education in critical care a fertile ground for simulation. Unfortunately, the practice of critical care has not received as much attention from the simulation community as anesthesiology or emergency medicine. This is due to a combination of factors. The fidelity of currently available simulators is limited, and improvements in fidelity are expensive. In addition, a shortage of critical care faculty and difficulties with reimbursement for critical care services limit the availability of critical care teaching in general and simulation teaching in particular. Nevertheless, simulation has some important instructional advantages for teaching critical care medicine. Basic and routine training is required for new groups of medical students, nurses, and residents throughout the year. Crisis recognition and management are important for physicians, nurses, respiratory therapists, and other unit personnel to learn and practice. Teamwork and crisis resource management (CRM) is particularly important in the critical care setting and can be taught and practiced effectively in a simulated environment.[1] Uncommon events can be presented as often as is needed for all caregivers to learn about them and know their role in management. Most simulation modalities have been used for teaching critical care skills, including computer screen-based simulation, actors, animals, human cadavers, partial-task trainers, videotape, and full-scale human patient simulators. Simulators have been effective for teaching multiple aspects of critical care medicine to all types of trainee without risk to patients.

Unique Aspects of Critical Care Favoring Simulation

Good psychomotor skills are essential for procedures commonly performed in the intensive care unit. Because these procedures are inherently dangerous to real patients, practice in a simulated environment is preferable. Placement of chest tubes and pulmonary artery catheters (PACs), percutaneous tracheostomies, and intubations can be practiced in the risk-free environment of the simulation lab, and good evidence indicates that practice of some procedures improves performance in real patients.[2,3] Other management techniques may also improve with practice, such as ventilator manipulations and treatment of shock. Decision-making is a cognitive skill that is an essential part of intensivist training, and with simulation the trainee can see the results of their decisions, even when they make inappropriate choices. Unlike human actors, the simulated human patient can become extremely ill or even die while the students learn to diagnose and treat a variety of problems commonly encountered in the intensive care unit (ICU).

It is possible to create a realistic environment for simulation that encourages students to suspend their disbelief. Since ICU patients are highly monitored and often unable to move about, speak, or even communicate, the plastic mannequin is not as much of a drawback in intensive care simulation compared with other specialties. A portable simulator such as the Laerdal SimMan or even a simple mannequin such as the Laerdal Resusci-Anne (Wappingers Falls, NY) can be taken to the ICU and placed in an empty bed for practice sessions (Fig. 1). This arrangement takes advantage of the equipment and monitors in the trainees' own hospital unit to create a realistic environment, although the capacity to mimic invasive monitors and shock states is limited. In order to use the more advanced full-scale simulators that are not so easily moved about, such as the METI Human Patient Simulator, the team at the Pennsylvania State University College of Medicine at Hershey Medical Center has used the simple technique of painting an ICU backdrop on curtains hung in the background (Fig. 2). These curtains, along with a few props such as an actual ventilator, ICU bed, and typical ICU monitor, help to create a highly realistic environment that allows trainees to forget that they are managing a mannequin rather than a real patient. This realistic environment is an essential component of teaching with simulation because it allows the instructor to observe the way trainees actually perform rather than what they say they would do in a given situation.

Initial Assessment of Critically Ill Patients

For many students, particularly those who are the least experienced, the recognition that a patient has become or is becoming critically ill is a major challenge. Intensivists typically learn to recognize impending deterioration by observing the natural course of

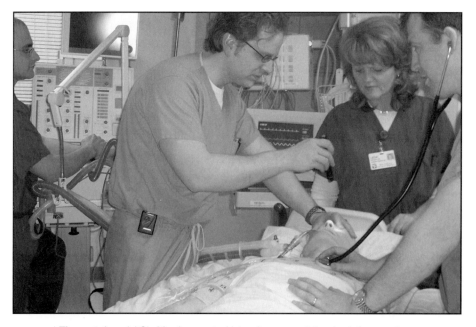

Figure 1. Laerdal SimMan in an actual intensive care unit for simulation practice.

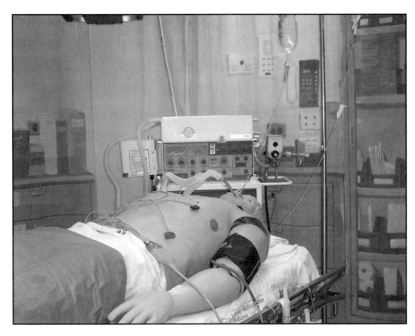

Figure 2. Addition of a painted backdrop to enhance the environment in the simulation laboratory with the METI Human Patient Simulator at the Pennsylvania State University College of Medicine, Hershey, Pennsylvania.

acute illness in many patients. Recognition is particularly important because early intervention may significantly reduce morbidity and mortality. Coates et al. compared simulator training with a problem-based learning (PBL) format for recognition and management of dyspnea by a group of medical students.[4] Dyspnea is one of the most common presenting signs of acute illness. In this study, medical students who were taught about shortness of breath in the simulator demonstrated improved patient management skills compared to those taught with the standard PBL format.

At the Hershey Medical Center, the simulation laboratory was used to teach floor nurses when to call the physician in various case scenarios. For example, a heart rate of 100 beats per minute in a previously healthy 20-year-old trauma victim may be considered acceptable, whereas a similar heart rate in a 90-year-old patient should trigger concern. Each nurse was given a history of the patient and his or her injury and then asked to make a decision. The group then discussed the decision. The teaching point emphasized in this example was, "When in doubt, call for help." The simulated patient "died" on multiple occasions when the call for help was delayed, making it clear that real patients may die if intervention is delayed. Although allowing a simulated patient to die during simulation exercises is controversial, it can be a highly effective teaching tool.

Use and Interpretation of Invasive Monitors

The use of invasive monitors is typically taught through lectures, reading assignments, and pictures or graphs of typical tracings seen on a monitor. However, students who do well on written exams may nevertheless have difficulty interpreting data as they are presented clinically. There has been a fair bit of controversy over the use of PACs, most likely due to the widespread misunderstanding of the measured and derived values that they provide.[5-11] For more than a decade, devices to practice placement of central lines and interpretation of waveforms have been available.[12]

A website dedicated to PAC education through the use of computer screen-based examples of PAC waveforms and self-assessment tests can be found at PACEP.org. A company based in Australia lists a commercially available PA catheter simulator at its website (Manbit.com) (Kingswood, Australia). The simulator includes hardware that looks and feels like a PA catheter when it is manipulated, along with software that mimics waveforms and values consistent with normal and abnormal physiology. Some full-scale simulators, such as the METI Standard Man (Sarasota, FL), can mimic typical waveforms and measurements of central venous pressure, pulmonary artery pressure, pulmonary capillary wedge pressure (PCWP), cardiac output via the thermodilution technique, urine output via a Foley catheter, and intracranial pressure. The pressure tracings can realistically mimic a variety of pathophysiologic alterations and can even accurately reflect the pressures achieved with chest compressions in a cardiac arrest. The use of simulated patients and PAC waveforms is one method to practice and improve the difficult cognitive skills of proper PAC use.

In a simple training exercise developed at West Virginia University,[13] a PAC waveform is displayed with the tip in an inappropriate location. Initially the patient is not acutely ill, but the nurse indicates that the PAC "numbers" are not what they had been earlier. In this exercise the student is required only to identify the position of the PAC based on the waveform and length of the catheter from the patient's skin to its tip. This is the type of manipulation required fairly often as the tip of the catheter changes position in response to patient movement or volume status changes. Despite adequate prior training, including demonstrated knowledge of waveforms and catheter markings, inexperienced students find this exercise to be exceedingly difficult in the context of critical illness. Only personnel experienced in the use of PACs have been able to make the appropriate adjustments efficiently and correctly.

Use of Vasoactive Medications and Inotropes

Many of the medications commonly used for critically ill patients have traditionally been demonstrated in a different type of simulation setting: the animal laboratory. Either livestock (e.g., pigs) or animals destined for destruction (e.g., homeless dogs or cats) have been administered a variety of vasoactive or inotropic medications to demonstrate the effects of these drugs. The animals are anesthetized for the demonstration and usually euthanized afterward. This approach involves several ethical concerns. From a teaching-learning perspective, the main problem with using animals is that they are expensive and may not appropriately demonstrate the points to be taught. The response of the animals is usually an excellent demonstration of how a healthy human might respond to the drugs; however, the human patients that receive these drugs are typically not healthy. In addition, the animal may have an adverse response to a medication and die before the entire demonstration has been completed. Residual effects from the last medication given may interfere with the demonstration of the next medication. Because there is no "reset" button for an animal, it is difficult to eliminate these problems.

In contrast, both computer-based simulators and full-scale human patient simulators respond consistently to a variety of medications. The medications can typically be administered as a single bolus or a continuous infusion, as in real patients. The response to the medication can be shown in real time, slow time, or fast time. This unique feature of simulators is not possible in real patients or animals. Depending on the level of sophistication of the trainees, the response to an intervention can be demonstrated in slow time, allowing the trainees to consult resources, to ask questions, or even to recognize that the situation is deteriorating. The simulator can even be stopped as information is reviewed or retrieved by the trainees, and then the simulation can be resumed from that point in time. The simulation can be completed in real time or in the same amount of time that changes would typically be observed in a real patient. In some demonstrations, it is most appropriate to use fast time, which entails advancing immediately to a later time point after an intervention to demonstrate what would be occurring. The simulator allows the students to see what happens if the wrong dose or wrong drug is administered. If the simulated patient dies, the program is simply restarted. This approach makes it possible for trainees to go back to the beginning and try something different; it gives them the "right to make mistakes."[14]

Intravenous Pumps, Monitors, and Other Equipment

The ICU is home to a wide variety of equipment, all of which may break or be misused, potentially leading to adverse patient outcomes. Various simulation environments allow the student to demonstrate and practice the use, repair, and maintenance of typical equipment, such as IV pumps, pressure transducers, and monitors. When trainees are asked actually to perform tasks rather than merely to describe them, knowledge deficits are often uncovered. The moment that trainees recognize that they do not know something they need to know may be the best time to teach this information; this concept is often referred to as the "teachable moment." Such an opportunity is often lost during clinical care due to the time pressure of completing the tasks required for the patient. In the simulation laboratory, the simulation can be stopped and the necessary teaching completed before moving on with the case—an example of "slow time."

The United States Army has used human patient simulators to test new equipment before using it for critically injured patients. In a study reported by Johnson et al.,[15] physicians and nurses using a human patient simulator as the critically ill "patient" tested the Life Support for Trauma and Transport (LSTAT) system. After learning how to use the new equipment, the volunteers were divided into two groups. Each clinician in the first group used the LSTAT equipment for the first two scenarios and conventional equipment for the second two scenarios. The clinicians in the second group followed a cross-over pattern so that they used conventional equipment for the first two scenarios and the LSTAT equipment for the second two scenarios. The time needed to reach the correct diagnosis and begin treatment was recorded as well as the number of times that the correct diagnosis could not be quickly determined using both types of equipment. The use of simulators allowed the new equipment to be tested in "critical" situations before it was put to use for the care of highly vulnerable patients, possibly under hostile conditions.

Airway Management

Airway management in a critically ill patient is somewhat different from the airway management of patients in the operating room. Typically, the critically ill patient is intubated due to acute deterioration. The algorithm for failed intubation is much simpler and does not include postponing the procedure. There is much less variety in the equipment available for alternative airway access in most ICUs compared with surgical suites. In addition, less time and expertise are available to use alternative means to secure the airway due to the type of patients as well as the variable backgrounds of intensivists with regard to airway training and experience. The self-inflating bag-mask is used for mask ventilation, and this technique is both more difficult to use and less effective than the typical anesthesia machine delivery system. A review of cases referred to the National Board of Patients' Complaints in Denmark[16] revealed a high rate of mortality and morbidity for patients who had adverse respiratory events in the ICU and operating room. The authors recommended better education and guidelines for managing the difficult airway, improvement in communication among personnel, and use of simulator training. In the United States, where most intensivists are not anesthesiologists, difficult airway management practice using simulation would seem to be even more beneficial. Schaeffer developed the airway technology incorporated into the Laerdal AirMan and SimMan to assist with airway training. It is particularly useful for practicing difficult airway algorithms, such as that developed by the American Society of Anesthesiologists. Schaeffer's group at the University of Pittsburgh Medical Center has shown that students can develop the cognitive skills and judgment needed to manage an airway crisis by training in the simulation lab.[17,18]

Ventilator Management

As far back as the early 1980s, computer models of the respiratory system were developed that could make reasonable predictions of a patient's response to alterations in ventilator settings.[19] By the late 1990s, the physiologic simulators were more accurate and consistent than experienced physicians at predicting the pH and pCO_2 changes in patients when ventilator adjustments were made.[20,21] Today computer-based simulators can demonstrate ventilator malfunctions and airway problems and allow trainees to practice interventions and adjustments. The trainees can experience a realistic representation of the outcome of blood gas analysis as well as changes in patient airway pressures, tidal volume, and respiratory rate. Airway waveforms, such as pressure-volume loops, also can be demonstrated and interpreted with devices such as the IngMar Ventilation Simulator (Pittsburgh, PA) (Fig. 3). Other types of ventilation dilemmas, such as tachypnea, bradypnea, occluded or kinked endotracheal tubes, dislodged endotracheal tubes, circuit leaks or disconnects, and loss of power or gas supply, can also be demonstrated realistically using partial-task trainers or full-scale human patient simulators.[22,23] These simulators give a realistic rendering of lung sounds, chest excursion, and respiratory rate. The monitors display physiologic changes in oxygen saturation, electrocardiograms, and blood pressure. To date, there is no realistic clinical representation of cyanosis, but several centers are currently working on this problem, particularly for use in pediatric simulators.

Human patient simulators are excellent tools for teaching the appropriate sequence to evaluate and safely manage an endotracheal tube cuff leak.[24] This deceptively simple and typical ICU management problem is best taught using a typical ICU ventilator

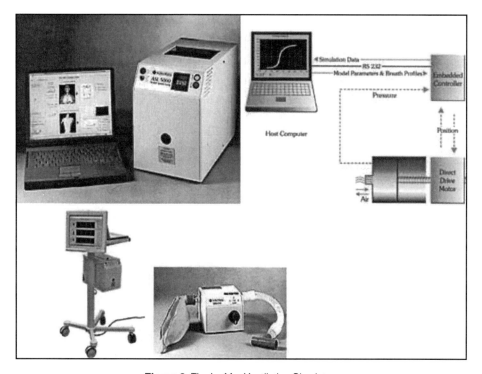

Figure 3. The IngMar Ventilation Simulator.

and a full-scale human patient simulator or an advanced airway trainer that includes realistic lungs. The students are introduced to a simulated patient who is already intubated. The ventilator's low pressure and/or low tidal volume alarms are sounding. The trainees are then asked to give a differential diagnosis for these alarms. They must then evaluate the cause, which in this scenario is an endotracheal tube cuff leak. Once they identify this problem, they must act upon it. Inexperienced trainees almost always remove the faulty endotracheal tube immediately and then attempt to replace it using direct laryngoscopy. If the trainee makes no assessment or preparation for a difficult airway, the instructor adjusts the airway so that the mannequin cannot be re-intubated. If trainees demonstrate any sort of preparation, such as direct laryngoscopy with the endotracheal tube still in place, use of a tube exchanger, passage of a fiberoptic scope beside the original tube, or asking for expert assistance ahead of time, they are able to exchange the tube without difficulty. No matter what the trainee does, the case is an excellent springboard for discussion of difficult airways in the ICU and different methods for safe management. During debriefing, all possible management options can be reviewed, including packing the throat to reduce the air leak and using continuous oxygen insufflation to match the cuff leak and maintain a seal. The point of this exercise is to demonstrate the danger inherent in removing an endotracheal tube before carefully planning the subsequent management of the airway. Unfortunately, this situation has actually occurred in countless ICUs, emergency departments, and operating rooms, sometimes resulting in no difficulty, sometimes in a near-miss, and occasionally in a patient's death. This scenario can be taught without a simulator, but it is much more dramatic with a simulator, particularly when a trainee can be shown the potential consequences of his or her own actions. It is another of example of how simulation creates an ideal "teaching moment" by allowing the students to make a potentially fatal mistake without risk to any patient.

A simple simulation exercise can be used to help trainees at all levels understand the principles of mechanical ventilation by allowing them to experience mechanical ventilation themselves. The only requirement is a working mechanical ventilator and some disposable bacterial filters that fit on the end of the ventilator circuit. The trainee breathes with the ventilator through the filter. The instructor or respiratory therapist allows each trainee to try a variety of ventilator modes and settings. This exercise is used in many teaching centers and is quite valuable for trainees. The Society for Critical Care Medicine has created a two-day course, called Fundamental Critical Care Support (FCCS), that covers the basics of critical care. In some centers, this experience is incorporated into the ventilator workshop of the FCSS course to simulate the experience of being on a ventilator.[25]

Emergency Procedures

Animals are still used to practice certain emergency procedures for which simulators do not yet provide a realistic feel. Live or dead animals, including primates,[26] dogs, and pigs, have been used to practice chest tube insertion, emergency cricothyrotomy, and diagnostic peritoneal lavage. The use of live animals is rapidly declining as improvements in simulator technology make simulators an acceptable alternative to the animal laboratory for teaching procedures.[27] Animal cadavers are still used, particularly if they are inexpensive and readily available.[28] The West Virginia University Department of Anesthesia uses deer heads from wild game after it is butchered for practice of emergency cricothyroidectomy and retrograde intubation

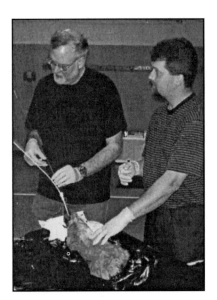

Figure 4. *A-C,* West Virginia University emergency airway practice workshop using discarded deer heads.

over a wire (Fig. 4), and the Emergency Medicine Department uses pig tracheas for the same purpose.

Bronchoscopy

Human cadavers have been used frequently for practice of procedures such as bronchoscopy. The airway anatomy is accurate in a human cadaver, and a ventilator can be used to mimic the movement of breathing. Cadavers, however, do not cough, have secretions, or provide variable pathology, and they are usually difficult to obtain. Technologic advances in the current generation of bronchoscopy simulators, such as the AccuTouch Endoscopy Simulator by Immersion Medical (San José, CA), make them so useful in this regard that they are likely to replace the use of cadavers (Fig. 5). In addition to providing realistic anatomy, the simulators exhibit movements such as vocal cord spasm, cardiac pulsations, and cough; various pathologies are also available. There is also a scoring system to evaluate the trainees on their performance and encourage continued practice. In a study by Ost et al., expert bronchoscopists scored better than intermediate-level bronchoscopists, who scored better than novices on this simulator.[29] Fellows who were trained on the simulator also performed better than their conventionally trained peers on their first actual bronchoscopies, as assessed by procedure time, bronchoscopy nurse assessment, and a quantitative bronchoscopy quality score.

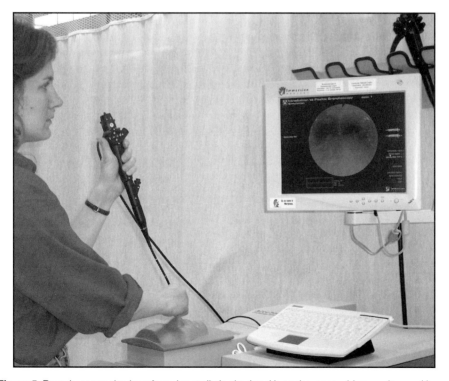

Figure 5. Bronchoscopy simulator featuring realistic simulated bronchoscope, video monitor, and haptic interface.

Traditionally, bronchoscopy has been taught in the course of performing this procedure on actual patients. Unfortunately, this approach may increase the risk of discomfort and complications. At risk of inducing temporary hypoxemia, a bronchoscope may be used to obtain lung specimens to determine the cause of pneumonia in critically ill patients or to remove mucous plugs from the large airways. Under these circumstances, time is of the essence, and trainees are often excluded from performing the procedure. Colt et al. found more evidence that bronchoscopy simulators allow trainees to improve their speed and accuracy.[30] Novices were trained and allowed to practice flexible bronchoscopy using a virtual reality simulator. Virtual reality is a computer-based, simulated environment that uses a high-performance computer, graphics, and specialized software and hardware to provide visual, tactile, and auditory feedback. This group used the PreOp Endoscopy Simulator by HT Medical Systems (Gaithersburg, MD) for teaching novice physician trainees to perform bronchoscopy. After training, novice performance equaled or exceeded that of skilled attending physician colleagues with several years of experience. This study did not assess skills during actual patient care, but the results were reproducible in a conventional inanimate-airway model. Another study found that pediatric residents who trained on an airway simulator were dramatically faster and better at pediatric intubations using a fiberoptic bronchoscope than those who had practiced by performing two consecutive intubations on children.[3]

Shock

Full-scale human patient simulation is well-suited for demonstrating shock physiology. The simulator can be programmed to demonstrate all four types of shock: cardiogenic, distributive, obstructive, and hypovolemic. At the request of the trainee, simulated invasive monitors can be placed, including arterial lines and central venous catheters that display either central venous pressure only or the full range of data obtainable with a PAC. This approach allows the student to make decisions about the diagnosis and management of the patient with the data that they choose and often provides an excellent beginning for discussion on the risks and benefits of invasive monitoring. Therapeutic interventions can be tried and the results demonstrated in real time, fast time, or slow time, depending on the level of the trainee. If management decisions are inappropriate, the student can see what the result would be. The scenario can either be started again from the beginning or continue, giving the trainee the opportunity to treat iatrogenic complications as well. Since it is all done with a simple keystroke with no risk to a patient and no additional cost, mistakes become learning opportunities without any negative consequences to patients or to trainees' egos.

Teamwork and Interactions

Crisis management and teamwork are particularly relevant in critically ill patients, who are cared for by a diverse team that may include physicians of different specialties, nurses, respiratory therapists, and others. Human patient simulators are widely used to study, practice, and ultimately improve the communication of medical teams, and critical care teams are starting to benefit from this approach as well. Some innovative plans to improve ICU communication have been suggested as a result.[31,32] Simulation can be incorporated into standardized courses that teach aspects of crisis re-source management, such as the FCCS course. At West Virginia University, we use full-scale simulation with a shock scenario to demonstrate aspects of crisis manage-ment and review resuscitation principles instead of the standard lecture on resuscita-tion principles.

Family Interaction and Breaking Bad News

Good communication skills are especially important during interactions with critically ill patients and their families. Whether the health care professional is obtaining informed consent for procedures, giving daily updates, or delivering bad news, the inherent stress of being ill or having an ill family member can create discord for the doctors, nurses, and fam-ily, despite good intentions by all. Critical care fellows at the Children's National Medical Center in Washington, DC, were taught to give bad news to a family through practice with actors simulating a patient's family members. These physicians' performance scores im-proved significantly between the first and second sessions.[33] In another study at the Euro-pean Donor Hospital Education Programme (EDHEP) workshop, doctors showed some improvement in breaking bad news, but the skills were not maintained.[34]

One Australian center uses a human patient simulator in combination with actors to teach new interns about many aspects of patient death. This group utilizes a full-scale human simulator as the "patient," and several actors play the roles of family members. In this scenario, the patient dies unavoidably but unexpectedly with a family member present. The team is unable to resuscitate the patient, even if they perform appropriately. The scenario then turns to the interaction between the medical team and the family members, one of whom was present throughout the attempted resuscitation and another of whom arrives unaware of the preceding events. The second family member is typi-cally the patient's husband, who has come to take her home but instead must be in-formed that she has died unexpectedly. The trainees learn about the proper steps for pro-nouncing the death of a patient. After interacting with the "family," the interns must fill out the appropriate medical and legal paperwork, including the death certificate. This scenario is used to teach about sudden death, including interaction with the patient, fam-ily, and staff. At the end of the scenario, the chaplains, social workers, and other end-of-life specialists, as well as psychologists and experienced physicians, are present to review the actions of the interns. The students have the opportunity to review their own feelings and responses to the events. Professional debriefing and adequate support are important aspects of this program due to the realism of the scenario. Trainees often be-come emotional during this exercise, an aspect that many believe contributes to reten-tion of the concepts learned.

Range of Trainees

Simulation is ideal in many ways for teaching inexperienced providers critical care skills. Rogers et al.[35,36] used simulation for both training and assessment of fourth-year medical students during their critical care rotation. During their month in the ICU, the students were exposed to a variety of teaching tools, including lectures, case discus-sions, and rounds. They also had the opportunity to practice on partial-task trainers and an adult full-scale simulator. Simulators are ideal for this group of students, who typically have a great deal of "book knowledge" but almost no integration of knowledge, skills, and behavior. Using a simulator, the students made decisions in real time and saw the effects of their decisions, good or bad. Students also made decisions in slow time, with the simulator paused so that they could take the time to gather resources not immediately available. Students are not allowed to work out problems in such a manner with real patients, who may further deteriorate or even die if treatment is delayed or inappropriate. Simulators allowed the students the opportunity to make mistakes, and benefit from seeing the outcome. In this course, the simulator was believed to have contributed to the students' ability to apply knowledge to problem-solving and was also believed to be useful as an evaluation tool. Others have used simulation to evaluate the critical care skills of graduating medical students.[37]

Surgery residents at the Robert Wood Johnson Medical School in New Brunswick, New Jersey,[38] were given three unknown scenarios using a human patient simulator. In this observational study, the residents were unsuccessful in the first scenario, but subsequent performance improved in areas previously neglected. The authors believed that the use of the simulator uncovered weaknesses in individual student performance as well as program content, an observation that has been echoed by others. Some validity is given to simulator training and assessment in a study by Marshall et al., which compared the performances of interns and senior residents in a full-scale trauma management simulation as part of an ATLS course.[39] The performance of the interns improved in trauma management skills, critical treatment decisions, and team behavior after simulation training. In addition, the performance of the more experienced senior residents was superior to that of the interns on the simulator, indicating some degree of validity.

Full-scale human patient simulators have been used to orient nurses to high-acuity areas, such as the emergency department or ICU. This is one of the few areas where the cost-benefit of simulation has been demonstrated. Because the trainees are exposed to acute events only, the training is consolidated into a shorter time than the traditional method of having a trainee "shadow" an experienced nurse during an orientation period. The new nurse is therefore able to begin working in the new environment more quickly. This benefit translates into a direct cost savings for nurse orientation. Such savings are much harder to document in the financial chaos surrounding payment for physician training. Jay Ober, RN, Director of Staff Development at Holyoke Hospital in Holyoke, Massachusetts, has demonstrated this cost savings with nurse orientees in the intensive care unit and emergency department (Table 1). He also has anecdotal evidence that the nurses oriented in the simulation laboratory are better prepared for high-acuity situations compared with those oriented in the traditional manner, despite the shorter orientation time (Table 2). In contrast, another study found that the level of anxiety in nursing students who attended a critical care simulation prior to their clinical exposure was not decreased compared with other nursing students, despite better familiarity with the required psychomotor skills.[40] However, others have found critical care simulation an effective means to achieve multiple competencies necessary for clinical nursing practice.[41]

Rare Events

Even experienced residents and physicians occasionally encounter events for which they may be ill prepared if they have had only traditional instruction. The so-called

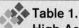

Table 1.
High-Acuity Nursing Orientation: Comparison of Traditional Orientation Method vs. Orientation Using Simulation

	Traditional Orientation	Orientation Using Simulation
Average training time*	6 weeks	3 weeks
Cost	$20/hr for 6 weeks	$20/hr for 3 weeks
Total cost per orientee	$7680	$3840

*Recommended orientation time of 6–9 months is rarely practical.

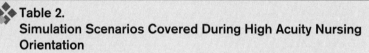

Table 2.
Simulation Scenarios Covered During High Acuity Nursing Orientation

Cerebral vascular accident	Shock
Subdural hemorrhage	Acute respiratory failure
Subarachnoid hemorrhage	Drug overdose
Emergency nurse challenge	Acute coronary syndrome
Diabetic emergencies	Arrhythmia management
Chest trauma	ACLS provider practical
Surgical emergencies	Sedation and analgesia practical

"rare" life-threatening event can be scripted and practiced using the simulator. Anaphylaxis, hyperthermia, thyrotoxicosis, malignant hyperthermia, and hyperkalemia after succinylcholine administration have been demonstrated, identified, and treated in simulator patients. If management is incorrect, the participants have the opportunity to review the case and see where their decision-making went wrong and possibly to try again. This approach is especially useful for cases that practitioners might see only rarely during their career. The benefit of such training has been particularly difficult to prove, but intuitively it seems to be helpful.

Other events are perhaps not so rare but nonetheless somewhat complex to understand and interpret. At the Simulation Center at the Johannes Gutenberg-University in Mainz, Germany, a full-scale human patient simulator is used to demonstrate advanced principles of apnea in testing for assessment of brain death.[42] For patients that have a severe lung injury, performing apnea testing by disconnecting the ventilator may cause a loss of positive pressure that rapidly leads to severe hypoxemia and cardiac arrest. The dilemma posed is how to conduct the test to allow the partial pressure of carbon dioxide (pCO_2) to increase above the required level of 60 without allowing the patient to become hypoxemic. Their group advocates changing the ventilator setting to continuous positive airway pressure (CPAP) rather than disconnecting the patient from the ventilator. This approach should allow for apneic oxygenation and prevent the patient from desaturating. Use of this type of simulation may help to preserve more organs for eventual donation.

Congestive heart failure is a common problem that requires the mastery of specific technical, judgmental, and interpretive skills by the time a student graduates from medical school. At Wake Forest University, a human patient simulator is used to demonstrate the variety of responses seen when different doses of several medications are given to treat this type of problem.[43,44] The simulated patient can dramatize complications such as hypotension, hypertension, tachycardia, myocardial ischemia, cardiac and respiratory arrest, and tension pneumothorax, giving students the opportunity to improve their skills in managing congestive heart failure.

There is even a program that radiologists can use to prepare for unusual critical events that are more likely to occur in a radiology suite.[45] This system uses an interactive computer screen-based simulator to train and evaluate radiologists' performance in case scenarios of acute deterioration due to oversedation, apnea, agitation, bronchospasm, hypotension, hypertension, bradycardia, tachycardia, myocardial ischemia, and cardiac arrest.

Testing, Assessment, and Accreditation

Skills assessment and credentialing using simulators are performed in divergent fields. In psychiatry, actors mimic psychiatric illness, and board examiners require candidates to correctly interview and diagnose these standardized patients. In courses such as ACLS and ATLS, participants are expected to appropriately manage cardiac arrest and acute trauma care using mannequins and/or standardized patients (actors). The premise is the same: the students are presented with a case history and then required to perform as they presumably would with a real patient. They are then graded on their performance. The use of simulators for testing is controversial due to their lack of fidelity in some cases, but some studies have demonstrated a correlation between better performance in a simulation exercise and a more advanced level of training.[37,46] For many however, simulation has been an accepted testing modality for some time. Critical care has not yet developed any high-stakes testing for credentialing or certification using simulators, but this approach may not be far off. Already the Australian Medical Board has used simulation as one tool in evaluating anesthesiologists who reportedly perform below the standard of care. Many are already looking to simulation as a tool to assist in assessment of competencies, as required by the newest ACGME guidelines for all types of medical training. In some reports, the "testing" of trainees has been most useful in uncovering deficits in the training program.[38]

Conclusion

The intensive care unit is one of the most challenging settings in which to teach. Simulation can be used to provide training and practice with both psychomotor and cognitive skills required to care for the sickest patients. Various tools, including computer-based simulators, partial-task trainers, and full-scale human patient simulators, provide a range of options to students. As virtual reality and haptics advance the field and the human physiology project gets under way, the fidelity of simulators will improve and the cost of devices should decrease. The major remaining barrier will be the availability of qualified instructor-clinicians who can provide excellent hands-on teaching and practice for the care of the most fragile patients without putting patients or trainees at increased risk of harm.

Acknowledgment
Special thanks to Kathleen Rosen, MD, and W. Bosseau Murray, MD, for editing assistance.

References
1. Howard SK, Gaba DM, Fish KJ, et al: Anesthesia crisis resource management training: teaching anesthesiologists to handle critical incidents. Aviat Space Environ Med 1992;63:763–770.
2. Seymore NE, Gallagher AG, Roman SA, et al: Virtual reality training improves operating room performance: results of a randomized, double-blinded study. Ann Surg 2002;236:458–463.
3. Rowe R, Cohen RA: An evaluation of a virtual reality airway simulator. Anesth Analg 2002;95:62–66.
4. Coates WC, Steadman RH, Huang YM, et al: Full-scale high fidelity human patient simulation vs. problem based learning: comparing two interactive educational modalities. Acad Emerg Med 2003;10:489.
5. Robin ED: Death by pulmonary artery flow-directed catheter. Time for a moratorium? Chest 1987;92:727–731.
6. Robin ED: Overuse and abuse of Swan-Ganz catheters. Int J Clin Monit Comput 1987;4:5–9.
7. Spodick DH: Flow-directed pulmonary artery catheterization. Moratorium vs. clinical trial. Chest 1989;95:957.
8. Trottier SJ, Taylor RW: Physicians' attitudes towards and knowledge of the pulmonary artery catheter: Society of Critical Care Medicine membership survey. New Horizons 1997;5:201–206.
9. Sprung CL, Eidelman LA: The issue of a U.S. Food and Drug Administration moratorium on the use of the pulmonary artery catheter. New Horizons 1997;5:277–280.
10. Vincent JL, Dhainaut JF, Perret C, Suter P: Is the pulmonary artery catheter misused? A European view. Crit Care Med 1998;26:1283–1287.
11. Cruz K, Franklin C: The pulmonary artery catheter: uses and controversies. Crit Care Clin 2001;17:271–291.
12. Saliterman SS: A computerized simulator for critical-care training: new technology for medical education. Mayo Clin Proc 1990;65:968–978.
13. Rosen KR, Sinz EH: Simulation Case Library: The case of the coiled cardiac catheter. J Educ Perioper Med 2002;IV(II).
14. Larbuisson R, Penderville P, Nyssen AS, et al: Use of anaesthesia simulator: initial impressions of its use in two Belgian university centers. Acta Anaesthesiol Belg. 1999;50(2):87–93.
15. Johnson K, Pearce F, Westenskow D, et al: Clinical evaluation of the Life Support for Trauma and Transport (LSTAT) platform. Crit Care 2002;6:439–446.
16. Rosenstock C, Moller J, Hauberg A: Complaints related to respiratory events in anaesthesia and intensive care medicine from 1994 to 1998 in Denmark. Acta Anaesthesiol Scand 2001;45:53–58.
17. Schaefer J, Gonzalez R: Dynamic simulation: A new tool for difficult airway training of professional healthcare providers. Am J Clin Anesthesiol 2000;27:232–242.
18. Schaefer JJ, Dongilli T, Gonzalez R: Results of systematic psychomotor difficult airway training of residents using the ASA Difficult Airway Algorithm & Dynamic Simulation. J Am Soc Anesthesiol 1998;89(3A):A60.
19. Hinds CJ, Roberts MJ, Ingram D, Dickinson CJ: Computer simulation to predict patient responses to alterations in the ventilation regime. Intens Care Med 1984;10:13–22.
20. Hardman JG, Bedforth NM, Ahmed AB, et al: A physiology simulator: validation of its respiratory components and its ability to predict the patient's response to changes in mechanical ventilation. Br J Anaesth 1998;81:327–332.
21. Bedforth NM, Hardman JG: Predicting patients' responses to changes in mechanical ventilation: a comparison between physicians and a physiological simulator. Intens Care Med 1999;25:839–842.
22. Arne R, Stale F, Ragna K, Petter L: PatSim—simulator for practising anaesthesia and intensive care. Development and observations. Int J Clin Monit Comput. 1996;13(3):147–152.

23. Fatta C, Moreles J, Skartwed RC, Wilks DH: The use of a whole body simulator to train respiratory therapy students in advanced application skills. Presented at the International Meeting for Medical Simulation, 2002, Santa Clara, CA.
24. Sinz EH: Workshop on endotracheal tube cuff leak. Presented at the International Meeting for Medical Simulation, 2003, San Diego, CA.
25. Sinz EH: Ventilator teaching tips. Beat: fundamental critical care support. Instruct Newslett 2002:1.
26. Sims JK: Advanced Trauma Life Support laboratory: pilot implementation and evaluation. JACEP 1979;4(8):150–153.
27. Block EF, Lottenberg L, Flint L, et al: Use of a human patient simulator for the advanced trauma life support course. Am Surg 2002;7(68):641–651.
28. Gardiner Q, White PS, Carson D, et al: Technique training: endoscopic percutaneous tracheostomy. Br J Anaesthesiol 1998;81:401–403.
29. Ost D, Rosiers AD, Britt EJ, et al: Assessment of a bronchoscopy simulator. Am J Respir Crit Care Med 2001;164:2248–2255.
30. Colt HG, Crawford SW, Oliver Galbraith I: Virtual reality bronchoscopy simulation: a revolution in procedural training. Chest 2001;120:1333–1339.
31. Renard JM, Bricon-Souf N, Geib JM, Beuscart R: A simulation of dynamic tasks routing to improve cooperation in intensive care units. Stud Health Technol Inform. 1999;68:31–36.
32. Bricon-Souf N, Renard JM, Beuscart R: Dynamic workflow model for complex activity in intensive care unit. Int J Med Inform 1999;2–3(53):143–150.
33. Vaidya VU, Greenberg LW, Patel KM, et al: Teaching physicians how to break bad news: a 1-day workshop using standardized parents. Arch Pediatr Adolesc Med 1999;153:419–422.
34. Morton J, Blok GA, Reid C, et al: The European Donar Hospital Education Programme (EDHEP): enhancing communication skills with bereaved relatives. Aneaesthesiol Intens Care 2000;28:184–190.
35. Rogers PL, Jacob H, Rashwan AS, Pinsky MR: Quantifying learning in medical students during a critical care medicine elective: a comparison of three evaluation instruments. Crit Care Med 2001;29:1268–1273.
36. Rogers PL, Jacob H, Thomas EA, et al: Medical students can learn the basic application, analytic, evaluative, and psychomotor skills of critical care medicine. Crit Care Med 2000;28: 550–554.
37. Murray D, Boulet J, Ziv A, et al: An acute care skills evaluation for graduating medical students: A pilot study using clinical simulation. Med Educ 2002;36:833–841. 38. Hammond J, Bermann M, Chen B, Kushins L: Human patient simulator in critical care training: a preliminary report. J Trauma 2002;53:1064–1067.
39. Marshall RL, Smith JS, Gorman PJ, et al: Use of a human patient simulator in the development of resident trauma management skills. J Trauma 2001;51:17–21.
40. Erler CJ, Rudman SD: Effect of intensive care simulation on anxiety of nursing students in the clinical ICU. Heart Lung 1993;22:259–265.
41. Morton PG: Using a critical care simulation laboratory to teach students. Crit Care Nurse 1997;6(17):66–69.
42. Heinrichs W, Moenk S, Depta A, Grass C: Apnoea testing in brain death—a field for simulation? Presented at the International Meeting for Medical Simulation, 2002, Santa Clara, CA.
43. Olympio MA, MacGregor D, Saunders I: Modeling congestive heart failure and its treatment using a full scale human patient simulator. Presented at the International Meeting for Medical Simulation, 2002, Santa Clara, CA.
44. Zvara DA, Olympio MA, MacGregor DA: Teaching cardiovascular physiology using patient simulation. Acad Med 2001;76:534.
45. Medina LS, Racadio JM, Schwid HA: Computers in radiology. The Sedation, Analgesia, and Contrast Media Computerized Simulator: a new approach to train and evaluate radiologists' responses to critical incidents. Pediatr Radiol 2000;30(5):299–305.
46. Reischman RR: Critical care cardiovascular nurse expert and novice diagnostic cue utilization. J Advanc Nurs 2002;39:24–34.

Chapter 13

SIMULATION IN EMERGENCY MEDICINE

James A. Gordon, MD, MPA, Steven A. McLaughlin, MD,
Marc J. Shapiro, MD, William F. Bond, MD, and Linda L. Spillane, MD

Mandate for Emergency Medicine Training

Although advanced skill in emergency care constitutes a unique medical specialty, basic competence in emergency medicine is expected of all physicians. According to a national consensus conference on the role of emergency medicine (EM) in the future of American medical care, sponsored in 1993 by the Josiah Macy, Jr. Foundation:

> State medical licensing boards, the national Board of Medical Examiners, the Liaison Committee on Medical Education (LCME), and medical school deans and faculty must ensure that every medical student has acquired the appropriate knowledge and skills to care for emergency patients. This education must be provided through educational experiences supervised by appropriately qualified emergency physicians.[1]

With over 100 million emergency department (ED) visits per year, emergency physicians are uniquely qualified to help bring instructive patient encounters or "good teaching cases" to life utilizing high-fidelity patient simulation.[2] In 2002, the Society for Academic Emergency Medicine (SAEM) convened an interest group dedicated to simulation-based technologies. A group of emergency medicine educators attending a Council of Residency Directors (CORD) meeting in Washington, DC, summarized their recommendations and began to set the simulation agenda for the field as follows:[3]

1. Simulation is a useful tool for training residents and can be used to assess competence. The core competencies best assessed with this method include patient care (decision-making, prioritizing, procedural skills), interpersonal skills (team leadership, communication), and systems-based practice (team structure and utilization, resource use).

2. Simulation is appropriate for performance assessment now, but there is a lack of evidence to support the validity of simulation for high-stakes assessment decisions such as promotion or certification.

3. Operational definitions of competence and tools to evaluate performance must be developed and tested. These include critical actions checklists, behavioral ratings, compliance ratings relative to algorithms, and simulated patient mortality.

4. Scenarios and evaluation tools should be formatted in a standardized way and shared among EM educators, perhaps using a website. Standardization allows testing of the reproducibility of simulated patient encounters using different simulator models and among different residency programs. It also permits assessment of the reliability and validity of the tools used to measure performance.

History of Simulation in Emergency Medicine

From the beginning of formal training programs in emergency medicine in 1970 through designation of emergency medicine as the twenty-third specialty of the American Board of Medical Specialties (ABMS) in 1979 with board-certification examinations, the field of emergency medicine has incorporated varieties of simulation into its training and testing methods. As in other fields, emergency physicians routinely use "case presentations" or "case scenarios" as the most basic method of representing the clinical encounter for educational purposes. In particular, the American Board of Emergency Medicine (ABEM) has used simulated patient encounters as part of an oral examination administered after completion of the written exam. These oral board modules are similar to standard objective structured clinical examinations (OSCEs) that use situated role-playing to recreate clinical scenarios and are now widely used in medical schools and emergency certification courses (e.g., Basic and Advanced Cardiac Life Support [ACLS], Pediatric Advanced Life Support [PALS], and Advanced Trauma Life Support [ATLS]).

Along with the founding anesthesia groups, emergency physicians have helped further develop simulator-based case scenarios and explore the feasibility of simulator-based teaching and testing. In 1999 the Josiah Macy, Jr. foundation funded a multiyear project entitled "Realistic Patient Simulation for Training in Critical Care and Emergency Medicine," with a grant to a multidisciplinary team at the Harvard-MIT Division of Health Sciences and Technology and the Center for Medical Simulation. This funding was designed to develop and disseminate educational materials (Appendix A),[4] conduct research on simulator-based teaching and testing, and establish training programs for the instructors in the field.

Simulation for Teaching in Emergency Medicine

High-fidelity patient simulators (full-body robot-mannequins) have many potential applications in emergency medical training. They promise to enhance the efficiency of the learning process in a safe environment, reliably allowing trainees to gain clinical experience without depending on chance encounters with real patients. The degree to which emergency simulation exercises are used varies by level of access to a simulator, location and characteristics of the trainees, and availability of instructors. This section describes the learners, teaching applications, and logistics involved with simulation-based training in emergency medicine, with particular attention to the development of overall clinical competence.

Defining the Learners in Emergency Medicine

Along with colleagues from across disciplines, emergency medicine faculty, residents, nurses, medical students, technicians, and prehospital providers can benefit from simulation-based training programs.[5-9] Pilot studies of such groups demonstrate a high-level of acceptance of simulation as an educational tool. Simulation-based experiences can be tailored to the needs of individual groups, or used to foster collaborative skills within interdisciplinary teams. Although improvement in team performance might be expected of real teams who practice together on a simulator, studies to evaluate the transfer of cognitive and teamwork skills to actual practice have been limited. For pure procedural skills, some data suggest that practice on a simulator improves operative performance.[10,11]

Teaching Applications in Emergency Medicine

EM shares with other critical care disciplines the need to manage rare but life-threatening events. The principles that make simulation an appealing modality for teaching crisis management in the operating room (Anesthesia Crisis Resource Management [ACRM])[12,13] also apply to emergency care in the ED. Simulation provides an opportunity to practice complex diagnosis and management skills in situations that are difficult to teach with real patients. For example, upper airway obstruction in the ED demands immediate decisions and action of an experienced physician, leaving limited time for real-time instruction. Just like a classic ACRM scenario, thoughtful clinical decision making and management of emergent ED cases can be effectively practiced and repeatedly debriefed in a simulator environment.

Because emergency care providers work at the intersection of myriad disciplines, systems, and patients, a high-quality ED encounter depends on effective communication and teamwork. In addition to critical thinking and management skills, simulation scenarios also allow a health care team to practice organization and multitasking skills. Through the debriefing process, team performance characteristics can be identified and improved. Although the basic modeling of communication skills has been incorporated into traditional standardized patient exercises, the unique challenges of communication in an emergency—to patients, family, and providers—can be remarkably reproduced by voices and actors in a fully mocked-up simulator environment.

The intersection of full-body simulators and procedural simulators will expand as technologies evolve to produce increasingly realistic and functionally integrated models.[14–16] In general, the strength of performing procedures on existing full-body simulators lies not in the tactile realism of the procedure itself, but in making the decision to perform the procedure, managing the equipment, and defining how the procedure fits into the care protocol. Because these machines were originally designed for use by anesthesiologists, the airway has a particularly high degree of functional realism; the most advanced models also reproduce realistic needle decompression of tension pneumothorax as well as various body fluids (urine, sweat, tears, blood). However, the quality of tube thoracostomy, cricothyroidotomy, and intravenous access in current full-body models is of marginal reality; other dedicated procedure models for thoracostomy and vascular access as well for laparoscopy, endoscopy, and cardiac catheterization can provide a much higher level of realism but lack a convincing mannequin-patient.

A Simulation-based Curriculum for Training in Emergency Medicine

McLaughlin et al. published a three-year curriculum for emergency medicine residents using human simulation to guide development within the six competency domains outlined by the Accreditation Council of Graduate Medical Education (patient care, medical knowledge, practice-based learning, interpersonal and communication skills, professionalism, and systems-based practice; Appendix B).[17] The curriculum was designed to teach EM residents how to function competently in the dynamic, uncertain, and high-stakes environment of the ED and to allow opportunities for self-assessment.[18,19] Fifteen different cases are presented with specific goals and objectives for each case. Simulation sessions are held weekly with each topic repeating multiple times during the year.

During first postgraduate year (PGY I), trainees are expected to develop competence in basic emergencies, learn how to function as a team, and refine their clinical assessment skills. Through the use of simulation, concepts of crisis management are incorporated alongside basic elements of patient care, medical knowledge, professionalism, and interpersonal skills. Residents begin the simulator curriculum with an introduction to the simulator and an orientation to the learning objectives. The initial scenarios outlined in Appendix B allow trainees to build familiarity with the technology and with each other. Groups of three residents work together as a crew, and role-play nurses, paramedics, or other physicians. This model offers some advantages including cross-training, a focus on team-specific dynamics, and simplified logistics.[20]

The simulator cases designed for second-year (PGY II) and third-year (PGY III) residents are more complex, incorporating equipment management, teamwork, communications, ethics, and systems-based practice. The underlying teaching model at this level gradually transitions to a "team" format, involving the coordinated effort of varied professionals working together. The team-training model allows for realistic interpersonal interactions, and is particularly suited for groups that actually work together.[21,22] Third-year residents are encouraged to participate as simulator instructors for junior residents, a role that models the progressive assumption of teaching responsibilities within the residency.

Throughout the curriculum, basic types of cognitive errors such as anchoring bias, confirmation bias, and prevalence bias are described alongside techniques to enhance clinical decision-making. Persuasive arguments have been made that the quality of decision-making is strongly influenced by "cognitive dispositions to respond" (CDRs), often consisting of heuristics—or shortcuts in thinking—that lead to diagnostic error;[23] thirty of these CDRs have been described. Such error may be mitigated by practicing "cognitive forcing strategies," a de-biasing technique that entails recognition of error-prone scenarios and application of corrective thinking.[24-26] Simulator scenarios can vividly demonstrate common pitfalls in decision-making as well as error-prevention strategies. During these sessions, participants can "cognitively walk through" correct and incorrect thought patterns to de-bias error-prone behavior.

Simulation and ACGME Competencies in Emergency Medicine

Below are examples of how simulation can enhance professional development in emergency medicine within each of the ACGME competency areas.

Patient Care

The simulator allows resident education and assessment of resident performance in clinical situations that may be infrequent but critical to emergency practice. During the simulation sessions the residents gather information, make decisions, develop a management plan, and provide directed care. The simulator allows residents to safely practice[27] procedures such as defibrillation, pacing, pericardiocentesis, intubation, needle thoracentesis, and chest compressions, among others. One of the biggest strengths of simulation is the ability to train residents to work well in a team by rehearsing and debriefing teamwork skills.[28] The realism of the simulator places real stress and time pressure on the teams,[29] allowing them to train for actual emergency care.

Medical Knowledge

Although simulations may improve the acquisition and retention of knowledge,[30-32] they are commonly used in emergency medicine to help trainees understand integrated clinical applications. Problems can be presented as poorly defined and changing, forcing residents to synthesize and apply prior training.[28] During debriefing sessions, gaps in medical knowledge can be identified and addressed by brief focused didactics.

Practice-based Learning and Improvement

During simulations residents may need to use reference material, bedside computers, or other resources to help make decisions. Faculty have the discretion to give trainees complete control of simulated patient care, allowing them to see the outcomes of their actions and learn from mistakes in real time.[33]

Interpersonal and Communication Skills, and Professionalism

Simulated encounters with family members, "difficult" patients, and diverse hospital personnel can be used to teach communication skills and professionalism.[20,34] Patients with varied social, economic, demographic, and personal characteristics can be incorporated. For example, a simulation scenario might include a multitrauma victim with pelvic fractures and significant ongoing blood loss who is opposed to receiving blood products. Because the patient requires immediate intubation during the initial resuscitation, the resident must discuss the patient's condition with a simulated "family" and determine preferences regarding transfusion therapy. This process occurs in real time with a patient who requires continuous treatment. Such a case is similar to standardized cases that have previously been developed to demonstrate resident professionalism and ethics, and showed good testing characteristics.[34] "Death" scenarios can also be used to place the participant in the position of breaking "bad news" to a family after completing a challenging and stressful resuscitation.[20]

Systems-based Practice

Effective functioning in a health care system is taught by observing diagnostic test utilization during the scenarios and helping the resident to choose among scarce resources. Occasionally, the simulated patient may have trouble getting a bed in the hospital, and the resident will have to talk to simulated insurance representatives or hospital managers by phone. Or an admitting physician may be unclear about the need to admit a patient to the hospital, and the resident will have to use effective communication and listening skills to negotiate an optimal outcome.

Developing and Running Emergency Medicine Simulations

Simulations generally include an orientation, introduction to the session, actual simulation, debriefing, and evaluation. The residents or the EM-based "team" of residents, nurses, and technicians begin with a review of the rules and operation of the simulator. The group may be introduced to the teaching objectives and briefed on the case, or the group may enter the simulation without any introduction for a truly spontaneous exercise.

A simulation scenario typically begins with a medic or nurse's report. When the resident enters the room, he or she must take a history from the patient (the mannequin has a radio-transmitted voice produced by a hidden facilitator) and proceed with routine evaluation and management. Caretakers must do everything as if they were seeing a real patient. Such realism is enhanced by having actors play family members; using actual radiographs, electrocardiograms, and lab reports; minimizing instructor input; presenting multiple patients; arranging for intermittent interruptions or pages; and generally replicating the ED working environment, chart, and equipment.[28]

Every simulation exercise should be debriefed to foster critical discussion and reflection.[35] The debriefing may occur in the simulation room or in a separate conference room and may be a concluding exercise or spread out during the case itself. Although the instructor usually facilitates the debriefing, the participants can also be in charge, especially if they are upper-level trainees or functional teams.[28] A videotape of the encounter is often reviewed before the discussion. The feedback and debriefing should be constructive, nonjudgmental, and supportive. During the debriefing, the facilitator guides the group to tasks that they did well and gives suggestions on areas that need improvement. The team often comes up with a global consensus that informs individual perspectives and guides future behavior. Participant evaluation and critique of the session are also important parts of the debriefing process.

Basic emergency medicine simulations (single patient) typically require at least one faculty member along with a technician-assistant. More people are required for ED-based teamwork scenarios, ideally including nurses, allied-health professionals, and additional technical staff. Development time includes several hours to write a case, program the simulator, design a rudimentary assessment tool, and conduct a practice run. Each case can take anywhere from 15–30 minutes to an hour, depending on the objectives of the session and level of teaching and debriefing. Case development should focus on constructing scenarios that meet the desired learning objectives in a reasonable time period. After initial development, cases should be peer-reviewed and piloted. Any possible opportunities for negative or erroneous learning should be identified.

Just as simulation provides a controlled opportunity for teaching and learning in emergency medicine, it can also provide a useful environment for performance assessment. The next section provides some context on simulator-based evaluation in emergency medicine.

Simulation for Evaluation in Emergency Medicine

Simulation promises to advance the field of assessment in emergency medicine by more accurately predicting the kind of dynamic performance capability captured neither by written nor oral-OSCE testing. Although it would be ideal to observe all residents taking care of actual patients with life-threatening conditions, this goal is nearly impossible, given the unpredictability of patient presentation and physician staffing. Indeed, most faculty have never observed individual residents throughout the entirety of a clinical encounter; instead, they sporadically monitor critical actions of a variety of residents during a busy shift. Moreover, many residents may never encounter certain cases unless they can be recreated in the simulation laboratory.

Utility of Simulator-based Evaluation in Emergency Medicine

Current state-of-the-art mannequin-simulators are perhaps the most effective way to mimic the complex hemodynamics of critically ill patients. Illnesses such as flash pulmonary edema with with hypertension, congestive heart failure (CHF) with cardiogenic shock, and adult respiratory distress syndrome (ARDS) with sepsis can be reproduced (including, for example, differential pulmonary artery catheter readings). Residents can administer fluid boluses, vasoactive medications, positive and negative inotropes, antiarrhythmics, and other therapies, while observing the effects of interventions in real time. Compared with direct clinical observation in the ED, simulation allows broad availability of standardized experiences, control of situational factors, close observation of procedural technique, and full debriefing of mistakes.

Although trainees are routinely able to "suspend disbelief" in a typical simulator scenario, evaluation schemes can be limited by the plastic and mechanical characteristics of the mannequin itself. Breath and heart sounds can have variable qualities, and the portals for performing procedures are obvious and unilateral. Although some simulators offer simulated bowel sounds and can mimic esophageal intubation, the abdominal exam is unrealistic. Pattern recognition on simulators is limited; important clinical cues such as mannerisms and general appearance cannot be reproduced. Although some models and techniques can be used to simulate diaphoresis and skin pallor, overall clinical presentation must be largely imagined.

Despite such limitations, high-fidelity simulators show great promise as evaluation tools in emergency medicine. The Model of Clinical Practice of Emergency Medicine, a consensus description of core elements of emergency medical practice, outlines a matrix of physician tasks by patient acuity.[36] Simulations can be an ideal way to assess the performance of most of the tasks described, including emergency stabilization, therapeutic interventions, pharmacotherapy, observation and reassessment, multitasking, and team management in critical care scenarios. As described in the previous section, all of the ACGME competency domains, ranging from interpersonal and action skills to overall competence, are well-suited for simulator-based assessment.

Simulator-based Assessment Tools in Emergency Medicine

To use simulation as an assessment tool, we must define levels of competence, design scenarios that allow demonstration of requisite skills, and develop robust measurement tools. Assessment techniques such as checklists and global rating scales can be used to gauge simulator-based performance.[37,38] Although checklists tend to reward structure and thoroughness, they can limit flexibility in evaluating patient interactions and management; they are, however, quite good for recording performance of objective management steps and can be used to assess certain aspects of affective and behavioral performance. Global rating scales are generally more subjective but allow the rater to capture alternative or "expert" approaches to a problem or interaction.

Integrated assessment tools that have been validated for use in traditional OSCE exercises may be transferable to simulator-based scenarios. For example, an OSCE-based assessment tool used for oral certification examinations in emergency medicine has shown a similar degree of validity in a simulator-based testing environment.[39,40] Consistent with ACGME criteria, the scoring tool consists of a wide range of eight competency domains (each scored on a scale of 1–8), including data acquisition, problem solving, patient management, resource utilization, health care provided (outcome), interpersonal relations, comprehension of pathophysiology, and clinical competence (overall).[41]

Another assessment tool that may transfer well to a simulator-based environment in emergency medicine is the SEGUE Framework for Teaching and Assessing Communication Skills (**s**kills needed to set the stage, **e**licit information, **g**ive information, **u**nderstand the patient, and **e**nd the encounter).[42] The SEGUE checklist can accommodate real-time and videotape assessment of interpersonal and communication skills and can evaluate nonverbal behavior as well. The checklist can be supplemented to assess critical elements of history, physical exam, and management, along with a global assessment of procedural competence, teamwork, and "flow" of the resuscitation. Other useful metrics may include measuring time to critical interventions or stabilization, self-assessment questionnaires, team-based "360-degree" assessments, and a variety of other validated scales and inventories.[42,43] Although each tool has different strengths and limitations in emergency medicine, most have not been tested on patient simulators.

Special Issues in Simulation and Emergency Medicine

This section discusses simulation and teamwork training for general emergency care, emergency-based simulation for general medical curricula, and the use of simulation to enhance disaster preparedness.

Teamwork Training in Emergency Medicine

Anesthesia Crisis Resource Management (ACRM) is a simulation-based workshop focusing on crisis management skills such as leadership, communication, prioritization, and situational awareness.[12,20] Although this pioneering work provides a foundation for simulation-based teamwork in other specialties, the single operative patient is not representative of emergency medicine practice. Operating room simulations have reiterated that some of the most serious human factor issues arise between professional disciplines.[44] Because of the dynamic nature of practice in a busy emergency department, teamwork training in emergency medicine must incorporate multiple patients and disciplines and simulate the coordination that is required, for example, of a trauma team.

MedTeams Project in Emergency Medicine

The MedTeams project is the most comprehensive research on teamwork in emergency medicine to date. Beginning in 1995, the U.S. Department of Defense embarked on a military and civilian research project to transfer successful team-training concepts from army aviation (Crew Resource Management [CRM]) to emergency medicine.[45] Estimated savings in lives and money, along with potential mitigation of human error,[46] provided a compelling argument to expand the program to healthcare. Because emergency medicine has numerous parallels to aviation—including the need to make quick decisions with incomplete information in a high-stakes environment—it was chosen as a logical candidate for a health care validation trial.

The MedTeams project began with a closed-claim needs analysis based on malpractice insurance records, which estimated the potential savings of implementing teamwork training in emergency medicine. Investigators concluded that approximately 40% of relevant cases involved preventable teamwork errors, the correction of which may have mitigated or prevented an adverse event. Based on this premise, a conservative estimate of savings from teamwork training was calculated at $3.45 per patient.[47] Advocating for cross-monitoring of team members and asserting corrective actions were identified as two "high-drivers" of corrective teamwork dynamics. Information gained from these data helped shape the Emergency Team Coordination Course (ETCC), which served as the curriculum for the validation study.[48]

The validation study consisted of a prospective multicenter trial (non-simulator-based) designed to assess the effectiveness of introducing optimal teamwork behaviors among emergency department staff.[45] The Behavioral Anchored Rating Score (BARS), a evaluation tool used in aviation for assessing teamwork performance,[46] was tailored to the ED environment (Appendix C). Using this tool, military and civilian investigators identified a significant improvement in quality of team behaviors in the ED after ETCC training and reported an accompanying decrease in the observed clinical error rate.

Simulation as a Tool to Promote and Sustain Emergency Teams

Although the results of the MedTeams validation were encouraging, the challenges of sustaining improvements in team performance are significant. Attempting to maintain ETCC-enhanced team behaviors by ongoing job training and mentoring in an actual ED is of value, but the workload and time pressures of such an approach make it less practical. Sustainment training, however, may be more easily accomplished in a simulated environment, which allows tailored scenario development (actual ED cases can improve "buy in" from staff), a consistent and reproducible training platform, and video debriefing. Because video taping is generally not possible in patient care areas, simulator-based video debriefing is an extremely powerful tool for peer assessment and often leads to behavior modification.

In response to the need for sustainment training, experts in anesthesia and emergency medicine, in collaboration with MedTeams researchers, undertook a joint effort to better define the cognitive, social, and system-based challenges faced in EM practice. This work explored the use of simulation as a primary tool for improving and sustaining effective team behaviors among ED staff.[28] Investigators found that effective ED simulations required multipatient scenarios conducted within facilities that can incorporate (and record) activity in all areas of an ED, including triage. Live actors and realistic distractions were also incorporated to effectively replicate and model optimal teamwork skills. Additional work to define the effectiveness of simulation in teaching ED-based teamwork, conducted by investigators from one of the original MedTeams sites,[49] suggested that simulation training can also produce improvement in ED team performance.

Emergency Simulations to Support General Medical Curricula

High-fidelity Simulation to Enhance Standardized Emergency and Prehospital Training

A natural application of high-fidelity simulation can be found within standardized emergency-based courses such as Advanced Cardiac Life Support (ACLS) and Advanced Trauma Life Support (ATLS). Although these courses already use basic simulation and mannequins for teaching and assessment, the realism of these scenarios is limited and may not predict competence;[50] history and physical findings are static and provided by the instructor rather than elicited by the trainee. In many ways high-fidelity simulation can portray more realistically didactic materials and assess basic competency.[51]

High-fidelity simulation has already been piloted and used as an adjunct to the traditional ACLS courses for teaching skills, assessing performance, and enhancing teamwork. Other pilot work has used simulation to teach and assess trauma team and ATLS skills, with favorable reactions among trainees.[52] Before and after a month-long trauma rotation, trauma team performance on the simulator was assessed based on critical actions and timed tasks in areas of airway, breathing, circulation, and disability; a small number of items on team organization were also included.[53] After the trauma rotation, team performance tended to improve on most of the identified outcome measures.

General emergency and prehospital provider training may also benefit from current generation of more portable and less expensive simulator-systems. Multiple systems can be used to create mass casualty or multiple patient scenarios within single centers. Some such centers already exist, concentrating on large-scale training of paramedics and other pre-hospital providers within both civilian and military emergency medical systems (EMS).

Emergency Simulations for Medical School Curricula

Because emergency medicine can effectively highlight instructional elements of generalist medical care, acute care simulations can be particularly useful at all levels of the medical school curriculum. Together with anesthesia colleagues at the Center for Medical Simulation in Boston, faculty and residents from the Harvard Division of Emergency Medicine have helped institute a simulator-based "medical education service"—like any other clinical teaching service but designed exclusively to help students "practice" medicine with a physician-mentor, on demand.[54] Established as part of the on-campus Gilbert Program in Medical Simulation at Harvard Medical School,[55,56] the medical education service assigns a dedicated pager to an on-call educator, including on-service teaching faculty and senior residents participating in a medical education elective.

Each year hundreds of medical students at all levels take advantage of the service. More than of 90% of the students feel that simulation exercises should be a mandatory component of their medical school curriculum,[57] and the program has become integrated into both basic science and clinical coursework. Not only do students enjoy the opportunity to practice medicine "on demand," but course directors like "bringing to life" basic teaching cases in the simulator. Creative use of the simulator-voice or standardized patient-actors within the simulation can provide even more memorable contrast between mild and severe pathology, highlighting the interdependence of laboratory work, office practice, and acute care. By offering a medical education elective for residents, we have not only provided a "resident as teacher" experience but also fostered additional opportunities for cross-disciplinary collaboration throughout the medical school community.

Disaster Medicine and Simulation

Another area of emergency medicine that can benefit from simulation-based training is disaster preparedness, a prominent component of current public health care policy and practice. The study of disaster medicine, focusing on pre-event planning, emergent medical care, and public health response, has matured rapidly through advances in networking, communications, and computer technologies. Examination of prior events and intercession with ongoing disasters have become much more sophisticated, timely, and pertinent. Implementation of preventive, preparatory, and training protocols has been avidly recommended in the hope of minimizing the consequences of such large-scale events.[58,59]

Educational training for those who may respond to disasters must be accurate, thorough, relevant, and up-to-date. The target audience includes prehospital and hospital-based health care providers, law enforcement and fire department personnel, and disaster relief organizations. The training needs to impart specialized medical knowledge as well as protocols for interagency cooperation. Basic tenets of disaster management—triage, decontamination, communications, incident command, and transport—have to be successfully conveyed. The ability to rapidly form effective multidisciplinary work teams and communication systems must be cultivated. Other areas of instruction beyond the scope of basic medical training include crisis psychology, tactical command, hazardous materials (HazMat), and "refugee medicine."

Current Disaster Training

Disaster training requires the transference of specialized but rarely used skills that must be employed in uncertain environments; a flexible and dynamic pedagogical approach is required. Rapid attrition of knowledge from training measures is expected, resulting in the need for ongoing training and refresher courses.

Lectures and seminars are currently used to present a large component of any disaster curriculum. Emergency medical technician (EMT) courses at all levels incorporate basic teaching in disaster response. However, such training is not uniform among emergency medicine residency training programs[60] and is generally not covered in medical or nursing schools. Moreover, an American College of Emergency Medicine (ACEP) task found that didactic courses for EMT, nursing and physician education in this area were unsatisfactory.[61] An effort by the federal Office of Emergency Preparedness (OEP) to create a uniform curriculum has led to an improved and comprehensive web-based course in disaster training, although access is currently limited to members of the National Disaster Medical System (NDMS).

Simulation can be a central instrument for meaningful disaster training, particularly given multi-casualty nature of the event. Disasters are chaotic events demanding multi-faceted reponses; simulation can be used effectively to teach, reinforce, and test critical concepts. By constructing dynamic and stressful situations that respond to participant actions, simulation can cultivate flexible problem-solving approaches for all aspects of disaster management. In particular, multidisciplinary simulations foster teamwork elements critical to any event response. Simulated disaster exercises vary in scale and nature from "table-top" computer re-enactments and full-scale field exercises[62,63] to more moderately scaled local disaster drills.[64,65]

Application of High-Fidelity Medical Simulation to Disaster Training

As with any form of simulation, the higher the fidelity of the disaster exercise, the greater the immersion in the training experience. Typical disaster simulations use actors and volunteers along with low-fidelity mannequins as victims. A recent advance in disaster training includes physicians posing as interactive "smart simulated casualties" to directly observe and debrief trainees.[66] Although low-fidelity mannequins are life-like in form and can withstand life-support maneuvers, they cannot exhibit physiologic behaviors such as breathing; conversely, of course, intubation and CPR cannot be practiced on actors. High-fidelity medical simulation technology can help overcome such disparities. Fully programmable to display acute physiologic responses and free of restrictions inherent to live patient-actors, high-fidelity patient simulators allow greater verisimilitude to "practice without risk." Such scenarios can bring the distressing, distracting sights and sounds of disasters and their victims to life, ultimately helping reconcile the theory with practice of disaster response.

As opposed to surgical re-enactments with a single operative mannequin-patient, a simulator-enhanced disaster exercise requires multiple moulaged, programmed, and strategically positioned mannequins within a mass-casualty environment. In addition to actors and low-fidelity mannequins, the number and location of simulator-victims—complete with realistic verbal responses and deteriorating vital signs—constitute a uniquely effective training platform:

> A major difference between scenario-based training and more traditional training is that in scenario-based training situations there is no formal curriculum; instead *the scenario itself is the curriculum*. This means that the scenario must be crafted, and the training executed around it, in a manner that accomplishes desired training objectives.[67]

After establishment of the credibility and urgency of the scenario, participants have to interact fully with the simulators in a manner and degree unlike any prior experience. Caring for multiple moaning and bleeding mannequin-victims, while wearing a hazardous materials (HazMat) suit, is powerful preparation for an actual event. Bradycardic and weak pulses have to be taken, and diagnoses need to be deduced from the most basic data. Resuscitative measures must be actively carried out, as opposed to simply verbalized. Identification of miotic pupils and wheezing in the proper setting, for example, may prove crucial to the initiation of advanced airway management, intravenous access, fluid administration, and aggressive atropine treatment in a simulated chemical attack. This level of integrative, action-driven, realistic instruction is impossible outside of the simulated environment.

Basic disaster response skills such as decontamination, transport, and treatment for traumatic or nuclear-biologic-chemical (NBC) events can also be incorporated into simulated exercises. Preparation for incident command, triage, and resource management in a mass casualty incident can be realistically modeled by high-fidelity simulations. Activities ranging from crowd control to assignment and attachment of triage tags become qualitatively different when mannequins can portray the full range of dynamic changes, personal animation, and treatment complications enabled by high-fidelity simulators. Field testing of protocols and equipment is another benefit of simulator-enhanced disaster training. For example, the level of personal protective equipment (PPE) necessary in a chemically contaminated area may preclude effective auscultation of rhonchorous breath sounds, and otherwise routine intubation might be precluded by a cumbersome HazMat suit.[68] Proactive real-time assessment and troubleshooting of a realistic disaster drill may very well help avert mismanaged rescue efforts in the real world.

With respect to objective measures of trainee performance, high-fidelity simulators are generally capable of logging interventions and changes in physiologic parameters so that debriefing can be tailored to individual caregivers or work teams. The time-critical nature of therapeutic actions can also be stressed; in conjunction with standard audiovisual logs, automated simulator records may assist in the determination of specific shortcomings or strengths and promote improved field performance.

Even though simulation-enhanced disaster exercises may be effective, they can be quite challenging. Large-scale disaster simulations require a simulation center that houses flexible work areas capable of multipatient scenarios. Typically, the level of personnel and equipment resources requires regional collaboration and support. Despite these obstacles, the benefits of this level of simulation training cannot be achieved through other methodologies. State agencies that are planning and conducting disaster drills would be well-advised to incorporate high-fidelity simulation into their strategic budgets and plans.

Case Study

A disaster exercise is outlined in Appendix D to demonstrate how simulator technology may be integrated into responder training, with particular focus on design and planning aspects of the exercise itself. Chemical agent exposure was chosen because of its medical complexity, tendency toward mannequin-enabled interventions, need to operate within PPE, and applicability to both civilian and military populations. The Israeli experience with simulator-enhanced training of medical personnel responding to a chemical warfare incident was instructive in defining the exercise outlined here.[69] The presence of high-fidelity simulator-mannequins in the exercise should accomplish the following goals:

1. Accurately simulate a weapons of mass sestruction (WMD) disaster with subsequent prehospital and hospital response to the exposure. Specific elements include:
    ◆ Incident command
    ◆ Communications
    ◆ Triage
    ◆ Decontamination
    ◆ Transport
    ◆ Treatment
    ◆ Resource management
    ◆ Debriefing
2. Provide clinical stimuli and generate a learning environment above and beyond what is attained with current disaster training.
3. Achieve maximal training yield with minimal risk to participant rescuers and "victims."
4. Observe and record in real-time, then evaluate and debrief participant actions in detail.
5. Allow participants to become familiar with simulator technology and its role in training.
6. Fine-tune simulator technology for the special needs of disaster exercises

These goals are in addition to the standard objectives of a traditional disaster drill, namely to assemble multidisciplinary teams for educational interaction and cooperation; to field-test and familiarize rescuers with communications equipment and PPE in the context of chemical WMD hazards; and to assess prehospital and hospital medical processes/systems under disaster conditions

Scenarios involving multiple simulator-mannequins have been carried out successfully, and extension to disaster exercises engaging more than ten victims is within reach. Rhode Island Hospital Medical Simulation Center is currently working with local disaster management agencies to realize enhanced disaster simulation based on the outline presented. In addition, simulation technology has been incorporated into Phase 2 of the Rhode Island Disaster Initiative, funded by the Department of Health and Human Services and the Department of Defense. Phase 2 evaluates potential solutions to vulnerabilities identified in Phase 1.

Conclusion

High-fidelity human patient simulation is a promising tool for teaching and demonstrating emergency medical skills. Together with colleagues from across all disciplines, emergency physicians will continue to work toward better understanding and utilization of this remarkable new technology.

Acknowledgments

Portions of this chapter are drawn directly from the material that originally appeared in the following publications, modified with permission: (1) Mclaughlin SA, Doezema DD, Sklar DP: Human simulation in emergency medicine training: A model curriculum. Acad Emerg Med 2002; 9:1310–1318; (2) Bond WF, Spillane L, for the CORD Core Competencies Simulation Group: The use of simulation for emergency medicine resident assessment. Acad Emerg Med 2002; 9:1295–1299; (3) Gordon JA: A simulator-based medical education service [letter]. Acad Emerg Med 2002: 9:865; and (4) Kobyashi L, Shapiro MJ, Suner S, Williams K: Disaster medicine: the potential role of high-fidelity medical simulation for mass casualty incident training. Medicine and Health Rhode Island 2003;86(7):196–200.

Funding to develop curricular materials in Appendix B was provided by a grant from the Josiah Macy, Jr. Foundation to the Harvard-MIT Division of Health Sciences and Technology and the Center for Medical Simulation.

References

1. Bowles LT, Sirica CM (eds): The Role of Emergency Medicine in the Future of American Medical Care. New York, Josiah Macy, Jr. Foundation, 1995.
2. Gordon JA: A simulator-based medical education service [letter]. Acad Emerg Med 2002;9:865.
3. Bond WF, Spillane L, for the CORD Core Competencies Simulation Group: The use of simulation for emergency medicine resident assessment. Acad Emerg Med 2002;9:1295–1299.
4. Gordon JA: Macy Cases for Realistic Patient Simulation in Critical Care and Emergency Medicine. Harvard Medical School, Boston: President and Fellows of Harvard College, 2002. [Sponsored by a grant from the Josiah Macy Jr. Foundation to the Harvard-MIT Division of Health Sciences and Technology and the Center for Medical Simulation (www.harvardmedsim.org). Presentation template adapted from Medical Education Technologies, Inc.].
5. Friedrich MJ: Practice makes perfect: Risk free training with patient simulators [news article]. JAMA 2002;288:2808–2812
6. Bond WF, Kostenbader M, et al: Prehospital and hospital-based health care providers' experience with a human patient simulator. Prehosp Emerg Care 2001;5:284–287.
7. Jacobsen J, Lindekar AL, Ostergaard HT, et al: Management of anaphylactic shock evaluated using a full-scale anaesthesia simulator. Acta Anaesthesthesiol Scand 2001;45:315–319.
8. Halamek LP, Kaegi DM, Gaba DM, et al: Time for a new paradigm in pediatric medical education: Teaching neonatal resuscitation in a simulated delivery room environment. Pediatrics 2000;106(4):E45.
9. Gordon JA, for the Medical Readiness Trainer Team: The Human Patient Simulator: Acceptance and efficacy as a teaching tool for students. Acad Med 2000;75:522.
10. Pittini R, Oepkes D, et al: Teaching invasive perinatal procedures: Assessment of a high fidelity simulator-based curriculum. Ultrasound Obstet Gynecol 2002;19:478–483.
11. Seymour NE, Gallagher AG, Roman SA, et al: Virtual reality training improves operating room performance: Results of a randomized, double-blinded study. Ann Surg 2002;236:458–463.
12. Gaba D, Fish K, Howard S: Anesthesia Crisis Resource Management. New York, Churchill Livingstone, 1994.
13. Holzman RS, Cooper, JB, Gaba DM, et al: Anesthesia crisis resource management: Real-life simulation training in operating room crises. J Clin Anesth 1995;7:675–872.
14. Resnek M, Harter P, Krummel T: Virtual reality and simulation: Training the future emergency physician. Acad Emerg Med 2002;9:78–87.
15. Dawson SL, Cotin S, Meglan D, et al: Designing a computer-based simulator for interventional cardiology training. Catheter Cardiovasc Interv 2000;51:522–527.
16. Center for Integration of Medicine and Innovative Technology: Program: simulation—VIRGIL chest tube insertion training simulator. Boston, CIMIT, 2003 (www.cimit.org/simulation.html).
17. McLaughlin SA, Doezema D, Sklar DP: Human simulation in emergency medicine training: A model curriculum. Acad Emerg Med 2002;9:1310–1318.
18. Klein G, Orasanu J, Calderwood R: Decision Making in Action: Models and Methods. Norwood, NJ, Ablex, 1993.
19. Croskerry P: The cognitive imperative: Thinking about how we think. Acad Emerg Med. 2000;7:1223–1231.
20. Gaba DM, Howard SK, Fish KJ, et al: Simulation-based training in anesthesia crisis resource management (ACRM): A decade of experience. Simul Gaming 2001;32(2):175–193.
21. Marsch S: Team oriented medical simulation. In Henson L, Lee A (eds): Simulators in Anesthesiology Education. New York, Plenum, 1998, pp 99–110.
22. Sexton B, Marsch S, Helmreich R, et al: Participant evaluation of team oriented medical simula-

tion. In Henson L, Lee A (eds): Simulators in Anesthesiology Education. New York, Plenum, 1998, pp 99–110.

23. Croskerry P: Achieving quality in clinical decision making: Cognitive strategies and detection of bias. Acad Emerg Med 2002;9:1184–1204.

24. Croskerry P: Cognitive forcing strategies in clinical decision making. Ann Emerg Med 2003;41:110–120.

25. Croskerry P: The importance of cognitive errors in diagnosis and strategies to minimize them. Acad Med 2003;78:775–780.

26. Bond WF, Detrick LM, Arnold DC, et al: Using simulators to instruct emergency medicine residents in cognitive forcing strategies. Acad Med 2004;79 [in press].

27. Cavanaugh S: Computerized simulation technology for clinical teaching and testing. Acad Emerg Med 1997;4:939–943.

28. Small SD, Wuerz RC, Simon R, et al: Demonstration of high-fidelity simulation team training for emergency medicine. Acad Emerg Med. 1999;6:312–323.

29. Gordon JA, Wilkerson WM, Shaffer DW, Armstrong EG: "Practicing" medicine without risk: Students' and educators' responses to high-fidelity patient simulation. Acad Med. 2001;76:469–472.

30. Issenberg SB, McGaghie WC, Hart IR, et al: Simulation technology for health care professional skills training and assessment. JAMA 1999;282:861–866.

31. Gaba DM, DeAnda A: Role of experience of the response to simulated critical incidents. Anesth Analg 1991;72:308–315.

32. Gordon, JA, Armstrong E: Effects of a single exposure to high-fidelity patient simulation in the preclinical curriculum: A pilot study [abstract A17]. Anesth Analg 2002;95(2S):S119.

33. Gaba DM: Anaesthesiology as a model for patient safety in health care. BMJ 2000;320:785–788.

34. Larkin GL: Evaluating professionalism in emergency medicine: Clinical ethical competence. Acad Emerg Med. 1999;6:302–311.

35. Center for Medical Simulation: Simulation instruction series: Debriefing I [course outline]. Cambridge, MA, CMS, 2003 (http://www.harvardmedsim.org/CMS%20SIC%20Outline.htm).

36. Hockberger RS, Binder LS, Graber MA, et al: The model of the clinical practice of emergency medicine. Ann Emerg Med 2001;37:745–770.

37. Regehr G, Freeman R, Robb A, et al: OSCE performance evaluations made by standardized patients: Comparing checklist and global rating scale. Acad Med 1999;74(10):S135-S137.

38. Hodges B, Regehr G, McNaughton N, et al: OSCE checklists do not capture increasing levels of expertise. Acad Med 1999;74:1129–1134.

39. Gordon JA, Tancredi DN, Binder WD, et al: Assessment of a clinical performance evaluation tool for use in a simulator-based testing environment: a pilot study. Acad Med 2003(10 Suppl);78:545–547.

40. Clyne B, Gutman D, Sutton E, et al: Oral board versus high fidelity simulation for competency assessment: senior emergency medicine resident management of an acute coronary syndrome [abstract]. Anesth Analg 2004 (Suppl) [in press].

41. Gossman W, Plante S, Adler J: Emergency Medicine Pearls of Wisdom: Oral Board Review. Watertown, MA, Boston Medical Publishing, 1998:3–4.

42. Boon H, Stewart M: Patient-physician communication assessment instruments: 1986 to 1996 in review. Patient Educ Couns 1998;35:161–176.

43. Byrne A, Greaves J: Assessment instruments used during anaesthetic simulation: Review of published studies. Br J Anaesth 2001;86:445–450.

44. Helmreich RL, Schaefer HG: Team performance in the operating room. In Bogner MS (ed): Human Error in Medicine. Hillsdale, NJ, Lawrence Erlbaum Associates, 1994, pp 225–253.

45. Morey JC, Simon R, Jay GD, et al: Error reduction and performance improvement in the emergency department through formal teamwork training: evaluation results of the MedTeams Project. Health Serv Res 2002;37:1553–1581.

46. Leedom DK, Simon R: Improving team coordination: A case for behavioral-based training. Mil Psychol 1995;7:109–122.

47. Risser DT, Rice MM, Salisbury ML, et al, for the MedTeams Consortium: The potential for improved teamwork to reduce medical errors in the emergency department. Ann Emerg Med 1999;34:373–383.

48. Risser DT, Simon R, Rice MM, Salisbury ML: A structured teamwork system to reduce clinical

errors. In Spath PL (ed): Error Reduction in Health Care. San Francisco, Jossey-Bass, 1999, pp 235–278.

49. Jay GD, Small SD, Langford V, et al: Teamwork training supported by high fidelity simulation training improves emergency department team behaviors [abstract]. Acad Emerg Med 2000;7:519.

50. Shapiro MJ, Kobayashi L, Morchi R: High-fidelity medical simulation and its role in evaluating fundamental advanced cardiac life support (ACLS) skills [abstract 194]. Acad Emerg Med 2003 [in press].

51. Shapiro M, Morchi R: High-fidelity medical simulation and teamwork training to enhance medical student performance in cardiac resuscitation [abstract]. Acad Emerg Med 2002;9: 1055c–1056c.

52. Marshall RL, et al: Use of a human patient simulator in the development of resident trauma management skills. J Trauma 2001;51:17–21.

53. Holcomb JB, et al: Evaluation of trauma team performance using an advanced human patient simulator for resuscitation training. J Trauma 2002;52:1078–1086.

54. Gordon JA, Pawlowski J: Education 'on-demand': The development of a simulator-based medical education service. Acad Med 2002;77:751–752.

55. Gordon JA, Oriol NE, Cooper JB: Bringing good teaching cases "to life": a simulator-based medical education service. Acad Med 2004;79(1):23–27.

56. Reynolds T: Patient simulator comes to life in TMEC. Focus: News from Harvard Medical, Dental, and Public Health Schools, May 4, 2001 (http://focus.hms.harvard.edu/2001/May4_2001/medical_education.html).

57. Takayesu JK Gordon JA, Farrell SE, et al: Learning emergency medicine and critical care medicine: What does high-fidelity patient simulation teach? [abstract 319]. Acad Emerg Med 2002;9:476–477.

58. American College of Emergency Physicians Terrorism Response Task Force: Positioning America's emergency health care system to respond to acts of terrorism. Irving, CA, American College of Emergency Physicians, 2002 (http://www.acep.org/library/pdf/TerrorismResponse.pdf).

59. Institute of Medicine and National Research Council: Chemical and Biological Terrorism: Research and Development to Improve Civilian Medical Response. Washington, DC, National Academy Press, 1999.

60. Pesik N, Keim M, Sampson TR: Do U.S. emergency medicine residency programs provide adequate training for bioterrorism? Ann Emerg Med 1999;34:173–176.

61. Waeckerle JF, Seamans S, Whiteside M, et al: Executive summary: Developing objectives, content, and competencies for the training of emergency medical technicians, emergency physicians, and emergency nurses to care for casualties resulting from nuclear, biological, or chemical (NBC) incidents. Ann Emerg Med 2001;37:587–601.

62. Tyre TE: Wake-up call: A bioterrorism exercise. Mil Med 2001;166(Suppl 2):90–91.

63. Inglesby TV: Observations from the Top Off exercise. Public Health Rep 2001;116(Suppl 2):64–68.

64. Hogan DE, Burstein JL: Disaster Medicine. Philadelphia, Lippincott Williams & Wilkins, 2002.

65. Tur-Kaspa I, Lev EI, Hendler I, et al: Preparing hospitals for toxicological mass casualties events. Crit Care Med 1999;27:1004–1008.

66. Gofrit ON, Leibovici D, Shemer J, et al: The efficacy of integrating smart simulated casualties in hospital disaster drills. Prehosp Disaster Med 1997;12(2):97–101.

67. Cannon-Bowers, Burns JJ, Salas F, Pruitt JS: Advanced technology in scenario based training. In Cannon-Bowers JA, Salas E (eds): Making Decisions Under Stress: Implications for Individual and Team Training. Washington, DC, American Psychological Association, 1998, pp 365–374.

68. Suner S, Williams K, Shapiro MJ, et al: Effect of personal protective equipment (PRE) on rapid patient assessment and treatment during a simulated chemical weapons of mass destruction (WMD) attack [abstract]. Acad Emerg Med 2004 [in press].

69. Vardi A, Levin I, Berkenstadt H et al: Simulation-based training of medical teams to manage chemical warfare casualties. Isr Med Assoc J 2002;4(7):540–544.

Appendix A

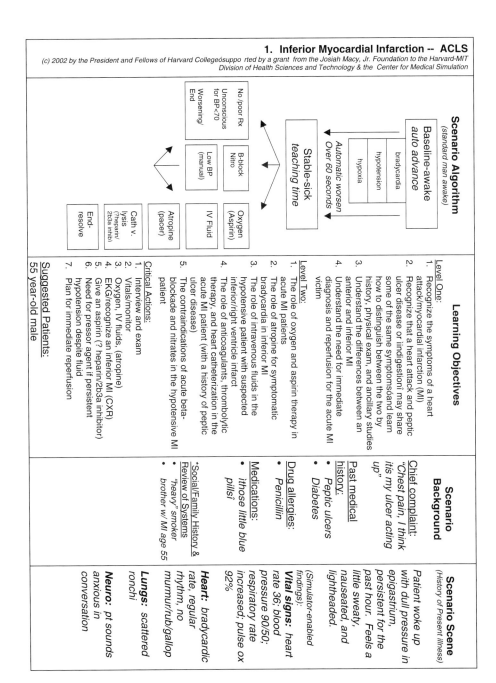

1. Inferior Myocardial Infarction -- ACLS

Scenario Algorithm
(standard man awake)

Baseline-awake
auto advance

- bradycardia
- hypotension
- hypoxia

Automatic worsen
Over 60 seconds

Stable-sick
teaching time

- No /poor Rx
- Unconscious for BP<70
- Worsening/ End

- B-block Nitro
- Low BP (manual)

- Oxygen (Aspirin)
- IV Fluid
- Atropine (pacer)
- Cath v. lysis (?heparin/ 2b3a inhib)
- End-resolve

Learning Objectives

Level One:
1. Recognize the symptoms of a heart attack/myocardial infarction (MI)
2. Recognize that a heart attack and peptic ulcer disease or lindigestion̂ may share some of the same symptomsoand learn how to distinguish between the two by history, physical exam, and ancillary studies
3. Understand the differences between an anterior and inferior MI
4. Understand the need for immediate diagnosis and reperfusion for the acute MI victim

Level Two:
1. The role of oxygen and aspirin therapy in acute MI patients
2. The role of atropine for symptomatic bradycardia in inferior MI
3. The role of intravenous fluids in the hypotensive patient with suspected inferior/right ventricle infarct
4. The role of anticoagulants, thrombolytic therapy, and heart catheterization in the acute MI patient (with a history of peptic ulcer disease)
5. The contraindications of acute beta-blockade and nitrates in the hypotensive MI patient

Critical Actions:
1. Interview and exam
2. Vitals/monitor
3. Oxygen, IV fluids, (atropine)
4. EKG/recognize an inferior MI (CXR)
5. Give an aspirin (? ? heparin/2b3a inhibitor)
6. Need for pressor agent if persistent hypotension despite fluid
7. Plan for immediate reperfusion

Suggested Patients:
55 year-old male

Scenario Background

Chief complaint:
"Chest pain, I think its my ulcer acting up"

Past medical history:
- Peptic ulcers
- Diabetes

Drug allergies:
- Penicillin

Medications:
- *those little blue pills*

Social/Family History & Review of Systems
- *"heavy" smoker*
- *brother w/ MI age 55*

Scenario Scene
(History of Present illness)

Patient woke up with dull pressure in epigastrium, persistent for the past hour. Feels a little sweaty, nauseated, and lightheaded.

(Simulator-enabled findings):
Vital signs: heart rate 36; blood pressure 90/50; respiratory rate increased; pulse ox 92%

Heart: bradycardic rate, regular rhythm, no murmur/rub/gallop

Lungs: scattered ronchi.

Neuro: pt sounds anxious in conversation

1. Inferior Myocardial Infarction -- ACLS

Scenario States	Equipment / Supplies Needed	Instructor Support Notes
1. Baseline *(Automatic advance)* **2. Bradycardia** *(Automatic advance)* **3. Hypotension** *(Automatic advance)* **4. Hypoxia** *(Automatic advance)* ***STABLE-SICK LEVEL*** *(auto advance if BP<70)* **5. Unconscious** *(manual advance)* **6. Resolution**	Case advances automatically to "stable-sick" level, where patient continues to get worse, but there is some time for reflection and instruction (instructor may manually make worse or better at anytime to fit custom objectives). At this point intervention may be guided by the instructor, or initiated by the student. Student interventions may or may not "work" depending on the instructor's preference and/or the state of the model. If severe hypotension progresses, patient automatically becomes unconscious. Manual progression to resolution improves patient state, but without reperfusion, the awake patient still complains of severe chest pain.	
	NIBP—yes Art Line—desired* ECG monitor—yes Temp—optional SpO2—yes EtCO2—optional PA line—optional CVP—optional Anest Machine–optional Pumps—optional Other Pacer/pads—desired Defibrillator—desired IV Pole/line—yes Ambu-bag—yes O2 mask/tank/line—yes Nebulizer—optional Intubat. Equip—desired CXR/viewer—desired EKG with inf. MI—yes *Pre-existing ECG monitor hookup and "arterial line" tracing for continuous blood pressure monitoring is often helpful for instructional purposes—if more realism is desired, the student must ask for/hook up monitor on own and use NIBP cuff.	*Note: this case represents a template/example for instructional purposes only. It is not an authoritative pathway or set of expert guidelines. Actual use of any case/scenario with trainees in the simulator should be supervised by an on-site medical expert to ensure accuracy and up-to-date conformance to applicable standards of care. Instructor will have to decide whether student-driven progression of the case produces the desired response, and may need to manually alter case programming/progression to provide the most appropriate instruction. The transmitted "voice" of the patient – simulator is critical to the exercise. Facilitators should reference the "chief complaint" & "scenario scene" to guide the patients verbalization and response to student interview (should mimic an actua patient encounter). When the patient becomes unconscious in a scenario (i.e. eyes close) remember that patient will stop "speaking." Students should elicit as much history as possible by interview with the "patient," otherwise the information is not provided. Student should perform an appropriate physical exam and the facilitator (or "patient") should verbalize physical findings that the student is seeking but are not enabled by the simulator (i.e. pain on palpation). Ancillary studies (i.e. EKG, CXR, labs) and equipment (i.e. IV/O2) are not initially provided until the student asks for them. They may be simulated (i.e. verbalized) or actual. Debriefing and instruction after the scenario (or during "stable-sick" state of algorithm) are critical (see "learning objectives"). Students/instructors may wish to view a videotape of the scenario afterward for instructional/debriefing purposes. *Case author: James A. Gordon, MD, MPA*

2. Anterior Myocardial Infarction -- ACLS

(c) 2002 by the President and Fellows of Harvard College ósuppo rted by a grant from the Josiah Macy, Jr. Foundation to the Harvard-MIT Division of Health Sciences and Technology & the Center for Medical Simulation

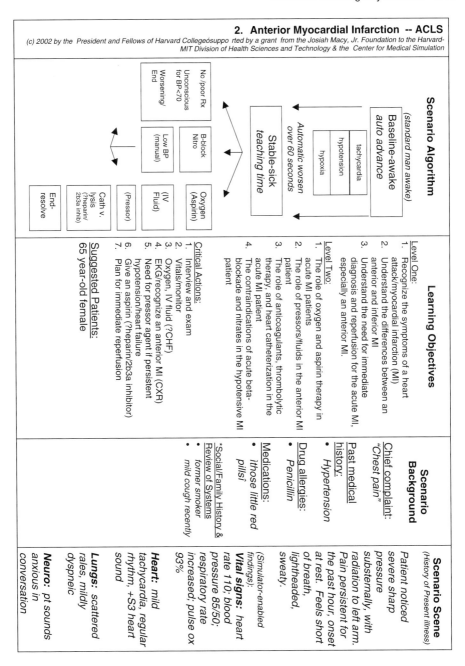

Scenario Algorithm

(standard man awake)

Baseline-awake
auto advance

Stable-sick
teaching time

Automatic worsen
over 60 seconds

No /poor Rx			
Unconscious for BP<70	B-block Nitro	Oxygen (Aspirin)	
Worsening/ End	Low BP (manual)	(IV Fluid)	Cath v. lysis (?heparin/2b3a inhib)
		(Pressor)	End-resolve

tachycardia
hypotension
hypoxia

Learning Objectives

Level One:
1. Recognize the symptoms of a heart attack/myocardial infarction (MI)
2. Understand the differences between an anterior and inferior MI
3. Understand the need for immediate diagnosis and reperfusion for the acute MI, especially an anterior MI.

Level Two:
1. The role of oxygen and aspirin therapy in acute MI patients
2. The role of pressors/fluids in the anterior MI patient
3. The role of anticoagulants, thrombolytic therapy, and heart catheterization in the acute MI patient
4. The contraindications of acute beta-blockade and nitrates in the hypotensive MI patient

Critical Actions:
1. Interview and exam
2. Vitals/monitor
3. Oxygen, IV fluid (?CHF)
4. EKG/recognize an anterior MI (CXR)
5. Need for pressor agent if persistent hypotension/heart failure
6. Give an aspirin (?heparin/2b3a inhibitor)
7. Plan for immediate reperfusion

Suggested Patients:
65 year-old female

Scenario Background

Chief complaint:
"Chest pain"

Past medical history:
• Hypertension

Drug allergies:
• Penicillin

Medications:
• ithose little red pills í

*Social/Family History & Review of Systems
• former smoker
• mild cough recently

Scenario Scene
(History of Present Illness)

Patient noticed severe sharp pressure substernally, with radiation to left arm. Pain persistent for the past hour; onset at rest. Feels short of breath, lightheaded, sweaty.

(Simulator-enabled findings):

Vital signs: heart rate 110; blood pressure 85/50; respiratory rate increased; pulse ox 93%

Heart: mild tachycardia, regular rhythm, +S3 heart sound

Lungs: scattered rales, mildly dyspneic

Neuro: pt sounds anxious in conversation

2. Anterior Myocardial Infarction -- ACLS

Scenario States	Equipment / Supplies Needed	Instructor Support Notes
1. Baseline *(automatic advance)*	NIBP—yes Art Line—desired* ECG monitor—yes Temp—optional SpO2—yes EtCO2—optional PA line—optional CVP—optional Anest Machine-optional Pumps—desired **Other** Pacer/pads–optional Defibrillator–desired IV Pole/line–yes Ambu-bag–yes O2 mask/tank/line–yes Nebulizer–optional Intubat. Equip–desired CXR/viewer–desired EKG with ant. MI–yes	*Note: this case represents a template/example for instructional purposes only. It is not an authoritative pathway or set of expert guidelines. Actual use of any case/scenario with trainees in the simulator should be supervised by an on-site medical expert to ensure accuracy and up-to-date conformance to applicable standards of care. Instructor will have to decide whether student-driven progression of the case produces the desired response, and may need to manually alter case programming/progression to provide the most appropriate instruction.
Case advances automatically to "stable-sick" level, where patient continues to get worse, but there is some time for reflection and instruction (instructor may manually make worse or better at anytime to fit custom objectives).		
2. Tachycardia *(automatic advance)*		
At this point intervention may be guided by the instructor, or initiated by the student. Student interventions may or may not "work" depending on the model. If severe hypotension progresses, patient automatically becomes unconscious. Manual progression to resolution improves patient state, but without reperfusion, the awake patient still complains of severe chest pain.		The transmitted "voice" of the patient –simulator is critical to the exercise. Facilitators should reference the "chief complaint" & "scenario scene" to guide the patients verbalization and response to student interview (should mimic an actual patient encounter). When the patient becomes unconscious in a scenario (i.e. eyes close) remember that patient will stop "speaking."
3. Hypotension *(automatic advance)*		
4. Hypoxia *(automatic advance)*		
STABLE-SICK LEVEL *(auto advance if BP<70)*		Students should elicit as much history as possible by interview with the "patient," otherwise the information is not provided. Student should perform an appropriate physical exam and the facilitator (or "patient") should verbalize physical findings that the student is seeking but are not enabled by the simulator (i.e. pain on palpation).
5. Unconscious *(manual advance)*	*Pre-existing ECG monitor hookup and "arterial line" tracing for continuous blood pressure monitoring is often helpful for instructional purposes—if more realism is desired, the student must ask for/hook up monitor on own and use NIBP cuff.	Ancillary studies (i.e. EKG, CXR, labs) and equipment (i.e. IV/O2) are not initially provided until the student asks for them. They may be simulated (i.e. verbalized) or actual.
6. Resolution		Debriefing and instruction after the scenario (or during "stable-sick" state of algorithm) are critical (see "learning objectives"). Students/instructors may wish to view a videotape of the scenario afterward for instructional/debriefing purposes.

Case author: James A. Gordon, MD, MPA

3. Unstable Angina with Cardiac Arrest – ACLS

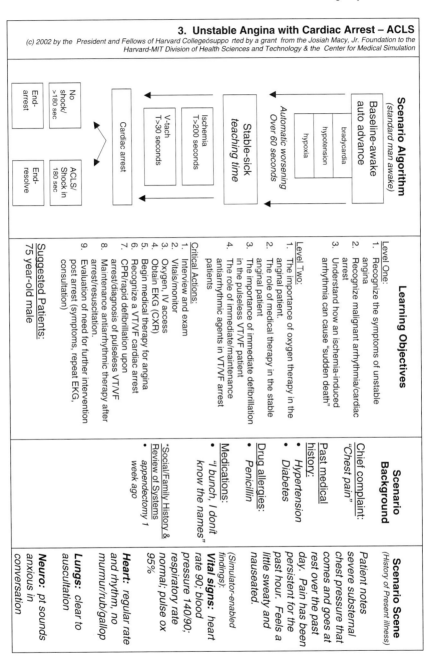

Scenario Algorithm
(standard man awake)

Baseline-awake auto advance
- bradycardia
- hypotension
- hypoxia

Automatic worsening
Over 60 seconds

Stable-sick *teaching time*

Ischemia T>200 seconds

V-tach T-30 seconds

Cardiac arrest

No shock/ >180 sec → End-arrest

ACLS/ Shock in 180 sec → End-resolve

Learning Objectives

Level One:
1. Recognize the symptoms of unstable angina
2. Recognize malignant arrhythmia/cardiac arrest
3. Understand how an ischemia-induced arrhythmia can cause "sudden death"

Level Two:
1. The importance of oxygen therapy in the anginal patient.
2. The role of medical therapy in the stable anginal patient
3. The importance of immediate defibrillation in the pulseless VT/VF patient
4. The role of immediate/maintenance antiarrhythmic agents in VT/VF arrest patients

Critical Actions:
1. Interview and exam
2. Vitals/monitor
3. Oxygen, IV access
4. Obtain EKG (CXR)
5. Begin medical therapy for angina
6. Recognize a VT/VF cardiac arrest
7. CPR/rapid defibrillation upon arrest/diagnosis of pulseless VT/VF
8. Maintenance antiarrhythmic therapy after arrest/resuscitation.
9. Evaluation of need for further intervention post arrest (symptoms, repeat EKG, consultation)

Suggested Patients:
75 year-old male

Scenario Background

Chief complaint:
"Chest pain"

Past medical history:
• Hypertension
• Diabetes

Drug allergies:
• Penicillin

Medications:
• "I bunch, I don't know the names"

Social/Family History & Review of Systems
• appendectomy 1 week ago

Scenario Scene
(History of Present Illness)

Patient notes severe substernal chest pressure that comes and goes at rest over the past day. Pain has been persistent for the past hour. Feels a little sweaty and nauseated.

(Simulator-enabled findings):
Vital signs: heart rate 90; blood pressure 140/90; respiratory rate normal; pulse ox 95%

Heart: regular rate and rhythm, no murmur/rub/gallop

Lungs: clear to auscultation

Neuro: pt sounds anxious in conversation

3. Unstable Angina with Cardiac Arrest -- ACLS

Scenario States	Equipment / Supplies Needed	Instructor Support Notes
1. Baseline *(automatic advance)* **2. Mild hypertension** *(automatic advance)* **3. Mild hypoxia** *(automatic advance)* **_STABLE-SICK LEVEL_** **4. Ischemia** *(auto advance after 200 sec)* **5. Ventricular tachycardia** *(auto advance after 30 sec)* **6. Cardiac arrest** *(auto advance to "late shock/arrest" if no defib at 200J in under 180 sec—to "resolution" if 200J under 180 sec)* **7. Late shock/arrest** **8. Resolution** *Case advances automatically to "stable-sick" level, where patient continues to get worse, but there is some time for reflection and instruction (instructor may manually make worse or better at anytime to fit custom objectives). After 200 seconds of "ischemia" the patient automatically progresses to symptomatic ventricular tachycardia (with pulse), regardless of student intervention. After 30 seconds of arrhythmia (regardless of intervention), patient will experience cardiac arrest and become unconscious. Resolution automatically proceeds if defibrillation at 200 J occurs in under 180 seconds, otherwise no recovery is programmed (ends at "late shock/arrest," although instructor can manually override).*	NIBP—yes Art Line—desired* ECG monitor—yes Temp—optional SpO2—yes EtCO2—desired PA line—optional CVP—optional Anest Machine-optional Pumps—optional Other Pacer—optional Defibrillator—yes IV Pole/line—yes Ambu-bag—yes O2 mask/tank/line—yes Nebulizer—optional Intubation equip—yes CXR/viewer—desired EKG w/ischemia—yes	*Note: this case represents a template/example for instructional purposes only. It is not an authoritative pathway or set of expert guidelines. Actual use of any case/scenario with trainees in the simulator should be supervised by an on-site medical expert to ensure accuracy and up-to-date conformance to applicable standards of care. Instructor will have to decide whether student-driven progression of the case produces the desired response, and may need to manually alter case programming/progression to provide the most appropriate instruction. The transmitted "voice" of the patient –simulator is critical to the exercise. Facilitators should reference the "chief complaint" & "scenario scene" to guide the patients verbalization and response to student interview (should mimic an actual patient encounter). When the patient becomes unconscious in a scenario (i.e. eyes close), remember that patient will stop "speaking." Students should elicit as much history as possible by interview with the "patient," otherwise the information is not provided. Student should perform an appropriate physical exam and the facilitator (or "patient") should verbalize physical findings that the student is seeking but are not enabled by the simulator (i.e. pain on palpation). *Pre-existing ECG monitor hookup and "arterial line" tracing for continuous blood pressure monitoring is often helpful for instructional purposes—if more realism is desired, the student must ask for/hook up monitor on own and use NIBP cuff. Ancillary studies (i.e. EKG, CXR labs) and equipment (i.e. IV/O2) are not initially provided until the student asks for them. They may be simulated (i.e. verbalized) or actual. Debriefing and instruction after the scenario (or during "stable-sick" state of algorithm) are critical (see "learning objectives"). Students/instructors may wish to view a videotape of the scenario afterward for instructional/debriefing purposes.

Case author: James A. Gordon, MD, MPA

4. Severe Young Asthmatic -- ALS

(c) 2002 by the President and Fellows of Harvard Collegeósuppo rted by a grant from the Josiah Macy, Jr. Foundation to the Harvard-MIT Division of Health Sciences and Technology & the Center for Medical Simulation

Scenario Algorithm

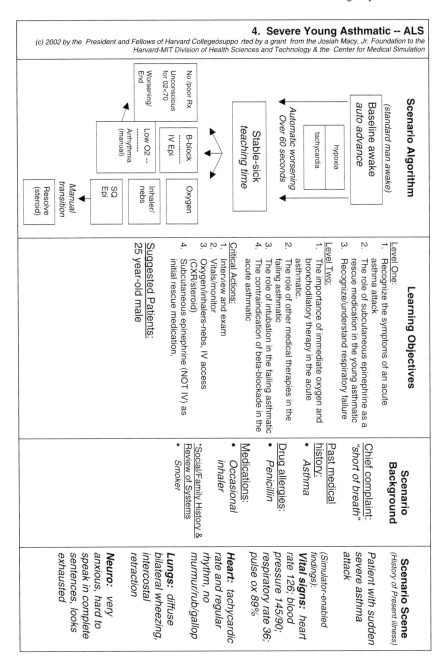

(standard man awake)

Baseline awake auto advance

Automatic worsening
Over 60 seconds

Stable-sick
teaching time

No /poor Rx
Worsening/
End

Unconscious
for 02<70

hypoxia

tachycardia

B-block   IV Epi

Low O2 --
Arrhythmia
(manual)

Inhaler/
nebs

Oxygen

SQ
Epi

Resolve
(steroid)

Manual
transition

Learning Objectives

Level One:
1. Recognize the symptoms of an acute asthma attack
2. The role of subcutaneous epinephrine as a rescue medication in the young asthmatic
3. Recognize/understand respiratory failure

Level Two:
1. The importance of immediate oxygen and bronchodilatory therapy in the acute asthmatic.
2. The role of other medical therapies in the failing asthmatic
3. The role of intubation in the failing asthmatic
4. The contraindication of beta-blockade in the acute asthmatic

Critical Actions:
1. Interview and exam
2. Vitals/monitor
3. Oxygen/inhalers-nebs, IV access (CXR/steroid)
4. Subcutaneous epinephrine (NOT IV) as initial rescue medication.

Suggested Patients:
25 year-old male

Scenario Background

Chief complaint:
"short of breath"

Past medical history:
• Asthma

Drug allergies:
• Penicillin

Medications:
• Occasional inhaler

*Social/Family History & Review of Systems
• Smoker

Scenario Scene

(History of Present Illness)

Patient with sudden severe asthma attack

(Simulator-enabled findings):
Vital signs: heart rate 126; blood pressure 145/90; respiratory rate 36; pulse ox 89%

Heart: tachycardic rate and regular rhythm, no murmur/rub/gallop

Lungs: diffuse bilateral wheezing, intercostal retraction

Neuro: very anxious, hard to speak in complete sentences, looks exhausted

4. Severe Young Asthmatic -- ALS

Scenario States	Equipment / Supplies Needed	Instructor Support Notes
1. Baseline *(automatic advance)*	NIBP—yes Art Line—optional* ECG monitor—yes Temp—optional SpO2—yes EtCO2—optional PA line—no CVP—no Anest Machine-optional Pumps—no	*Note: this case represents a template/example for instructional purposes only. It is not an authoritative pathway or set of expert guidelines. Actual use of any case/scenario with trainees in the simulator should be supervised by an on-site medical expert to ensure accuracy and up-to-date conformance to applicable standards of care. Instructor will have to decide whether student-driven progression of the case produces the desired response, and may need to manually alter case programming/progression to provide the most appropriate instruction.
2. Hypoxia *(automatic advance)*		
3. Tachycardia	Other Pacer—no Defibrillator—no IV Pole/line—yes Ambu-bag—yes O2 mask/tank/line—yes Nebulizer—yes Intubation equip—yes CXR/viewer--desired EKG—optional TB syringe/subQ inj—yes	The transmitted "voice" of the patient – simulator is critical to the exercise. Facilitators should reference the "chief complaint" & "scenario scene" to guide the patient's verbalization and response to student interview (should mimic an actual patient encounter). When the patient becomes unconscious in a scenario (i.e. eyes close) remember that patient will stop "speaking."
STABLE-SICK LEVEL		
4. Unconscious *(auto advance to unconscious for pOx<70)*		Students should elicit as much history as possible by interview with the "patient," otherwise the information is not provided. Student should perform an appropriate physical exam and the facilitator (or "patient") should verbalize physical findings that the student is seeking but are not enabled by the simulator (i.e. pain on palpation).
5. Resolution *(manual advance to resolution if SQ epinephrine)*	*Pre-existing ECG monitor hookup and "arterial line" tracing for continuous blood pressure monitoring is often helpful for instructional purposes—if more realism is desired, the student must ask for/hook up monitor on own and use NIBP cuff.	Ancillary studies (i.e. EKG, CXR, labs) and equipment (i.e. IV/O2) are not initially provided until the student asks for them. They may be simulated (i.e. verbalized) or actual. Debriefing and instruction after the scenario (or during "stable-sick" state of algorithm) are critical (see "learning objectives"). Students/instructors may wish to view a videotape of the scenario afterward for instructional/debriefing purposes.

Scenario States descriptions:

1. Baseline *(automatic advance)*
Case advances automatically to "stable-sick" level, where patient continues to get worse, but there is some time for reflection and instruction (instructor may manually make worse or better at anytime to fit custom objectives). At this point intervention may be guided by the instructor, or initiated by the student. Student interventions may or may not "work" depending on the instructor's preference and/or the state of the model. If severe hypoxia progresses, patient automatically becomes unconscious. Manual progression to resolution (after subcutaneous epinephrine) improves patient state.

(auto advance to unconscious for pOx<70)

Case author: James A. Gordon, MD, MPA

5. COPD Exacerbation with Respiratory Failure ñ ALS

(c) 2002 by the President and Fellows of Harvard Collegeósuppo rted by a grant from the Josiah Macy, Jr. Foundation to the Harvard-MIT Division of Health Sciences and Technology & the Center for Medical Simulation

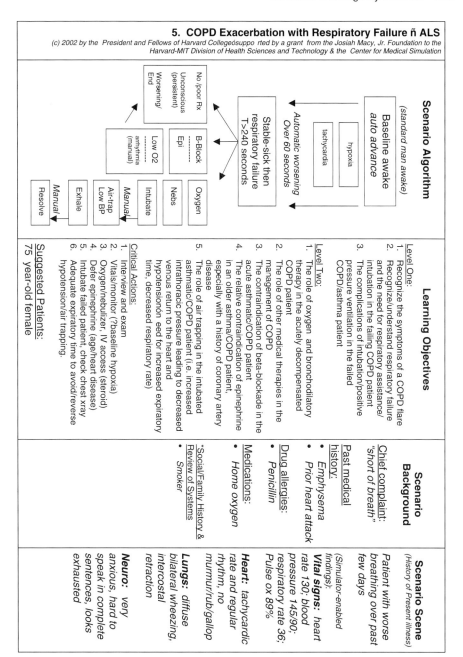

Scenario Algorithm

(standard man awake)

Baseline awake
auto advance

*Automatic worsening
Over 60 seconds*

Stable-sick then
respiratory failure
T>240 seconds

- hypoxia
- tachycardia

- No/poor Rx
- Unconscious (persistent)
- Worsening/ End

- B-Block
- Epi
- Low O2
- arrhythmia (manual)

- Oxygen
- Nebs
- Intubate
- Air-trap Low BP   *Manual*
- Exhale   *Manual*
- Resolve

Learning Objectives

Level One:
1. Recognize the symptoms of a COPD flare
2. Recognize/understand respiratory failure and the need for respiratory assistance/ intubation in the failing COPD patient
3. The complications of intubation/positive pressure ventilation in the failed COPD/asthma patient

Level Two:
1. The role of oxygen and bronchodilatory therapy in the acutely decompensated COPD patient
2. The role of other medical therapies in the management of COPD
3. The contraindication of beta-blockade in the acute asthmatic/COPD patient
4. The relative contraindication of epinephrine in an older asthma/COPD patient, especially with a history of coronary artery disease
5. The role of air trapping in the intubated asthmatic/COPD patient (i.e. increased intrathoracic pressure leading to decreased venous return to the heart and hypotensionón eed for increased expiratory time, decreased respiratory rate)

Critical Actions:
1. Interview and exam
2. Vitals/monitor (?baseline hypoxia)
3. Oxygen/nebulizer, IV access (steroid)
4. Defer epinephrine (age/heart disease)
5. Intubate failed patient, check chest xray
6. Adequate expiratory time to avoid/reverse hypotension/air trapping.

Suggested Patients:
75 year-old female

Scenario Background

Chief complaint:
"short of breath"

(Simulator-enabled findings):

Past medical history:
- *Emphysema*
- *Prior heart attack*

Drug allergies:
- *Penicillin*

Medications:
- *Home oxygen*

Social/Family History & Review of Systems
- *Smoker*

Scenario Scene
(History of Present illness)

Patient with worse breathing over past few days

Vital signs: *heart rate 130; blood pressure 145/90; respiratory rate 36; Pulse ox 89%*

Heart: *tachycardic rate and regular rhythm, no murmur/rub/gallop*

Lungs: *diffuse bilateral wheezing, intercostal retraction*

Neuro: *very anxious, hard to speak in complete sentences, looks exhausted*

5. COPD Exacerbation with Respiratory Failure -- ALS

Scenario States		Equipment / Supplies Needed	Instructor Support Notes
1. Baseline *(automatic advance)*	Case advances automatically to "stable-sick" level, where patient continues to get worse, but there is some time for reflection and instruction (instructor may manually make worse or better at anytime to fit custom objectives). After 240 seconds (or sooner if severe hypoxia or hypotension) patient	NIBP—yes Art Line—desired* ECG monitor—yes Temp—optional SpO2—yes EtCO2—yes PA line—no CVP—optional	*Note: this case represents a template/example for instructional purposes only. It is not an authoritative pathway or set of expert guidelines. Actual use of any case/scenario with trainees in the simulator should be supervised by an on-site medical expert to ensure accuracy and up-to-date conformance to applicable standards of care. Instructor will have to decide whether student-driven
2. Hypoxia *(automatic advance)*			
3. Tachycardia	unconscious, regardless of student intervention. Manual advance to "airtrap/hypotension" is designed to demonstrate hypotension that	Anest Machine-optional Pumps—optional	progression of the case produces the desired response, and may need to manually alter case programming/progression to provide the most appropriate instruction.
STABLE-SICK LEVEL *(automatic advance for T>240 sec or pox<70 or BP<70)*	would accompany airtrapping after intubation if not adequate expiratory time on ventilation (but may be skipped based on student performance and/or instructor preference). Manual progression to	**Other** Pacer—no Defibrillator—desired IV Pole/line—yes Ambu-bag—yes O2 mask/tank/line—yes Nebulizer—yes	The transmitted "voice" of the patient --simulator is critical to the exercise. Facilitators should reference the "chief complaint" & "scenario scene" to guide the patients verbalization and response to student interview (should mimic an actual patient encounter). When the patient
4. Failure *(manual advance if want to demonstrate air n trap/hypotens after intubation if not adequate expiratory time).*	resolution improves patient state (if airtrapping/hypotension pathway, resolution would occur after patient is allowed sufficient expiratory time).	Intubation equip—yes CXR/viewer—desired EKG—desired TB syringe/subQ inj—optional	becomes unconscious in a scenario (i.e. eyes close) remember that patient wi stop "speaking." Students should elicit as much history as possible by interview with the "patient," otherwise the information is not provided.
5. Airtrap/Hypotension *(manual advance for resolution)*		*Pre-existing ECG monitor hookup and "arterial line" tracing for continuous blood pressure monitoring is often helpful for instructional purposes—if more realism is	Student should perform an appropriate physical exam and the facilitator (or 'patient') should verbalize physical findings that the student is seeking but are not enabled by the simulator (i.e. pain on palpation).
6. Resolution		desired, the student must ask for/hook up monitor on own and use NIBP cuff.	Ancillary studies (i.e. EKG, CXR, labs) and equipment (i.e. IV/O2) are not initially provided until the student asks for them. They may be simulated (i.e. verbalized) or actual. Debriefing and instruction after the scenario (or during "stable-sick" state of algorithm) are critical (see "learning objectives"). Students/instructors may wish to view a videotape of the scenario afterward for instructional/debriefing purposes.

Case author: James A. Gordon, MD, MPA

6. Asthmatic with Pneumothorax -- ALS

Scenario Algorithm

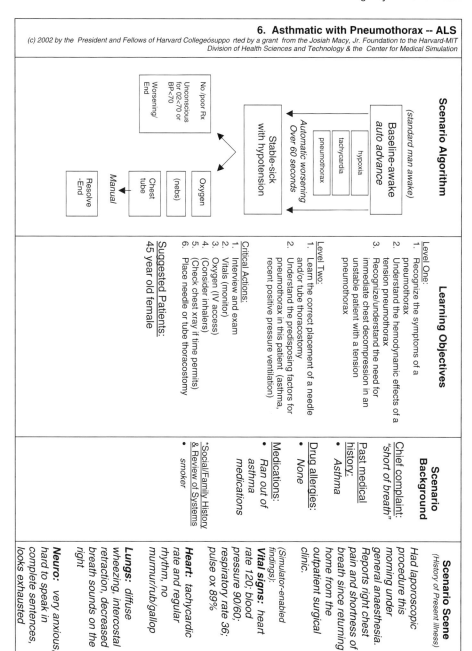

Baseline-awake auto advance *(standard man awake)*

- hypoxia
- tachycardia
- pneumothorax

No /poor Rx

Unconscious for O2<70 or BP<70

Worsening/ End

Stable-sick with hypotension

Automatic worsening Over 60 seconds

Oxygen

(nebs)

Chest tube

Resolve -End

Manual

Learning Objectives

Level One:
1. Recognize the symptoms of a pneumothorax
2. Understand the hemodynamic effects of a tension pneumothorax
3. Recognize/understand the need for immediate chest decompression in an unstable patient with a tension pneumothorax

Level Two:
1. Learn the correct placement of a needle and/or tube thoracostomy
2. Understand the predisposing factors for pneumothorax in this patient (asthma, recent positive pressure ventilation)

Critical Actions:
1. Interview and exam
2. Vitals (monitor)
3. Oxygen (IV access)
4. (Consider inhalers)
5. (Check chest xray if time permits)
6. Place needle or tube thoracostomy

Suggested Patients:
45 year old female

Scenario Background

Chief complaint: "short of breath"

Past medical history: Asthma

Drug allergies: None

Medications: Ran out of asthma medications

*Social/Family History & Review of Systems
- smoker

Scenario Scene
(History of Present Illness)

Had laparoscopic procedure this morning under general anaesthesia. Reports right chest pain and shortness of breath since returning home from the outpatient surgical clinic.

(Simulator-enabled findings):

Vital signs: heart rate 120; blood pressure 90/60; respiratory rate 36; pulse ox 89%

Heart: tachycardic rate and regular rhythm, no murmur/rub/gallop

Lungs: diffuse wheezing, intercostal retraction, decreased breath sounds on the right

Neuro: very anxious, hard to speak in complete sentences, looks exhausted

6. Asthmatic with Pneumothorax -- ALS

Scenario States	Equipment / Supplies Needed	Instructor Support Notes
1. Baseline *(automatic advance)* **2. Hypoxia** *(automatic advance)* **3. Tachycardia** *(automatic advance)* **4. Pneumothorax** *(automatic advance)* *STABLE-SICK LEVEL* *(automatic advance to unconscious if BP<70 or pOx<70)* **5. Unconscious** *(automatic advance to resolution)* **6. Resolution** *(Manual advance to resolution)*	*Case advances automatically to "stable-sick" level, where patient continues to get worse, but there is some time for reflection and instruction (instructor may manually make worse or better at anytime to fit custom objectives). At this point intervention may be guided by the instructor, or initiated by the student. If severe hypoxia progresses, patient automatically becomes unconscious. Manual progression to resolution (after decompression of pneumothorax) improves patient state.*	
	NIBP—yes Art Line—desired* ECG monitor—yes Temp—optional SpO2—yes EtCO2—optional PA line—no CVP—optional Anest Machine-optional Pumps—optional Other Pacer—no Defibrillator—yes IV Pole/line—yes Ambu-bag—yes O2 mask/tank/line—yes Nebulizer—yes Intubation equip—yes CXR w/PTX—yes EKG—desired TB syringe/SQ inj—yes Chest tube—yes Needle for PTX decompress—yes	*Note: this case represents a template/example for instructional purposes only. It is not an authoritative pathway or set of expert guidelines. Actual use of any case/scenario with trainees in the simulator should be supervised by an on-site medical expert to ensure accuracy and up-to-date conformance to applicable standards of care. Instructor will have to decide whether student-driven progression of this case produces the desired response, and may need to manually alter case programming/progression to provide the most appropriate instruction* The transmitted "voice" of the patient—simulator is critical to the exercise. Facilitators should reference the "chief complaint" & "scenario scene" to guide the patients verbalization and response to student interview (should mimic an actual patient encounter). When the patient becomes unconscious in a scenario (i.e. eyes close) remember that patient will stop "speaking." Students should elicit as much history as possible by interview with the "patient," otherwise the information is not provided. Student should perform an appropriate physical exam and the facilitator (or "patient") should verbalize physical findings that the student is seeking but are not enabled by the simulator (i.e. pain on palpation). Ancillary studies (i.e. EKG, CXR, labs) and equipment (i.e. IV/O2) are not initially provided until the student asks for them. They may be simulated (i.e. verbalized) or actual.
	Pre-existing ECG monitor hookup and "arterial line" tracing for continuous blood pressure monitoring is often helpful for instructional purposes—if more realism is desired, the student must ask for/hook up monitor on own and use NIBP cuff.	Debriefing and instruction after the scenario (or during "stable-sick" state of algorithm) are critical (see "learning objectives"). Students/instructors may wish to view a videotape of the scenario afterward for instructional/debriefing purposes. **Case author: James A. Gordon, MD, MPA**

OUTLINE OF THREE-YEAR EM SIMULATION CURRICULUM

(See Note for abbreviations)

PGY I Curriculum

A. Goals:
1. Introduction to the simulation environment and to simulated patient management skills.
2. Demonstrate respect and compassion for patients.
3. Demonstrate effective communication skills with patients, families and team members.
4. Demonstrate effective application of medical knowledge to clinical situations.
5. Observe your performance/skills/attitudes and team members' behavior performance/skills/attitudes and provide effective self/other directed feedback.

B. Description of Simulation Cases with Objectives:
1) Acute myocardial infarction progressing to cardiac arrest
   a) Recognize patient deterioration as rhythm changes to ventricular tachycardia (PC)
   b) Demonstrate management of ventricular tachycardia (MK/PC)
   c) Recognize problem with debifrillator and reconfigure defibrillator paddles (PC)
   d) Demonstrates empathy for wife of patient (PR)
   e) Appropriate explanation of events to wife (IC)
   f) Demonstrate the ability to give specific and constructive feedback to self and others (IC/PL)*
2) Blunt trauma patient with difficult airway
   a) Coordinate the roles of trauma team (PC/IC)
   b) Recognize and manage the difficult airway (PC)
   c) Demonstrate basic steps in management of increased intracranial pressure (MK)
   d) Order appropriate lab and imaging tests (PC/SB)
3) Severe anaphylaxis presenting as an "asthma" attack
   a) Recognize an acute allergic emergency (MK/PC)
   b) Direct team to perform simultaneous evaluation and management (PC/IC)
   c) Perform a complete history and physical to ascertain cause of reaction(PC)
   d) Recognize error in triage of patient as "asthma" and address triage system (SB)
4) Adult male with fatal gastrointestinal bleeding
   a) Develop a broad differential diagnosis of pulseless electrical activity (MK)

     b) Demonstrate application of differential diagnosis to patient care through actions (PC)

     c) Inform family about patient's death, and answers questions with compassion (IC)

     d) Recognize limitations of self and system as demonstrated by ending resuscitation(PL)

   5) Adult patient with tricyclic antidepressant and acetaminophen overdose

     a) Stabilize patient and obtain appropriate history and physical exam (MK/PC)

     b) Order appropriate tests for unknown overdose (MK/PC/SB)

     c) Obtain psychiatric evaluation and poison center consultation (SB)

     d) Demonstrate empathy and compassion in communication with patient (IC/PR)

PGY II Curriculum

A. Goals:

   1) Successful management of complex medical cases and equipment failures.

   2) Analysis and improvement of systems performance as well as individual performance.

   3) Demonstrate respect and compassion for a diverse patient population.

   4) Demonstrate effective communication skills with patients, families and team members in more challenging environments.

   5) Demonstrate effective tools for obtaining medical knowledge and applying to new clinical situation.

   6) Observe your performance/skills/attitudes and team members' behavior performance/skills/attitudes and provide effective self/other directed feedback.

B. Description of Simulation Cases with Objectives:

   1) Unstable atrial fibrillation with congestive heart failure

     a) Recognize unstable patient and demonstrate appropriate initial management (MK/PC)

     b) Explain cardioversion procedure to patient and family (IC/PC)

     c) Demonstrate empathy to patient about fears regarding procedure (IC/PR)

     d) Demonstrate ability to perform synchronized cardioversion (PC)

     e) Demonstrate ability to identify areas of possible improvement in self, team and in the system, provides and accepts appropriate feedback* (PL/IC)

   2) Multi-trauma patient with splenic injury and hypotension

     a) Demonstrate initial management of hypovolemic shock (MK/PC)

     b) Respect patient's request for withholding blood products (PR)

     c) Communicate with family about patient's wishes (IC)

     d) Advocate for patient and family with trauma surgeon (IC/PR)

   3) Pediatric non-accidental trauma patient with head injury and extremity fracture

     a) Recognize "shaken baby" syndrome (MK/PC)

     b) Demonstrate management of head injury and screen for other injuries (MK/PC)

     c) Consult law enforcement and social work (SB)

     d) Explain situation to distraught mother of child (IC)

     e) Demonstrate accurate and complete documentation in chart (IC)

4) Pediatric patient with sepsis, dehydration, and hyponatremia
   a) Identify and manages all three primary medical problems (MK/PC)
   b) Demonstrate alternative techniques for vascular access (PC)
   c) Recognize nursing medication error and addresse issue appropriately (SB/IC)
   d) Arrange transfer of patient to another facility due to ICU availability (SB)
   e) Demonstrate cultural sensitivity to families wish for a traditional healer (PR)
5) Adult patient with diabetic ketoacidosis, substance abuse, and poor social support system
   a) Demonstrate medical management of DKA (MK/PC)
   b) Addresses social situation and substance abuse non-judgmentally with patient (IC/PR)
   c) Recognize patient's wish to leave but bargain with patient to stay in hospital (IC)
   d) Demonstrate ability to constructively interact with consultant who is reluctant to admit (IC/SB)

PGY III Curriculum

A. Goals:
   1) Continued analysis and improvement of systems performance as well as individual performance.
   2) Assist junior residents with successful management of complex medical cases and equipment failures.
   3) Demonstrate a high level of sophistication in interpersonal skills, professionalism and interaction in complex medical system.
   4) Simultaneously manage multiple patients in realistic ED setting.
   5) Develop personal strategies for self-improvement, error reduction and life-long learning.
   6) Transition to instructor/preceptor role in simulation environment.
B. Description of Simulation Cases with Objectives:
   1) Multiple patient encounter
      a) Pediatric patient presenting with cough, and issue of consent (PR/PC)
      b) Admitted chest pain patient with wrong ECG on chart (SB)
      c) Patient with rare neuromuscular disorder requesting information (PL)
      d) Phone call with issue of inappropriate transfer of a patient (SB)
      e) Demonstrate ability to identify areas of possible improvement in self, team and in the system, provides and accepts appropriate feedback* (PL/IC)
   2) Routine conscious sedation with oversedation and vomiting
      a) Follow guidelines for conscious sedation (MK/PC)
      b) Demonstrate ability to manage complications of conscious sedation (PC)
      c) Appropriate informed consent obtained (PR/PC)
      d) Appropriate and honest explanation of complication to family (PR/IC)
   3) Delirious and combative patient from an unknown cause
      a) Demonstrate appropriate and respectful use of physical and chemical restraint (PC/PR)

    b) Assess patients decisional capacity and recognize need for consult (MK/IC/PR/SB/PC)

    c) Develop a broad differential diagnosis and correct sequencing of plan of care (MK/PC)

    d) Interacts effectively with hospital administrator to advocate for ICU bed (IC/SB/PR)

4) Simulated "check-out" of hypothermic patient with incorrect information

    a) Reexamines and repeats history when inconsistencies noted (PC/PR)

    b) Changes management to reflect new information (PC/MK)

    c) Corrects documentation in chart with additional note (PR/IC)

    d) Creates an open dialogue with initial caregiver about source of incorrect information (PR/IC)

5) Cases from PGY I and II

    a) May be repeated with additional equipment or teamwork challenges (PC/MK/IC)

    b) Increased role as bedside teacher, supervisor and facilitator during simulation (PR/IC)

    c) Lead role as facilitator during debriefing session (IC)

    d) Identify learning opportunities and techniques for self-education (PL)

* *This objective is part of every scenario for this year.*

Note: *Patient Care (PC), Medical Knowledge (MK), Practice-Based Learning and Improvement (PL), Interpersonal and Communication Skills (IC), Professionalism (PR), Systems-Based Practice (SB)*

(This outline originally appeared in McLaughlin, Acad Emerg Med 2002;9:1310–1318.)

TEAM DIMENSIONS RATING FORM

Clearly print in the boxes the date, time, observation code, and ratings. Place an X in the box to identify the evaluator. Use the instructions in the ETCC® Measures Guide to complete the team ratings. If you witness one or more errors while observing for team-work ratings, complete the necessary Observed Error Records.

Date: _____   **Time:** _____   **Observation Code:** _____

    Mo   Day   Hr   Min   Level of   Chief
   01–12   01–31   (Use 24 hour clock)   Effort   Complaint

Evaluator: **Physician**   **Nurse**

No	Team Dimension	Descriptors	Rating
1	Team Structure and Climate	Establish the leader, assemble the team, assign roles and responsibilities, communicate essential team information, acknowledge contributions of team members to team goals, demonstrate mutual respect in all communication, hold each other accountable for team outcomes, address professional concerns directly, resolve conflicts constructively	_____
2	Apply Problem Solving Strategies	Engage members in planning process; identify established to be used or develop a plan; engage team members in decision making process; alert team to potential biases and errors; report slips, lapses, and mistakes to team; advocate and assert a position or corrective action, invoke the Two-Challenge rule when an initial assertion is ignored	_____
3	Communicate with the Team	Request situation awareness updates, provide situation awareness updates, use ED common terminology in all communications, call out critical information during emergent events, use check backs to verify information transfer, systematically handoff responsibilities during tea transitions, offer information to support planning and decision making, communicate decisions and actions to team members, seek information for planning and decision making	_____
4	Execute Plans and Manage Workload	Execute protocol or team-established plan, integrate individual assessments of patient needs, replan patient care in response to overall caseload of team, prioritize tasks for individual patients, cross monitor actions of team members, balance workload within team, request assistance for task overload, offer assistance for task overload, constructively use periods of low workload	_____
5	Improve Team Skills	Engage in situational learning and teaching with the team, engage in coaching with team members, conduct shift reviews of teamwork, conduct event reviews of teamwork, include teamwork considerations in educational forums, review teamwork as part of clinical case reviews	_____

Notes: Consult the behaviorally anchored rating scales for details. Enter a summary rating (1, 2.. 7) in the rating block for each Team Dimension. Refer to the rating scale below.

			Rating Scale			
Very Poor	Poor	Marginal	Acceptable	Good	Very Good	Superior
1	2	3	4	5	6	7

Check the box if you have completed one or more Observed Error Records on this observation. ☐

SIMULATOR-ENHANCED DISASTER EXERCISE SCENARIO (SARIN EXPOSURE)

1. Preparation:

1.1 Personnel
◆ Exercise Controller: 1
◆ Exercise Directors: 3 (1 scene, 1 triage / decontamination, 1 hospital)
◆ Evaluators / Observers: 3
◆ Simulator Controllers: 3
◆ Scenario Assistants: 3–5 (runners, scenario setup)
◆ Live "Victims": 5

1.2 Participants
◆ Incident Command – Incident Commander (IC)
◆ Prehospital
  ✓ Hazmat: 5–7
  ✓ Police / Security: 3–5
  ✓ EMS: 10–12 (teams of 2; at least 1 EMT-I/C or EMT-P per team)
◆ Hospital
  ✓ Physicians: 2
  ✓ Nurses: 4–5

1.3 Equipment
◆ high-fidelity mannequin × 3
◆ low-fidelity mannequin × 7 (including at least 1 with airway and EKG capabilities)
◆ perimeter / disaster scene containment equipment (tape, markers)
◆ triage equipment (tags)
◆ personal protective equipment (PPE − level B)
◆ decontamination equipment (washdown / showering)
◆ communications
  ✓ portable radios + cell phones with PPE-compatible headsets
  ✓ central phone #'s for dispatchers; incident command; hospital triage; poison control
◆ ambulance stretchers × 4
◆ hospital stretcher × 6
◆ resuscitative medical equipment (gloves, shears, stethoscopes, airway/IV equipment, medications)

1.4 Orientation
◆ ground + safety rules

- orientation to Simulation Center grounds
- orientation to simulators (characteristics / capabilities of low- and high-fidelity mannequins)
- participant equipment distribution and check

2. Background:

- Location: City Hall
- Time: <u>10:00 am</u>
- Setting: odorless white vapor leaking from outside 2nd floor Mayor's Clerk's office;
- Source canister containing oily substance
- Exposure: 10–20? victims

3. Incident Notification / Command (<u>10:11 am</u>)

- First responders / EMS
- HazMat
- Police / Fire
- Hospital
    - ✓ turnout gear / PPE utilization
    - ✓ establishment of scene security
    - ✓ establishment of Hot Zone perimeter and quarantine area
    - ✓ identification of IC, institution of command structure (e.g. identifying clothing)
    - ✓ creation of upwind staging area
    - ✓ communications

4. On-scene:

- Location: plaza outside of City Hall
- Time: <u>10:18 am</u>
- 15 victims as described in diagrams
    - ✓ actors and low-fidelity mannequins wearing cards identifying key symptoms and vital signs
    - ✓ high-fidelity mannequins displaying key symptoms and vital signs

CONTAMINATED ZONE

- Disaster area
- Triage
- Decontamination
    - ✓ minimization of further exposure by PPE-wearing HazMat technicians
    - ✓ identification and triage of victims by PPE-wearing prehospital providers
    - ✓ attempts to identify toxic agent
    - ✓ on-scene initial / basic life support treatment
    - ✓ transportation of victims to decontamination area
    - ✓ proper decontamination of victims
    - ✓ clothing removal
    - ✓ decontamination on scene (with water, showers)
    - ✓ stabilizing measures
    - ✓ basic airway management

✓ atropine
✓ +/−IV
✓ triage / decontamination of "wandering" victims
✓ "crowd control"
✓ decontamination of HazMat and field personnel

NON-CONTAMINATED ZONE
◆ Treatment area
   ✓ continued stabilization of victims
   ✓ transfer arrangements / communications

5. Hospital
◆ *Location: Receiving Community Hospital*
◆ *Time: 10:35 am–11:20 am*
◆ *5 chemical exposure victims as described in diagrams*
◆ communication with IC and EMS, acceptance of victims—2 RED and 3 YELLOW
◆ hospital emergency response plan activation [Hospital Emergency Incident Command System (HEICS)]
   ✓ staff safety
   ✓ incident command
   ✓ evacuation
   ✓ air monitoring
◆ if incomplete or absent field decontamination, in-hospital decontamination and use of PPE
◆ treatment
   ✓ airway management
   ✓ IV
   ✓ atropine
   ✓ pralidoxime / 2-PAM
   ✓ acquisition and resupply of pharmaceuticals, ventilators
◆ definitive disposition
   ✓ ICU
◆ integration of non-disaster cardiac arrest patient care with disaster patient treatment

6. Debriefing
◆ Incident command
◆ Scene security
◆ Toxic agent identification
◆ PPE utilization
◆ Communications
◆ Triage procedure
◆ Decontamination procedure
◆ Prehospital medical treatment
◆ Hospital medical treatment / integration
◆ Supply management

Incident Control:	—Coordination of Hazmat, police, security for institution of Hot Zone perimeter around disaster area
	—establishment of upwind staging area, command hierarchy, and communications
Disaster Scene:	—15 victims scattered in parking lot outside City Hall (5 bold patients to be transported to hospital)

	age/sex	*responsive**	*airway/ lungs*	*resps*	*pulse*	*heart rate*	*pupils*	*sim***
2 BLACK (dead or expectant dead)								
A.	64 f	U	secretions	0	absent	0	pinpoint	low
B.	56 m	U	secretions	2	absent	<10	pinpoint	low
3 RED (acute / immediate)								
C.	**45 m**	**U**	**secretions**	**26**	**weak**	**50**	**pinpoint**	**high**
D.	**32 m**	**P**	**vomiting**	**30**	**weak**	**40**	**pinpoint**	**high**
E.	36 f	V	secretions	30	weak	40	pinpoint	high
5 YELLOW (urgent, delayed)								
F.	**29 f**	**A**	**wheeze**	**26**	**strong**	**40**	**2 mm**	**actor**
G.	**22 f**	**A**	**wheeze**	**26**	**strong**	**40**	**2 mm**	**actor**
II.	**54 f**	**A**	**rhonchi**	**24**	**irregular**	**100**	**2 mm**	**actor**
I.	28 f	A	wheeze	28	strong	50	2 mm	actor
J.	12 m	A	wheeze	24	strong	60	3 mm	actor
5 GREEN (nonurgent)								
K.	48 m	A	clear	18	strong	80	3 mm	low
L.	58 m	A	clear	20	strong	80	3 mm	low
M.	45 f	A	clear	16	strong	60	2 mm	low
N.	33 f	A	clear	12	strong	58	5 mm	low
O.	35 m	A	clear	18	strong	70	4 mm	low

* "responsive" column indicates awake (A), responsive to verbal stimulation (V), responsive to painful stimulation (P), or unresponsive (U)

** "sim" column indicates whether victim is an actor, low-fidelity simulator (low), or a high-fidelity simulator (high)

Triage:	—use of standard triage protocols to "tag" victims and determine disposition
	—initiation of basic life support interventions to stabilize
Decontamination:	—use of appropriate level of personal protective equipment (PPE)
	—clothing removal from victims (no washdown)
	—minimization of further exposure
Treatment:	—attempts at identification of toxic agent
	—supportive and stabilizing BLS, ACLS interventions
Communication:	—effective communication with and between Hazmat, EMS, fire, and police personnel
	—effective communication between IC and personnel

	—requests for further assistance as needed
	—notification of receiving hospitals of incoming patients and status
	—hospital disaster plan activation
Transport:	—determination of victims to be transported, mode and destination of transfer
	—physical transfer of victims from field location to hospital setting
Definitive treatment:	—identification and management of cholinergic toxicity with atropine infusion / antidotes
	—stabilization and ICU admission
Integration:	—coordination of disaster care with standard medical procedures for following patients
	—2 RED high-fidelity manikins (2 controllers) and 3 YELLOW actors
	—1 non-disaster ACUTE low-fidelity manikin — 83y female, acute MI, unresponsive, intubated, in ventricular fibrillation with no pulses
Incident Debriefing:	—small-group audiovisual-enhanced review of events and actions with moderators
	—general discussion

(This scenario originally appeared in Kabayashi, Medicine and Rhode Island 2003;86:196–200.)

SURGICAL SIMULATION: AN OVERVIEW

Carol L. Lake, MD, MPH, MBA

Demands from the many consumers of surgical services of all types, including general and specialty surgery, have revolutionized the approaches to the teaching and learning of future surgeons. Accreditation agencies expect that the education of surgical residents will occur within strictly controlled work hours; third-party payers expect time-efficient, expert surgical procedures for their clients; and patients themselves no longer accept being "guinea pigs" for fledgling surgical trainees. Among the new approaches is the use of a variety of simulated techniques that may range from a simple piece of fabric for practicing suturing to a sophisticated virtual reality device that simulates laparoscopic surgery or joint replacement.

Thus, ethical issues, patient safety, regulatory rules, and economics are driving the change from surgical education as an apprenticeship or mentorship to a trainee progression from novice to expert with documentation of performance at regular intervals. The subspecialties of orthopedic and urologic surgery have been using simulated techniques for at least several decades. Surgical subspecialties with better defined procedures, such as prostatic resection or joint replacement, may be more amenable to use of a simulated environment than general surgery, in which traumatic injuries and anatomy may be more unique and patient-specific.

In Chapter 15, three general surgeons from the University of Kentucky's Center for Minimally Invasive Surgery, led by Dr. Adrian Park, describe the stages of learning and transfer of training to trainees and the variety of mechanical simulators that are currently available. Examples include laparoscopic models, high-fidelity patient simulators, computer-based simulators, the Minimally Invasive Surgery Training System (MIST), and the future need for real-time interaction with three-dimensional datasets and haptics.

Chapter 16 describes the extensive use of simulation in orthopedic surgery. Simulation in orthopedic surgery has advanced because of the interest of the Association for the Study of Internal Fixation (ASIF) in maximizing restoration of anatomic form and function in injured limbs and their regular dissemination of new developments at annual meetings since the 1960s. ASIF was the first to use simulation in training orthopedic surgeons. Orthopedic simulators are available for the teaching of arthoscopy, total joint surgery, and repair of fractures. Significant research in orthopedic simulators is also ongoing with the support of the national specialty organization, the American Academy of Orthopedic Surgeons.

Chapter 17 discusses the use of physical model-based, computer-based, and hybrid simulators for the training of novices in procedures ranging from digital rectal examination of the prostate through transurethral resection of the prostate to endoscopy and procedures in the upper urinary tract and kidney. Laguna and colleagues detail the learning of psychomotor skills required for genitourinary procedures as well as the educational goals of simulation in urology.

In all of the surgical subspecialties, the state of the art presented in this chapter as a whole should be viewed as only a beginning. As technology continues to advance, more realistic simulators will become available. The ultimate goal may be that all medical students, surgical residents in all specialties, and nonsurgical trainees who perform limited surgical procedures will be initially trained in a simulated environment and demonstrate their competence and skill in a simulated environment before touching a real patient. In addition, fully trained experts eventually will recertify their skills with a simulator. Surgical practitioners in isolated environments will use simulators to learn new techniques and to refresh their skills in infrequently performed procedures. In teaching future surgeons, the best is yet to come.

Chapter 14

SIMULATION IN GENERAL SURGERY

Alejandro Gandsas, MD, Gina L. Adrales, MD,
and Adrian E. Park, MD

Innovation in surgical education has been spurred by increasing concern for patient safety, issues of physician competence and credentialing, and overwhelming cost and time constraints on resident training. It is evident that surgical education should evolve, particularly as technologic advances continue to eclipse traditional clinical therapies. Teaching highly technical skills in the operating room (where surgeons have traditionally been mentored) to trainees who have not previously demonstrated relevant knowledge and visuomotor skills raises significant ethical and safety concerns. Surgical simulation is a response to these needs and concerns, offering a safe, low-stress venue for learning and evaluation. The basis of surgical simulation is multifactorial, as is the variety of available methods of simulation for education and assessment.

Scope of the Problem: Safety, Economics, Ethics

Surgical training is based on clinical need. The issue of patient safety underlies the great need for surgical simulation, with the intent to improve operative performance and patient management through directed practice and assessment. The number of medical errors contributing to patient injury and death is alarming. According to a 1999 Institute of Medicine report, medical errors are responsible for 44 to 98 thousand patient deaths each year.[1,2] In addition, the latest Center for Disease Control (CDC) National Vital Statistics Report (NSVR) identified medical error as the eighth cause of preventable death, ahead of vehicular accidents, breast cancer, and AIDS.[3] Although most surgical errors have been categorized as clerical or administrative, the accidents and errors attributed to individual providers are substantial.[1] Experts have estimated that 2.9–3.7% of patients admitted to U.S. hospitals will suffer injuries caused by medical management, 55% of which will be attributed to medical errors.[4] These errors represent considerable patient morbidity but also contribute to significant economic losses. The financial burden that medical error carries in terms of lost income, lost household production, disability, and health care cost is as high as 30 billion dollars per year.[4] Costs of this magnitude motivate widespread efforts to streamline patient management, adopt clinical care pathways, and increase efficiency in the operating room. Quality of care and operative efficiency should increase with practice and experience. These are all areas in which surgical simulation may play an important role.

The negative effects of medical errors attributed to surgeons make it clear that more surgical education needs to take place outside the arena of patient care. The bottom line is the doctor-patient relationship, and when surgical education is viewed from this perspective, the ethical implications are clear. Responsibility to the patient not only pertains to direct care but also to the proper education of those who are learning through caring for the patient at hand and who will be the practicing surgeons of tomorrow. A high level of skill requires practice. Countless studies have researched the number of cases that represent the learning curve of various procedures.[5-8] As Atul Gawande noted in *The Learning Curve*, "Like everyone else surgeons need practice. That's where you come in."[9] Shocking as this may sound, it is true that surgical education has been based largely on an "apprenticeship" approach. Although our current residency system is more formally organized than its historical predecessor and is now based on graded responsibility, surgery is still largely taught by example and mentorship in the operating room and on the wards. Surgical simulation can and should change this approach by removing considerable learning and practice from the operating room.

Basis of Surgical Simulation

Lessons from the Aviation Industry

Simulation is not new to other professions. Training devices have been implemented in aviation since the early twentieth century. The aviation industry has shown that simulators can reduce the number and type of flight errors by allowing pilots to rehearse different flight scenarios in a controlled environment.[10] Different sources, including the Institute of Medicine, have speculated that surgical simulators may afford similar outcomes if implemented in surgical training.[11] In their 1970 study of aircraft cockpit training, Prophet and Boyd presented a number of conditions under which training devices are justified: (1) high difficulty level of skills, (2) high criticality of skills or tasks, (3) infrequent practice of skills, (4) difficulty of teaching in the operational equipment, (5) safety factors, and (6) cost of using operational equipment for training.[12] It is clear that the practice of general surgery, particularly laparoscopic surgery, meets these criteria for the justification of "training devices."

Stages of Learning and Transfer of Training

Knowledge, cognitive skills, and psychomotor skills are central to surgical education. As outlined by Kopta, the acquisition of motor skills occurs in three stages: (1) cognition, (2) integration, and (3) automation.[13] To master a task, it must first be understood. The specific motor skills are then applied to the task. After time, the skill becomes "automatic" and can essentially be performed efficiently and precisely without prerequisite thinking or evaluation of external cues. As Hamdorf and Hall have shown, the retention of motor skills seems to be more dependent on the degree to which the skill was mastered rather than the environment in which it was learned.[14] In addition, learning is optimized when feedback is incorporated.[15] These principles are the foundation for surgical simulation: basic surgical skills can be attained outside the operating room in a dry lab setting where individualized instruction and feedback are available.

Fidelity and Transfer of Training

Surgical training devices should not only develop desired skills but also should result in transfer of skills to the operating room. Specific task repetition results in better performance than broad training in a number of different skills.[16] The simulator should target specific skills in an environment that will foster their acquisition. However, it is not mandated that the simulation correspond exactly with the actual surgical procedure to result in transfer of the learned skills to the operating suite. In other words, the optimal level of fidelity to the actual surgical procedure for transfer of training (TOT) may be variable, according to the level of expertise of the trainee and the type of exercise (i.e., skill training vs. assessment).

The fidelity of surgical simulators can be examined with respect to several dimensions, including haptic and tactile features, visual cues, and ergonomics. Both high- and low-fidelity models have roles in surgical training. Surgical trainees with little experience may demonstrate significant educational gain from low-fidelity models, such as laparoscopic placement of pins into a pegboard. In contrast, participants with more advanced laparoscopic surgical skills may learn little from these basic tasks but benefit from simulated laparoscopic procedures on porcine models. Novice trainees may be overwhelmed by the complexity and dynamics of such high-fidelity simulations, which incorporate a number of visual and tactile cues and multiple levels of decision-making.

If young surgeons have their initial experience in the operating room, the diversity among the actual patient population may detract from their learning process due to the wide variability in patient presentation for various illnesses and the constellation of prior surgeries and medical problems. This phenomenon is well studied in the aviation literature. The total fidelity of an actual flight environment may be detrimental to the performance of a novice pilot.[16] However, transfer of learned skills by expert pilots to the conduct of real flights is improved with higher-fidelity simulator training. The effectiveness of simulation TOT can be calculated as a transfer effectiveness ratio or (TER).[17] For example, previous studies have established that the TER in aviation is approximately 0.48, suggesting that each hour of flight simulator training is equivalent to approximately a half-hour on an actual aircraft.[18]

As proposed by Alessi and Trollip in 1991,[19] there are four stages of effective instruction: presentation, guidance, practice, and assessment. The level of fidelity of the training simulation should increase with each stage. When these concepts are applied to surgical simulation, it appears that trainees with little surgical experience should be introduced to low-fidelity simulations, such as simple knot-tying exercises[20] (Fig. 1). The law of diminishing returns applies in that these low-fidelity simulations may fail to motivate the expert learner and the rate of learning and TOT become limited.[13] Simulation should also have high fidelity when used to assess trainees as expert performers, whereas training and assessment simulations for instructing and distinguishing novice to intermediate trainees need not be. Simulation fidelity in surgical education should be graduated in accordance with the level of training.

Similarly, part-tasks rather than complex simulations closely resembling entire actual procedures (whole-tasks) are more appropriate for novice surgeons. Part-tasks allow the learner to attend to a limited set of perceptual cues and focus on the acquisition of specific skills. This approach also facilitates repetitive task performance. It follows that a curriculum of part-tasks with increasing complexity, eventually leading to whole-tasks with high fidelity, could be incorporated into surgical resident training. The curriculum should be tailored to the specific skill set desired. Very little TOT from open surgical procedures to laparoscopy seems to occur.[20,21] This finding underscores the need for specific training in laparoscopic skills and runs counter to the expectation that surgeons skilled in advanced open cases will immediately be proficient in laparoscopic procedures.

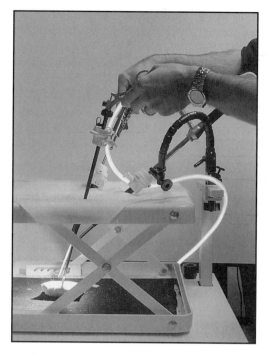

Figure 1. Relationship between simulation fidelity and level of training.

Demonstrated Transfer of Training in Surgery

Demonstration of skill transfer from surgical simulators to the operating room justifies the utility of such training exercises. TOT to the operating room has been shown for a variety of surgical simulators, from inanimate virtual reality systems to animate porcine lab exercises. Skills learned in inanimate bench training models have transferred to performance on porcine models and human cadaver models.[22] Skill transfer to the operating room has also been shown in select studies. Scott et al. provided evidence that intense training in a standard laparoscopic trainer does improve video-hand-eye skills that translate into improved surgery performance for junior residents.[23] The outcome of this study was based on comparing the time that it took for two different groups—a group practicing on the trainer-boxes with operating room (OR) experiences vs. a group experiencing training only in the OR—to accomplish a given task.[23]

With new advances in digital imagery and the development of virtual reality-based computer simulators, Seymour et al. investigated the feasibility of transfer of training from virtual reality training simulator (MIST VR; Fig. 2) to the operating room.[24] Surgical residents exposed to the VR simulator showed a 29% increase in dissection speed and were significantly less likely to fail in making progress or injure the gallbladder. They concluded that VR trainers significantly improve the OR performance of surgical residents in conducting a laparoscopic cholecystectomy.[24] Similar findings have been shown in other studies of both computer-based laparoscopic simulators (LapSim; see Appendix) and virtual trainers.[25–27]

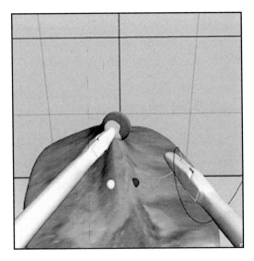

Figure 2. The Minimally Invasive Surgery Training System (MIST) is used to train laparoscopic basic skills to students and residents.

Current State of Surgical Simulation

Many surgical simulators have been developed for training and assessment. They range in design from mechanical task models to mannequin patient simulators and highly sophisticated computer-generated virtual environments. Some simulators focus on part-tasks, others on whole-tasks; some are designed primarily for instruction, others primarily for assessment. The selection of a particular surgical simulator must be made with consideration of the level of experience of the targeted user and thus the requisite level of simulation fidelity.

In the following section, examples of a mechanical model simulator, a patient simulator, and a virtual reality training system will be discussed. Appendix A gives a brief overview of a number of currently available surgical simulators.

Mechanical Simulators

This group of training models is characterized by its nonelectronic and simple, yet effective approach. The most elementary mechanical simulators include tasks such as dropping beans into a cup or inserting pins into a peg-board to develop the basic perceptual-motor skills required for laparoscopic surgery.[28–33] Knot-tying, bowel anastomosis, and vascular anastomosis simulations are examples of open surgery mechanical simulators. More complex mechanical models are directed to more comprehensive procedural skills, such as laparoscopic appendectomy, that combine several basic skills.

University of Kentucky Laparoscopic Models

The University of Kentucky Laparoscopic Models (UKLM) were developed as part of a resident curriculum to teach laparoscopic skills.[34] These mechanical models are part-task simulations, representing key portions of the corresponding laparoscopic procedures (Fig. 3). For example, the laparoscopic cholecystectomy and cholangiography simulation targets cystic duct dissection and cholangiocatheter insertion. The UKLM

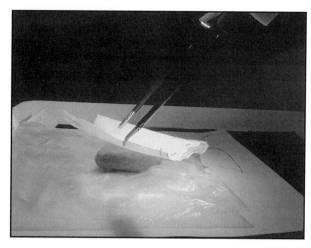

Figure 3. University of Kentucky Training Model uses puppet-like organs to teach basic and advanced laparoscopic skills.

include simulations of laparoscopic inguinal herniorrhaphy, appendectomy, cholecystectomy, splenectomy, bowel mobilization and enterotomy repair, and Nissen fundoplication. Increasingly complex models are incorporated into the residency curriculum to match a rising level of surgical experience.

The materials and design of these models are carefully selected to maintain at least a moderate level of fidelity to the actual procedure in terms of appearance, tissue characteristics, and handling. Inclusion of actual laparoscopic images into the background environment for these models has also contributed to the face validity.[34]

The UKLM shares a cost advantage with other mechanical models when compared with advanced technology, computer-based systems. This advantage contributes to the widespread accessibility of mechanical models for surgical residency programs. The majority of materials used in these models can be purchased at a nominal cost, and several other items are reusable or renewable.

The UKLM may be used for assessment in addition to training. Performance is videotaped and assessed by trained faculty evaluators on a global scale grading five items: (1) clinical judgment or respect for tissue, (2) dexterity, (3) serial/simultaneous complexity (flow of the operation), (4) spatial orientation, and (5) overall competence in each simulation. In addition, a checklist assessment for errors and completed models assessments (e.g., accuracy of clip and tack placement) can be performed by nonclinicians.

Patient Simulator

This type of surgical simulator, generally an inanimate human form, trains the student by using a familiar interface (the patient). The incorporation of one of the best-known patient simulators, the Harvey cardiac simulator, into a skills course at the University of Michigan resulted in significantly improved cardiac examination skills as measured by pre- and post-tests.[35] Patient simulators offer the benefit of practice of physical diagnosis skills in a safe, controlled environment—skills that can then be applied to patient care.

Medical Education Technology Inc. (METI) Simulator

The METI simulator (Fig. 4) is a full-size mannequin that integrates sophisticated electronic and mechanical mechanisms to emulate physiologic cardiopulmonary responses. This mannequin is connected to a customized monitoring system capable of displaying EKG, blood pressure, temperature, cardiac output, and oxygen saturation among other routine parameters usually seen in the intensive care unit. The METI unit allows the user to practice airway and ventilator management while monitoring the resultant physiologic changes. More than 50 common drugs used in advanced cardiac and advanced trauma life support (ACLS/ATLS) courses can be administered to the mannequin while the student assesses the response. Trainees are also able to practice cardiopulmonary resuscitation (CPR) techniques, endotracheal intubation, chest tube insertion, pulse palpation that varies according to the current simulated hemodynamic status, and neurologic assessment by checking pupil size and reactivity to light. Although the METI unit is a significant advancement in simulation technology, it lacks real-time feedback. Assessment is usually provided by an onsite instructor.[36]

Computer-based Simulators

Computer-based simulators are responsible for creating virtual worlds using two-dimensional structures named polygons. By combining multiple polygons together, a smooth three-dimensional object can be generated.[37] In order for the viewer to experience the three-dimensional effect of an image, the object must be perceived by each eye individually and the final image regenerated in the brain using both pieces of information. This phenomenon is known as stereopsis.[38,39] The liquid crystal display (LCD) of a head-mounted display unit can achieve this effect by having the display screens slightly offset from each other. Three-dimensional video monitors with special glasses can accomplish the same effect by including an active shutter.[40]

Most three-dimensional images are obtained through a process called segmentation, in which the anatomic structure represented in the simulator is taken from computerized scanners, MRIs, or other raw input. One of the most commonly used datasets comes

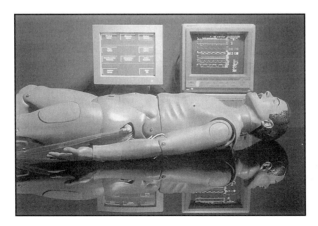

Figure 4. The METI–Human Patient Simulator. (courtesy Randy S. Haluck, MD. PennState, Director of Surgical Simulation).

from the Visible Human Project, which consists of 1-mm frozen slice images photographed and scanned in the transverse plane.[41]

Following segmentation, each organ's properties (e.g., elasticity, density) are calculated so that they can be rendered accurately. This step, known as tissue modeling, adds realism to organ manipulation. Adapted surgical instruments are often used as the user input interface to interact with the organs, programmed to reflect mathematical computations of collision forces between the tissue and the instruments (i.e., tissue-tool interaction). By integrating both tissue modeling and tissue-tool interaction, the simulation allows the user to "feel" the tissue being manipulated. This phenomenon, known as haptics, is one of the most exciting areas under development, since the technology can be used in conjunction with robotics for telemedical applications in the battlefield or in space.

Computer-based simulators can be categorized as immersive or nonimmersive, depending on how the information is displayed to the user. Although both types of simulators use virtual reality technology to create objects in three dimensions, they differ in the way those images are delivered. Immersive virtual reality systems generally use a head-mounted display connected to the computer output, therefore isolating the user from the real world. The nonimmersive simulator outputs are mainly based on monitors or holographic images. Both types have advantages and disadvantages; the appropriate choice depends on their intended purpose.[17]

The construct validity and reliability of virtual reality trainers have been established in recent studies. Gallagher et al. reported that a virtual reality simulator was able to distinguish novice, junior, and senior laparoscopists when differences in speed, economy of movements, and use of diathermy were measured.[42] In another study by Gallagher and Satava, experienced laparoscopic surgeons performed tasks faster with less error and greater efficiency and consistency. The reliability for the performance measures was consistently high ($\alpha = 0.89$ to 0.98).[43] As mentioned, transfer of training from virtual reality simulators to the operating room has also been demonstrated.

Minimally Invasive Surgery Training System

The Minimally Invasive Surgery Training System (MIST) uses high-end virtual reality software to teach and assess basic laparoscopic skills (see Fig. 2). Desktop computers can be customized to interface with two laparoscopic instruments through an electronic link. The system is adequate to train students in simple laparoscopic tasks. Training on the MIST VR may help students acquire laparoscopic psychomotor skills faster than they would without such training.[44] Although MIST VR does not provide any haptic information, the system is able to record and keep a log of the time employed for each task, efficacy of movements, and number of errors. These datasets can be used to compare individuals or for self-assessment.[45] Currently, researchers using the MIST-VR simulator have demonstrated construct validity in the assessment of skill level.[45]

Hybrid Simulators

Hybrid simulators combine the sophistication of computer-based simulation with the flexibility, expandability, and cost benefits of a mechanical trainer. The optimal hybrid simulator allows the use of any type of laparoscopic, thorocoscopic, or arthroscopic instruments. The tips of the instruments are tracked and either displayed directly on the video screen (as they interact with mechanical models) or reconfigured to appear and respond, in real time, in a virtual environment.

An example of such a hybrid is the Pro MIS Surgical Simulator. Trainees practice with real instruments in a mechanical trainer with normal laparoscopic degrees of freedom and haptic feedback. Trocar positions in the "body form" trainer box are not fixed or limited. Ports can be inserted according to surgeon preference. Real tissues or mechanical models can also be placed within the trainer. Conversely the surgeon can elect to use his or her real instruments in the trainer to interact with a virtual model. While the surgeons complete a task, their performance can be tracked and analyzed in real time against metrics established for that particular task. Immediate feedback is then offered to the surgeon.

Residency Training

Surgical residency training is becoming increasingly stressed by financial pressures, liability issues, and time restrictions caused by work-hour limits and overwhelming noneducational responsibilities in the workplace. Surgical simulation may address these problems by allowing practice of skills in a protected environment—practice that may increase operative and clinical management efficiency and patient safety. Procedural techniques that have a steep learning curve and require repeated practice are particularly suited to simulator training. However, for simulation technology to make a real impact in surgical education, it should be incorporated into an educational curriculum as opposed to stand-alone training devices without appropriate guidance and feedback.[8] Virtual reality systems may continue to evolve to higher-fidelity simulators with improved haptic feedback, but the role of lower-cost, accessible mechanical simulators should not be diminished. As previously emphasized, the simulation should be directed to the experience level of the trainee for optimal transfer of training. A continuum of surgical simulators, from low to high fidelity, part- to whole-task, and training and/or assessment simulations in various surgical procedures (laparoscopic and open) may represent the ideal curriculum applicable to all levels of training.

The Future of Surgical Simulation

Over the past ten years there have been significant advances in simulation technology. From inanimate models to sophisticated machines that integrate computer robotics and state-of-the-art digital imaging, surgical simulators promise a change in the paradigm of surgical training and planning. Incorporating simulators into a residency curriculum can enhance a surgery program by providing residents with exposure to a variety of cases, including infrequent but important procedures and surgical complications. Surgical simulators may also play a role in assessing surgical competency, obtaining hospital privileges, and certification and recertification by a specialty medical board. Surgical simulation will address the current financial and ethical dilemma of teaching surgical skills solely in the operating room. In addition, simulation technology can overcome the decreasing availability of and limited interest in animal or cadaveric models for surgical training.[46]

Despite significant advances in simulation technology, more training challenges await us in the future. It is crucial for simulation technology to achieve real time interaction with three-dimensional datasets without losing graphics resolution. Moore's Law predicted in 1965 that computational power availability would double every 18 months; thus, it is likely that real-time interaction with realistic visual imagery will eventually be achieved.[47] Unlike flight simulators, surgical simulators and surgical teaching rely on force feedback, the ability to "feel" the tissue while it is being handled. By "touching" the organs and their surroundings, the surgeon obtains definitive information necessary to plan the strategy of an operation. Surgical simulation research should develop more precise haptic interfaces that will allow better response to virtual manipulation and tissue handling.

To gain acceptance from the medical community, simulation technology needs to become more readily available to training institutions, most of which struggle with budget limitations. If the industry's goal is widespread medical use of its more costly technology, the industry must find a way to make it available in academic venues. In addition, transfer of training should continue to be studied. Strong demonstration of its validity is crucial if simulation is to fulfill its potential for enhancing both surgical training and patient safety. Only convincing evidence that performance on simulators is relevant to performance in the operating room will clear the way for incorporating simulators into educational, training, and credentialing curricula for surgeons.

Conclusion

The role of surgical simulation in training, assessment, and credentialing will continue to expand as new technologies emerge, enhancing both surgical skills and patient safety. Skill development and assessment via simulators can supplement established avenues of surgical education, such as directed didactic sessions, bedside teaching, procedural instruction in the operating room, and faculty evaluation and mentorship. Yet it should be remembered that the most advanced technical skills cannot replace good surgical judgment, based on solid knowledge and understanding of surgical principles.

Acknowledgments

Donald B. Witzke, Ph.D., of the University of Kentucky College of Medicine, provided key sources for this chapter.

References

1. Roscoe LA, Krizek TJ: Reporting medical errors. Bull Am Col Surg 2002;87(9):12–17.
2. Kohn LT, Corrigan JM, Donaldson MS: To Err Is Human: Building a Safer Health System. Washington, DC, National Academy Press, 1999, p 1.
3. Centers for Disease Control and Prevention (National Center for Health Statistics): Deaths: Final Data for 1997. National Vital Statistics Reports 1999;47(19):27.
4. Thomas EJ, Studdert DM, Newhouse JP, et al: Costs of medical injuries in Utah and Colorado. Inquiry 1999;36:255–264.
5. Liem MS, van Steensel CJ, Boelhouwer RU, et al: The learning curve for totally extraperitoneal laparoscopic inguinal hernia repair. Am J Surg. 1996;171:281–285.
6. Watson DI, Baigrie RJ, Jamieson GG: A learning curve for laparoscopic fundoplication. Ann Surg 1996;224(2):198–203.
7. Schauer P, Ikramuddin S, Hamad G, Gourash W: The learning curve for laparoscopic Roux-en-Y gastric bypass is 100 cases. Surg Endosc. 2003;17:212–215.
8. Park A, Witzke D, Donnelly M: Ongoing deficits in resident training for minimally invasive surgery. J Gastrointest Surg 2002;6:501–507; discussion, 507–509.
9. Gawande A: The learning curve: Like everyone else, surgeons need practice. That's where you come in. New Yorker 2002;Jan. 28:52–56.

10. Croft JW: Refuse-to-crash: NASA tackles loss of control. Aerosp Am 2003;41(3):42–45.
11. Rosser JC Jr : Minimally invasive surgical training solutions for the twenty-first century. Surg Clin North Am 2000;80:1607–1624.
12. Prophet WW, Boyd HA: Device-task fidelity and transfer of training: Aircraft cockpit procedures training. 1970.
13. Kopta JA: An approach to the evaluation of operative skills. Surgery 1971;70:297–303.
14. Hamdorf JM, Hall JC: Acquiring surgical skills. Br J Surg 2000;87:28–37.
15. Fischman MG, Oxendine JB: Motor skill learning for effective coaching and performance. In Williams JM (ed): Applied Sport Psychology, 3rd ed. Mountain View, CA, Mayfield, 1998, pp 11–24.
16. Noble C: The relationship between fidelity and learning in aviation training and assessment. J Air Transport 2002;7(3):33–54.
17. Edmond CV Jr, Wiet GJ, Bolger B: Virtual environments: Surgical simulation in otolaryngology. Comput Otolaryngol 1998;31:369–381.
18. Johnston R, Bhoyrul S, Way L, et al: Assessing a virtual reality surgical skills simulator. Stud Health Technol Inform 1996;29:608–617.
19. Alessi SM, Trollip SR: Computer-based Instruction: Methods and Development. Englewood Cliffs, NJ, Prentice Hall, 1991.
20. Figert PL, Park AE, Witzke DB, Schwartz RW: Transfer of training in acquiring laparoscopic skills. J Am Coll Surg 2001;193(5):533–537.
21. Grantcharov TP, Bardram L, Funch-Jensen P, et al: Learning curves and impact of previous operative experience on performance on a virtual reality simulator to test laparoscopic surgical skills. Am J Surg 2003;185:146–149.
22. Fried GM, Derossis AM, Bothwell J, Sigman HH: Comparison of laparoscopic performance in vivo with performance measured in laparoscopic simulator. Surg Endosc 1999;13(11): 1077–1081; discussion, 1982.
23. Scott DJ, Bergen PC, Rege RV, et al: Laparoscopic training on bench models: Better and more cost effective than operating room experience? J Am Coll Surg 2000;191:272–283.
24. Seymour NE, Gallagher AG, Roman SA, et al: Virtual reality training improves operating room performance: Results of a randomized, double-blinded study. Ann Surg 2002;236: 458–463; discussion, 463–464.
25. Hamilton EC, Scott DJ, Fleming JR, et al: Comparison of video trainer and virtual reality training systems on acquisition of laparoscopic skills. Surg Endosc 2002;16:406–411.
26. Hamilton EC, Scott DJ, Kapoor A, et al: Improving operative performance using a laparoscopic hernia simulator Am J Surg 2001;182:725–728.
27. Hyltander A, Liljegren E, Rhodin PH, Lönroth H: The transfer of basic skills learned in a laparoscopic simulator to the operating room. Surg Endosc 2002;16(3):1324–1328.
28. Rosser JC, Rosser LE, Savalgi RS: Skill acquisition and assessment for laparoscopic surgery. Arch Surg 1997;132:200–204.
29. Rosser JC, Rosser LE, Savalgi RS: Objective evaluation of a laparoscopic surgical skill program for residents and senior surgeons. Arch Surg 1998;133:657–661.
30. Melvin WS, Johnson JA, Ellison EC: Laparoscopic skills enhancement. Am J Surg 1996;172:377–379.
31. Chung JY, Sakier JM: A method of objectively evaluating improvements in laparoscopic skills. Surg Endosc 1998;12:1111–1116
32. Derossis AM, Fried GM, Abrahamowicz M, et al: Development of a model for training and evaluation of laparoscopic skills. Am J Surg 1998;175:482–487.
33. Risucci D, Cohen JA, Garbus JE, et al: The effects of practice and instruction on speed and accuracy during resident acquisition of simulated laparoscopic skills. Curr Surg 2001;58:230–235.
34. Adrales GL, Chu UB, Witzke DB, et. al: Evaluating minimally invasive surgery training using low-cost mechanical simulations. Surg Endosc 2003;17:580–585.
35. Woolliscroft JO, Calhoun JG, TenHaken JD, Judge RD: Harvey: The impact of cardiovascular teaching simulator on student skill acquisition. Med Teach 1987;9:53–57.
36. Schwid HA, Rooke GA, Carline J, et al: Evaluation of anesthesia residents using mannequin-based simulation: A multiinstitutional study. Anesthesiology 2002;97:1434–1444.

37. Coleman J, Nduka CC, Darzi A: Virtual reality and laparoscopic surgery. Br J Surg 1994;81: 1709–1711.
38. Chan M, Lin W, Zhou C, Qu JY: Miniaturized three-dimensional endoscopic imaging system based on active stereovision. Appl Opt. 2003;42:1888–1898.
39. Passmore PJ, Read OJ, Nielsen CF, et al: Effects of perspective and stereo on depth judgements in virtual reality laparoscopy simulation. Stud Health Technol Inform 2000;70: 243–245.
40. Kourambas J, Preminger GM: Advances in camera, video, and imaging technologies in laparoscopy. Urol Clin North Am 2001;28:5–14.
41. Temkin B, Acosta E, Hatfield P, et al: Web-based three-dimensional Virtual Body Structures: W3D-VBS. J Am Med Inform Assoc 2002;9:425–436.
42. Gallagher AG, Richie K, McClure N, McGuigan J: Objective psychomotor skills assessment of experienced, junior and novice laparoscopists with virtual reality. World J Surg 2001; 25:1478–1483.
43. Gallagher AG, Satava RM: Virtual reality as a metric for the assessment of laparoscopic psychomotor skills. Learning curves and reliability measures. Surg Endosc 2002;16:1746–1752.
44. Jordan JA, Gallagher AG, McGuigan J, McClure N: Virtual reality training leads to faster adaptation to the novel psychomotor restrictions encountered by laparoscopic surgeons. Surg Endosc 2001;15:1080–1084.
45. Taffinder N, Sutton C, Fishwick RJ, et al: Validation of virtual reality to teach and assess psychomotor skills in laparoscopic surgery: Results from randomised controlled studies using the MIST VR laparoscopic simulator. Stud Health Technol Inform 1998;50:124–130.
46. Satava RM: Surgical education and surgical simulation. World J Surg 2001;25:1484–1489.
47. Moore GE: Electronics. 1965;38 (8):114–117.
48. Macmillan AI, Cuschieri A: Assessment of innate ability and skills for endoscopic manipulations by the Advanced Dundee Endoscopic Psychomotor Tester: Predictive and concurrent validity. Am J Surg 1999;177:274–247.
49. Schijven MP, Jackmowicz J, Schot C: The Advanced Dundee Endoscopic Psychomotor Tester (ADEPT) objectifying subjective psychomotor test performance. Surg Endosc 2002; 16:943–948.
50. Martin JA, Regehr G, Reznick R, et al: Objective structured assessment of technical skill (OSATS) for surgical residents. Br J Surg 1997;84:273–278.
51. Derossis AM, Antoniuk M, Fried GM: Evaluation of laparoscopic skills: A 2-year follow-up during residency training. Can J Surg 1999;42(4):293–296.
52. Shapiro MJ, Kobayashi L, Morchi R: High-fidelity medical simulation and its role in evaluating advanced cardiac life support (ACLS) skills. Acad Emerg Med 2003 10(5):488.
53. Sedlack RE, Kolars JC: Colonoscopy curriculum development and performance-based assessment criteria on a computer-based endoscopy simulator. Acad Med 2002;77:750–751.
54. Reznek MA, Rawn CL, Krummel TM: Evaluation of the educational effectiveness of a virtual reality intravenous insertion simulator. Acad Emerg Med 2002;9(11):1319–1325.
55. Weale AR, Mitchell DC: A do-it-yourself vascular anastomosis simulator. Ann R Coll Surg Engl 2003;85(2):132.
56. Arezzo A, Ulmer F, Weiss O, et al: Experimental trial on solo surgery for minimally invasive therapy: comparison of different systems in a phantom model. Surg Endosc 2000;14: 955–959.
57. Knudson MM, Sisley AC: Training residents using simulation technology: experience with ultrasound for trauma. J Trauma 2000;48:659–665.
58. Gordon MS, Ewy GA, Felner JM, et al: Teaching bedside cardiologic examination skills using "Harvey", the cardiology patient simulator. Med Clin North Am 1980;64(2):305–313.
59. Jones JS, Hunt SJ, Carlson SA, Seamon JP: Assessing bedside cardiologic examination skills using "Harvey," a cardiology patient simulator. Acad Emerg Med 1997;4:980–985.

Appendix

SIMULATION SYSTEMS

1. ADEPT (Advanced Dundee Endoscopic Psychomotor Tester): This system, designed by Sir Alfred Cuschieri, objectively evaluates mainly psychomotor skills and ability rather than task performance during simulated endoscopic procedures.[48] The ADEPT system is thought to be able to identify individuals with the necessary psychomotor skills required to perform laparoscopic procedures.[48]
2. OSATS (Objective Structured Assessment of Technical Skill): Designed by Carol R. Hutchison, M.D., and supported by the Academy's Council on Education and by the Orthopaedic Research and Education Foundation, the OSATS is a multi-station performance-based examination designed to measure the effectiveness of surgical education activities.[50]
3. MISTELS (McGill Inanimate System for Training and Evaluation of Laparoscopic Skills): Designed by McGill University to evaluate laparoscopic technical skills through a series of tasks, taking into account precision and speed of movements.[51]
4. UK-CMIS (University of Kentucky–Center for Minimally Invasive Surgery): These models for training and assessing surgical performance consist of inexpensive mechanical model simulations that resemble abdominal organs[34] (see Fig 3).
5. Laerdal SimMan — Universal Patient Simulator: This simulator assesses the student on different clinical and decision-making skills during realistic patient care scenarios. The SimMan is the most common simulator used during the ATLS/ ACS courses and anesthesia training programs.[52]
6. LapSim (Surgical Science): High-end software that relies on three-dimensional modeling to simulate a laparoscopic procedure. The LapSim is integrated to a virtual laparoscopic interface that tracks the motion of a pair of laparoscopic graspers that navigate through three-dimensional space. Each instrument allows 5 degrees of freedom, including pitch and yaw motions. With the LapSim, the student has an opportunity to acquire basic laparoscopic skills, including camera navigation, grasping and transferring objects, and intracorporeal knot tying. The company's latest software version, LapSim Dissection, simulates an entire laparoscopic cholecystectomy. The student dissects and divides the cystic duct between clips and may even use suction irrigation if the surgical field becomes obscured with bleeding. The LapSim is able to track student performance and generate a report after each exercise.
7. Accutouch Endoscopy Simulator: This system offers three types of simulated endoscopic procedures: flexible bronchoscopy, flexible sigmoidoscopy, and colonoscopy. The module consists of a human-shaped mannequin, customized for upper and lower endoscopic procedures only. The input interface is a scoped-shape module that interacts with a computer in real time. During the simulation, a navigation map of the bronchial tree and the upper or lower gastrointestinal tract can be displayed for

orientation purposes. One of the main advantages of this system is the ability to provide the trainee with instructional information and anatomy tutorials before hand, real-time feedback while the simulation is in progress, and constructive feedback after the simulation has been completed.[53]

8. CathSim Vascular Access Simulator: This simulator was developed to teach the technique of intravenous catheterization. A sophisticated haptic device provides the "pop" force-feedback that results when the operator pierces the lumen of the vessel. This simulator uses virtual reality (VR) technology as a visual aid and provides outcomes feedback at the end of the exercise.[54]

9. The Minimally Invasive Surgery Training System or MIST uses high-end virtual reality software to instruct on basic laparoscopic skills (see Fig. 2). Desktop computers can be customized to interface with two laparoscopic instruments through an electronic link. The system is able to instruct trainees in simple laparoscopic tasks. It is able to record and keep a log of time employed for each task, efficacy of movements and number of errors. These datasets can be used to compare individuals or be used as self assessment.[45]

10. Endoscopic Sinus Surgical Simulator: This is a nonimmersive type simulator developed by Madigan Army Center in collaboration with several academic centers for training surgeons in endoscopic sinus surgery.[17] The rigidity of the anatomy of the sinus region allows a steady and nondeformable environment easy to replicate within the simulator. The main goal is to make the user familiar with anatomical landmarks rather than develop psychomotor skills.

11. Anastomosis Simulator (Boston Dynamics Inc.): This simulator allows students and residents to rehearse the complexity and the choreography of movements involved in performing a vascular anastomosis. One of the main features of this machine is that the computer gives the trainee a continuous assessment of his/her skills performance in real time, indicating the amount of pressure or accuracy of the hand motion.[55]

12. The Phantom (Sensable Technologies, Cambridge, MA): The Phantom arm is an external piece of hardware that is connected into the serial port of a personal computer, usually running VR applications. The arm is capable of providing the user with 6 degrees of freedom input and 3 degrees of freedom output combined with a high-fidelity three-dimensional force-feedback that allows the trainee to feel the collision and reaction forces and torques of an object.[56]

13. UltraSim: An ultrasound simulator machine that stores patient data in three-dimensional images. Students are able to reconstruct such images in real time by scanning on the mannequin.

14. Promis (Haptica Ltd., Dublin): A laparoscopic simulator that combines real-world and virtual training exercises and environments. Real-time tracking of performance allows immediate feedback to the surgeon.

Chapter 15

SIMULATION IN ORTHOPEDIC SURGERY

Joseph A. O'Daniel, BS, Craig S. Roberts, MD, and David Seligson, MD

Simulators have long been used to train pilots. When stakes are high and the costs of errors are loss of life or expensive equipment, simulators have an important niche for training novices. They allow complicated maneuvers and dangerous situations to be rehearsed without facing the consequences of failure. Feedback can be provided when mistakes are made during a simulated task, and progression of the learning curve can be charted.

Because of the level of difficulty involved in orthopedic surgery and the consequences of surgical errors, simulators are attractive and potentially useful. In fact, simulated operations are routinely performed on cadavers in many orthopedic residency programs. Over 50% of orthopedic residency training institutions report using cadaveric wet labs.[1] However, cadaver training is usually limited to 2–3 days before the specimen becomes unusable. Surgical simulation ranges from cadaveric wet labs to purely computer simulation or physical model simulators incorporating actual surgical instruments with computer virtual reality displays.

An example of a successful simulator program with 45 years of proven success is the teaching of fracture surgery.

Association for the Study of Internal Fixation

After World War II, many new surgical techniques, especially in the fields of gastrointestinal and lung surgery, were developed. However, orthopedic surgery lagged behind for several reasons. According to Urs Heim in *The AO Phenomenon*, "Fractures at the time were rarely life-threatening because the polytraumatized generally died before reaching the hospital."[2] Traction and casting were the preferred techniques, with patients remaining in the hospital for months. The concept of open reduction with internal fixation was accepted, but surgical equipment lacked development and the technique remained largely conceptual. As Heim observes, "There was a consensus that the prognosis for articular fractures could only be improved by open reduction and fixation, but this was rarely attempted due to lack of technical experience and fear of infection or the operation was only performed after many weeks of procrastination. Poor results were attributed to the method."[2] Heim noted three elements that were lacking in developing orthopedics: "Reliable instrument sets, asepsis appropriate for the implantation of metal foreign bodies, and specially trained surgeons."[2]

Maurice Müller, a Swiss Orthopedist, created the concept of a school of operative technique, which he named Association pour l'Osteosynthese (AO). The concept was inspired through a combination of friendship, requisite military training in the Swiss Army, and courses about nonorthopedic surgical instruction. The resulting conference,

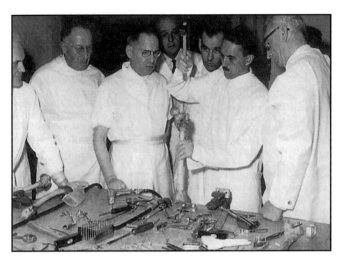

Figure 1. One of the first AO Courses, held in 1960. Dr. Müller demonstrates the insertion of a femoral nail during practical exercises. (From Heim U: The AO Phenomenon. Seattle, Hogrefe and Huber, 2001, with permission).

held 15–17 March 1958, marked the first instance of simulation training in orthopedic technique (Fig. 1). Held in Chur, Switzerland, the conference became regarded as the "first extended AO conference because of its structure and content. In three working days, the whole known spectrum of traumatology and related problems had been discussed."[2]

AO, also known as the Association for the Study of Internal Fixation (ASIF), grew through yearly conferences with hands-on workshops. The first conference in 1958 established the need for the development of specially designed orthopedic instruments, which Müller undertook with a Swiss metallurgist named Robert Mathys. Ensuing conferences included instruction on the "four advocated methods of internal fixation on human bones," including the newly developed instruments.[2]

The initial goals of ASIF were (1) to allow a privileged level of working together toward a definite objective; (2) to offer operative treatment to patients who would benefit; (3) to inform members about the current status and further developments of instruments and implants; (4) to allow maximal restoration of anatomic form and function of the injured limb (osteosynthesis that permits immediate mobilization); (5) to promote the shortest socially and economically justifiable hospital stay, with rapid return to work; and (6) to preserve soft tissues, and especially the vessels.[2] ASIF holds the distinction of being the first organization to use simulation in orthopedic training.

Orthopedic Simulator Objectives

ASIF sets the standard in orthopedic simulation because of its highly focused objectives, proven history, and rigorous scientific examination of surgical technique and outcome. For any orthopedic simulator to be successful, its purpose must be clearly identified. Potential surgical simulator objectives include the following: (1) to improve surgical outcomes or patient satisfaction; (2) to teach procedural technique and repetitive movements; (3) to provide feedback on surgical technique; (4) to maintain existing surgical skills not routinely used; (5) to validate skills such as certifying graduating residents or recertifying licensed physicians; (6) to aid in presurgical planning; and (7) to decrease costs by decreasing operating room time.

Simulators face numerous challenges in filling the above objectives, all centering on the artificiality of virtual reality training. Ultimately, surgical simulators are not real surgery; a patient's life is not at risk. The attendant stresses of operating on live persons cannot be adequately simulated. Complications that arise in the operating room during procedures are numerous and difficult to simulate. Whereas a simulator or virtual reality trainer can always be reset, the operating room is much less forgiving. Simulation development should strive to address these issues as well as anatomic correctness and feedback on technique.

This chapter examines simulators currently under development for arthroscopy, total joint surgery, and fracture applications. The focus is on what makes each simulator unique and the objectives that it attempts to fulfill. Simulators currently in use are then reviewed, and the future of orthopedic simulation is discussed.

Simulators Under Development

Virtual reality (VR) surgical training aims to improve the education of surgeons by offering a realistic experience, teaching basic skills of navigation with surgical equipment, and helping the surgeon learn the ordered steps of both arthroscopic examination and surgical repair.

VR also provides the opportunity to learn surgical technique and operation sequences without incurring operating room costs or risks to patients. The American Academy of Orthopaedic Surgeons (AAOS) believes that VR can be superior to traditional surgical instruction because (1) the simulator user can see and feel everything that surgical instruments are doing; (2) simulators are available on demand and are not dependent on operating room time or specimen availability; (3) medical education can become more uniform; and (4) no risk is incurred by patients.[3]

To produce the desired results, VR must achieve several goals. First, it must provide good simulation of reality, of actual surgery. Second, training on a simulator must be validated or deemed time worthy and somewhat lifelike by experienced surgeons. Third, the training system has to be cost-effective and ideally, PC-compatible. The simulator must provide objective assessment based on established task lists. Finally, the VR experience needs to have sensory realism, including tactile (haptic) feedback, audio reality, and visual reality.

Arthroscopic Surgery

The word arthroscopy comes from the Greek words *arthro,* (joint) and *skopein* (to look). This minimally invasive surgical procedure allows an orthopedic surgeon to "look within joints" through small incisions. Slender, pencil-sized instruments are inserted into the joint through dime-sized incisions, using a fiberoptic camera. This allows the inside of a joint to be viewed under magnification and displayed on a video monitor.[4]

Arthroscopic surgery demands skills that are different from traditional, open surgery.

With the scope one triangulates the position of instruments in a joint by following on a two-dimensional video monitor. To learn this skill, training can be done on cadavers, animals, or physical models.

Knee Arthroscopy Simulators

The Sheffield Model. The University of Sheffield in England has developed a PC-based knee arthroscopy simulator system. This system uses replicas of surgical instruments and a virtual camera, along with a three-dimensional model of the knee, to simulate core features of arthroscopy.[5] The goal of this project is to teach basic elements of arthroscopic technique and offer specific instruction and feedback on four common orthopedic procedures.

The simulated surgical procedures include trimming of meniscal tears, suturing of the patella tendon, cauterization of blood vessels, and reconstruction of the anterior cruciate ligament. Both experienced and trainee surgeons used the model to test the simulator's realism. Valuable lessons were learned from initial trials, the most prominent being that "an optimal training environment should be task-driven and not simulation-driven." Basic skills training and assessment were determined to be the primary objective. System and model improvements have focused on the following objectives: (1) modifications to lighting and field of view, improved update rate, improved design of the replica of the lower limb, and intersection testing for the soft tissue components; (2) emphasis on forming tasks to develop core psychomotor skills rather than procedure simulation alone; (3) evidence that skills developed on the simulator are similar to those used in real-world arthroscopy; and (4) inclusion of simulation of deformation of menisci.[5]

Through surveys and questionnaires, essential skills were identified for both arthroscopic diagnosis and surgical treatment: (1) triangulation (bringing the instrument into field of view of the camera); (2) orientation within the joint; (3) identification of anatomic landmarks; (4) appropriate limb manipulation; and (5) visual-guided control of the camera and instruments.[5]

The Sheffield project determined that the best way to maintain system cost effectiveness is to design the simulator to run on a standard personal computer. System requirements include a Pentium Pro 200MHz with 128Mb RAM and 550 graphics card. Software employed includes World Toolkit (WTK) Release 7 from EAI Sense8 with Visual C++.[5]

Medical Physics and Clinical Engineering created the knee model through the Knees Up EU Project. MRI scan slices were incorporated into a three-dimensional reconstruction of the knee. To create feedback on position and location within the knee joint, visual orientation was provided via computer display. However, touch sensation was not simulated.

To stimulate the feeling of moving medical instruments inside a joint space requires force feedback as part of the virtual reality experience. The virtual reality term for force feedback is haptic, which literally means "of or relating to the sense of touch; tactile." Without the sensation of resistance from skin, muscle, joint fluid, and even delicate joint surfaces, training on a model of any joint lacks a high degree of reality. Because the Sheffield model lacked haptic feedback, collisions were indicated by visual and auditory simulation.[5]

The model not only needs to sense lifting of the meniscus; it must also provide timely feedback to the surgeon to make the experience life-like. Developers used World Toolkit software to allow movement of the meniscus, followed by remodeling of the visual presentation to the viewer. This software has allowed real-time update rates to be achieved.

A study of the system was conducted to verify whether the simulator had the potential to "train core skills." This study involved simulating a joint inspection and triangulation exercise. The object was to locate ten yellow spheres within the joint capsule while minimizing collisions. Once located, the spheres had to be triangulated with the virtual probe tip. A fat pad was created that "imposed a penalty on non-optimal entry pathways by occluding the joint view."[6] The test assessed the total time required to complete the task as well as the number of collisions incurred.

Results demonstrated that the system was able to distinguish between experienced and novice surgeons as well as a control group. Greater surgical experience correlated with shorter simulation time and fewer collisions. Both novices and experienced surgeons reported the simulation to be worthwhile.

Experienced arthroscopic surgeons reported that the major drawback of the experiment was the lack of haptic feedback. Haptics place the user's motion into a computer, which then provides the sensation of tactile feedback. Current plans call for future developments to incorporate haptic feedback to increase the reality of the simulation experience.

The benefits of the Sheffield Model include training surgeons in minimally invasive techniques before they operate on patients. In addition, the model provides objective assessment of surgical skills.

Virtual Reality Arthroscopic Knee Simulator (VR-AKS) Project. The American Academy of Orthopedic Surgeons (AAOS) began investigating virtual reality for orthopedic surgery training in 1997. The AAOS believes that virtual reality can be superior to traditional training in four ways: (1) VR involves no risk to the patient; (2) the simulator user can see and feel what surgical instruments are doing, mimicking reality; (3) simulators are not dependent on operating room time or case presentation to the hospital; and (4) VR can make medical education more uniform. In addition, VR has the potential to reduce the time, effort, and money required to train residents in anatomic relationships.[3]

Virtual reality surgery can also teach difficult arthroscopic techniques to residents, especially "triangulation, spatial relationships, and eye-hand control."[7] In a study conducted by the AAOS in 1999, "time savings" was seen as the largest benefit of a VR arthroscopic simulator. Other benefits included the value of the learning experience and a reduction in the cost of cadaver training.

The American Board of Orthopaedic Surgery (ABOS) is interested in the VR arthroscopic knee simulator to test candidates' surgical skills, especially arthroscopic, and for certification. Robert Poss stated, "ABOS interest grew out of the fact that there was no effective way to evaluate skills proficiency for certifying and recertifying exams."[7] Research for the Virtual Reality Arthroscopic Knee Simulator (VR-AKS) began in 1997 with development of a prototype by Boston Dynamics (Table 1). The ABOS project demonstrated that "virtual reality could be applied to teaching techniques in arthroscopic surgery" (AAOS, Febuary 2002). However, as the scope of the project became apparent, the ABOS turned development over to the AAOS. "The Academy's arthroscopic knee surgery simulator project is based upon the work of the ABOS."[8] As Poss stated, "We knew this effort would have to be one of the entire orthopedic community. Before a simulator could be used as a testing tool, it would first have to be used as an educational and training tool."[7]

Table 1.
Virtual Reality Arthroscopic Knee Simulator (VR-AKS)

1. Surrogate leg model can be stressed in varus, valgus, flexion, and extension.
2. Internal knee structures are anatomically correct, including synovium and fat pad.
3. A screen depicts internal anatomic structures, taken from actual arthroscopic surgical procedures.
4. Procedural instructions go into the model for verification by surgeons.
5. User interface allows triangulation and surgical imitation, including feedback about surgical sequencing and technique.
6. Validation study will be conducted in early 2004.

The AAOS created a Virtual Reality Task Force to examine current technology and the requirements for arthroscopic simulation. Because the research and development of a prototype trainer would cost millions, the AAOS searched for a partnership with companies already involved in orthopedic simulator development. The AAOS found a partner for the simulation project with Touch of Life Technologies (TOLTech, Aurora, Coloroado). This research and development company was created by the University of Colorado Center for Human Simulation after completion of work on the NIH Visible Human Dataset Project.[9]

The partnership has received funding through the National Institutes of Health (NIH) Small Business Innovation Research Grant Program. In 2000 AAOS formed an Academy Content Development Group, which was responsible for developing a simulator educational program. The first program requires a complete diagnostic arthroscopy of the knee, "identifying pathologies with and without a probe." The hardware for simulation includes a knee joint capable of various orthopedic manipulation techniques, including manipulation of the knee in varus, valgus, flexion, and extension. Evaluation consists of "time, thoroughness of the examination, tissue injury, pathology identification, and manipulation of the leg."[9]

To test the simulator's effectiveness as a training device, the AAOS will perform a study that incorporates the simulator into various residency programs and test it at the Orthopaedic Learning Center in Rosemont, Illinois. Incorporation of the simulator into residency programs will include training attending staff on the best methods to teach residents the methodology of knee arthroscopy that are "consistent with the simulator program." In addition, the AAOS will determine the number of simulated surgeries residents must complete before actual patient experience and create a standardized checklist to evaluate resident performance.

To assess the reality of the simulator in both display and tissue deformation (in response to mechanical knee manipulation in both varus and valgus), the AAOS Content Development Group has asked approximately 50 academy members to perform this assessment. In addition to visual display and tissue deformation, surgeons will rate the haptics of the simulation in creating "the feel of an instrument sliding along tissue, including display of cartilage damage from excessive force."[9]

The VR-AKS project consists of two stages. The first stage, described above, teaches residents how to perform an arthroscopic examination of the knee joint. The second stage will focus on developing software to teach surgical protocol for various knee pathologies.[7]

The AAOS has also begun work on a VR surgical anatomy project. The goal of this project is to teach orthopedic residents the structure of the acetabulum and pelvis on a three-dimensional level so that they can provide better care for trauma patients. The VR surgical anatomy project uses a unique hardware and software device developed by the University of Illinois and known as the "immersadesk." This device is composed of a 4 by 5 foot projection screen that can shift orientation from "large-screen TV to that of a drafting desk" to enhance three-dimensional effects.[7]

Feedback between user and display is accomplished by tracking the user's head position with respect to the computer image; three-dimensional imagery is changed based on the user's head movements. The end result provides the sensation of being completely immersed within the computer-generated image. The project uses a series of CT scans of a complex pelvic fracture, including a posterior wall fracture and transverse component. The user can compare anatomy on the injured side with the anatomically intact contralateral side.[7]

Shoulder Arthroscopy

Mentice Corporation (Gothenberg, Sweden) has created a computer-based arthroscopic shoulder simulator with haptics and video display. The simulator uses two LapIE manipulators (Immersion Corp.) with supporting software from Mentice that incorporates graphics with haptics. The simulator's physical model consists of "cartilage, labrum, ligaments, biceps tendon and rotator cuff."[10]

To test whether simulators can actually help with surgical education and training, two research groups at Stanford University (the Stanford University Medical Media and Information Technologies [SUMMIT] and the Center for Advanced Technology in Surgery at Stanford) have formed a reviewing body, the SurgSim group. To assess the arthroscopic shoulder simulator by Mentice Corp, SurgSim performed a study to determine whether the simulator can be used to distinguish varying levels of proficiency in arthroscopic technique. Three groups were tested, including medical students, orthopedic residents applying for sports medicine fellowship training, and attending faculty with experience in teaching arthroscopic techniques. Tasks that were tested included locating and contacting a sphere in 11 different locations throughout the joint with an arthroscopic probe. As soon as a sphere was located, the device immediately placed another sphere in a different location in the joint.

Test results indicated that total test time for location of all 11 spheres and "path ratio (percent of measured path length relative to the ideal path)" correlated directly with surgical experience. The study also analyzed collisions and injuries, defined as "collisions beyond a set threshold force." Results of the study demonstrated that surgical simulators can be used to teach shoulder arthroscopic techniques. Based on a standardized skills assessment, "arthroscopy simulation facilitates discrimination of arthroscopic skills. Computer-based simulation technology provides a major opportunity for surgical skills development without morbidity and operating room inefficiency."[10]

Total Joint Applications

Knee Replacement Simulators

Orthopedic surgeons have performed total hip and knee replacement for more than 40 years. Material advances and improvements in surgical technique have led to success rates close to 90% after 20 years. However, current surgical techniques of joint replacement rely on surface anatomy for preoperative planning, assuming a standard or normal anatomy. Computer-assisted surgery is improving total joint replacement through more precise modeling of individual patient anatomy.

Total knee replacement (TKR) surgery offers a great opportunity for computer simulator instruction due to the complex nature of the surgery. TKR involves a sequence of surgical steps with precision bony cuts that is difficult to learn.

Researchers at the University of California, San Francisco, have developed a computer simulation "to provide immediate, constructive feedback while reinforcing the specific protocol of the operative procedure."[11] The project involves three-dimensional modeling with wire-modeled surgical instruments. The tutorial requires the user to select surgical instruments in proper sequence and teaches surgical protocol through repetition.

The TKR simulator evaluates the user's performance by grading the sequence of the procedure and the total time to complete the simulation. The simulator was evaluated by a study in which one group of medical students learning the protocol of TKR by studying a surgical protocol manual and a second group of medical students learned the protocol by practicing on the TKR simulator. The students were then tested using bone models with real surgical instruments. Overall, students who learned the technique using TKR simulation completed the modeled operation with less error and in shorter time than students who had studied the surgical protocol manual.

This study of the TKR simulator demonstrates that simulators have much to offer with respect to learning orthopedic surgical skills. Simulators "provide a linear, sequential method of skill acquisition and direct feedback which is ideally suited for learning stepwise surgical protocols."[11] The TKR simulator directly involves students and residents in the learning process and provides interactive feedback about skill acquisition from the first moments of skill acquisition.

Simulators have also been developed to teach physical examination to medical students and residents. The Technical University of Munich developed a knee joint simulator capable of teaching both normal anatomy and pathologica states of the knee. The simulator provides haptic, acoustic, and visual feedback to the user while he or she is working on a modeled knee. "Users move a virtual shank, bones or muscles within the leg, and simultaneously observe the generated movement, feel the contract force, and hear sounds."[12]

The multimodel virtual human knee joint also allows students to test for joint laxity or end-point stiffness in six degrees of motion by "grasping and pulling at muscles, rupturing ligaments or changing muscle/ligament paths." The simulator can also imitate any pathologic process within the knee, which makes it ideal for teaching physical examination and evaluation techniques for diagnosis and therapeutic planning.[12]

Hip Replacement Simulators (HipNav)

In 1993, the Centers for Medical Robotics and Computer Assisted Surgery (MRCAS) were founded at Carnegie Mellon University in conjunction with the University of Pittsburgh Medical Center's Shadyside Hospital. In 1997, as a way to commercialize the byproducts of this research, Dr. Anthony DiGioia (director of the Center for Orthopaedic research at Shadyside Hospital and codirector of MRCAS), along with Dr. Branislav Jaramax, founded CASurgica, Inc. This company uses its research to create computer-assisted tools and technologies to improve surgical procedures and minimize invasiveness.

Initially CASurgica aimed to produce image-guided systems to aid orthopedic surgeons in reconstructive hip, knee, and joint procedures. Currently the company is working on the following: (1) preoperative surgical planners and simulators for patient-specific surgical plans; (2) image-guided surgical navigation systems; (3) sensors, actuators, and robotic assistive devices used during surgical interventions as well as preoperative and postoperative clinical evaluations; and (4) less invasive and minimally invasive surgical techniques, along with new surgical tool designs to support these techniques.[13]

CASurgica developed a Hip Navigation System (HipNav) in a combined effort with Shadyside Hospital and Carnegie Mellon University. HipNav makes use of computers to achieve hip replacement as precisely as possible, with the intention of increasing joint longevity by minimizing wear and tear (Fig. 2). HipNav intends to decrease the risk of dislocation, a common complication after total hip replacement that is usually related to malposition of the acetabular component.

HipNav has the potential to ensure precise positioning of the acetabular component, thereby decreasing the incidence of postoperative dislocations. HipNav accomplishes precise positioning by aiding surgeons in determining exact acetabular placement. The HipNav includes a preoperative planner, a range of motion simulator, and an intraoperative tracking and guidance system.

Based on patient CT scans, a surgeon can use the preoperative planner "to specify alignment of the acetabular component within the pelvis" (Fig. 3). Instead of relying on a two-dimensional x-ray for preoperative surgical planning, a three-dimensional image developed from CT scans allows the surgeon to create a more accurate representation of the patient's pelvis on the computer. This, in turn, allows more accurate placement of the acetabular component.

An intraoperative tracking and guidance system with an optical camera tracks the position of particular light-emitting diodes (LEDs). The tracking is accurate (0.1 mm) and

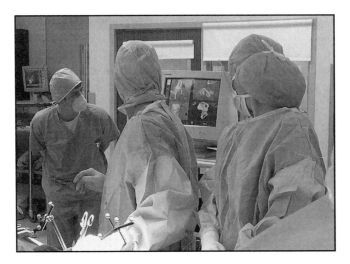

Figure 2. Surgeons use HipNav to ensure precise anatomic alignment during a hip replacement operation.

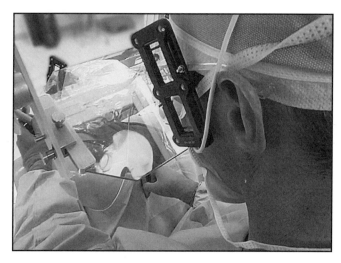

Figure 3. Surgeons use HipNav image overlay as a preoperative and intraoperative planning tool to ensure precise cup alignment.

high-speed (100 Hz), since both the pelvis and surgical tools are attached to the LED targets. The tracking measurements enable the surgeon to determine acetabular implant position in relation to the patient's pelvis, which is displayed on a computer. This technique allows correct orientation and position of the implant. DiGioia believes that the increased accuracy of placement of the acetabular component will translate into smaller incisions and decreased patient recovery time. Therefore, HipNav will not only allow more precise implant placement but will also be a learning tool for "critically examining common assumptions concerning range of motion, bone motion and optimal implant alignment."[13,14]

Applied Simulators

Computer-assisted Surgery

During presurgical planning virtual simulators are used to maximize the opportunity for success in orthopedic surgery. Researchers in Taiwan are working to design a three-dimensional VR simulator that provides preoperative simulation "to verify that osteotomy and fusion procedures chosen to treat musculoskeletal defects are appropriate."[15] The system can also be used to train surgeons in new orthopedic procedures without incurring risk to patients and to teach procedures to students and residents. This project differs from previously described simulators in that it is actually used as a surgical planning tool.

In contrast to many VR training devices, which build a surface model from video data, x-rays, or synthetic surfaces, this simulator creates a volume model of structures by stacking two-dimensional images. The volume is then partitioned into small cuboids known as voxels to simulate relations between tissues and simulated surgery.

CT or MRI images are placed into the system computer, which recreates a three-dimensional structure. The system runs on Visual C++ version 5.0 through Microsoft

Windows. The computer has fairly standard specifications: Pentium III 800 MHz CPU with 256M RAM. Users wear a "shuttle eyeglass," an image device that fits over the eyes like a large pair of glasses, and manipulate images presented on the computer display with a surgical instrument that "tracks motion in six dimensional degrees to simulate surgical procedures."[16]

The primary advantage of this system lies in allowing CT or MRI images of actual patients to be fed into the simulator, which recreates a three-dimensional model of the site of interest. Time from input of two-dimensional images to recreation and display of the three-dimensional model takes less than three seconds. Furthermore, volume modeling allows much faster mathematical representation and graphic display of structure manipulation in a three-dimensional environment. As a result, surgeons can simulate tissue sectioning, exposure, repositioning, suturing, and prosthesis placement with minimal time delay. The simulator results in a preoperative system that models specific patient data for any orthopedic procedure, including arthroplasty and osteotomy.[15,16]

Presurgical Planning Software: Singapore General Hospital

In cooperation with the School of Applied Science at Nanyang Technological University (NTU), orthopedic surgeons at Singapore General Hospital (SGH) are developing a virtual orthopedic surgical training software program. The goals of this program are to lower costs (synthetic bones used to train orthopedic students are expensive) and to allow both students and surgeons to work with as many bones as possible, especially those in which synthetic models are unavailable. Furthermore, because bone structure and shape may vary slightly within given races, computer simulation based on CT scans will provide more realistic training than traditional synthetic bones in current use. Students can be trained using virtual models of true fractures from CT and MRI information. Virtual training is not intended to replace completely the traditional methods of preparing students for orthopedic surgeries; rather, it is intended to correct traditional training weaknesses.

In developing the virtual surgical training program, surgeons at SGH realized that creating a program accessible from both hospital and home would be most beneficial. Therefore, the goal was to develop a realistic virtual training software program able to run on PCs without expensive accessories such as head-mounted displays. The goals of the project are (1) to store in the computer every single bone of different sizes and specific features that might be difficult and expensive to obtain using synthetic models; (2) to create models of fractured bones from real patients using data form CT and MRI images; and (3) to perform surgical operation planning before undertaking the actual operation.[17]

With these goals in mind, surgeons developed a program that allows realistic three-dimensional images to be created along with real-time simulation, including collision detection and sounds. After CT images were obtained, workstations were used to process the two-dimensional images. They were then converted into three-dimensional models using the free-ware software NUAGES by Bernhard Geiger, which creates three-dimensional polygonal meshes from two-dimensional contours. Once a three-dimensional model was created, surgeons developed an editing program that enables removal or addition to the contour lines of the three-dimensional image, thereby making the model appear more realistic.

Surgeons next created a geometric database of fractured bones, using "geometric models of broken bones created from standardized geometric models." All of the tools that surgeons use to fix fractures were also geometrically modeled and stored in a database. The actual fixation of bones on the computer simulation involves preset data that the user must choose in proper sequential order. Since internal fixation of bone fractures often involves standardized surgical technique, surgeons at SGH analyzed techniques to develop sequential procedures for generic virtual fixation techniques. These techniques were implemented internally; the user chooses familiar procedural names and commands at the user interface.

Once the geometric database was created, surgeons then considered collision detection, an important component of VR surgery. Collision detection programs had to be developed for each surgical procedure. For instance, insertion of a screw into a bone can be simulated with the program making use of sensors; proper screw alignment will depend on the surgeon's choice of the proper location. The screw will not be inserted more deeply than it would be in reality, since the correct sizes of instruments and tools are stored in the geometric database.

Once a surgeon has begun the virtual surgery and is examining a three-dimensional model of the bone of interest, several commands can be chosen, depending on the fracture. First, instruments are used and surgical procedures are simulated, complete with collision detection and realistic sounds. Users may move, rotate, and zoom the scene and objects contained within; they may also "look at the assembly through the x-ray lens, examine seated implants from inside the bone for education and control purposes, reverse the process, and set the lights and the background." Therefore, the surgeon still makes his or her own decisions, using the software as a guide. As the surgeon fixes the fracture, scenes can be saved for later use and review, and implants can be created if they are not already in the database.

Software for the project, the "Virtual Bone-Setter," was developed at the School of Applied Science, Nanyang Technological University. It runs on personal computers, preferably not less than 150 MHz, 64 MB extended RAM, with video card supporting three-dimensional polygon rendering and real transparency. A normal mouse may be used; however, three-dimensional mice or graphic pads may make the experience more realistic. The project continues internationally with collaboration among SGH, the Moscow Institute of Physics and Technology, and the Institute of Computing for Physics and Technology, Russia.[17]

Spine Surgery

The ability to visualize patient anatomy in real time using virtual fluoroscopy helps surgeons with implant insertion, placement of pedicle screws in spinal surgery, and treatment of orthopedic trauma. However, conventional fluoroscopy poses certain disadvantages, including provision of real-time images in only one plane and radiation exposure to personnel in the operating room. Furthermore, the C-arm has to be repositioned each time that images are required in different planes. Movement fo the C-arm in and out of the surgical field increases the potential for infection.[18]

Computer-assisted virtual fluoroscopy has been developed to address the disadvantages of traditional fluoroscopy. This system combines intraoperative fluoroscopic imagery with computer-assisted surgical navigation software to provide real-time, multiplanar imagery without the need for extensive fluoroscopic exposure to the patient, surgeon, or operating room personnel. Virtual fluoroscopy takes about ten minutes to set up and appears to improve the accuracy of surgery. The system imposes surgical instrument position onto multiplanar virtual fluoroscopic images in real time (Fig. 4).

Computer-assisted virtual fluoroscopy uses a standard fluoroscopy unit, a calibration grid with light-emitting diodes (LEDs), surgical instruments with LEDs, a dynamic reference array (DRA), a light-sensing camera, and supporting computer software. C-arm images of the patient are taken and sent to the computer, along with images of the position of the C-arm and relative patient position. The computer constructs a mathematical model of the patient by sensing the DRA, the operating field, and C-arm fluoroscopic unit. C-arm images are correlated with patient position through a calibration grid. Surgical instrument position is sensed via LEDs and recorded. The position of the instrument is then superimposed onto the fluoroscopic images in multiple planes and in real time."

Physicians at the Tulane University School of Medicine have used virtual fluoroscopy to perform 1039 pedicle screw emplacements. Computer-assisted virtual fluoroscopy resulted in correct placement of 99.3% of screws, which compares favorably with reported rates of misplaced pedicle screws of 10–40%.

Virtual fluoroscopy allows multiplanar imaging in real-time, with a set-up time under ten minutes. Spine screw placement time is dramatically decreased from the usual

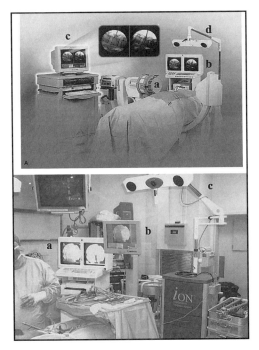

Figure 4. Typical operating room set-up for virtual fluoroscopy (VF). A, VF equipment includes (a) fluoroscope with calibration grid; (b) fluoroscope monitor; (c) computer monitor showing virtual images; and (d) light-sensing camera. B, VF in use: (a) fluoroscope monitor; (b) computer monitor showing virtual imagery; and (c) light-sensing camera. (Reprinted with permission from the University of Pennsylvania Orthopaedic Journal, 2002).

range of 20–65 seconds using traditional fluoroscopic methods to 2–9 seconds. Radiation exposure is limited, and the accuracy of virtual fluoroscopy provides significant improvement over traditional methods. However, these systems are not completely dependable. Improvements in both software and hardware reliability are needed before virtual fluoroscopy is adopted as a mainstream orthopedic technique.[18]

The Future of Orthopedic Simulation

Haptics

The future of orthopedic simulation is exciting because of the nearly limitless possibilities of emerging technologies. Haptics provides a case in point and can radically affect the design of future VR projects. In VR, a close resemblance to the "real world" determines the degree to which the experience seems real. The more closely VR models the real world, the more it begins to have the feel of and thereby to teach actual experience. Thus, feedback to the user is of paramount importance. Images portrayed in VR must be realistic in terms of shape and color, but they also need to be updated based on the actions of the user. For example, if the user is focused on the medial meniscus in a surgical field and then quickly moves the fiberoptic camera back out to just below the surface of the skin, the VR experience would quickly lose the sense of reality if the image presented to the user remained the surgical field of the medial meniscus. The actions of the user have to be relayed to a computer, which can mathematically model the actions and then create appropriate feedback to the user based on his or her movement. Image update rates are equally important. Continuing the same scenario, if the operator quickly moved the fiberoptic camera to another structure within the knee and the field of vision presented to him or her lagged behind by just 4 or 5 seconds, the sensation of reality would be destroyed.

To further increase the sensation of the "real world" in VR simulation, other senses besides vision need to be incorporated. For example, how does a drill bit coursing through the femoral condyle sound? How can a trainee develop "a surgeon's touch" if the VR device on which he or she is training offers no resistance in spatial orientation?

To address these issues, the field of haptics is being developed. According to the Naval Operations Office of Training and Technology, "A haptic interface is a force reflecting device which allows a user to touch, feel, manipulate, create, and/or alter simulated three-dimensional objects in a virtual environment."[19] Haptics provides a computer interface that allows training of physical skills "such as those jobs requiring specialized hand-held tools (e.g., surgeons, astronauts, or mechanics)."[19] This skill is different from procedural training. Although learning the steps of a procedure is vitally important, haptics is concerned with the specifics of the surgeon's hand motion, creating the sensation of surgical instruments moving through a joint. Haptic devices "track movement (head-trackers, eye-trackers, magnetic or optical motion trackers) and then provide force-reflecting feedback to the user."[19] Incorporation of this technology into developing VR projects will greatly enhance simulated reality.

VOEU Project

Six European nations are jointly developing a Virtual European Orthopaedic University (VOEU), bringing together computer system designers, researchers, engineers, educators, and physicians from Italy, France, Germany, Switzerland, the Netherlands, and the United Kingdom. VOEU holds much promise in furthering the future of VR because it is attempting to unify orthopedic standards and practice throughout Europe, utilizing Internet-based sharing of information and ideas (Fig. 5).

Traditional apprenticeship learning has created numerous problems that the VOEU is attempting to address. Foremost is variation in orthopedic techniques and practice across Europe, followed by absence of a qualitative gold standard for different procedures and wide variation in surgical skills. VOEU attempts to unify teaching, research, and surgical skills by combining knowledge, experience, virtual surgical training, interactive multimedia learning, real data, and new technologies in a widely distributed virtual class. The end result is enhanced student-teacher interaction in orthopedics.[20]

Project goals include (1) enhanced learning material, accessible on-line (via the Internet) or off-line; (2) multimedia educational orthopedic modules; (3) review of expertise in image-guided orthopedic surgery (IGOS) through a virtual, multicentric, and permanently updated observatory of ICT in orthopedics; (4) virtual classes that enable distant interaction between surgical residents and experts; and (5) development of surgical simulators designed to facilitate skill acquisition and evaluation. Four surgical simulators are being developed by VOEU: shoulder, iliac, hip surgery, and knee arthroscopy. The ultimate goal of these surgical simulators has been described as shortening the learning curve for surgical techniques.

VOEU has four educational objectives with surgical simulators. The first focuses on a "user-centered design" that facilitates simulators for the teaching of various surgical procedures. This first objective is to teach trainees the necessary skills, requisite background knowledge, and familiarity with procedures and equipment and to acquaint them

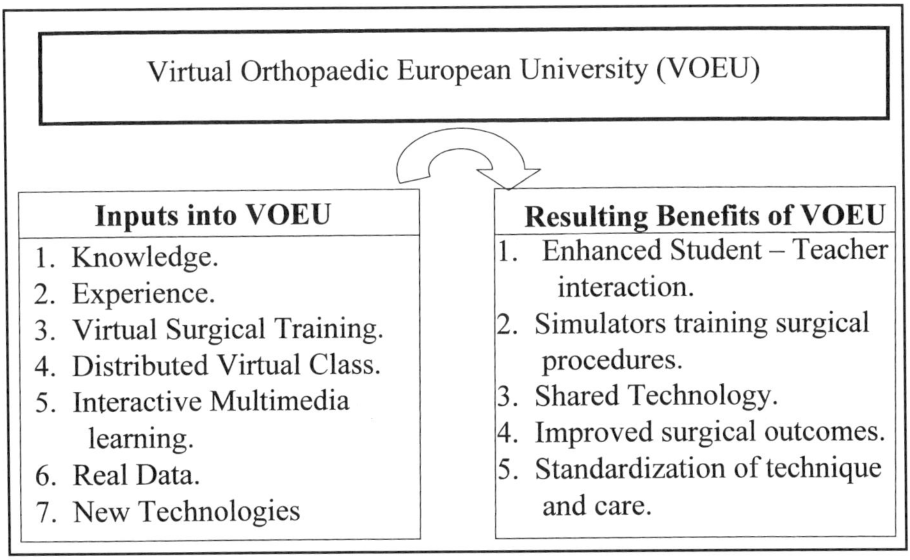

Figure 5. Advantages of the Virtual Orthopaedic European University.

with the basics of computer-assisted surgery. The second objective is to enable trainees and trainers to quantify the skill acquisition process. Third, simulators may allow residents to gain procedural knowledge in line with conceptual knowledge. Finally, simulator training can replace training on cadavers and animals.

Surgical simulators also focus on the skills required to perform difficult surgical procedures. Specific operations must be identified in which simulators will enhance learning the steps of the surgical procedure. Appropriate visual and haptic devices must be chosen that can most closely model actual surgery experience. These devices can teach visual integration, defined as "the capacity to recognize a complex anatomical environment from partial and potentially distorted images." Once the user is spatially oriented, manual dexterity with surgical instruments can be taught. Finally, simulators must be evaluated to verify educational value. Eventually the inclusion of interactive training may provide guidance in the form of pop-up messages and instruction.[20,21]

Knee Stress Modeling Simulation

Over 250,000 Americans undergo total knee replacement (TKR) each year. The Department of Mechanical and Aerospace Engineering at the University of Florida is spearheading a project focused on enhancing longevity of TKR by applying mechanical engineering technology to the human body. The project is creating more effective methods of testing knee implant designs by developing "computational models that make quantifiable predictions of deterioration of artificial knees."[22] Research integrates motion data from artificial knees with computer simulations of walking that use "physiological loads and speeds." This project is unique because it utilizes simulators for scientific analysis of joint placement and attempts to improve implant design.

Fregly states that the aim of the research is not only to prolong artificial knee lifespan, which lasts on average 15–20 years, but also "to prolong a patient's enjoyment of life." Present technology is not highly efficient in evaluating the designs of implants. Current stress simulators that study TKR failure do not accurately model what happens in vivo. Furthermore, existing simulators may cost up to $40,000 and take three months to produce an assessment.

The University of Florida project tests artificial knee implants in patients in a simulated environment to determine stress and wear specific to each patient. First, the patient walks on a treadmill and stair-climber with reflective markers at various locations on skin and clothing. The motion data recorded are specific to each patient and stored in a computer. Motion data are then enhanced with fluoroscopy. Scott Banks (Biomotion Foundation, West Palm Beach Florida) has developed a fluoroscopic procedure that measures the movement of both knee implants and natural knees. Banks uses two-dimensional fluoroscopic images of the artificial knee and creates a three-dimensional computer-aided design (CAD) of the implant. The matched images are then used to measure three-dimensional motion of a patient's knee under realistic conditions, such as walking and stair-climbing.

Evaluation of natural knees is a more challenging endeavor because of the lack of computer-aided design models of actual bones. The process, although similar to artificial joint simulation, is a bit more complex. First, CT scan produces two-dimensional images of a patient's knee. Data are manipulated with sliceOmatic image-processing software from TomoVision (Montreal, Quebec, Canada), which stacks two-dimensional slices to create a three-dimensional model. The data from the three-dimensional model are collected in coordinates termed "point clouds." Point cloud data are used to create exact three-dimensional computer models that can be studied for contact stress with Geomagic Studio software (Raindrop Geomagic, Research Triangle Park, North Carolina). Lastly, Greg Sawyer, a specialist in wear and friction at the University of Florida, combines precise knee motion data with the contact stress indicators to develop a knee model that pinpoints exact sites within individual patients where an artificial knee is likely to fail.

The research hopes to gain a better understanding of the exact points at which stress is likely to occur in the knee, which can lead to advances that enhance the longevity and effectiveness of artificial knee replacement surgery. Eventually, the project aims to develop a whole-body model to simulate movement data collected from individual patients. The project will then remodel surgery to determine critical areas of stress. This research may lead to implant placement that is most beneficial to each patient.[22]

Conclusion

Major projects related to arthroscopy, knee, and hip replacement simulators are ongoing. Current applications of simulation in orthopedic surgery have several objectives. First and foremost is enhanced patient safety. Computer-assisted virtual fluoroscopy decreases ionizing radiation exposure for both patients and surgeons. Surgical simulation focuses on outcomes research in orthopedics, which links surgical technique with results. Individual patient modeling may prevent surgical outliers by identifying patients with slightly unique anatomy or conditions that do not conform to normal operational parameters.

As VR surgical simulation and computer-assisted surgery become more widespread, increasingly creative techniques and procedures will be developed that greatly enhance both patient care and surgical resident training. The field is changing rapidly. Future challenges for VR are to define what niche the simulator is attempting to fill and to improve surgical technique, teaching, or outcome through innovations in VR. As DiGioia has stated, "The only limitations we currently have in the application and adoption of these technologies is our imagination and understanding of what we can accomplish in the future."[23]

References
1. O'Neill PJ, Cosgarea AJ, Freedman JA, et al: Arthroscopic proficiency: A survey of orthopaedic sports medicine fellowship directors and orthopaedic surgery department chairs. Arthroscopy 2002;7:795–800.
2. Heim U: The AO Phenomenon: Foundation and the Early Years of the Association for the Study of Internal Fixation (ASIF). Seattle, Hogrefe & Huber, 2001.
3. Rogers C: Surgical training gets virtual. Am Acad Orthop Surg Bull 2001;49(6):43.
4. American Academy of Orthopedic Surgeons: Your Orthopaedic Connection. American Academy of Orthopaedic Surgeons website at http://orthoinfo.aaos.org/.
5. McCarthy AD: A multimedia arthroscopic simulator of surgical procedures. SKATS final report.doc 1 20/12/99. A multimedia arthroscopic simulator of surgical procedures. Grant reference: GR/L28692. Available at http://www.shef.ac.uk/~mpce/rsch/SKATS.pdf.
6. McCarthy AD, Hollands RJ: Human factors related to a virtual reality surgical simulator: The Sheffield knee arthroscopic training system. Available at http://www.brunel.ac.uk/faculty/tech/systems/groups.

7. Rogers C: Surgical VR gets real. Am Acad Orthop Surg Bull 1999;47(5):43.
8. ABOS role in VR-AKS devt. Am Acad Orthop Surg Bull 2002;(1):11.
9. Cannon WD, Mabrey JD: Virtual reality simulator—on track to reality. Am Acad Orthop Surg Bull 2002;50(6):62.
10. Pedowitz RA, Esch J, Snyder S: Evaluation of a virtual reality simulator for arthroscopy skills development. Arthroscopy 2002;18(6):E29.
11. Gunther SB, Soto GE, Colman WW: Interactive computer simulations of knee-replacement surgery. Acad Med 2002;77:753–754.
12. Riener R, Hoogen J, Burgkart R, et al: Development of a multi-model virtual human knee joint for education and training in orthopaedics. Stud Health Tech Inform 2001:81;410–416.
13. CASurgica website. http://www.casurgica.com/general.htm.
14. Ostendorf K: Hip replacement combined computers, surgery to make Sal Sirabella a new man. Pittsburgh Post Gazette1999;(Feb):23.
15. Hsieh MS, Tsai MD, Chang WC: Virtual reality simulator for osteotomy and fusion involving the musculoskeletal system. Comput Med Imag Graph 2002;26(2):91–101.
16. Hsieh MS, Tsai MD, Jou SB: Virtual reality orthopedic surgery simulator. Comput Biol Med 2001;31(5):333–351.
17. Sourina O, Sourin A: Virtual orthopedic surgery training on personal computer. Int J Inform Technol 2000;6(1):16–29.
18. Eyke JC, Ricciardi JE, Roesch W, Whitecloud TS: Computer-assisted virtual fluoroscopy. Univ Penn Orthop J 2002;15:53–59.
19. Chief of Naval Operations Office of Training and Technology website: http://www.ott.navy.mil/index.cfm?RID=TTE_OT_1000022.
20. VOEU Project website: http://www-crim.sssup.it/research/cas/default.htm.
21. Vadcard L., Zimolong A, Grange S: Specific surgical course model. Available at http://lotus5.vitamib.com/hnb/voucaos/vouaos.nsf/All/EDBB0A9F675AD0BEC1256C37005A2A33.
22. Versweyveld L: University of Florida research team to develop computational wear models for knee joints. Virt Med Worlds Month 2002;Nov.
23. Breisch SL: Future is here: Does it work? Am Acad Orthop Surg Bull 1998;46(4):35.

Chapter 16

SIMULATION IN UROLOGIC SURGERY

M. P. Laguna, MD, PhD, D. N. Mitropoulos, MD, FEBU,
J. J. M. C. H. de la Rosette MD, PhD

Surgical specialties are facing great changes. Beside the fact that a case performed by a trainee lasts longer and is more expensive than a case performed solely by a staff surgeon,[1] current economic constrictions, increasing demands in health care, fiscal constraints, and medical and legal considerations limit the time available in the operating room and the opportunities for the trainee to "practice and learn" while operating on patients.[2] At the same time operating approaches are changing. In urology open surgery is increasingly replaced by endoscopy and laparoscopy. Because endoscopy is essentially a "one-person" procedure, teaching an assistant during the procedure is more difficult than in open surgery.[3] Laparoscopy, on the other hand, is a difficult technique—difficult to teach and difficult to learn. These are among the many reasons that is becoming more difficult for trainees to acquire adequate experience in a time-efficient manner.

As the number of minimally invasive procedures increases, urologic teaching centers face the challenge of providing residents with the surgical training that optimizes learning. Furthermore, teaching advanced skills such as endourology or laparoscopy—in which even the location of the monitor significantly influences performance—can lead to technical difficulties.[4]

The 1999 report of the Institute of Medicine offers further evidence of the urgent need for reform in surgical education. Entitled "To Err Is Human," the report estimates that at least 44,000 Americans die every year from medical error, with surgical error accounting for a greater proportion than pharmaceutical mistake.[5] It seems clear that with a living patient on the table, learning by trial and error is no longer an option.

Bench models are used as a surrogate for human patients with increasing frequency to simulate real procedures without health or safety issues. During recent years some inanimate or bench simulators for laparoscopy have incorporated a pulsate perfusion system (POP, Optimist, Bregenz, Austria) that allows realistic simulation of bleeding in "in block" animal organs.

Advances in mimetic technology and development of the three-dimensional integration system and virtual reality computer-based systems have led to the development of the virtual reality simulators (VR simulators). By incorporating tissue properties and force feedback mechanisms that make the models more realistic, virtual simulation has emerged in the past decade as a promising tool for helping in the acquisition of technical skills.[6]

A previously described classification system divides the simulators into three categories: physical model-based or inanimate simulators, computer-based simulators, and hybrid simulators, a combination of the two models. In urology the available simulators are model-based and hybrid (VR simulators).

EDUCATIONAL OBJECTIVES

Surgical training has traditionally been a true apprenticeship in which trainees learned as they performed under the guidance of an experienced surgeon. Like other surgical specialties, urology has long faced the conflict between the imperative to give the patient the best possible care and the need to provide novices with experience.[7] The educational literature refers to three domains of competence: knowledge, attitudes, and skills. In addition, the individual neuropsychological attributes of surgeons include complex visual-spatial organization, stress tolerance, and psychomotor abilities. Visual-spatial ability seems to be related to competence and quality of results in complex surgery. Visual-spatial ability may potentially be used in residents' selection and career counseling.[8]

Trainees with higher visual-spatial scores seem to do significantly better in surgical procedures than those with lower scores. Nevertheless, after practice and feedback, trainees with lower scores achieve a comparable level of competence.[8] Practice is thus the basis of surgical skills. However, for the above-mentioned reasons, manual and technical skills must be acquired before invasive procedures can be performed in a competent manner. Surgical simulators have a great potential in mitigating the surgical risk related to the educational process. They also give the opportunity for supervised and constructive feedback from experienced trainers.

Because urologists, even more than other surgical specialists, perform endoscopic procedures in three-dimensional views while looking at a two-dimensional magnified screen, one may think that urologic surgeons require special spatial awareness for endoscopic and laparoscopic surgery. A recent comparison of the innate spatial awareness among three groups—consultant urologists, urologic trainees, and controls not trained in surgery—showed that urologists do not differ from the general population in terms of innate spatial ability. About 10% of people in each of the three groups appeared to have deficient spatial awareness skills without further evidence that this deficiency hinders surgical training or performance.[9]

Learning a new psychomotor skill includes three different phases.[10] In the **cognitive phase**, the basic steps of the procedure are didactically taught. After understanding these steps, the novice progresses to the second phase or **integration**, in which a mental inventory of the different steps is translated into psychomotor action. Performance remains erratic until the novice reaches the **automatic phase**, in which, as a result of repetitive practice, the required motor skills are executed automatically with little cognitive input. The importance of the cognitive component has been fully recognized in the learning process of a new surgical skill. It is clear now that, after a didactic session only, trainees significantly improve their performance.[11]

A surgeon should and must be able to practice new procedures repeatedly until he or she is judged proficient without endangering patients. During the training process it is desirable to face cases of increasing complexity to measure progress and improvement. The learning curve is defined not only by the time needed to achieve a definite performance (quickness) but also by the number of cases (trials) necessary to attain proficiency.[12]

Simulators have a potential impact in all stages of a surgeon's carrier and can be used for assessment, training, and possible certification. Simulated training should be helpful for teaching the required skills and preparing trainees for emergency situations and can even be used as a selection or counseling tool. More precisely the educational objectives of a simulator in urology can be summarized as follows:

◆ To familiarize the trainee with the anatomy of the urogenital system and the various steps of different endoscopic procedures
◆ To teach the trainee to replace the two-dimensional diagrammatic representation of the urinary collecting system with a three-dimensional spatial model.
◆ To make the trainee knowledgeable about various landmarks of the urinary tract and how to adapt behavior according to these landmarks
◆ To teach the trainee to identify and correct major and minor technical defects in manipulation of different instruments
◆ To allow the trainee to practice individual maneuvers to the point of automatism and thus develop a general sense of "being at home" in the endourology field
◆ To help the trainee gain the hand-eye coordination, spatial awareness, and other skills necessary to perform endourologic procedures without risk for the patient
◆ To shorten the learning curve of endourologic procedures
◆ To help maintain "currency" and thus improve performance of a particular procedure

Simulators in Lower Urinary Tract

Digital rectal examination (DRE) is a fundamental technique in the assessment of the prostate gland. In fact, a rubber prostate model has been widely used in all urologic departments, representing the most primitive and probably the first of the currently available simulators in urology. Four different types of prostate glands are available: normal, enlarged, incipient malignancy (single tumor), and advanced malignancy. The biggest disadvantage of this simple simulator is the absence of an objective way to follow the improvement in DRE when the technique is repeated by an experienced urologist. Even in this setting assessment remains highly subject-dependent.

The recently developed prototype for a VR-based simulator consists of a phantom haptic interface that provides feedback to the trainee's index finger, a motion-restricted board, and a workstation that represents the patient's anatomy.[13] As in the inanimate simulator, four types of prostate are modeled. After only five minutes of training, non-medical students had a 67% correct diagnosis rate for malignant vs. nonmalignant cases. This finding compared with 56% for urology residents in the same trials. Nevertheless, this VR simulation of palpation of different prostate conditions needs significant improvement in both model realism and haptic interface hardware.[13]

Urethrocystoscopy and electroresection of the prostate and bladder tumors are the most commonly performed endourologic procedures in every day practice. Despite advances in audiovisual and optics technology that offer trainees the opportunity to visualize recorded and actual diagnostic and therapeutic endourologic procedures, performing them safely and effectively still depends on long-term practical experience. Phantoms were long ago recognized as necessary and efficient teaching instruments and vary from animal models to human or animal cadaver organs, synthetic organ models and mechanical simulation systems.

Historically, the first endoscopic training models were cadavers.[14–16] Particular interest has been focused on using this model, primarily for prostatic resection and secondarily for ureterorenoscopy. The performance of the procedures is similar to the clinical situation, but cadaver models are restricted by the lack of bleeding. Cadaver models represent a poor approximation to living tissue and are expensive; consequently, they have an even more limited use. In the past several attempts were initiated to overcome these problems. Habib et al.[17] proposed the use of cow's udder to teach transurethral surgery. Again the procedures were restricted by the lack of bleeding, although the authors found that the structure resembles that of the male urogenital system. To overcome the problems encountered with human or animal cadaver tissues, a canine model was introduced more than two decades ago.[18] Ethical issues and high maintenance costs limit the use of animals for learning purposes. Furthermore, although biologic conditions are emulated, animal anatomy is not always sufficiently close to human anatomy.

For prostatic procedures, several inanimate models, including an apple representing the gland[19] and a wax model of the prostate and bladder,[20] have been used through the years (Fig. 1). A simulator for transurethral resection of the prostate (TURP), introduced in 1996[21] and currently marketed by Limbs and Things (http://www.limbsandthings.com), includes a model prostate with bladder neck. The simulator is made of a resectable material that has electrical and cutting characteristics similar to those of the human prostate. A simulated bladder is provided as a reservoir for the insufflating fluids and chippings while excessive fluid drains through the base to which the model is secured. TURP is performed using a standard resectoscope and electrosurgical diathermy. The boundary of resection is marked by a color change within the model that reveals excavation of the bladder neck or perforation of the prostatic capsule. The performance of the entire procedure closely approximates the clinical setting, but realism is restricted by the lack of bleeding.

A computer simulation of TURP was envisioned in 1990,[22] but the first realistic computer-generated interactive simulator for TURP was published by Ballaro et al.[23] in 1999. The system consists of a personal computer, resectoscope, and magnetic position sensor attached to the resectoscope. Images of the lumen of the prostatic urethra, in-

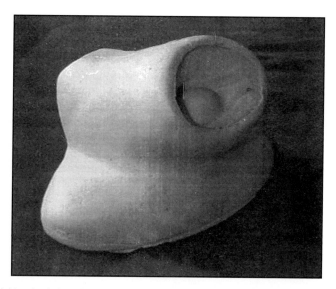

Figure 1. Model for simulation of transurethral resection of the prostate (Limbs and Things, Bristol, UK).

cluding standard anatomic landmarks, are created by specifically developed software using a mesh framework that is colored and textured realistically. Lighting parameters represent views through a 30^0 resectoscope lens with a point light source. The same software is used to create the image of the cutting loop of a resectoscope; to cause movements of the resectoscope and its handle; to control the image of the cutting loop; to recognize collisions between the loop and the prostate; to eliminate tissue when the loop occupies the same virtual space as the prostate, creating a furrow; and to cause a series of red points to move away from the "cut" surface, simulating bleeding. The simulator is limited by delayed images and the absence of haptic feedback and awaits further development and upgrading.

Another computer-assisted TURP trainer was published by Kumar et al.[24] in 2002. A disposable latex polymer prostate model provides the dimensional data to build nonuniform, rational B-spline surfaces, which are a mathematical description of complex surfaces, and to create a three-dimensional image, stored as a standard-format IGES (International Graphics Exchange Standard) file. The position of the resectoscope with respect to the prostate model is monitored by an optical tracker with 12 infrared-emitting diodes housed in a 100-mm diameter ring at 30^0 intervals. The tracker is attached to the resectoscope. Movement of the loop is detected through a potentiometer attached to the working element. The computer monitor shows the endoscopic view of the prostatic urethra, a three-dimensional image of the prostate model with the current resectoscope position superimposed in real time, a two-dimensional cross-sectional view coinciding with the current area of resection, and two-dimensional, cross-sectional thumbnail images of the prostate at constant intervals. The software incorporated into the system is programmed to highlight the cross-sectional image closer to the current position of the loop in real time and to provide information about resection progress and proximity to the capsule. A warning highlights resection distal to the verumontanum or proximal to the bladder neck. Haptic feedback is provided by deformation and resection of the physical phantom. Again, the lack of bleeding limits trainer realism, and several problems, mainly with model movement and permanent deformation of the model, were encountered during resection.

The URO Mentor simulator (Simbionix, Tel Aviv, Hashomer, Israel) allows the simulation of cystoscopic and upper urinary tract endoscopic procedures with simultaneous real-time fluoroscopic control (Fig. 2). The software includes a proprietary visualization engine, the Simbionix Visualization Engine (SVE), which allows real-time simulation by offering a high-level object-oriented application program interface. The simulator includes general procedures that allow two- and three-dimensional rendering, collision correction, three-dimensional morphing, two-dimensional image manipulation, texture mapping, "bump" mapping, video texture, x-ray rendering, special effects (blood, smoke, stone fragments), and reflections. The endoscopic texture of the urinary tract was created from videotapes taken during actual endoscopic procedures. The information about the location and movements of the endoscope is transmitted from a sensor on the endoscope and three sensors in the workstation to the computer to create a three-dimensional geometric model used for the real-time simulation process.[25] Although the URO Mentor system is mainly designed to simulate upper urinary tract endoscopic procedures, it has been successfully used in teaching flexible cystoscopy to inexperienced subjects.[26, 27] The simulator allows assessment of the subjects' level of

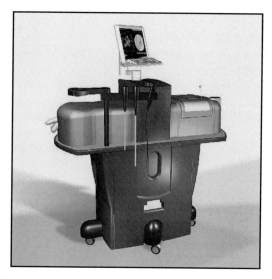

Figure 2. URO Mentor virtual reality simulator for endoscopy of lower and upper urinary tract.

experience in flexible cystoscopy, and the repetitive practice on the simulator leads to an improvement in the objective parameters recorded by the simulator. Consequently, one can conclude that the device has construct validity. Nevertheless, the transfer to real practice was never evaluated.[26, 27] Simulations of TURP and transurethral resection of bladder tumor (TURBT) are currently under development and will be integrated into the system in the future.[25]

Simulation of lower urinary tract endoscopic procedures, using a computer-based system that incorporates a surgical tool interface with haptic feedback, has been the subject of two other research teams. Manyak and coworkers[28] constructed a surgical interface device that allows users to vary the angle of the endoscope in the pitch and yaw directions and to advance or retract the instrument in a linear fashion, thus providing four degrees of freedom in simulation. The sense of resistance to linear push is provided in real-time by a computer-controlled linear braking device; the resistance is proportional to the video image (tissue or lumen) and the spatial orientation of the cystoscope. Graphic simulation of the lower urinary tract was developed on a Silicon Graphics Visual Workstation using surface-based geometric data generated from the National Library of Medicine Visible Human dataset and textural data from recorded endoscopic video procedures. The system was found to be adequate in coordinating virtual perception with appropriate feedback in all normal ranges of motion of the cystoscope within an actual cystoscopy.

Mitropoulos and coworkers also developed an interactive virtual reality urethrocystoscopy simulator with haptic feedback.[29–31] The interface haptic device allows the cystoscope to rotate 360 degrees about the x axis and 30 degrees about the y and z axes, respectively. It also allows a translational motion along both the x and y axes, thus providing five degrees of freedom (two translational and three rotational). It consists of a five-bar linkage with two degrees of freedom and a spherical joint with three degrees of freedom. To reproduce very small forces and moments, the mechanism has low friction, inertia, and mass; is statically balanced; and has a simple mass matrix. Roll-pitch-yaw motions of the surgical tool result in motions of the corresponding actuator (base-mounted DC motors). Force feedback transmission is achieved via capstan drives, pulleys, and miniropes. The graphic models of the urethra and the bladder were created using splines-modelling techniques and digitized textures whose imaging quality was enhanced with specialized photo-editing software. A specially designed synchronization module is used to communicate rapidly the graphic engine with the haptic device. The system is currently under evaluation.

Realistic haptic feedback and rapid as well as precise control of the interaction between the virtual reality environment and the movements of the surgical tool are essential for a surgical simulator. In addition, realistic graphic depiction of both the normal and abnormal urinary tract and simulating issues related to tissue resection, bleeding, and hemostasis add significantly to the realistic simulation of the various endourologic procedures. Initially bleeding was modelled mathematically by representations of blood flow over tissue surfaces[32] or within vessels.[33] However, another approach that focuses on macroscopic visualization of bleeding in a fluid environment was recently reported.[34,35] Blood flow movies of bleeding vessels, with different severity and position, were generated under variable fluid flow conditions and after the appropriate process to separate the blood flow from the background anatomy was organized into a parametric database. The movies can be mapped as textures onto a virtual surface, and the playback (representing a bleeding event) can be triggered by "resection" of the particular texture. This approach seems to provide the necessary realism of bleeding during tissue resection without investing in the computational power necessary to use a particle-based modeling approach. Implementation of several other forms of interactions, such as probing, piercing, cauterising, and ablating virtual tissues, will enhance modeling of different procedures and the educational value of all available and still to be developed simulators.

Currently under development are various VR simulators for TURP with appropriate bleeding and irrigation effects, haptic feedback, and realistic interplay of visual, tactile, and auditory cues as well as metrics of the performance.

Simulators of the Upper Urinary Tract

Advanced endourology or endourology of the upper urinary tract is relatively new and still evolving. Dexterity and high accuracy are needed for endoscopic techniques in the ureter and kidney. As for the lower urinary tract, the animal cadaveric urinary tract has been used for upper urinary tract simulation purposes. A complete urinary tract dissected from the retroperitoneum of freshly slaughtered pigs has been successfully used by Strohmaier et al.[36] in training courses for endoscopy of the upper urinary tract. This porcine urinary tract model allows practice of all aspects of diagnostic and therapeutic ureteroscopy, including lithotripsy and "stenting" in a way that is almost identical to the clinical situation in humans.

Inanimate model-based and virtual reality computer-based simulators are available to practice skills in upper urinary tract manipulation, whether in the retrograde (ureteroscopy) or antegrade (percutaneous renal puncture) approach. Currently two inanimate simulators, or high-fidelity bench models, for endoscopy of the upper urinary tract have become popular and are widely used in training facilities: the Ureteroscopy trainer (Limbs and Things, Bristol, UK) (Fig. 3) and the Mediskills Scope trainer (www.mediskills.com). These inanimate simulators include reproduction of the urethra, bladder, ureter, renal pelvis, and calices in a rubber or silicon model. The external genitalia are also simulated, allowing external manipulation during the initial endoscopic maneuvers. Different conditions, such as diverticula or tumors and various stone locations, can be simulated not only in the bladder but also in the collecting system. Both simulators are used in a real practice environment with actual instruments, lubricating jellies, and water as irrigating fluid. The scope trainer from Mediskills has also a distendable bladder and fluoroscopic properties. These simulation models have evolved enormously in the past few years and now possess a high degree of realism that fully allows the trainee to practice with flexible and rigid instrumentation and to become familiar with the endoscopic maneuvers to access the upper urinary tract. However, these nonbiologic models still lack reality, especially in biofeedback.

There is also a percutaneous model (Perc Trainer, Mediskills) that simulates endoscopic percutaneous procedures and techniques of access. This simulator can reproduce the ultrasonographic and fluoroscopic features of the human kidney.

Surprisingly, despite the fact that they are frequently used in hands-on training sessions and systematic training of novices, very little literature is available on this subject. In acquiring surgical skills, training in bench models seems to be superior to the classical didactic sessions.

In a longitudinal study Matsumoto et al.[11] investigated the effects of didactic teaching and supervised hands-on practice on endourologic skills using a high-fidelity genitourinary bench model from Limbs and Things. Seventeen right-handed urologic residents (11 junior and 6 senior) participated in a two-day study in which their ability to remove a mid-ureter stone was checked on three occasions. At the beginning of the study, all of the residents completed a questionnaire about their past endoscopic experience that was cited as pretest status. Before starting the training sessions, all residents received a manual about cystoscopy, guidewire insertion, ureteroscopy, and mid-ureter stone extraction. The training session was then performed under camera control. After

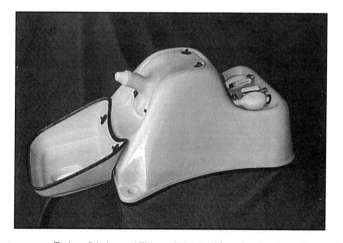

Figure 3. Ureteroscopy Trainer (Limbs and Things, Bristol, UK), an inanimate endourologic simulator.

a didactic teaching session was given by an experienced endourologist, the trainees completed a postdidactic test. Afterward a 1-hour, hands-on, supervised session took place. Finally, the third phase of the study consisted of a bench performance evaluated by two staff urologists and two fellows. A global rating scale and a checklist were used for evaluation. In addition, a pass-rating test and the time required to complete the task were assessed to determine performance. As expected, previous experience with cystoscopy, stent insertion, and ureteroscopy was a significant predictor of the pretest global rating score and time to complete the task but not of the checklist score. There was a significant difference between junior and senior pretest scores with respect to the global rating score, pass-rating, and time needed to complete the task, but the difference in the checklist score was not significant. A significant effect of training was noted on the global rating and checklist scores; the pass-rating also improved. However, the authors found no significant difference between the pretest and postdidactic tests or between the postdidactic and post hands-on practice tests.

In a second phase of the same study, the beneficial effects of hands-on training with a bench model compared with conventional didactic teaching [37] were assessed. During the same study the efficiency of low- vs. high-fidelity bench models for complex ureteroscopy was explored.[37] Forty medical students in the final year of surgical rotation without experience in endoscopy participated in the study. All of them received a manual detailing the procedure that they were going to be asked to perform. All of them watched a 15-minute video about the procedure on a high-fidelity bench model and were subsequently randomized into three arms: didactic teaching session only, hands-on training in a low-fidelity (home-made) model, and hands-on training in a high-fidelity (commercialized) model.

Before and after didactic teaching alone or practice for one hour with the bench models, the students were given a pretest and a posttest to assess baseline endoscopic ability. Finally, all students were asked to remove a mid-ureteral stone from the high-fidelity bench model. The student's ability was assessed by two staff examiners blinded to the randomization. Performance was assessed using the same instruments as in the previous study. No significant differences in the pretest global rating scores, checklist scores, pass-rating, or time needed to complete the procedure were found among the three groups. Hands-on training had a significant effect on performance, and the group trained for one hour in the low-fidelity bench model did significantly better than the group trained for one hour solely by didactic teaching. However, no significant differences in performance were found between the groups trained in the low- or high-fidelity bench models, despite the significantly lower costs of the home-made model. The authors concluded that practical training had a significant effect on performance and that the low-fidelity model was more cost-effective than the high-fidelity model.

Brehmer and Tolley attempted to validate a bench model (Scope Trainer, Mediskills) for ureteroscopy by comparing the performances of 14 urologists (trainees and consultants) in the simulator with their performance in real patients.[3] As in the former studies, performance was assessed by a global score and a task-specific checklist (maximal score = 19 points); both assessments were done by an expert endourologist. All urologists had equal scores on the simulator and with patients (mean score in both cases = 17.6 points). No differences in scoring were found between trainees and consultants. All participants considered the procedure on the model similar to real surgery.

Although the authors concluded that the model is realistic and consequently valid for training, this assertion is based on the subjective perception of the experienced urologist, as demonstrated by the high median scores with both the simulator and the patients. In fact, due to the design of the study, no information can be extracted about the validity of the bench model as a training tool. Nevertheless, it is worthwhile to mention that urologists who subspecialized in endourology scored significantly higher with both patients and model, indicating that experience or practice is of crucial importance for better performance.

Virtual reality simulators that replace the patient with expandable pixels also have been recently developed for the upper urinary tract. The first VR simulator for ureteroscopy was developed in 1995.[38] All of the concepts previously described about VR are fully applicable to simulation in the upper urinary tract. To the authors' knowledge, only one VR simulator is currently available for practicing endourologic procedures of the upper urinary tract. The previously mentioned URO Mentor[25–27] offers an excellent opportunity for hands-on-training in diagnostic and therapeutic procedures in the upper urinary tract. Flexible and rigid real instruments are available for practice and provide the opportunity to become familiar with many of the currently used tools (Fig. 4). Different guidewires, baskets, endoscopic forceps, lithotriptors, electrodes, stents, and even a dilatation balloon can be found among the features of this VR simulator (Fig. 5). Simulation of x-ray control is also available in the integrated platform, and foot pedals for instrumentation make the procedure close to reality by allowing hand-eye-foot coordination (Fig. 6). Furthermore, the simulator can objectively measure the performance with a large number of quantitative parameters. Preliminary studies show that the URO mentor can be a useful tool for training purposes. Endourologic training in a VR simulator seems to improve the repetition of a given procedure and facilitates the performance of basic endourologic tasks that might translate into better performance in the operating room.[39]

Wilhem et al. evaluated the effect of supervised training using a VR simulator in 21

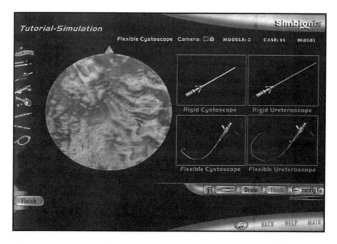

Figure 4. Hybrid, computer based simulator for endourology with flexible and rigid instruments (URO Mentor).

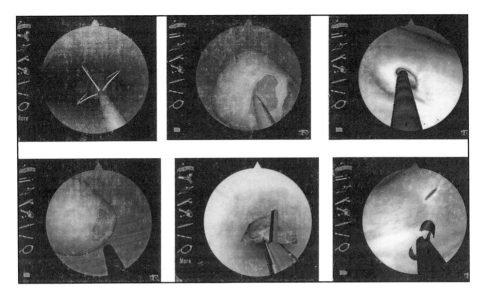

Figure 5. A sample of the currently available endourologic instruments in the URO Mentor simulator. From left to right and top to bottom: stone retrieval basket, rigid lithotripsy probe, guidewire, laser fiber, grasper, biopsy forceps.

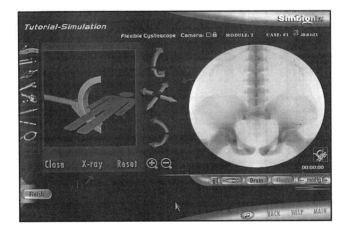

Figure 6. Fluoroscopic control is included among the features of the URO Mentor virtual reality simulator.

medical students who performed an initial VR case scenario requiring rigid cystoscopy and flexible ureteroscopy with laser lithotripsy and basket retrieval of a proximal ureter stone. Performance was assessed using the objective parameters available in the VR simulator (Fig. 7); furthermore, two experienced evaluators used a global scale rating. After the pretest (first performance) students were randomized to a control group receiving no further training or a training group that received five supervised training sessions using the VR simulator. The initial case scenario was used to re-evaluate the students. In the nontrained group no major differences were found between pre and posttest

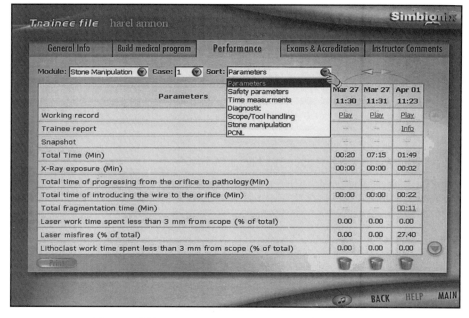

Figure 7. Objective assessment of performance (URO-Mentor).

performances. In the trained group posttest results showed a statistically significant improvement from baseline in the following parameters: total procedure time, time to introduce a ureteral guidewire, self-evaluation, and evaluator assessment. The comparison of the posttest results between the nontrained and trained groups also favored the trained group in ability to perform the task, overall performance, and total examiner score.

Working with the same VR simulator Watterson et al.[40] performed a similar study with 20 second-year medical students who had no previous experience in endourology and were randomized into two groups (training and control group). After receiving didactic teaching, including a video with a ureteroscopy performed in the VR simulator, all students performed the procedure once in the simulator. An experienced urologist, blinded to the randomization, evaluated their performances subjectively by means of a modified global rating scale.[11] For an objective assessment, the parameters recorded by the simulator were used (e.g., time required to perform each step of the procedure, number of attempts at cannulation of the ureter, number of times that the student needed reorientation, and rate of complications). Subsequently the test group received 10 minutes of individualized practice in the URO Mentor simulator, whereas the control group received no additional training. Then all students repeated the task in the simulator, and objective and subjective measurements were reassessed.

Although the prepractice test demonstrated equivalence between the two groups in the objective parameters measured by the simulator, the subjective global rating and pass-rating were higher for the untrained group. Posttest assessment revealed a significant improvement in the trained group in both objective and subjective assessment. These results not only confirm the usefulness of a model as a potential training tool but also stress the fact that significant improvement can be achieved in a short time. Currently integrated in the same platform of the URO Mentor is a PERC Mentor VR simulator, a commercial device for the practice of percutaneous procedures under fluoroscopy.

Simulators for Urologic Laparoscopy

Hand in hand with the development of modern endourology and following a universal trend, urologists have focused also on other minimally invasive techniques, among them laparoscopy. As in endourology, the main drawback of laparoscopy is a steep learning curve. Although the training in laparoscopic urology can be considered equal to the training needed for general surgery or other specialities, urologic laparoscopy has two specific differences: (1) the procedure has evolved from a excisional to a reconstructive technique,[41] and (2) the most challenging of the laparoscopic urologic procedures, radical prostatectomy, takes place in a deeper and more difficult anatomic field than that in which general surgeons are accustomed to work: the small pelvis.[42] A further disadvantage for urologic surgeons involved in laparoscopy is the lack of an organ that is easily accessible by laparoscopy (such as gallbladder for general surgeons).

Testing basic laparoscopic skills on inanimate models, becoming familiar with the principles of dissection and hemostasis in living animals, and studying surgical anatomy in cadavers should be considered indispensable and complementary elements for laparoscopic training.[43] Nevertheless, the use of living animals is expensive, requires sophisticated venues, and is subject to legal restrictions. In addition, cadaver models involve several problems and cannot be widely used as a training model for laparoscopy.

Although the use of simulators for laparoscopic training has already been broadly treated in the chapter of General Surgery, some considerations are worthy of mention. In reconstructive urologic laparoscopy, suturing is a basic skill; yet laparoscopic suturing is probably the most difficult of the laparoscopic tasks.

An adequate degree of rotation of the human wrist is needed to direct the needle effectively, and a large surgical field is necessary for proper positioning and actual performance of the suture. Because this rotation is hampered by long and awkward instruments and the fixed position of the trocars, laparoscopic suturing requires special dexterity and considerable practice in the training bench.[44]

The most popular inanimate model is the PelviTrainer, but a simple training bench can be hand-constructed, and some training facilities work with home-made bench models (Fig. 8). Dexterity and suturing models have been already described and validated for general surgery.[45] The same models are applicable to urologic laparoscopic training. Using precisely standardized and previously validated dexterity and suturing models, some studies in laparoscopic skills training have been published with special focus on urology.[46]

The impact of laparoscopic skills training on the operative performance of urologic surgeons inexperienced with laparoscopy has been assessed by Traxer.[46] Twelve residents (third to fifth year) were randomly assigned to either training or control groups. At baseline and after completion of the study, residents completed questionnaires about laparoscopic experience and perceived competence. At baseline and after 2 weeks, each resident performed a porcine laparoscopic nephrectomy. Each surgical procedure was

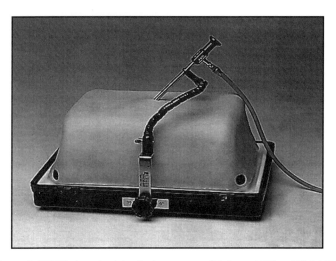

Figure 8. MAT Trainer simulator for laparoscopy (Limbs and Things,Bristol, UK).

intraoperatively evaluated by two experienced laparoscopic urologists who were blinded to the randomization status of the students. At baseline and two weeks later the residents also were tested on an inanimate simulator. The cumulative time needed to complete five tasks was recorded. After baseline evaluation the residents assigned to a training group practiced the same tasks alone on the bench trainer for 30 minutes/day for 10 days; the control group did not receive this training.

At baseline no statistical differences were noted in laparoscopic experience, inanimate training, or overall operative assessment between the two groups, but after training the cumulative time to perform the tasks decreased significantly in the group assigned to daily training. Although assessment improved significantly in both groups, training did little to improve overall performance of the laparoscopic nephrectomy. Essentially the most important factor for improvement in operative performance was the baseline "in-vivo laparoscopic nephrectomy."[46] This paradoxical result can be justified by the fact that only dissection skills are needed for a nephrectomy, whereas more advanced laparoscopic skills are needed for urologic laparoscopy.[44] It is nevertheless a universal consensus that hands-on training is an essential part of the acquisition of laparoscopic skills.[44, 47, 48]

A second generation of simulators between inanimate and VR simulators is the recently marketed Pulsate Organ Perfusion (POP) (Fig. 9). As mentioned previously, "in block" organs with the correspondent blood supply and venous drainage can be used in this simulator. A perfusion pump allows fluid circulation, and dye simulates the color of blood. All in all, a realistic simulation of bleeding and sealing and coagulative procedures can be achieved.

VR simulators for laparoscopy have been described extensively in previous chapters. All of them digitally recreate the procedures and environment of minimally invasive surgery, including extensive tasks, tailoring of functions, and advanced features for the recording and processing of training results. Despite their broad availability, new models with better interfaces and realistic haptic feedback are currently under development.

Based on the recognized need for laparoscopic training and the availability of bench

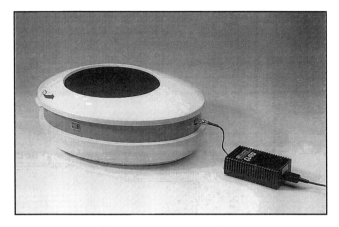

Figure 9. Pulsate Organ Perfusion (Optimist, Bregenz, Austria) simulator for laparoscopy training skills.

model, fellowships for training urologists in laparoscopic surgery are currently available[49] in specialized centers. Basically they consist of three steps: (1) a course of variable length that includes 2–3 days of hands-on experience with pelvic trainers and animal models; (2) observation of a clinical mentor performing a minimal number of major renal laparoscopic procedures; and (3) performance of a minimal number of major renal laparoscopic procedures under the direct guidance of the mentor.

Role of Robots in Laparoscopic Training

It has been hypothetisized that robot-assisted laparoscopy may decrease operative times and shorten the learning curve. Robots provide a three-dimensional visualization of the operative field and a larger range of instrument articulation (degrees of freedom), both of which help to optimize suturing tasks. However, there is still a lack of tactile feedback Yohannes et al.[50] compared the learning curves for robot-assisted and manual laparoscopic suturing in eight physicians (categorized as novice and experienced laparoscopist). Two skills—dexterity (passing a suture through seven needles mounted in a wooden block in a P configuration) and free-hand suturing (placement of three sutures through a thick sponge fixed to a Pelvitrainer)—were compared in a series of five trials each.

A conventional pelvic trainer was used to assess the learning curve with manual laparoscopy, and the da Vinci Robotic Surgical System (Intuitive Surgical, Mountain View, California) was used to assess the learning curve with robot-assisted laparoscopy. For the first skill (dexterity), both novice and experienced groups showed steady statistically significant improvement during the timed trials, although in manual laparoscopy a longer time was needed to achieve an end-point similar to that with robot-assisted laparoscopic skill performance. For the second skill (free-hand suturing), robot-assisted and manual laparoscopy could be compared only for the experienced group. The difference in learning curve was not statistically significant. The authors postulated that the same results can be achieved using manual laparoscopy at the expense of time.[50]

At present no conclusive data affirm that robots shorten the learning curve and have a role in the training process. Economical considerations also have to be taken into account before definite conclusion will be drawn.[51]

Validation of Current Simulators

Surgical simulation is considered with increasing frequency for training, testing, and possibly credentialing in medicine and surgery. Beside the fact that 97% of U.S. medical schools use mannequins as "standardized patients" for instruction and 85% use them for assessment, standardized patients are expected to be used for the U.S. Medical Licensing Examination in 2003.[5]

The important issue of validation needs to be addressed before inanimate or virtual reality simulators become widely accepted or used for training and accreditation purposes. Simulators, especially the sophisticated VR ones, are expensive tools that need to prove their effectiveness and reability.[40] Their usefulness depends on the extent to which they possess a number of features: credibility, comprehensiveness, reliability, and feasibility.[52] In fact, performance measurement has been severely neglected and ignored in many applications of simulators.[53] Two different aspects must be considered in discussions of validation. On one hand, the simulation device must be validated as a proper model to improve performance; thus a tool to measure performance is needed. The second and most important goal of any validation process is to answer the crucial question: Can the use of the simulator ultimately improve performance in a real patient and a real environment? Thus *validation means effective transfer of lab skills to real performance in the operating room.*

Despite abundant literature about the use of simulators, little has been done to validate urologic simulators, and tension often exists between the design and evaluation of surgical simulators.[54] The lack of high-quality published data is compounded by the difficulties of conducting longitudinal studies in such a fast moving field.[54]

Appropriate measuring instruments have been developed to validate simulators in other surgical fields. Two tests are currently used:

1. Advanced Dundee Psychomotor Test (ADEPT), which reflects innate psychomotor ability.[54]

2. OSATS (Objective Structured Assessment of Technique Skills (OSATS), which measures technical ability by means of specific checklists and a global rating score. This test is highly reliable and has construct validity.[45]

In endourology the few attempts to validate different simulators have led to the development of at least two structured checklists and score ratings.[3, 11] The checklist is intended to itemize important steps during the surgical procedure, whereas the global rating score captures the overall process, taking advantage of examiner expertise.[11] The global rating scale for assessing endourological performance was adapted from Anastakis[55] by Matsumoto et al.,[11] and the checklist was developed using a modified Delphi process.[56] Seven domains are evaluated:

1. Respect for tissue
2. Time and motion
3. Instrument handling
4. Handling of scope
5. Flow of procedure and forward planning
6. Use of assistants
7. Knowledge of procedure

Each domain has a 5-point Likert-type scale to assess generic aspects of ureterorenoscopy (URS) performance, including the necessary previous bladder maneuvers

Table 1.
The Seven Domains Evaluated in a Ureteroscopic Global Rating Scale and the Specific Part of the Procedure That They Evaluate

Domain	Evaluates
Respect for tissue	Trauma to urinary system tissue with the scope or other instruments
Time and motion	Unnecessary moves and time
Instrument handling	Number and quality of maneuvers needed to insert instrument
Handling of scope	Relationship of the scope with the anatomic landmarks
Flow of procedure and forward planning	Plannning and sequence of the procedure
Use of assistants	Ability to use assistant properly
Knowledge of procedure	Knowledge of and familiarity with the procedure

Adapted from Matsumoto ED, Hamstra SJ, Radomski SB, Cusimano MD: A novel approach to endourological training: Training at the surgical skills center. J Urol 2001;166:1261–1266.

(Table 1). In addition, the examiner has to fill out a pass-rating intended to respond to the ultimate goal of the training process: Would you be confident in allowing this trainee to perform the procedure in the operating room? The checklists and global score have internal validity and seem to fulfil the basic knowledge requirements for an efficient endoscopic urologic performance. These instruments have been used by other groups for the same purpose.[40] The checklist and global score used by Brehmer et al. are simpler, with the aim of making them useful and flexible,[3] but they have not been properly validated.

Although the word *validation* is used in the title of some articles about endourologic simulators,[3, 26, 27, 40] in fact what has been compared is the effect of the training on repeated performance in the same simulator or the features of the simulator in relation to the real procedure. In endourology the effect of training on transfer rate from simulator to real patient has never been measured. Although the design of some of these reports as well as their measurement tools allow the conclusion that the studied device is valid as a simulation tool, *to date no real validation or measurement of the transfer from simulator to patient has been done in urology.*

Conclusion

Different types of simulators have emerged in the past few years to help in the acquisition of surgical skills by bridging the gap between theoretical learning and real practice. In urology the bench models for the practice of endourology and, in some instances, VR simulators have been fully integrated in hands-on training courses. Most of the currently available models have been tested and proved to have construct validity, although little evidence attests to their beneficial effect. Simulation may play a crucial role not only in the training of surgeons but also in certification and accreditation programs.

Before generally accepting simulation skills training as a crucial educational step and as a tool for accreditation and selection, this technology must be properly assessed and validated. The educational value of simulation requires not only assessment and comparison with current methods of training but also measurement of reality transfer. This issue remains unanswered.

References
1. Bridges M, Diamond DL: The financial impact of teaching surgical residents in the operating room. Am J Surg 1999;177:28–32.
2. Vela Navarrete R, Andersen JT, Borowka A, et al: The future of urology in Europe: An overview from the European Association of Urology. Eur Urol 2001;39:361–368.
3. Brehmer M, Tolley DA: Validation of a bench model for endoscopic surgery in the upper urinary tract. Eur Urol 2002;42:175–180.
4. Hanna GB, Shimi SM, Cuschieri A: Task performance in endoscopic surgery is influeced by location of the image display. Ann Surg 1998;227:481–484.
5. Kaufmann CR: Computers in surgical education and the operating room. Ann Chirurg Gynaecol 2001;90:141–146.
6. Laguna MP, Hatzinger M, Rassweiler J: Simulators and endourological training. Curr Opin Urol 2002;12:209–215.
7. Friedrich MJ: Practice makes perfect: Risk-free medical training with patient simulators. JAMA 2002;288:2808–2812.
8. Wanzel KR, Hamstra SJ, Anastakis DJ, et al: Effect of visual-spatial ability on learning of spatially-complex surgical skills. Lancet 2002;359:230–231.
9. Gallagher HJ, Allan JD, Tolley DA: Spatial awareness in urologists: Are they different? Br J Urol Int 2001;88:666–670.
10. Kopta JA: The development of motor skills in orthopaedic education. Clin Orthop 1971;75:80–85.
11. Matsumoto ED, Hamstra SJ, Radomski SB, Cusimano MD: A novel approach to endourological training: Training at the surgical skills center. J Urol 2001;166:1261–1266.
12. Cadeddu JA: Comparison of robotic versus laparoscopic skills: Is there a difference in the learning curve? [editorial]. Urology 2002;60:39–45.
13. Burdea G, Patounakis G, Popescu V, Weiss RE: Virtual reality-based training for the diagnosis of prostate cancer. IEEE Transact Biomed Eng 1999;46:1253–1260.
14. Cervantes L, Keitzer WA: Endoscopic training in urology. J Urol 1960;84:585–586.
15. Fiddian RV: A method of training in perurethral resection. Br J Urol 1967; 39:192–193.
16. Narwani KP, Reid EC: Teaching transurethral prostatic resection using cadaver bladder. J Urol 1969;101:101.
17. Habib HN, Berger J, Winter CC: Teaching transurethral surgery using a cow's udder. J Urol 1965;93:77–79.
18. Trindade JCS, Lautenschlager MFM, de Araujo CG: Endoscopic surgery: A new teaching method. J Urol 1981;126:192.
19. Pirkmajer B, Leusch G: A bladder-prostate model on which to practice using transurethral resection instruments. Urologe A 1977;16:336–338.
20. Baumrucker GO: TUR—Transurethral Prostatectomy: Teaching, Hazards and Pitfalls. Baltimore, Williams & Wilkins, 1969.
21. Cooper M, Elves A, Feneley RCL: Preliminary evaluation of a TUR training model [abstract 348]. Eur Urol 1996;Suppl.
22. Lardennois B, Clement T, Ziade A, Brandt B: Simulation of endoscopic resection of the prostate. Ann Urol 1990;24:519–523.
23. Ballaro A, Briggs T, Garcia-Montes F, et al: A computer generated interactive transurethral prostatic resection simulator. J Urol 1999;162:1633–1635.
24. Kumar PVS, Gomes MPSF, Davies BL, Timoney AG: A computer assisted surgical trainer for transurethral resection of the prostate. J Urol 2002;168:2111–2114.
25. Michel MS, Knoll T, Koehrmann KU, Alken P: The URO Mentor: Development and evalu-

ation of a new computer-based interactive training system for virtual life-like simulation of diagnostic and therapeutic endourological procedures. Br J Urol Int 2002;89:174–177.

26. Shah J, Darzi A: Virtual reality flexible cystoscopy: A validation study. Br J Urol Int 2002;90: 828–832.

27. Shah J, Montgomery B, Langley S, Darzi A: Validation of a flexible cystoscopy course. Br J Urol Int 2002;90:833–835.

28. Manyak MJ, Santangelo K, Hahn J, et al: Virtual reality surgical simulation for lower urinary tract endoscopy and procedures. J Endourol 2002;16:185–190.

29. Mitropoulos D, Dounavis P, Papageorgiou S, et al: Virtual urethrocystoscopy simulator with haptic feedback. Eur Urol 2002;Suppl 1:7.

30. Papadopoulos E, Vlachos K, Mitropoulos D: Design of a 5-dof haptic simulator for urological operations. Proceedings of the 2002 IEEE International Conference on Robotics and Automation, 2002.

31. Papadopoulos E, Vlachos K, Mitropoulos D: On the design of a low-force 5-dof force-feedback haptic mechanism. Proceedings of the DETC'02 ASME 2002 Design Engineering Technical Conferences and Computers and Information in Engineering Conference, 2002.

32. Friedman CP: Anatomy of the clinical simulation. Acad Med 1995;70:205–209.

33. Bricken M: Virtual reality learning environments: Potential and challenges. Comput Graph 1991;25:178–184.

34. Oppenheimer P, Gupta A, Weghorst S, et al: The representation of blood flow in endourological surgical simulations. Stud Health Technol Inform 2001;81:365–371.

35. Sweet R, Porter J, Oppenheimer P, et al: Simulation of bleeding in endoscopic procedures using virtual reality. J Endourol 2002;16:451–455.

36. Strohmaier WL, Giese A: Porcine urinary tract as a training model for ureteroscopy. Urol Int 2001;66:30–32.

37. Matsumoto ED, Hamstra SJ, Radomski SB, Cusimano MD: The effect of bench model fidelity on endourological skills: A randomized controlled study. J Urol 2002;167:1243–1247.

38. Preminger GM, Babayan RK, Merril GL, et al: Virtual reality surgical simulation in endoscopic urologic surgery. Stud Health Technol Inform 1996;29:157–163.

39. Wilhelm DM, Ogan K, Roehrborn CG, et al: Assessment of basic endoscopic performance using a virtual reality simulator. J Am Coll Surg 2002;195: 675–681.

40. Watterson JD, Beiko DT, Kuan JK, Denstedt JD: Randomized prospective blinded study validating acquisition of ureteroscopic skills using computer based virtual reality endourological simulator. J Urol 2002;168:1928–1932.

41. Turk IA, Davis JW, Winkelmann B, et al: Laparoscopic dismembered pyeloplasty: The method of choice in the presence of an enlarged renal pelvis and crossing vessels. Eur Urol 2002;42:268–275.

42. Guillonneau B, el-Fettouh H, Baumert H, et al: Laparoscopic radical prostatectomy: Oncological evaluation after 1.000 cases at Montsouris Institute. J Urol 2003;169:1261–1266.

43. Hozneck A, Katz R, Gettman M, et al: Laparoscopic and robotic surgical training in urology. Curr Urol Rep 2003;4:130–137.

44. Rassweiler J, Frede T, Guillonneau B: Advanced laparoscopy. Eur Urol 2002;42.

45. Reznick R, Regehr G, MacRae H, et al: Testing technical skill via an innovative "bench station" examination. Am J Surg 1997;173:226–230.

46. Traxer O, Gettman MT, Napper CA, et al: The impact of intensive laparoscopic skills training on the operative performance of urology residents. J Urol 2001;166:1658–1661.

47. Seymour NE, Gallagher AG, Roman SA, et al: Virtual reality training improves operating room performance: Results of a randomized, double-blinded study. Ann Surg 2002;236: 458–464.

48. Kneebone R: Simulation in surgical training: Educational issues and practical implications. Med Educ 2003;37:267–277.

49. Shalhav AL, Dabagia MD, Wagner TT, et al: Training postgraduate urologists in laparoscopic surgery: The current challenge. J Urol, 2002;167:2135–2137.

50. Yoannes P, Rotariu P, Pinto P, et al: Comparison of robotic versus laparoscopic skills: Is there a difference in the learning curve? Urology 2002;60:39.

51. Guillonneau B: What robotics in urology?. A current point of view. Eur Urol 2003;43: 103–105.
52. Berg D, Raugi G, Gladstone H, et al: Virtual reality simulators for dermatologic surgery: Measuring their validity as a teaching tool. Dermatol Surg 2001;27:370–374.
53. Sanders AF: Simulation as a tool in the measurement of human performance. Ergonomics 1991;34 :995–1025.
54. Schijven MP. Jakimowicz J, Schot C: The Advanced Dundee Endoscopic Psychomotor tester (ADEPT) objectifying subjective psychomotor test performance. Surg Endosc 2002;16: 943–948.
55. Anastakis DJ, Regehr G, Reznick RK, et al: Assessment of technical skills transfer from the bench training model to the human model. Am J Surg 1999;177:167–170.
56. Stewart J, O'Halloran C, Harrigan P, et al: Identifying appropriate tasks for the preregistration year: Modified Delphi technique. BMJ 1999;319:224–229.

Chapter 17

SIMULATION IN LIFE SUPPORT PROTOCOLS

Glen A. Franklin, MD

The use of simulator technology, human patient simulation, and "standardized" (practice) patients has recently become increasingly popular for the training of allied health personnel, medical students, residents, and physicians.[1–4] With increasing demands on educational time and quality, the introduction of advanced patient simulation offers new avenues of educational instruction in a controlled environment. For many years advanced training has been offered in the areas of airway management, intubation, cardiopulmonary resuscitation (CPR), intravenous access, and injury assessment and management. The American College of Surgeons (ACS), American Heart Association (AHA), and the American Burn Association (ABA) have sponsored additional training courses for specific skill maintenance. These courses have been developed for training at both basic and advanced levels. They are relatively portable and are offered at a number of sites nationwide. Specific course information can be found at the website of each of these organizations (Table 1).

In the broadest sense, patient simulation can incorporate a number of different training modalities. Simulation can be as simple as the use of a standardized patient as well as mannequins. With technologic advances, full patient and disease simulation can be achieved with advanced mannequins, computer simulation, and virtual reality. There are many advantages to the routine use of simulators. The experience can be standardized to help minimize the course-to-course variation. Likewise, identical experiences can be recreated to allow correction of previous mistakes and review of key principles. This chapter discusses four different advanced training courses: advanced trauma life support (ATLS), advanced cardiac life support (ACLS), pediatric advanced life support (PALS), and advanced burn life support (ABLS). The chapter reviews the general scope of each course and the current use of simulation technology. A brief discussion of possible future adaptations of advanced simulation techniques for each course is also included.

Table 1.
Course Links to ATLS, ACLS, PALS and ABLS

Organization	Website	Course
American College of Surgeons	www.facs.org	ATLS
American Heart Association	www.americanheart.org	ACLS, PALS
American Burn Association	www.ameriburn.org	ABLS

Advanced Trauma Life Support

Following its development in 1978, ATLS was readily approved by the American College of Surgeons Committee on Trauma (ACS-COT) in 1979 as a standard in initial assessment and trauma management. The course was first offered nationally in 1980. Worldwide promulgation of ATLS began in 1986, and currently more than 40 countries have adopted this course. It is offered at 1,087 sites worldwide; two-thirds of the courses are provided in the United States.

Of interest, this physician-only course had its roots in an airplane tragedy. In 1976, an orthopedic surgeon was piloting a private aircraft over rural Nebraska. During an emergency crash landing the pilot's wife was killed. He sustained major injuries, as did three of his four children. They were transported to a local hospital where the medical care delivered was less than adequate. Dr. Steiner made this now infamous statement: "When I can provide better care in the field with limited resources than what my children and I received at the primary care facility, there is something wrong with the system and the system has to be changed." Focused on the "golden hour" of trauma care, ATLS seeks to provide a standard framework for the initial assessment and care of the trauma victim.[5]

From its inception, ATLS has used a combination of didactic and skills stations to review the initial phase of care for the injured patient. Each skills station is designed to train and reinforce a particular technique or procedure. Many of the stations review the principles of patient immobilization and physical exam by using patient volunteers for cervical collar placement, spine board use, and log-roll techniques. Mannequins are used for Gardner-Wells tongs placement and for the head and neck exam. The mannequin, "Mr. Hurt", has several simulated head and neck injuries (Fig. 1). This model provides a fairly accurate simulation of a complex neck laceration, open skull fracture, zygomatic fracture, hemotympanum, Marcus Gunn pupil, alveolar ridge fracture, and Battle's sign. Through the use of simulations, the student may also practice common procedures on standard mannequins such as intubation and central catheter placement (Fig. 2). These devices are similar to those commonly used in ACLS and PALS training courses.

Large animal models have been used for the simulation of key surgical procedures in the ATLS course. The surgical skills laboratory typically uses a canine or porcine model for venous cut-down, chest tube placement, cricothyrotomy, pericardiocentesis, and diagnostic peritoneal lavage (DPL) training. Animal models for these procedures offer many advantages, including the handling of living tissues, similar anatomic relationships, and required control of bleeding. They have also been shown to improve resident performance.[6] However, there are limitations to the routine use of animals for training purposes. Associated costs include purchase of the animals as well as maintenance of an approved animal research facility. With increasing concerns from animal rights activists and governmental regulations, these facilities are highly complex to maintain and present a barrier for smaller training centers.

Fresh tissue laboratories with minimally preserved cadavers have also been used by some centers for surgical skills training.[7] While providing the appropriate anatomic experience, they often lack the true feel of living tissue. The ready access to adequate facilities and number of cadavers is available at only a few centers. However appealing the use of actual human tissue may seem, the expense and limited availability makes the routine use of cadavers highly impractical for a course that requires such widespread promulgation.

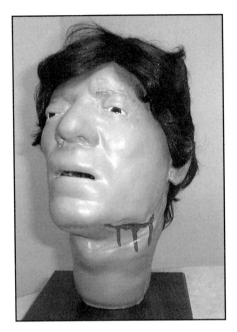

Figure 1. ATLS "Mr. Hurt": a mannequin used for training providers to identify head and neck injuries.

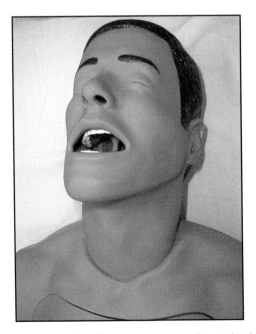

Figure 2. Mannequin used for practicing airway management and central catheter placement skills.

The recent momentum for development of advanced patient simulators is most likely due to advances in microprocessor technology and the increasing difficulty in offering live animal or cadaver training. Societal and economic pressures have also helped to advance the development of alternatives to these common models. ATLS has traditionally been more procedure-weighted than other courses of its type. The need for efficient, cost-effective, reproducible patient simulation has always been important to the objectives of ATLS. Perhaps a hallmark of the course is the surgical skills station where students are trained in the indications and techniques for needle and open cricothyrotomy, chest tube placement, DPL, pericardiocentesis, and venous cut-down. Currently only one device is approved by the ACS-COT Subcommittee on ATLS as an alternative to the traditional live animal or cadaver laboratory section of the course. This device is the TraumaMan system provided by Simulab Corporation (Seattle, WA). Details about the device can be found at the company's website (www.simulab.com).

The TraumaMan system is a self-contained, life-sized torso covered with a pliable elastomeric polymer that mimics human skin. The polymer contains multiple layers to simulate the natural layers of the abdomen and contains a capillary system that "oozes" red dye when cut (Figs. 3 and 4). The device uses "skin" overlays for multiple-use applications. It provides a realistic representation of multiple surgical procedures and allows the simultaneous involvement of several students (Figs. 5 and 6). This type of technology is gaining popularity and momentum as a viable alternative to traditional animal or cadaver models. Of the 438 ATLS teaching sites in the United States (civilian and military), 150 currently use the TraumaMan system for training.

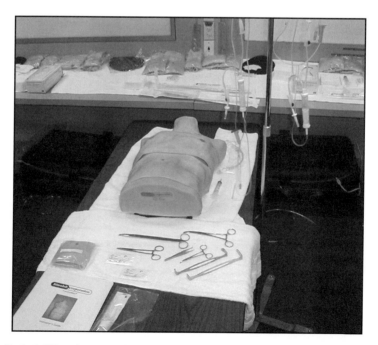

Figure 3. Typical skill station set-up for use of the TraumaMan system for the surgical skills station of ATLS.

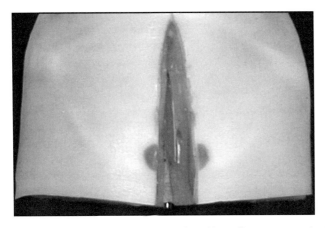

Figure 4. Abdominal layers on the TraumaMan skin overlay with capillary system to simulate bleeding.

As an educational tool little has been reported about this or any other system. Block et al. used the TraumaMan with 14 participants in a standard ATLS course as an experimental station in addition to the traditional surgical skills station with live animal models. Overall the participants felt that the simulator was quite useful and even superior to the animal model in the teaching of surgical airway management and chest tube insertion.[8] Conversely, computer-based trauma simulation training showed no significant difference with students trained in a seminar-based fashion, but both methods were

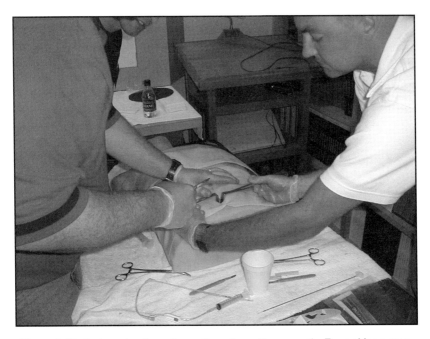

Figure 5. Students performing a diagnostic peritoneal lavage on the TraumaMan system.

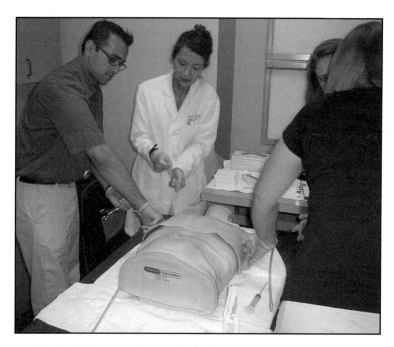

Figure 6. Placement of a closed tube thoracostomy on the TraumaMan.

superior to the control group that lacked additional focused trauma training.[9] Others have noted an enhancement of trauma management skills when an advanced human patient simulator is used.[10] These type of simulators have been used not only to teach ATLS and trauma management courses but also to evaluate the outcomes of these courses. Jameel et al. found that the simulator was a good way to assess student skills following ATLS training and provided a good standard for comparison of different training groups.[11]

Not all simulator technology requires the use of a mannequin. Software-driven simulation of how to perform a DPL is available and has been shown to be superior to animal training for teaching the procedure to medical students.[12] Albeit data are preliminary, there may be some procedures that can be effectively taught using a software self-study module alone. Because limited time is available for any simulation training, the ability to have a training program packaged on a CD-ROM that can be used at a student's own pace does have some advantages. This avenue of alternative training warrants further investigation both as a primary skill training modality and as an adjunct to hands-on experience.

Recently ultrasound has started to replace DPL and CT scan for evaluation of the trauma patient's abdomen. The current edition of the ATLS student manual (1997) provides a discussion of this procedure as well as an instructional video. However, skills stations to train physicians in the appropriate technique are not yet included in the course. With access to ultrasound simulation, it is not hard to imagine the addition of such technology and training to the course. Most ultrasound courses that are currently sponsored by the ACS use human models for live action training. The availability and cost of models continue to limit some course size and access. However, an ultrasound simulator has been shown equivalent to models for the training of residents in the standard exam for trauma—focused abdominal sonogram for trauma (FAST).[13] The UltraSim (MedSim, Ft. Lauderdale, FL) ultrasound eliminates the need for finding normal and abnormal models. The exam can be stored digitally and then recalled for review and critique.

The testing phase of the ATLS course uses volunteer patients who are given basic training in how to mimic several types of injury. The "patients" are placed in moulage to provide a more realistic experience. Typically the student and examiner enter an evaluation room with the standardized patient. The student is given a basic scenario and allowed to begin the work-up. In addition to moulage injuries, radiographs of the patient case are provided. Depending on the facility and desire of the examiner, the moulage tests can be fairly realistic and are designed to cover key course concepts. An advanced human patient simulator could easily be adapted for this portion of the course and would allow an experience that tests both diagnostic and technical skills in a single provider or multi-provider environment.

Advanced Cardiac Life Support

The ACLS course was developed by the American Heart Association (AHA) with the intention of improving basic and advanced emergency cardiac care by providing standard algorithms for treatment. The current course includes 10 case scenarios, including four types of cardiac arrest, four types of prearrest emergencies, respiratory failure, and stroke. Mannequins are provided at skills stations to assist with the use of bag-valve-mask with oral airway, CPR, and intubation (Fig. 7). One course objective is to provide a thorough familiarization with all the types of drugs and equipment used during a cardiopulmonary arrest. Examples of each piece of equipment are demonstrated during the skills stations. A thorough knowledge of this equipment is needed for its proper use. Simulated (low-voltage) defibrillations allow the student to train on an acutal defibrillator.

Because the course focuses heavily on cardiac events, it includes demonstrations of various cardiac rhythms (normal sinus, stable tachycardia, unstable tachycardia, bradycardia, ventricular fibrillation/tachycardia, pulseless electrical activity, asystole, and torsade de pointes). Rhythm strips and EKG cards can be used for initial training and review, but most training sites use a programmable defibrillator with the ability to alter type of rhythm and rate for a truly dynamic experience. This simulation helps provide the student with use of an actual cardiac monitor, the rapid changes that can occur when the heart switches rhythm, and further education on the use of a defibrillator.

Testing during ACLS involves the infamous "megacode." The student interacts with the instructors in a simulated cardiopulmonary emergency. The thought process, adherence to standard algorithms, and proper use of equipment are evaluated during this simulation. Rhythms are programmed to respond to the student's action and allow the testing of several different scenarios during one session. As sites gain access to an advanced patient simulator, the training and testing phases of ACLS are becoming more realistic. There are several advantages to the use of this technology, particularly with regard to a course such as ACLS. Of all the courses discussed in this chapter, ACLS may be the best example for widespread use of an advanced device.

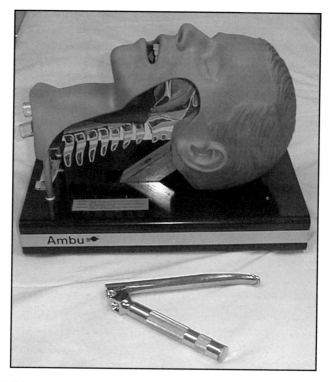

Figure 7. Adult airway trainer demonstrating anatomic landmarks for intubation teaching.

Algorithms are easy to memorize and easy to test, but the practical delivery of the medicines and procedures must also be mastered. In this regard, experience with a human patient simulator would be second to none. As the "code" develops, the student must demonstrate proficiency with the equipment and the correct delivery of the medication (including use of the correctly dosed syringe). An immediate physiologic response can be observed. This interactive and dynamic situation allows the instructor to observe several aspects of a student's ability. The addition of several students at once will allow evaluation team response, interaction, and leadership. With little effort, this experience can become totally immersive and provide a nearly realistic patient crisis. Most laboratories of this type include the ability to videotape the experience, which further enhances the educational process by allowing a period of post-testing debriefing and criticism. The military is already evaluating this type of team interaction for resuscitation training.[14]

Pediatric Advanced Life Support

Given the success of the ACLS course, in 1983 the AHA recommended the development of a resuscitation course specific to the needs of children. The first PALS manual was completed in 1988, and the first course was offered to providers later that year.[15,16] Like its predecessor, the PALS course offers advanced resuscitation training specific for children with a focus on airway control, fluid resuscitation, and cardiac support. This training is accomplished through the use of didactic lectures and skills sta-

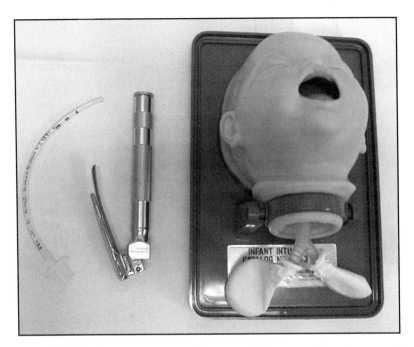

Figure 8. Pediatric airway mannequin used for demonstration and practice of airway control.

tions. The pediatric "megacode" is very similar to that of ACLS, with a combination of practical demonstration of technical skills and simulated code resuscitation.

Simulation technology is also used in the PALS course. Of key importance to the objectives of the course are familiarity with the unique features of pediatric anatomy and recognition of the signs and symptoms of cardiopulmonary collapse. Models of the pediatric airway have been used for many years to allow training and practice with endotracheal tube selection and placement (Fig. 8). Programmable defibrillators are also used during the megacode section to evaluate rhythm identification and treatment. Lower limb models are used for demonstration of intraosseous catheter placement, and most models have a fairly realistic feel to the advancement of the needle through the periostium. Models are also available for saphenous cut-down and IV placement.

Advanced human patient simulators are available for pediatric simulation and are used for training of emergency medical technicians, medical students, nurses, and residents. Although the cost of these facilities can be high ($250,000), they can be adapted to a variety of patient scenarios and provide an authentic experience.[10] Given the limited experience that many nonpediatric providers have with children, the use of simulation technology can greatly improve provider skill and confidence.

Advanced Burn Life Support

The ABLS course is a one-day course that focuses on the initial management of burn injury. Developed by the American Burn Association (ABA), ABLS provides training for physicians, physician assistants, nurses, and paramedics in the treatment and resuscitation

402 PRACTICAL HEALTH CARE SIMULATIONS

of burns during the first 24 hours. A shorter version of the course is available for prehospital providers. This course includes both didactic and skill modules. As with ACLS, PALS, and ATLS, a section of the course reviews the ABCs and airway control. The airway station utilizes mannequins to simulate the oral pharynx for intubation practice. These basic intubation simulators have been used for years to train young medical professionals in the technique of intubation. Anyone who has used this technology knows its limitations; however, the key anatomic landmarks are in place and offer good practice for those with little intubation experience.

The course contains an assessment module that uses simulated patients with moulage to demonstrate different types of burn wounds. Standard patients include a burn with inhalation injury, a burn with trauma, a burned pediatric patient, and an electrical burn. This method of education and assessment has been used in many types of patient interaction training. It has the advantage of using real human subjects to "augment" the simulated experience. It is time-consuming to place the patients in moulage, particularly in trying to provide a good simulation of thermal injury. Additional personnel are required with some level of medical knowledge to enact appropriately the symptoms of the disease process. Finally, experiences are not consistent from course to course and depend on the moulage volunteer.

Recent advances in "skins" or overlays provide a more realistic wound simulation and shorten the time traditionally needed for elaborate make-up. These prostheses can be made of standard sizes and depth to allow the instructor to provide many different total body surface area burns that are consistent from student to student and course to course.[17] The military and firefighting services often stage mass casualty simulations with both thermal and chemical burns. The ease with which latex prostheses can be placed on multiple "patients" makes them ideal for large demonstrations. Many vendors offer moulage kits with both burn wounds and traumatic injuries. Examples can be found at the following websites:

1. www.safetyprograms.org/images/simulaids/simcas.htm
2. www.drmass.com/casulty-simulation-deluxe-casualty-simulation-kit.html
3. www.flemingmedical.ie/simul-kits.htm
4. www.moulage.net/IPCat.htm
5. www.global-technologies.net/ShopSite/W44522_I.html

Advanced moulage kits of this type and a technologically advanced human patient simulator lab allow a highly realistic simulation of airway control, resuscitation, patient response to resuscitation, and wound assessment/treatment. Continued emphasis on disaster preparedness, bioterrorism training, and mass casualty management only helps to drive the innovations needed in this area to further train medical professionals in initial burn management.

Conclusion

All of the advanced training courses discussed in this chapter have used some type of patient simulation technology to augment the learning experience. From the most basic mannequins to the advanced human patient simulator, we continue to strive toward an experience to prepare young health care professionals for real life emergency situations. As technology advances, the cost associated with simulator laboratories will con-

Table 2.
Online Resuscitation and Code Simulators

Website	Course/Training Simulation
www.madsci.com/physicians.html	ACLS
www.acls.net	ACLS
mdchoice.com/cyberpt/acls/acls.asp	ACLS
www.anesoft.com/Products/acls.asp	ACLS
www.mdchoice.com/cyberpt/pals/pals.asp	PALS
www.netmedicine.com/cyberpt/pals/p1/p1-01.htm	PALS
www.trauma.org/resus/moulage/moulage.html	ATLS
www.lessstress.com	CPR, EMS, First Aid
www.ecglibrary.com/ecghome.html	ECG Library
www.mdchoice.com/cyberpt/cyber.asp	Acute MI
www.nyerrn.com/simulators.htm	ACLS, PALS, ATLS, BLS, Pediatric Trauma, Acute MI, TNCC

CPR = cardiopulmonary resuscitation, EMS = emergency medical services, ECG = electrocardiogram, BLS = basic life support, TNCC = trauma nurse core course.

tinue to decrease and access to these facilities will become more widespread. Several centers, especially the military, are already using simulators and standardized patients for disaster preparedness training, procedural training and proficiency, and resident education and evaluation.[18-22] The use of advanced simulators in endoscopy and laparoscopy is a growing field in surgical education,[23-25] and the addition of virtual reality technology will further advance minimally invasive procedural training.

These devices have multiple applications that help to drive the need for widespread availability. As medical educators continue to "think outside the box" of traditional didactic and observational methods, the access to advanced human patient simulation facilities will grow. Injury assessment and initial resuscitation continue to be at the center of discussions on bioterrorism and disaster planning. ATLS, ACLS, PALS, and ABLS have unique roles to play in the training of health care professionals—a role that will only increase the demand for these courses. The increased demand will create increased costs for the models, mannequins, and animals. Large simulation centers used for a variety of training modalities may decrease the duplication of resources commonly found at medical centers offering these four courses. Whatever the training modality, at the center of our discussion is the best method to prepare health care workers for the intimate interactions and emergencies found in the daily care of patients. Simulation technology allows mental and technical preparation prior to patient encounters. The old adage of "see one, do one, teach one" may well be replaced with "see one, simulate many, do one, simulate again, and grow in experience."

References
1. Macedonia CR, Gherman RB, Satin AJ: Simulation laboratories for training in obstetrics and gynecology. Obstet Gynecol 2003;102:388–392.

2. Brown A, Anderson D, Szerlip HM: Using standardized patients to teach disease management skills to preclinical students: A pilot project. Teach Learn Med 2003;15:84–87.
3. Berkenstadt H, Ziv A, Barsuk D, et al: The use of advanced simulation in the training of anesthesiologists to treat chemical warfare casualties. Anesth Analg 2003;96:1739–1742.
4. Kneebone R: Simulation in surgical training: Educational issues and practical implications. Med Educ 2003;37:267–277.
5. Course overview: The purpose, history and concepts of the ATLS program for doctors. In Advanced Trauma Life Support for Doctors, Instructor Course Manual, 199, pp 9–19.
6. Custalow CB, Kline JA, Marx JA, Baylor MR: Emergency department resuscitative procedures: Animal laboratory training improves procedural competency and speed. Acad Emerg Med 2002;9:575–586.
7. Available from URL: http://www.pcrm.org/resch/PDFs/med_trauma.pdf (accessed 2003 October 3).
8. Block EFJ, Lottenberg L, Flint L, et al: Use of a human patient simulator for the advanced trauma life support course. Am Surg. 2002;68:648–651.
9. Gilbart MK, Hutchison CR, Cusimano MD, Regehr G: A computer-based trauma simulator for teaching trauma management skills. Am J Surg. 2000;179:223–228.
10. Marshall RL, Smith S, Gorman PJ, et al: Use of a human patient simulator in the development of resident trauma management skills. J Trauma 2001;51:17–21.
11. Jameel A, Cohen RJ, Gana TJ, Al-Bedah KF: Effect of the advanced trauma life support program on medical students' performance in simulated trauma patient management. J Trauma. 1998;44:588–591.
12. Bowyer MW, Liu AV, Bonar JP: Validation of a diagnostic peritoneal lavage simulator for trauma skills training. Poster presentation, Sixty-second Meeting of the American Association for the Surgery of Trauma, September 11–13, 2003, Minneapolis, MN.
13. Knudson, MM, Sisley, AC: Training residents using simulation technology: experience with ultrasound for trauma. J Trauma 2000;48:659–665.
14. Holcomb, JB, Dumire, RD, Crommett, JW, et al: Evaluation of trauma team performance using an advanced human patient simulator for resuscitation training. J Trauma 2002;52:1078–1085.
15. Bardella IJ: Pediatric advance life support: A review of the AHA recommendations. www.aafp.org/afp/991015ap/1743.html (accessed 2003 Sept 14).
16. Quan L, Seidel JS (eds): Pediatric Advanced Life Support: Instructor's Manual. Dallas, American Heart Association, 1997.
17. Lindsey J: Moulage magic! Injury simulations so real they'll amaze you. J Emerg Med Serv 2003;28:122, 124, 126.
18. Bruce S, Bridges EJ, Holcomb JB: Preparing to respond: Joint Trauma Training Center and USAF Nursing Warskills Simulation Laboratory. Crit Care Nurs Clin North Am 2003;15:149–162.
19. Gofrit ON, Leibovici D, Shemer J, et al: The efficacy of integrating "smart simulated casualties" in hospital disaster drills. Prehosp Diaster Med 1997;12:97–101.
20. Serwint JR: The use of standardized patients in pediatric residency training in palliative care: Anatomy of a standardized patient case scenario. J Palliat Med 2002;5:146–153.
21. Halamek LP, Kaegi DM, Gaba DM, et al: Time for a new paradigm in pediatric medical education: Teaching neonatal resuscitation in a simulated delivery room environment. Pediatrics 2000;106:E45.
22. Lane JL, Ziv A, Boulet JR: A pediatric clinical skills assessment using children as standardized patients. Arch Pediatr 1999;153:637–644.
23. Prasad SM, Maniar HS, Soper NJ, et al: The effect of robotic assistance on learning curves for basic laparoscopic skills. Am J Surg 2002;183:702–707.
24. Dunkin BJ: Flexible endoscopy simulators. Semin Laparosc Surg 2003;10:29–35.
25. Hoznek A, Katz R, Gettman M, et al: Laparoscopic and robotic surgical training in urology. Curr Urol Rep 2003;4:130–137.

Chapter 18

SIMULATION IN OBSTETRICS AND GYNECOLOGY

Brigitte Bonin, MD, FRCS(C), and Glenn D. Posner, MDCM

Pregnant women seldom walk through the front door of the hospital with an inkling that they may never leave. Thankfully, due to advancements in medicine and obstetric care over the past century, maternal mortality is indeed a rare event. Therefore, despite adequate theoretical knowledge, trainees in obstetrics and gynecology may complete their residency without encountering in vivo some of the life-threatening conditions that befall pregnant women. However, 5–10 women per 100,000 continue to die each year due to hemorrhage, sepsis, thromboembolic disease, uncontrolled hypertension, and amniotic fluid embolism. The use of clinical simulators may present learners in this specialty with the only opportunity to face such challenging scenarios.

Status of Current Uses in Obstetrics and Gynecology

The study of medicine is largely an apprenticeship, with inexperienced learners practicing on patients. However, learners sometimes encounter more obstacles in the birthing unit than in the rest of the hospital. Compounding the usual apprehension is the idea that obstetric care usually involves a healthy woman and her healthy baby; pregnancy is a natural process that many people believe should require no medical intervention. For this reason, and due to the delicate nature of the examinations required in gynecology, obstetrics and gynecology have needed to employ models as an educational tool more often than the average discipline.

There are many commercially available models of the female pelvis with which students can practice bimanual examinations and speculum exams. These plastic models are often used in objective, structured clinical examinations of medical students and residents and have been described at a military university.[1,2] Many medical schools hire women who offer to be model patients. These women teach what they call the "sensitive" pelvic exam, demonstrating to small groups of students how to approach a patient for a pelvic exam, explain to her what they will be doing, and how to perform the exam. The students then take turns performing speculum exams and bimanual exams while receiving feedback about their bedside manner and technique.

Inanimate models are adequate for teaching physical examination skills, but demonstration of management and communication skills requires either a living and breathing patient or a reasonable facsimile: a simulation that responds to different stimuli and on which procedures can be performed. Examples of simulators currently used in obstetrics and gynecology and described in the literature can be found in Canada, the United States, and the United Kingdom.

Attempts have been made at simulating the amniotic sac to rehearse amniocentesis and other infrequent and potentially complicated invasive perinatal procedures. The goal is to teach technical skills to novice physicians by practicing on a model, thereby shifting the learning curve from the patient to the "classroom." In Toronto, a study was conducted in which trainees received a course about the practice of amniocentesis that involved a lecture, a syllabus, and a hands-on training session with a simulated patient.[3] The authors describe their simulator as "high-fidelity," referring to the ability to produce a realistic recreation of an actual amniocentesis. Pre- and posttraining performances were evaluated, and scores improved significantly as a result of the hands-on session. The study's demonstration of a positive effect of the hands-on session on the performance of trainees provides evidence that simulator-based education can be a valuable method of instruction that protects patients' safety.

The University of Pittsburgh School of Medicine recognized that residents in obstetrics and gynecology might miss out on managing certain rare cases during their training.[4] In 1996, a course was developed that employs a high-fidelity simulator to teach residents to manage critical events. In an arrangement similar to our own at the University of Ottawa, the simulations take place in a makeshift operative suite, complete with anesthesia machine, monitors, and a mannequin that acts as the patient. This mannequin is an elaborate, computer-operated replica of a human; it includes a mouth, airway, lungs, palpable pulses, and heart and breath sounds. Scenarios were generated to depict critical events that the residents would be asked to manage. The scenarios included pre eclampsia, amniotic fluid embolus, postoperative acute myocardial infarction, and anaphylaxis. The residents stated that the simulator training "allowed them to manage critical events in a realistic setting and improved their knowledge about their management of critical events."

In the United Kingdom, a program called Managing Obstetric Emergencies and Trauma (MOET) has been developed to respond to the need for improved maternity care and specifically to reduce the number of avoidable deaths.[5] This new training method employs animal cadavers, an assisted delivery model, and a symphysiotomy model (in case of a trapped after-coming head or severe shoulder dystocia). This course received accolades from the participating residents, who believed that they were better equipped to manage many critical conditions.

The simulator at the University of Ottawa was first used by the Department of Obstetrics and Gynecology in the spring of 2001; it was evaluated as a pilot project before being implemented as part of the residency training program. When the project was conceived, the anesthetists were using simulations extensively, but their use in educating obstetrics and gynecology residents had been limited. The objectives of the pilot study were (1) to assess the suitability of a simulator as a teaching aid in obstetrics and gynecology; (2) to use this teaching tool to provide exposure to rare and/or critical life-like events; and (3) to improve communicative interactions among team members during critical events.

Ten residents visited the simulator and participated in the project. The simulator is located in an operating room that contains a fully functioning anesthesia machine as well as appropriate monitors connected to a computer-operated, life-like mannequin. A model of a female pelvis is attached to the mannequin to aid in the simulation of cesarean sections and vaginal deliveries. As described previously, these computerized mannequins have palpable pulses, airways that can be intubated, and audible breath and heart sounds. The room is equipped with cameras and a two-way mirror to capture the subject on film and allow the technicians to monitor the scenario and adjust the vital signs of the "patient" in response to varying stimuli.

During this pilot project, residents arrived in pairs and were exposed to two scenarios. One involved a pregnant woman who had been involved in a high-speed motor vehicle accident, and the second scenario involved a molar pregnancy. A checklist specifically designed for each scenario was used to assess the residents' performance. The mean was 73% (ranging from 46% to 100%) for the first scenario and 79% (ranging from 65 to 85%) for the second scenario. A preceptor's feedback form was used to assess collaboration/cooperation, communication skills/overall behavior, and response to feedback. All three outcome measures were judged to be adequate in most cases (8/10).

From this pilot project, it was concluded that it was possible to adapt the simulator to the needs of trainees in obsterics and gynecology and to use it as an educational tool in their training. Based on this experience, plans were implemented to develop more scenarios, improve the adjustments made to the mannequin, and integrate this learning aid into the obstetrics and gynecology residency training program at the University of Ottawa.

Target Audience

Our simulations are targeted at residents in their third, fourth, and fifth year of training. Due to the time-consuming and costly nature of the exercise, our resources allow us to run the simulation with ten residents per year, during five half-day sessions. In this manner, residents benefit from the project during the final three years of their training and participate either directly or indirectly in six different scenarios. Second-year residents are invited to watch the simulation so that they may benefit from the experience of observation and allay their anxiety for the subsequent years. A senior resident from the department of anesthesia is present at each session to fulfill the role of the anesthetist, thereby benefiting from the simulations as well.

Educational Goals

General Purpose of the Simulation Exercise

For Students

At the University of Ottawa, residents are exposed to several formative and summative evaluation processes in each academic year. In an attempt to prepare trainees for both the specialty examination and real life, there are two structured oral examinations and written tests; the simulator is a recent addition to our armamentarium. Although oral exams with actors as patients can test a physician's communication skills and knowledge base, the simulator offers the additional opportunity for learners to demonstrate crisis management skills in unfamiliar clinical situations and to test their mettle. During a structured oral exam the resident takes a history, describes a physical exam, and orders investigations while being informed by the examiner of the pertinent findings.

Compare this approach to the sights and sounds of a real operating room with monitors, assistants, and a scenario that is played out in real-time. The goal of the simulator for the trainee is to provide a comfortable environment in which challenging clinical scenarios are encountered and managed, followed by timely, constructive feedback. The feedback session provides an opportunity for intense teaching around a difficult case in the realms of both content and process. Because the residents visit the simulator in pairs, they are exposed to two different situations, once as the primary physician and once in a supportive role. This approach allows residents to benefit from the experience of others, imagining what they might have done differently if they were in the spotlight, and provides peers with a review of their communication skills. The experience simultaneously provides an education in rare events, promotes teamwork, and offers an opportunity for constructive feedback from colleagues on the residents' medical expertise, collaborative efforts, and communication skills.

For Instructors

The goal for instructors is complex. One might think that, as playwright and director of a scenario, they have little to gain from the exercise. However, as a given clinical situation grows from an idea to reality, nursing and anesthesia considerations and the best management strategies need to be fully elucidated. Throughout this process, the instructor lives through the situation and gains a better appreciation for the decisions involved. Moreover, we have recruited a resident who once participated at the simulator to become involved in the orchestration of future simulations. This strategy allows the project to keep in touch with the needs of trainees and allows one resident a taste of the challenging work needed to construct a riveting scenario.

Teachers are also provided with an environment in which suggestions can be made in a nonconfrontational way. It is easier to analyze the details of a difficult case and tell residents what they could have done better when an actual patient's health is not at stake. The debriefing session after completion of the scenario, therefore, provides an opportunity for one-on-one teaching with the resident. This session provides a rare moment away from clinical responsibilities when staff and trainees can interact and discuss a case thoroughly.

For Institutions

Any academic institution should strive to produce physicians who are well equipped to deal with whatever their specialty demands of them. Unfortunately, despite many years of training, rare events remain rare. A resident may graduate and become a consultant without facing the reality of performing an emergency cesarean-hysterectomy, managing a severe shoulder dystocia, or controlling a seizure in an eclamptic patient. Simulation may be the only way to adequately prepare young physicians for such rare emergencies.

The medicolegal environment in obstetrics and gynecology in the twenty-first century is also a cause for concern. Lawsuits in this field render massive settlements when obstetric outcomes are suboptimal. Although such outcomes are unfortunate and inevitable, if exposing residents to simulated scenarios can effect a reduction in their occurrence, institutions and physicians would be exposed to less legal liability claims. In Canada, obstetricians face the highest malpractice insurance fees of any specialty. It is, therefore, in an institution's best interest to prepare its staff for the worst-case scenario. The simulator can be used in a risk-reduction program aimed at limiting exposure to liability from mismanaged obstetric cases. If a specific case is poorly handled at our institution, we can construct a scenario addressing this issue in a subsequent year. Some institutions, such as Harvard University, have actually started to offer malpractice insurance rebates to physicians who attend courses using the simulator. The simulator is to the obstetric emergency what the fire drill is to the fire. Rehearsal will never reduce the adverse outcomes in obstetrics to zero, but it can reduce the number of incidents attributable to suboptimal care.

In 2001, the Royal College of Physicians and Surgeons of Canada established a mandatory continuing medical education credit-reporting system. Fellows of the College, which represents the large majority of the specialists in Canada, can be dismissed from the college or be asked to retake the qualification exam if they are unable to provide proof of maintenance of competence through continuing medical education (CME) activities. At the end of 2002, the Royal College approved the simulator as a valid educational tool for anesthesiologists and practicing physicians. Participants who attend sessions at the simulator can now obtain official CME credits recognized by the college. It is, therefore, in the interest of all institutions to encourage physicians to consider this option as an enjoyable way to maintain their skills.

General Goals for the Simulation

The general goals of the simulation exercise are to expose future consultant obstetricians/gynecologists to rare or grave situations that call for immediate attention. By reenacting a particular crisis, the trainee can apply theoretical knowledge, display the necessary behaviors, and demonstrate the proper skills needed to manage the situation. In this manner, the simulation acts as both an educational device and a method of evaluation.

As described above, simulation can also be adapted to different needs and different levels of trainees. The general goals of the simulations vary according to the audience at which it is directed. For example, medical students can use the simulator and the pelvis to acquire the necessary skills to perform a procedure as simple as a normal vaginal delivery. Ideally, everyone would be guaranteed enough experience during the undergraduate years to obtain these skills. However, because of the difficulties inherent in obstetrics and gynecology, the simulator can serve as a surrogate teaching method in the event that the exposure to real births is deficient. Scenarios of the highest complexity can be reserved, of course, for practicing consultants and subspecialists. Even among residents, one can argue that the level of difficulty of the scenarios should vary according to the year of training. However, as long as we provide yearly exposure to the simulator and as long as expectations are commensurate to the residents' level of training, it is reasonable to expose all residents to the same scenario and still be able to assess the progress made by each individual over time.

Knowledge Acquisition

Although much of the knowledge needed as a consultant can be gathered from textbooks or the latest journals, simulations allow residents to learn from one another and from the other support staff in the room. They have an opportunity to find out what information the anesthetist will want the obstetrician to communicate when they are called to an emergency. The instructors provide practical feedback about the optimal management of the situation, which may not be obvious when the case is rare. More than just a practical run-through of a crisis, simulation allows the opportunity to learn about uncommon clinical conditions. For example, during a simulation involving a molar pregnancy, most of the participants, including one staff anesthetist, were interested to find out that evacuation of the uterus during surgery may precipitate a thyroid storm. Furthermore, in observing the choices that the trainee makes (the tests ordered and the management strategies employed), the trainee's level of expertise and knowledge base can be assessed. At an oral exam it is easy to decide to make a vertical skin incision in a particular situation, but the incision is harder to do when you are standing in an operating room in front of a patient. It is knowledge put into action that lends itself to assessment at the simulator.

Behavioral Changes

Medical students quickly realize that medicine is not practiced in a vacuum. During a written exam, the ideal answer is always available, and time constraints, human resources, and financial issues are hardly considered. Conversely, in real life, there are few moments more tense than an emergency or "crash" cesarean section when both mother and baby are at risk. The simulation requires learners to plan ahead, call for help, notify operating room staff, and communicate with the anesthetist, all the while reassuring the patient and obtaining informed consent for invasive procedures. This sounds like a daunting task to complete in 20 minutes, yet it is a simulation of real life. Few people actually know that the attention span of a person in a crisis situation is *a sentence and a half*. This means that we have a sentence and a half in which to transfer essential information about a case to someone—for instance, an anesthesiologist—who walks into a crisis situation. After that point, the person is already thinking of his or her own management plan and hears very little of what we say. This point is easy to emphasize at the simulator and important for trainees to learn; knowing how to effectively describe a crisis situation to someone from whom we are seeking help is a crucial communication skill. Behavior is sometimes hard to evaluate in trainees, because much of their interaction with patients, nurses, and colleagues takes place away from the watchful eye of attending physicians. Through this simulation, albeit artificial and nerve-wracking, the trainee's bedside manner and overall communication skills can be appraised.

Sometimes the simulation is set up in a manner that guarantees a poor outcome; in such cases it is the resident's reaction that is assessed and practiced. Conveying bad news, obtaining informed consent, and dealing with death can be practiced at the simulator.

Skill Acquisition

Attending physicians have the opportunity to watch residents perform vaginal deliveries and assist them in surgery every day. However, uncommon events such as shoulder dystocia and cesarean-hysterectomy involve technical skills that may be understood theoretically but less often used. During calm questioning, residents know the maneuvers that they should use in an attempt to dislodge the shoulders of a large baby. However, under pressure, with a model baby that refuses to be born, the simulator provides an opportunity to put these underused skills to the test. Every obstetrician fears the uterus that refuses to stop bleeding at the time of cesarean section. It is one thing to know that one can tie off the internal iliac artery or throw a stitch around the uterine arteries but quite another one to demonstrate how one would do so while up to the elbows in strawberry Jell-O. Simulation allows trainees to perform operative vaginal and cesarean deliveries, to demonstrate use of forceps and vacuum, and to make appropriate suture choices.

Learning Objectives

The basic goal of medical education is to train the future physician to diagnose and treat disease. Whereas the early years of medical school are occupied with providing a theoretical background in physiology, the latter years serve as an introduction to patho-physiology. During the time spent in the hospital at the patient's bedside, students learn to elicit an appropriate history, practice physical examination, and order investigations—a process that transforms them from scientists to diagnosticians. As the trainee moves into residency, diagnostic skills are honed and therapy is the focus.

Throughout this process, higher-level learning takes place at each stage. A graduating consultant needs to be able to process information quickly, arrive at a diagnosis with the benefit of a few probing questions and a focused physical examination, and rapidly institute therapy. The simulator provides an atmosphere in which these higher-level skills can be mastered.

Diagnosis Parameters

The simulator is set up in such a way that a history can be taken from the mannequin and a physical exam performed. Monitors provide vital signs, and laboratory test results are available to the physician. In this manner, an appropriate diagnosis, or a short list of differential diagnoses, can be arrived at quickly. Thankfully, few obstetricians are called on to make the diagnosis of an amniotic fluid embolus, which is a rare event. However, given this fact, a simulator scenario built around such a case can call on the trainee to manage respiratory collapse in an obstetric patient and to consider this diagnosis. The differential diagnosis at the back of every physician's mind lists rare conditions, but the simulator provides the chance to actually make the physician consider these diagnoses seriously and rule them out or manage them appropriately.

Medical Management Parameters

The real value of the simulator is its ability to provide a real-time model for patient management. The objective is for the resident to consider the given scenario and institute the appropriate therapy. This process includes considerations for consultants and nurses as well as communication with the patient. The resident can practice making medical decisions with authority and without the guidance of an attending physician looking over his or her shoulder.

Equipment Failures/Personnel Availability

Residency in the twenty-first century in a tertiary hospital rarely simulates real life as a general obstetrician/gynecologist in the community. Instead of using clinical acumen, residents begin to rely on portable ultrasound units to assess placental location or fetal presentation in the middle of the night. It is easy to call the neonatologist or anesthetist in case of emergency, but real life may call for difficult decisions to be made when consultants are not readily available. A simulated environment can be used to allow residents an opportunity to live life as a community practitioner without the benefit of technology or easy access to consultants. For example, the traditional "double set-up" refers to bringing a bleeding patient to the operating room (in preparation for urgent cesarean section) for pelvic examination in an attempt to diagnose or rule out placenta previa. This archaic practice has been rendered obsolete by the routine use and availability of ultrasound. But what if ultrasound is not available due to technical failures or lack of accessibility in the community? During a simulation, trainees can face this reality and manage the situation accordingly without depriving actual patients of the benefits of ultrasound. During a simulation, residents can be placed in a situation in which they need to perform a difficult operative vaginal delivery because the anesthetist is too far away or a neonatal resuscitation because the neonatologist is unavailable. These scenarios are real possibilities that generalists may encounter in practice but that residents may never face.

Crisis Management

As indicated, the diagnostic dilemmas and management challenges that serve as the most compelling simulated scenarios are usually the most infrequent crises. The greatest strength of simulator exercises is that they may be the only time that a resident is faced with atypical presentations of common diseases or rare emergencies. Few residents are called to assess an eclamptic patient with seizures, make the decision that a patient needs a postpartum hysterectomy, or co-ordinate the resuscitation of an obstetric patient who has experienced cardiac arrest during labor. Residents who participate in a multitude of simulator exercises will be better equipped to deal with these rare instances. The communication and collaborative skills of the trainee are tested most stringently during a crisis.

Problem Solving

The higher learning demanded of consultants sometimes involves unraveling a clinical puzzle, the solution to which is not readily obvious. At the University of Ottawa, we have used the simulator more often for crisis management scenarios than for diagnostic dilemmas. However, one case, which involved the diagnosis of a molar pregnancy based on hypertension and hemorrhage during dilatation and curettage, did pose a challenge to both obstetric and anesthesia residents.

Competencies

The Accreditation Council for Graduate Medical Education (ACGME) has developed six core competencies, or spheres of medical expertise in which trainees must demonstrate proficiency to be certified as consultants. Rather than simply being vessels of medical knowledge and skill, physicians need to display strong communication skills, professionalism, and teamwork; they must also have a life-long dedication to learning while managing their practices efficiently. The CanMeds roles are the equivalent of the competencies in Canada. Residents need to demonstrate proficiency not only as medical experts but also as communicators, collaborators, professionals, scholars, managers, and health advocates. They are evaluated accordingly.

It is easy for attending physicians to comment on a trainee's judgment and medical expertise, including surgical skill and management decisions. However, because most residents interact with nurses, patients, and consultants when the attending staff is not present, it is more difficult to comment on communication skills, professionalism, and collaborative efforts. The simulator allows observation and direct assessment not only of management decisions and skills but also the trainee's interaction with other health care providers and patients. Simulation exercises may offer the only opportunity for attending staff to observe how residents talk to support staff in an emergency, how they communicate difficult information to a worried patient, and how they handle themselves under stress. The simulator provides an opportunity for constructive criticism of a resident's performance in these areas.

As the core competencies weave their way into the fabric of medical education, the challenge faced by training programs is how to assess these intangible qualities adequately. The simulator provides one solution to this problem.

Functional Requirements

Optimal Size of Audience for Simulation Experience

The optimal number of people participating in a simulation session remains unclear and probably varies depending on the educational objective of the particular session. It makes intuitive sense that a smaller number of participants is preferable so that attention can be focused on the learning experience of individual trainees. As previously described, our sessions have several objectives. The first is to expose residents to rare but critical situations. To accomplish this objective, a minimum core of support staff is required. With the mannequin, a few actors, and one or two people behind the scenes to work the computer, we can easily get the job done.

The second objective implies a multidisciplinary approach and requires the presence of a different set of players. Because we strive to observe directly the communication skills of residents in crisis situations and to assess their ability to work with other health care staff, our sessions include one anesthesia resident as well as two staff anesthesiologists. Although the scenarios pose a challenge to both specialty residents, they also require good communication between the team members.

In the past each session has been attended by two residents in obstetrics and gynecology. While the first resident acted as the primary player, the second resident was recruited to be an actor in the scenario or remained in the background as an observer. Their roles were then reversed in the second scenario. These sessions have been attended by residents in their final three years of training. To expose junior residents to the simulator, in the future a resident in his or her second year of training will be invited to observe. There is inherent value to involving trainees early in their education without applying undue pressure to perform. This exposure allows them to "learn by osmosis," familiarize themselves with the simulator environment, and perhaps relieve some of their apprehension as well as increase their level of comfort when their turn comes to be in the spotlight.

The presence of two staff obstetricians/gynecologists was viewed as preferable, not only to create a good balance but also to allow a more complete assessment of the residents' performance by two separate observers. In addition, creating workable and original scenarios requires imagination and it is much more enriching for the instructors to bounce ideas off each other.

Our experience with the simulator, therefore, asked for the participation of an average of nine people: three trainees (two in obstetrics/gynecology, one in anesthesia), four attending physicians (two in obstetrics/gynecology, two in anesthesia), and two technical assistants. We were careful to keep the numbers small because we wanted to foster a nonthreatening environment to allow good and honest feedback sessions, and we believed that increasing the number of participants might jeopardize this goal. Any additional observers (e.g., junior residents, program director) invited to the sessions are tucked away out of sight in the adjacent conference room, where they watch through a two-way mirror. Of course, the number of attending staff can be reduced to one in each specialty.

Equipment and Space Requirements

The combined sessions for obstetrics/gynecology and anesthesia take place at the simulation center at our university. The simulator uses a realistic mock-up of an operating room that contains a fully functioning anesthesia machine as well as appropriate monitors connected to a computer-operated, life-like mannequin. The main room can be set up either as an emergency department cubicle, an intensive care unit (ICU) bed, or an operating room and easily switched from one to the other. In this room is a table on which the mannequin is installed. The anesthesia machine is found adjacent to this table. A drug cart is also in place, and all equipment necessary for the management of difficult and unusual anesthesia situations is provided. Commonly used operating room instruments are set up on a tray table. As previously stated, one of the walls in the room is set up as an ICU unit with all of the usual hook-ups available. Other necessary equipment and instruments specific to obstetrics and gynecology, such as a fetal monitor and a dilatation and curettage kit, are also added.

Adjacent to but separated from the main room by a two-way mirror is a second room where all of the computers and microphones are located. The main microphone is hooked up directly to the mannequin, giving it an actual voice and making communication with the trainee possible. This feature truly adds to the realism of the situation, and we have found it to be one of the most powerful ways to make the resident forget that the simulation is an artificial recreation of a real clinical situation and to facilitate the resident's complete immersion into the scenario. Instructors in the main room wear headsets to obtain information about the progress of the session as well as the amount of time remaining. The headset allows them to quickly adjust their interventions according to the situation (Fig. 1).

The main room is also equipped with two video cameras that are hooked up to the ceiling and pointed at different areas. These cameras are connected to monitors located in the computer room. The action in the main room can be seen from different angles by the people working the mannequin, again allowing the technicians and instructors to monitor the scenario and adjust the vital signs of the "patient" in response to varying stimuli.

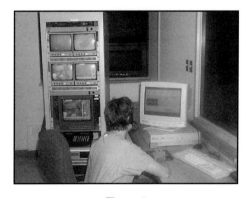

Figure 1

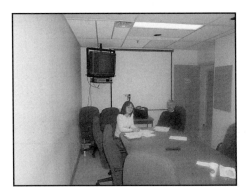

Figure 2

The scenario can be captured on video, and the tape can be used during the debriefing session to illustrate keys points. Recently, the anesthetists at our center have included time at the end of each debriefing session for residents to view the video in private and learn from their experience. Although sometimes disconcerting in that people may find it difficult to watch themselves in action, this strategy has been well received by residents and found to be quite useful. Videos are kept in a cupboard at the simulator to avoid divulgence of the scenarios among trainees and are re-used at the next session.

A third room equipped with a large table and chairs as well as a monitor and a video cassette recorder (VCR) is used for the debriefing sessions (Fig. 2). This arrangement allows some privacy as well as frees the two other rooms, giving the technicians the opportunity to set up the next scenario. The third room also serves as a conference room in which we hold business meetings when the simulator is not in use.

Two smaller rooms are available. One is used for storage of material and equipment. The other contains lockers and serves as a changing room. Operating room scrubs, gowns, masks, and hats are available, and all attendees are asked to wear them. This last room is also equipped with a sink.

The entire simulation center is located on the top floor of a research wing in one of our teaching hospitals. Access is restricted, and the center is closed when unattended by one of the technicians or instructors.

Technical Setting (Simulator Type)

An Eagle-MedSim simulator was used in the pilot project. As previously described, it consists of a life-size mannequin, hooked up to a fully functioning anesthesia machine. The simulator hardware and software provide inputs to actual clinical monitors (electrocardiography, invasive arterial and central venous pressure monitoring). All pieces of equipment are hooked up to a personal computer located in a separate room equipped with a two-way mirror. Over fifteen different variables can be modified. Scenarios are written before the sessions and may be run in either manual or automatic mode. Even in the automatic mode, the operator can override the computer and modify the script according to the trainee's actions.

Although this simulator offers numerous possibilities, it also has serious limitations. Among others, it cannot be moved from one teaching center to the other and, once installed, has to remain in a controlled area. Access, therefore, is somewhat limited. The simulator is also fairly rigid, and leg movements are quite limited. This limitation is somewhat of a problem during simulation of vaginal deliveries and gynecologic procedures. Seizures cannot be simulated other than through blood gas modification and perhaps brief twitching; thus, the ability to recreate eclampsia, a typical obstetric emergency, is also limited.

Another issue is gender. The mannequin looks like a male but lacks genitalia. Its appearance poses a minor problem in obstetrics and gynecology. To adapt the existing mannequin to our specific needs, a female pelvis model was purchased (S500 Advanced Childbirth Simulator). During the sessions, this model is attached to the mannequin to aid in the simulation of cesarean sections and vaginal deliveries. The anterior wall of the add-on model is detachable, and the pelvic cavity can contain a uterus and one or two fetuses as well as placentas and umbilical cords. All of these accessories were provided with the model except the uterus. We fabricated different types of uteri and cervices, depending on the requirements of the scenarios. The uterus used for simulations of cesarean sections allows the resident to choose the type of incision that is most appropriate for the situation. The pelvis makes a major difference in the types of challenges that we can present to trainees and allows simulations of the majority of obstetric situations encountered clinically. Its use remains somewhat limited in gynecology, although it worked quite well for simulating a dilatation and curettage and suction evacuation in the molar pregnancy scenario. Laparoscopic procedures, however, pose a challenge, and other solutions may have to be sought if they are to be simulated in the future. As for the rest, there is nothing that a bit of make-up and a wig cannot fix!

Of course, this pelvic model was designed to stand alone, and we have used it in different settings and found it to be an excellent teaching and evaluation tool. It can be used to illustrate deliveries during workshops or lectures. We have also used it during objective structured clinical examinations (OSCEs) to assess residents' management of shoulder dystocia as well as their ability to perform a breech delivery—something that is now rarely seen.

A new portable simulator was recently purchased from Laerdal. Although it may not have all of the bells and whistles of the original MedSim model, the complexity of the accompanying software makes it very useful in many ways and much easier to handle. Despite the fact that the new model does not have a pelvis that renders our current add-on model obsolete, it does feature interchangeable genitalia, making it easier to represent our patient population. A combination of the two types of simulators is probably ideal because they complement each other well. In one of our most recent simulations, the new model represents the patient in the obstetrical assessment unit, and the old model, equipped with the add-on pelvis, acts as the patient in the operating room.

Personnel

In the early days of simulation at our center, the department of anesthesia asked two staff anesthesiologists to coordinate all of the teaching sessions for anesthesia residents and to take charge of the simulation center. They were freed from their clinical responsibilities to fulfill this new mandate. In so doing, the department of anesthesia created ideal conditions to ensure that the project would get off the ground while sending a strong message that they considered this project of great importance. The anesthesiologists invested time and energy not only in writing scenarios but also in learning how to run the mannequin and the computer. They became self-sufficient but at the same time realized that, to attract other participants, the concept had to be made more accessible.

Although several departments and health care fields expressed an interest in making use of the simulator, it quickly became clear that not all of them could afford to invest as much time as the two anesthesiologists. In fact, just the need to understand the functioning of the simulator may deter some educators from using the center. A decision was made to hire two technicians, who were provided with the necessary training to help the instructors. These technicians are present during the entire session, work the computer, set up the rooms before the arrival of the participants, and store all equipment appropriately after each session. They identify problems, including technical ones, and order parts when necessary. They ensure that the simulators are properly maintained to avoid unnecessary malfunctions and expenses. The hiring of the two technicians, although an additional cost, has contributed to the smooth functioning of the simulator and has made everyone's life easier. More importantly, the techncians have made the simulator more accessible, thereby allowing an increase in the number of participating instructors. To cover this extra cost, a sessional fee is now charged to all participating groups. This fee takes care of salaries as well as maintenance fees and repair costs.

Simulation Construction

Each year, two new scenarios are developed to explore different diagnostic or management dilemmas in obstetrics and gynecology. During one half-day session, both simulations are enacted and two residents take turns acting as the primary physician.

Simulation construction involves inventing a patient with her own detailed history, physical exam findings, and laboratory values, along with a detailed script of the fluctuations in vital signs based on the trainee's performance. The script dictates the behavior of the supporting actors as well as the vital signs, which are presented at every moment. This complicated algorithm needs to be dynamic; it must be able to compensate for and respond to any anticipated course of action that the trainee may take. If the physician strays from the script too drastically, the support staff may nudge him or her back on track, guiding the physician toward a natural conclusion. The algorithm can also react to mismanagement on the part of the physician by precipitating deterioration of the patient's status. The foolhardy resident who elects to examine the patient with undiagnosed bleeding is suddenly faced with torrential hemorrhage from a placenta previa. The script itself is intended to guide the physician in a specific direction in an attempt to back him or her into a difficult corner. For example, if the intention of the simulation is for the physician to practice a difficult vaginal delivery, the trainee who decides to perform a cesarean section is told that the anesthetist is unavailable.

Residents enter the simulator environment with no advanced knowledge of the clinical dilemma that they are about to encounter. During a brief orientation the characters are introduced and participants are informed of the roles that they will assume. They are told that the scenario will last approximately fifteen to twenty minutes and will be followed by a debriefing session. They are encouraged to relax and treat the mannequin and allied health personnel as they would in "real life."

The specific clinical dilemma remains a medical mystery until the trainee steps into the simulation and is presented with the case. The simulation may begin with the resident being called to the emergency department to assess a patient who has been in a motor vehicle accident or to a patient's room because of a deceleration in fetal heart rate. When the resident enters the room, the situation becomes clear as a nurse or colleague explains the patient's presenting complaint. At this moment, the resident assumes the role of the primary physician and behaves as if faced with the situation in real life. The simulation plays out in real time, with the physician taking a history, performing the required physical exam, ordering the appropriate tests, and taking the necessary action. When blood work or intravenous lines are ordered, time is needed for the "nurse" to perform the procedure, thereby simulating real-time management of the situation.

The resident is presented with monitors displaying vital signs and fetal heart-rate tracings as dictated by the case. As the scenario unfolds, the resident responds to the stimuli offered and directs the supporting staff while moving toward resolution of the problem. Depending on the actions taken by the physician, a pre-set script directs the technician in the control booth to adjust the mannequin's vital signs accordingly. In this manner, the simulation can adapt to each resident's management style and pace. The plot of the script is constructed in such a way as to bring the case to an expected conclusion, and the supporting cast is instructed to nudge the physician gently toward the finish line. The simulation is nothing if not adaptable. The resident who speeds through the management of a placenta previa with time to spare may find himself or herself managing a severe postpartum hemorrhage that requires a hysterectomy, whereas the junior resident who manages the case more slowly will find that the bleeding responds to medical management (for the sake of time). This arrangement is not meant to imply that the efficient resident is "punished" for acting quickly, but if time allows, the scenario can accommodate different pathways. Similarly, the scenario can be truncated for the "unhurried" physician.

Because the simulations are designed to last fifteen to twenty minutes, they need to be succinct—focused on a particular emergency and resolved within that time frame. Alas, the fact is that many of the significant emergencies in obstetrics, such as shoulder dystocia or antepartum hemorrhage, can indeed begin and end within this short period.

Simulation Examples

The following two scenarios were used in the pilot project. The cases are presented along with the specific checklist of steps that are expected to be completed in the management of each scenario. These lists were designed according to what the Royal College of Physicians and Surgeons, the national licensing body of Canada, would expect of graduating residents. These objectives serve as a guide to the instructors during the debriefing sessions and facilitate the feedback process by providing structure to the discussion as well as ensuring that all important points are addressed.

Case No. 1: Motor Vehicle Accident in Pregnancy

A 26-year old G_2T_1 at 30 weeks of gestation is brought to the emergency department after a motor vehicle accident. She is conscious and oriented but very anxious. Her vital and neurologic signs are as follows:

◆ Pulse: 120 beats/min
◆ Blood pressure (BP): 110/50 mmHg
◆ Respiratory rate (RR): 25 breaths/min

♦ Neurologic status: adequate level of consciousness and responsiveness

In addition, the following observations are made:

♦ The neck is immobilized in a collar.

♦ The patient has a scalp lesion of approximately 5 cm at the left temple that requires stitches.

♦ The heart is in sinus tachycardia; there are no other sounds or murmurs.

 ˙ lungs are clear, with good air entry, and the trachea is midline.

  ˙ᵈᵒmen is bruised, showing marks from the seat belt that extend to the lower

   ˙ᵓᵉneralized bruising is also seen.

♦ On palpation the abdomen is diffusely tender, and guarding is present. Palpation of the uterus reveals a symphysis fundal height (SFH) of 32 cm and tenderness with occasional contractions.

♦ The pelvic exam is deferred.

♦ Examination of the limbs reveals an open fracture of the right femur, which is treated with immobilization and pressure dressing; no active bleeding is present. [This feature is optional].

♦ Fetal monitoring reveals occasional contractions (irregular); reactive fetal heart with occasional mild, variable decelerations; and a baseline fetal heart rate (FHR) of 140 beats/min.

The general practitioner gives a quick history to the resident and is then called away urgently to manage a cardiac arrest.

Management

♦ Airways, breathing, circulation; 2 large-bore intravenous lines; replacement of losses; RL wide open.

♦ Ensure that the airway is clear.

♦ Foley catheter in bladder, blood in urine.

♦ Continuous monitoring (only when asked).

Tests ordered

♦ Complete blood count (CBC)

♦ Prothrombin time (PT), partial thromboplastin time (PTT), international normalized ratio (INR), fibrin degradation products (FDPs), D-dimer

♦ Asparate aminotransferase (AST), alanine aminotransferase (ALT), lactate dehydrogenase (LDH)

♦ Electrolytes, blood urea nitrogen (BUN), creatinine, glucose

♦ Kleihauer-Betke status

♦ Blood group and Rh status

♦ Blood on hold

♦ X-rays: face, skull, neck, spine (all), pelvis

♦ Ask for antenatal records

Results (provided to trainee only if tests are ordered)

♦ Hemoglobin, 90 g/L (N = 115–155 g/L); platelets, 90 × 10 Eq/L (N = 145–400 × 10 Eq/L); leukocytes, 25,000 (N = 4.0–11.0 × 10 Eq/L)

♦ PTT, 31 sec (N = 24–36 sec); INR, 3.0 (N = 0.90–1.20); D-dimer < 300 μg/L; FDPs, 0

♦ AST, 30 U/L (N = 10–40 U/L); ALT, 25 U/L (N = 14–54 U/L); LDH, 100 U/L (N = 98–192 U/L)

♦ Electrolytes: sodium (Na), 136 mmol/L (N = 137–146 mmol/L); potassium (K), 5.0 mmol/L (N = 3.6–5.1 mmol/L); chloride (Cl), 100 mmol/L (N = 99–100 mmol/L)

♦ BUN = 6 mmol/L (N = 2.8–7.3 mmol/L); creatinine, 57 μmol/L (N = 35–88 μmol/L); glucose, 5.2 mmol/L

♦ Blood group: O negative

♦ Kleihauer-Betke status: pending

♦ X-rays done; no report yet

Additional orders

♦ Fresh frozen plasma (FFP)

- Cryoprecipitate
- Packed red blood cells (how much?)

Ask for transfer of patient to labor and delivery (L&D). After transfer, the patient is reassessed:

- Vital signs: pulse, 140 beats/min; BP, 90/50 mmHg; RR, 30 breaths/min.
- Fetal monitor: baseline FHR, 165 beats/min; variable decelerations more frequent, deeper; contractions more frequent and stronger, slow to relax.
- Patient starts bleeding from IV sites; more blood in urine; nose bleed.
- Resident asks about status of FFP and cryoprecipitate; starts replacing.
- Patient suddenly complains of increased abdominal pain. Examination reveals increased guarding; uterus hard, with no relaxation; vaginal exam reveals closed cervix (verbalized to resident if he or she asks).
- Fetal monitor: sudden bradycardia; cannot find fetal heart. Ultrasound confirms fetal bradycardia [optional].
- Start of vaginal bleeding

Management

- Immediate request for neonatology and anesthesia consultants.
- Crash cesarean section; call for other obstetrician to help.
- Anesthesia to manage airway with collar in place.
- Vertical incision at skin.
- Opening of abdomen reveals blood in peritoneal cavity.
- Steps
  1. Intraoperative consultation with surgery.
  2. Couvellaire's uterus.
  3. Bulging lower segment; transverse incision.
  4. Bloody amniotic fluid (+++).
  5. Baby delivered (with placenta); handed over to neonatology.
  6. Complete abruption.
  7. Close uterus quickly; oozing (++) observed.
- Uterus: boggy even after closing; not responding to massage
- Obstetric resident to ask for:
  1. IV oxytocin (How much? How fast?): no response.
  2. May advise anesthesia of possible hysterectomy.
  3. Hemabate injected into myometrium: good contractions.
- During surgery: patient still oozing; advise anesthesia about probable disseminated intravascular coagulation (DIC).

Wrap-up of Scenario

- No more significant oozing from uterine incision.
- Exploratory surgery reveals ruptured spleen; splenectomy.
- Orthopedics consulted to repair fracture.
- Scalp lesion to be repaired.

Checklist

	Complete	Partial	Not Done
(1) Assessment of the situation	☐	☐	☐
◆ Level of consciousness			
◆ ABC			
◆ Vital signs			
◆ Quick exam of the patient (wounds, abdomen, uterus, limbs)			
(2) Initial steps	☐	☐	☐
◆ Two large-bore IVs			

	Complete	Partial	Not Done
◆ Foley catheter			
◆ Fetal heart and uterine contractions monitoring			
(3) Request for lab tests and x-rays	☐	☐	☐
◆ CBC, coagulation, Kleihauer-Betke status			
◆ Blood group + blood on hold			
◆ Rh status, anti-D			
◆ Cryoprecipitate			
◆ Fresh frozen plasma			
◆ X-rays (at least of cervical spine)			
(4) Gathering of antenatal history	☐	☐	☐
◆ History taking			
◆ Request for patient's chart			
(5) Reaction to changes in clinical situation	☐	☐	☐
◆ Appearance of fetal heart decelerations			
◆ Increased contractions			
◆ Note: high suspicion of placental abruption			
◆ Steps			

1. Advises the following of possible cesarean:
   ◊ Neonatology
   ◊ Anesthesia
   ◊ Operating room
2. Calls for help

(6) Initiation of transfer of patient	☐	☐	☐
(7) Treatment of DIC	☐	☐	☐
◆ Acts promptly and adequately			
◆ Calls for help, if not already done			
◆ Starts replacement with FFP			
(8) Periodic assessment of patient's status	☐	☐	☐
(9) Timely call for urgent cesarean section and concise information provided to the newly arrived team members (namely, anesthesia and neonates) about the situation	☐	☐	☐
(10) Steps taken during surgery	☐	☐	☐
◆ Vertical skin incision			
◆ Surgery consult in view of blood in abdomen			
◆ Quick delivery of baby			
(11) Communication with team members (anesthesiologist in particular)	☐	☐	☐
◆ Continuous information about findings			
◆ Possibility of hysterectomy			
(12) Response to uterine atony	☐	☐	☐
◆ Uterine massage			
◆ Oxytocin			
◆ Hemabate or ergot			

Case No. 2: Molar Pregnancy and Thyroid Storm

You are paged by the emergency department for a gynecologic consultation. The patient is an 18-year old gravida 1 at a gestational age of 12 weeks. She presented to the emergency department because of vaginal bleeding. A molar pregnancy is suspected on ultrasound.

History

The patient reports that the bleeding started approximately 2 days ago. Its volume is comparable to heavy menses but progressively increasing. She has used 1 sanitary napkin every hour for the past 4 hours. She is also experiencing mild cramping in the lower abdomen. In the past two weeks, the patient has also suffered from nausea and occasional vomiting.

Her menstrual cycles are irregular, and currently she is not using contraceptive methods. She also claims that she suffers from headaches and reports experiencing panic attacks for about a month. She was recently started on rivotril, as needed, by her family physician. She was just informed by the physician in the emergency department that she is pregnant. She just broke up with her boyfriend and does not care about this pregnancy. She is quite upset and wants to leave.

Physical examination

The patient appears nervous. Her pulse is 116 beats/min; blood pressure is 140/100 mmHg. On chest auscultation, she is found to be tachycardic, but the heart beat is regular and no murmur is heard. The lungs are clear.

Gynecologic exam: Bleeding is clearly coming from the cervix; the cervix is otherwise normal. The digital exam reveals that the uterus is approximately 16 weeks in size. The ovaries are enlarged and tender.

Laboratory findings

Urine pregnancy test	Positive
Blood type	O +
Beta human chorionic gonadotropin	300,000 IV
Hemoglobin	104 g/L (N = 115–155)
Platelets	350,000 10^9/L (N = 125–400)
White blood cells (WBCs)	16,000 10^9/L (N = 3.0–10.5)
Biochemistry	Normal
Creatinine, electrolytes and liver function	Normal
Urinanalysis	2+ proteins
Chest x-ray	Normal

Ultrasound

You are handed an ultrasound report and some pictures. The uterus appears to contain a large amount of echogenic material that has a snowstorm appearance. You suddenly remember that this pattern is typical of a molar pregnancy. In fact, this possibility is clearly stated in the report. Large theca lutein cysts are also present bilaterally and measure 6 cm on the right and 8 cm on the left.

Management plan

◆ Convince the patient to stay for observation.
◆ Investigate signs and symptoms relating to pre-eclampsia and hyperthyroidism.
◆ Call operating room and book urgent D&C with suction.
◆ Consultation with anesthesia.
◆ Monitor vital signs.
◆ Start IV and ensure that blood is on hold.
◆ Start patient on IV magnesium sulfate ($MgSO_4$): bolus of 4 gm, then infusion of 1.5–2 gm/hr.
   Note: If resident does not start $MgSO_4$, patient begins to seize.

Reassessment

◆ The patient continues to bleed heavily.
◆ Her vital signs are as follows: pulse, 120 beats/min; BP, 150/100 mmHg.

Management plan

◆ Transfer of patient to the operating room
   1. Induce general anesthetic (to be decided by anesthesia resident).

  2. Start high-dose IV oxytocin.

  3. Proceed with D&C and start suctioning (Berkeley suction machine) (Fig. 3).

◆ After induction and beginning of procedure

  1. Patient suddenly goes into atrial fibrillation.

  2. Body temperature elevates to 38.6°C.

  3. BP rises to 200/120 mmHg.

◆ Treatment for thyroid storm (by anesthesia resident)

  1. Fast-acting IV beta blockers (best option: propranolol)

  2. Propylthiouracil (PTU)

  3. Lowering of body temperature

  4. IV hydration

  5. Oxygen

  6. IV antibiotics

  7. Iodine administration (not appropriate in urgent setting)

  8. Glucocorticoids

◆ After a short period, the phone in the operating room rings to inform the physicians that the T_4 level ordered by the emergency physician is so low it is impossible to measure (below 0.1).

◆ The Berkeley suction machine breaks down. The gynecology resident is to continue procedure with curette until the uterus is completely evacuated.

◆ If anesthesiologist asks to terminate procedure, gynecology resident should insist that evacuation of the uterus will help treat thyroid storm.

Wrap-up of scenario

◆ Uterus is completely evacuated, well contracted, with no further bleeding.

◆ Resolution of thyroid storm.

Checklist

	Complete	Partial	Not Done
(1) Assessment of the situation	☐	☐	☐

  ◆ Brief history

  ◆ Vital Signs, ABCs

  ◆ Physical exam

  ◆ Importance of vaginal bleeding

| (2) Request for laboratory tests and ultrasound | ☐ | ☐ | ☐ |

  ◆ Beta human chorionic gonadotropin

  ◆ Complete blood count

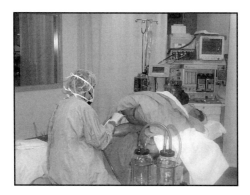

Figure 3

	Complete	Partial	Not Done

◆ Biochemistry
◆ Hepatic enzymes
◆ Blood type
◆ Urinalysis
◆ Ultrasound

| (3) Specific signs and symptoms | ☐ | ☐ | ☐ |

◆ Pre-eclampsia
◆ Hyperthyroidism

| (4) Convince patient to stay | ☐ | ☐ | ☐ |

◆ Remain calm
◆ Discuss importance of staying
◆ Discuss possible risks of molar pregnancy

| (5) Preparation for operating room | ☐ | ☐ | ☐ |

◆ Call operating room
◆ Prepare for blood transfusions
◆ Appropriate IV access
◆ Serial vital signs

| (6) Communication | ☐ | ☐ | ☐ |

◆ Call anesthetist
◆ Explain situation
◆ Explain risk for bleeding, pre-eclampsia
  and thyroid storm

| (7) Pre-eclampsia | ☐ | ☐ | ☐ |

◆ Reacts to high blood pressure and proteinuria
◆ Diagnosis of pre-eclampsia
◆ Start $MgSo_4$ IV
◆ If diagnosis not made, when seizures begin, start
  $MgSO_4$ or other anticonvulsants

| (8) Operating room | ☐ | ☐ | ☐ |

◆ Be sure to have blood available
◆ Oxytocin IV
◆ Ask for general anesthesia if not the case
◆ Dilatation of cervix
◆ Suction with large-caliber cannula

| (9) When suction machine stops | ☐ | ☐ | ☐ |

◆ Continue with sharp curette
◆ Remain calm

| (10) Persistence | ☐ | ☐ | ☐ |

◆ Continues the D&C even if anesthesiologist
  suggests stopping or if thyroid storm occurs
◆ Be sure that D&C is the treatment

As previously stated, the scenarios had to present challenges to both residents. In the first scenario, the challenges for anesthesia were to proceed with the intubation of a pregnant patient with a possible cervical spine injury as well as to manage the DIC while the obstetrics resident was proceeding with the cesarean section and controlling the hemorrhage. The second scenario required that the anesthesia resident recognize the thyroid storm and manage it appropriately. This scenario poses a particular challenge because it mimics malignant hyperthermia quite closely. Although the gynecology residents knew that a thyroid storm could be provoked by the evacuation of a molar pregnancy, it was interesting to note that the anesthesiologist was unaware of this possibility. As intended, this clinical vignette provided everyone involved with the opportunity to review the management of this rare presentation. Moreover, both scenarios called for excellent communication among team members at all times. This is a valuable learning experience for all!

Feedback and Evaluation

Immediately after resolution of the problem or conclusion of the simulation, the participants retire to an adjoining conference room for debriefing. The case is discussed openly among both staff and residents with the input of both anesthetists and obstetricians. Firstly, the residents are asked to comment on their own behavior and explain what they might do differently if faced with a similar situation in the future. The other residents are also asked what they learned from the scenario and what positive or negative feedback they have for the primary participant.

The attending staff who are administering and supervising the simulation, including both anesthetists and obstetricians/gynecologists, then provide constructive feedback relating to both content and process. They provide guidance rather than just the right answers, rendering this interaction an occasion for one-on-one teaching between trainees and staff. They help the participants explore the finer details of the case, the historical or physical elements that may have been missed, and different management decisions that could have been made. Unfortunately, in the current medicolegal climate, when emergencies occur, especially in near-miss cases, it is the rare clinician who takes the time to process the experience with the residents involved and to explore what could have been done better. The suggestion that there may be room for improvement may be construed as an admission of guilt if the outcome of the case is less than ideal. The simulator may be the only opportunity to dissect a case gone awry and to receive constructive criticism on how it could have been handled differently.

Even when outcomes are good, the debriefing session allows residents to hear what other options were available and to learn about management strategies that may not have occurred to them. In a busy specialty, this may be one of the only occasions for individual teaching around a difficult case. The take-home message is that at the simulator, regardless of the outcome, understanding how one can improve performance in the future is the ultimate objective. Furthermore, putting aside management issues and outcome measures, the resident receives feedback on communication skills, from the other members of the team as well as the patient.

Residents are then given a checklist with points for both content and process, outlining what was done satisfactorily and what was believed to be lacking. Residents are then given an opportunity to watch a video of the session in a private setting to witness first hand what they look like in action.

Thus far, summative evaluation has not been the goal of the simulation experience. The exercise is not meant to identify the resident in trouble or the dangerous physician and does not serve to recognize which residents are excelling in the program. The feedback session is meant to provide constructive criticism and guidance; it is not meant to be reproachful or judgmental. An evaluation form is completed by the instructors, ensuring that the resident performs the tasks expected, but this evaluation is only an aid for the feedback session and is not submitted to the program director. One expects that a resident who flounders at the simulator will gain insight into his or her situation and strive to improve. Indeed, all of the structured oral examinations and written tests administered during the residency program are meant as preparation for sitting for the final licensing examination. One might say that the simulator provides preparation for real life.

Expert Analysis vs. Self-Analysis

Different types of evaluation grids were designed for the pilot study based on an article by Holzman et al.[6] (see Appendix). As mentioned above, residents are given a self-assessment grid to evaluate their own experience with the simulator. In the pilot project, nine of the ten residents graded their global performance during the session as "good." Specific issues were addressed in the form of statements with which the residents totally agreed, partially agreed, partially disagreed, or totally disagreed. These statements asked for self-assessments of how they communicated with the rest of the team; whether they had responded in a timely fashion to the emergency at hand, prioritized well, and delegated tasks appropriately; and whether they felt in control of the situation and listened to the opinions of others. We believe that this self-assessment allows instructors to check the level of insight that residents have into their own performance and also indicates what types of behavior is expected of them. Although resident physicians are usually notorious for self-criticism and probably underestimate their performance, our residents were typically fair with themselves; most of them at least partially agreed with the self-evaluative statements.

The experts fill out an evaluation form that involves questions about the cooperative and collaborative skills of residents, their communication skills and overall behavior, and their response to feedback. The debriefing session then unfolds as described earlier, with the attending physicians using the evaluation key as a guide to their comments.

After the Simulation

Assessment of Validity

It is difficult to document the validity of the simulator as an educational tool that improves health care delivery. One would have to demonstrate that participating residents become better physicians and have lower rates of complications. Unfortunately, the practice of medicine, which involves both art and science, has far too many variables, and even exam marks cannot correlate with performance at the bedside. In Toronto, Pittini et al. were able to demonstrate that performance of amniocentesis improved after the simulation experience, but their study involved a discrete skill, not the holistic management of a difficult case.[3] As our experience grows, we may be able to demonstrate that our residents are better prepared to deal with challenges, but it will always be difficult to prove that any improvement is an effect of participation at the simulator. We prefer to say that the simulator is yet another valuable modality used by our department in fulfilling its mandate to produce competent and compassionate consultant obstetricians/gynecologists.

Evaluation of Simulation Experience

The ten residents in the pilot project completed an evaluation of the simulation experience. Presented with the statement, "I felt comfortable with the simulator environment," two residents totally agreed, seven residents partially agreed, and only one resident partially disagreed. Seven residents found it easy to treat the mannequin as a real patient and thought that the environment and team members were realistic. All of them found the debriefing sessions useful and well organized, and all indicated an interest in other sessions, finding the simulator to be a good educational tool. Above and beyond these general statements, residents were asked specifically about distractions (camera, instructor) and whether the simulation and debriefing session contributed to their knowledge base. It is important to solicit feedback from the residents about their experience, for such comments can help guide future improvements to the simulator.

Once the initial awkwardness of the simulation is overcome, we suspect that the residents will look forward to their time at the simulator even more. Nobody likes to perform under the scrutiny of others and feel judged, but as the simulator becomes part of the culture of our residency program, we anticipate that all residents will feel comfortable with this environment. To this end, we reiterate that inviting junior residents to observe the proceedings is a nonthreatening way of allaying their anxiety about future participation.

Conclusion and Recommendations

The simulation of obstetric and gynecologic situations has added a new dimension to the simulator center and is beneficial to more than just our residents. The simulator experience has especially enhanced our relationship with the department of anesthesia and has given each group insight into the particular challenges that the other group faces. Participating at the simulator allows us to be creative and to go beyond our limits. It fosters teamwork and makes us appreciate the importance of good communication skills. We are also provided with an evaluation tool that can help assess these skills—a problem with which educators are constantly struggling. Regarding this experience, we agree with the sentiments expressed by Pittini and his group:

> This shift [from the patient to the laboratory] provides a safe, standardized setting that fosters important learning concepts such as experiential learning, contextualization and immediate directive feedback. It encourages collaboration between peers and capitalizes on the expertise of faculty members as demonstrators and evaluators... without subjecting trainees to the stress of learning on actual patients.[3]

Our experience has also confirmed that "simulator training is especially useful for teaching the management of complex clinical situations that occur infrequently and are emergent, critical and unfamiliar."[4]

Our latest idea has been to involve a senior obstetric/gynecologic resident with a special interest in medical education in the design of future scenarios. The resident will have the unique opportunity to experience the simulator as an instructor after originally participating in the pilot study as a trainee. Other future directions include extending our multidisciplinary approach to involve other health care workers, such as nurses and respiratory therapists, as well as other groups of physicians (emergency physicians, surgeons).

As previously discussed, the crisis management and emergency drill types of exercises may help reduce the number of adverse outcomes as well as help employees recuperate faster from a traumatic experience. This aspect is becoming increasingly interesting to institutions and administrators to the point that future financing of the center may be directed partly toward those goals.

In the current medicolegal context, it is increasingly important for practicing consultants to maintain their skills beyond residency and to participate in recognized continuing medical education (CME) activities such as simulations. Governing bodies in Canada have already implemented a mandatory recording of CME credits, and these new regulations are unlikely to disappear any time soon. One might as well have fun while accumulating valuable credits!

Having established its value in educating residents, the application of the simulator in an undergraduate curriculum is the next logical step. Of course, the earlier we can expose future physicians to the concept of the simulator, the more comfortable they will feel in this environment and the more it will become second nature for them. Medical students can benefit from the simulator in a variety of ways. Teachers can use the simulator to help medical students grasp basic physiologic and pharmacologic principles during the junior year; the simulator helps illustrate key concepts and makes the learning experience much more enriching. By practicing on the simulator, students can see how their interventions directly affect patient outcomes.

More importantly, in this simulated environment we may have found the means to remove some of the obstacles often encountered by clinical clerks, including an opportunity to learn how to perform exams and practice deliveries away from the highly stressful and pressured milieu of the labor room. As indicated previously, models have traditionally been used in the instruction of the sensitive pelvic examination. The simulator takes this experience to the next level.

Of interest, the simulator can be used to help empower students to make medical decisions. Medical students, who are customarily in a position to make very few life-altering medical decisions in the hospital, can benefit greatly from doing so safely in a simulated situation. Allowing them, even in larger groups, an opportunity to visit the simulator can improve their knowledge base while giving them experience and confidence when they face similar challenges in the hospital with real patients. Once again, the simulator can be a valuable tool in training tomorrow's physicians and improving the quality of health care provision.

Finally, the first time that students experienced objective structured clinical exams (OSCEs), they most likely felt uneasy and remained skeptical about the whole idea. However, this skepticism did not dampen the enthusiasm of the true believers, and OSCEs are now among the most widely used evaluative techniques in medicine. Medical students probably do not even remember the days before this relatively new type of exam was initiated. It is our hope that the same principle will apply to the simulator in the future and that it will become an integral part of medical school curricula.

References

1.   Zedek IJ, Hines JF, Thomas AR, et al: Development and use of military-unique standardized gynecology patients for military residents in obstetrics and gynecology training programs. Mil Med 163:767–769, 1998.
2.   Hines JF, Thomas AR, Call R, et al: Development and use of military-unique standardized

gynecology patients in military undergraduate medical education. Mil Med 164:280–282, 1999.

3. Pittini R, Oepkes D, Macrury K, et al: Teaching invasive perinatal procedures: Assessment of a high fidelity simulator-based curriculum. Ultrasound Obstet Gynecol 19:478–483, 2002.

4. Patel RM, Crombleholme WR: Using simulation to train residents in managing critical events. Acad Med 73:593, 1998.

5. Johanson R, Cox C, O'Donnell E, et al: Managing obstetric emergencies and trauma. Obstet Gynecol 1(2):46–52, 1999.

6. Holzman RS, Cooper JB, Gaba DM, et al: Anesthesia crisis resource management: Real-life simulation training in operating room crises. J Clin Anesth 7:675–687, 1995.

Appendix: Evaluation Grids

PRECEPTOR FEEDBACK FORM

Student _____

COLLABORATION/COOPERATION

Grading Scale
1   2   3   4

1. Works towards the achievement of team goals

2. Demonstrates effective interpersonal skills

3. Effectively performs a variety of roles in a team

COMMUNICATION SKILLS AND OVERALL BEHAVIOR

Grading Scale
1   2   3   4

4. Is aware of available (necessary) resources

5. Evaluates the effectiveness of own actions (during scenario)

6. Communicates clearly his/her needs

7. Remains calm in situations of stress

8. Comfortably assumes leadership role when necessary

9. Is sensitive to the feelings and level of knowledge of others

10. Engages intensely in tasks even when answers or solutions are not immediately apparent

11. Demonstrates adequate self-assessment skills (ability to objectively evaluate own performance)

RESPONSE TO FEEDBACK

Grading Scale
1   2   3   4

12. Is receptive

13. Is open-minded

1 = Always, 2 = Most of the time, 3 = Sometimes, 4 = Rarely

SELF-ASSESSMENT FORM

Student _____

**PERSONAL EXPERIENCE IN THE
SIMULATOR ENVIRONMENT**

Grading Scale

1   2   3   4

1. I felt comfortable with the simulator environment

2. I felt in control of the situation

3. I felt well briefed prior to the scenario

4. I recognized abnormal events in a timely fashion

5. I notified the anesthetist promptly of a problem

6. I communicated clearly and specifically to those individuals from whom I needed help

7. I listened well to the opinions of others

8. I delegated tasks well

9. I was able to remain free of distractions

10. I was able to prioritize problems easily

11. I declared the emergency early

12. I called for help promptly

13. My overall performance was good

1 = Totally agree, 2 = Partially agree, 3 = Partially disagree, 4 = Totally disagree

STUDENT FEEDBACK FORM

Student _____

EVALUATION OF THE SIMULATOR EXPERIENCE   Grading Scale
                                                     1   2   3   4

1. I found it easy to treat the mannequin as a simulated human

2. The presence of the scenario director detracted from the realism

3. The team members were realistic and believable in the simulator environment

4. The video cameras interfered with the simulator experience

5. The debriefing session was logically organized and clarified important issues of the scenario

6. The debriefing session enhanced my fund of knowledge

7. The feedback I received in the debriefing session was useful and was provided adequately

8. I expect that the knowledge gained from the scenarios will be helpful to me in practice

9. I expect that the knowledge gained from crisis management will be helpful in practice

10. I felt that the simulation environment and scenarios prompted realistic responses from me

11. This scenario was adequate for my level of training

12. The simulator is a valuable teaching tool for OB/GYN residents in general

13. I would personally like to come back for other sessions

1 = Totally agree, 2 = Partially agree, 3 = Partially disagree, 4 = Totally disagree

Did you find the simulator valuable?   Yes ❑   No ❑

To what frequency should these sessions be held?

   Every 6 months   ❑

   Every 12 months   ❑

   Every 24 months   ❑

   Once during the residency program   ❑

   Never   ❑

Should we have sessions aimed at junior residents?   Yes ❑   No ❑

Starting at what level? _____

Do you find the video is a valuable teaching tool?   Yes ❑   No ❑

If so, would you like to keep it for future referencing?   Yes ❑   No ❑

Suggestions for future scenarios:

_____

_____

_____

_____

Chapter 19

SIMULATION IN PEDIATRICS

Gary E. Loyd, MD, MMM

Many health care professionals have their first experience with a pediatric mannequin during Basic Life Support courses or parental training classes. Unlike adult patients, children are less likely to allow strange adults to touch them in a learning environment, and even if they do, there are ethical considerations about the number and intensity of such encounters. Even though it seems intuitive that pediatric simulation should be developed before adult simulation, such has not been the case. Centers devoted to pediatric medical education are just now appearing, such as the Center for Advanced Pediatric Education at Stanford University.[1]

The history of pediatric simulation is covered by Dr. Rosen in the first chapter of this book. In a related article in 2003, Stewart described the evolution of medical training in the United Kingdom over the past 10 years, culminating with a brief overview of the current state of human patient simulators in pediatric medical training.[2] As early as 1979, Schreiner et al. described the use of an independent abdominal mass simulator to teach pediatric physical diagnosis skills related to ovarian cysts, neuroblastomas, and hepatic tumors. He also described a device used to simulate either congenital hip dislocation or subluxation of the hip in a newborn.[3] Gaba provided a 1992 editorial on how to improve performance with simulating reality. Most of his comments are still accepted as truths.[4] This chapter is intended to provide an overview of what has been reported in pediatric simulation.

PALS and NALS

As in adult life support courses, simulation gives teams of health care workers the opportunity to practice resuscitation of pediatric patients and Pediatric Advanced Life Support (PALS). The Center for Advanced Pediatric Education at Stanford University is a leader in this area. Halamek et al. reported the use of computer-based programs along with hands-on neonatal and maternal simulations in effectively teaching Neonatal Advanced Life Support (NALS).[5] There are online, virtual computer-based simulators for recertification in PALS, but they do not allow the development of crisis management skills, which must augment the knowledge base of these programs if resuscitation is to be optimal.[6] Simulators have allowed the assessment of providers of PALS. Cowie and Story studied the ability of different levels of anesthesia providers to perform PALS correctly on simulators and found that a significant number could not adequately manage the patient.[7] Palmisano et al. found that when pediatric cardiac arrest was simulated in a patient care area, the pediatric resident was the first to respond.[8] At the University of Louisville, PALS training routinely occurs with hospital and physician staff in the patient simulation laboratory, but the program is not reported in the literature. A similar situation may be true throughout the country.

Critical incidents and crisis management are important aspects of tertiary health care. Medina et al. reported the use of a computer-based simulation program to recreate critical event scenarios for radiologists providing conscious sedation to pediatric patients.[9] Blike et al. found that different sets of providers had very different outcomes in simulated critical events involving pediatric patients sedated for radiologic procedures.[10] Moyer described the use of a pediatric simulator in a pediatric emergency department to provide training in managing critical events.[11]

Respiratory System

Although airway management is an integral part of PALS and NALS, it has other applications and has been reported outside the PALS and NALS protocols. In 2002 Stringer et.al. described the different airway simulators available for training in airway management.[12] At the University of Louisville, pediatricians from both the pediatric intensive care unit and the pediatric emergency department provide regular instruction to their students and residents in the patient simulation laboratory, using numerous airway scenarios. In an interesting finding, Kanter, et al. used different simulators to evaluate the effectiveness of residents in mask ventilation of the different simulators and found that physician incompetence was the only factor in failure to ventilate.[13] In 2002 Rowe and Cohen reported how a virtual reality flexible bronchoscopy simulator improved resident skills in performing fiberoptic intubation of pediatric patients.[14]

In addition to providing skills training and assessment, pediatric simulation has added the ability to evaluate the effectiveness of medical tools that physicians use to ventilate their patients. A lung simulator with variable compliance and resistance components was used to evaluate the dynamic compliance of the three common pediatric ventilators.[15] Kain et al. used a lung simulator to evaluate the effectiveness of bag ventilation devices.[16] Simulation has been used to assess risk to children for aspirating small objects. In 1998 Stool et al. reported the use of computer models of anatomy to assess the ability of small items to become impacted in a child's airway.[17]

Decision Making and Problem Solving

Decision making is an essential skill for all primary care physicians. There are reports of complementing this skill with simulation among physicians, health care workers, and even patients. In 1999 Wilson wrote an editorial about the development of diabetes simulators and their role in the education of patients as well as other health care providers.[18] Lehmann et al. reported the improvements to a free software program about diabetes, called AIDA, in which patients can interactively learn about their disease and the principles of successful management.[19] In 2001 Tegtmeyer et al. discussed how computers can be used to assist in learning decision-makings skills in the pediatric critical care setting. The authors reviewed the use of computers in relation to problem-based learning, physiologic models, and the media lab.[20] In 1988 Klaassens reported the successful use of computer simulation in teaching critical decision-making skills to pediatric nursing students.[21] In 1985 Bidwell et al. reported the use of computers in simulating vital signs during patient management problems for teaching pediatrics at the University of Alberta.[22] Kamin et al. described the effective use of computer-based simulation as an adjunct to problem-based learning spread among different locations. Such developments can help eliminate the confining structure in which medical education now finds itself.[23]

Assessment by using simulation is another area under development. Kamin, et al. compared critical thinking among three groups of medical students during their pediatric rotation PBL at the University of Colorado School of Medicine. The three groups were (1) text-based in a face-to-face environment, (2) video-based in a face-to-face environment, {3) and a digital video case in a virtual reality environment. The virtual reality group performed significantly better than the video-based group, which performed significantly better than the text-based group.[24] Schwartz used a computer-based, clinical-choice simulation program to evaluate the performance of students on a pediatric rotation and found that a significant number of students who performed poorly on the simulator were judged to be very good clinically.[25] This report confirms the findings of similar studies using adult simulators, suggesting that medical teachers may have been using imprecise tools in the assessment of student and resident performances.

Procedural Skills

In addition to decision-making skills, psychomotor skills are necessary in providing effective health care. Nakajima et al. reported that using a virtual computer-based simulation program can effectively increase the skills of pediatric surgeons with few laproscopic experiences to the level of those with more than ten laparsocopic experiences.[26] Weber et al. reported the use of simulators in developing microsurgical proficiency.[27] Williams et al. reported the use of simulators in teaching and evaluating the skills of pediatric emergency physicians.[28] Millette et al. described the use of a cardiopulmonary bypass (CPB) simulator to teach students how to manage CPB in pediatric patients. This development was necessitated by the decreasing number of pediatric patients requiring CPB.[29]

Simulation in the pediatric population has also been described as an assessment tool. Gaskin et al. used a Harvey simulator to evaluate the diagnostic skills of pediatric residents and found a trend toward improvement as they progressed throughout their residency, but an overall inadequacy in detecting certain common murmurs compared with pediatric cardiologists.[30] Simulation has been shown to be an effective adjunct in assessing pediatricians' skills in performing otoscopy to differentiate acute otitis media from otitis media with effusion.[31,32]

References

1. Stanford University, Center for Advanced Pediatric Education: http://www.lpch.org/cape/about/about.html. Last accessed 2-12-2004.
2. Stewart D: Medical training in the UK. Arch Dis Child 88:655–658, 2003.
3. Schreiner RL, and et al: Simulators to teach pediatric skills. J Med Educ 54(3):242–243, 1979.
4. Gaba DM: Improving anesthesiologists' performance by simulating reality. Anesthesiology 76:491–494, 1992.
5. Halamek LP, Kaegi DM, Gaba DM, et al: Time for a new paradigm in pediatric medical education: Teaching neonatal resuscitation in a simulated delivery room environment. Pediatrics 106(4):E45, 2000.
6. MDchoice Pediatric Advanced Life Support Simulator: http://www.mdchoice.com/cyberpt/pals/pals.asp. Last accessed 2-12-2004.
7. Cowie DA, Story DA: Knowledge of cardiopulmonary resuscitation protocols and level of anaesthetic training. Anaesth Intens Care 28:687–691, 2000.
8. Palmisano JM, Akingbola OA, Moler FW, et al: Simulated pediatric cardiopulmonary resuscitation: Initial events and response times of a hospital arrest team. Respir Care 39:725–729, 1994.

9. Medina LS, Racadio JM, Schwid HA: Computers in radiology. The sedation, analgesia, and contrast media computerized simulator: A new approach to train and evaluate radiologists' responses to critical incidents. Pediatr Radiol 30(5):299–305, 2000.
10. Blike G, Cravero J, Nelson E: Same patients, same critical events—different systems of care, different outcomes: description of a human factors approach aimed at improving the efficacy and safety of sedation/analgesia care. Qual Manag Health Care 10:17–36, 2001.
11. Moyer M: Simulating the pediatric patient. Emerg Med Serv 32(7):66–69, 2003.
12. Stringer KR, Bajenov S, Yentis SM: Training in airway management. Anaesthesia 57:967–983, 2002.
13. Kanter RK, Fordyce WE, Tompkins JM: Evaluation of resuscitation proficiency in simulations: The impact of a simultaneous cognitive task. Pediatr Emerg Care 6:260–262, 1990.
14. Rowe R, Cohen RA: An evaluation of a virtual reality airway simulator. Anesth Analg 95:62–66, 2002.
15. Binda RE Jr, Cook DR, Fischer CG: Advantages of infant ventilators over adapted adult ventilators in pediatrics. Anesth Analg 55:769–772, 1976.
16. Kain ZN, Berde CB, Benjamin PK, et al: Performance of pediatric resuscitation bags assessed with an infant lung simulator. Anesth Analg 77:261–264, 1993.
17. Stool D, Rider G, Welling JR: Human factors project: Development of computer models of anatomy as an aid to risk management. Int J Pediatr Otorhinolaryngol 43:217–227, 1998.
18. Wilson DM: Diabetes simulators: Ready for prime time? Diabetes Technol Ther 1:55–56, 1999.
19. Lehmann ED: Experience with the Internet release of AIDA v4.0—http://www.diabetic.org.uk.aida.htm—an interactive educational diabetes simulator. Diabetes Technol Ther 1:41–54, 1999.
20. Tegtmeyer K, Ibsen L, Goldstein B: Computer-assisted learning in critical care: From ENIAC to HAL. Crit Care Med 29(8 Suppl):N177-N182, 2001.
21. Klaassens EL: Exploring the use of computer simulation to teach critical decision-making skills to pediatric nursing students. J Pediatr Nurs 3: 202–206, 1988.
22. Bidwell CM, et al: Multidisciplinary team production of computer-based simulations to teach pediatrics. J Med Educ 60(5):397–403, 1985.
23. Kamin C, O'Sullivan P, Deterding R: Does project L.I.V.E. case modality impact critical thinking in PBL groups? In Proceedings of the Annual Meeting of the American Educational Research Association, New Orleans, 2002.
24. Kamin C, O'Sullivan P, Deterding R, et al: A comparison of critical thinking in groups of third-year medical students in text, video, and virtual PBL case modalities. Acad Med 78: 204–211, 2003.
25. Schwartz W: Documentation of students' clinical reasoning using a computer simulation. Am J Dis Child 143:575–579, 1989.
26. Nakajima K, Wasa M, Takiguchi S, et al: A modular laparoscopic training program for pediatric surgeons. JSLS 7:33–37, 2003.
27. Weber D, Moser N, Rosslein R: A synthetic model for microsurgical training: A surgical contribution to reduce the number of animal experiments. Eur J Pediatr Surg 7(4):204–206, 1997.
28. Williams CL, Bricker JT, Hofschire PJ, et al: Teaching preventive cardiology in the pediatric setting. Am J Prev Med 6(2 Suppl):84–92, 1990.
29. Millette G, Weerasena N, Cornel G, et al: A reusable training circuit for cardiopulmonary bypass. J Extra Corpor Technol 34(4):285–288, 2002.
30. Gaskin PR, Owens SE, Talner NS, et al: Clinical auscultation skills in pediatric residents. Pediatrics 105:1184–1187, 2000.
31. Pichichero ME, Poole MD: Assessing diagnostic accuracy and tympanocentesis skills in the management of otitis media. Arch Pediatr Adolesc Med 155:1137–1142, 2001.
32. Sorrento A, Pichichero ME: Assessing diagnostic accuracy and tympanocentesis skills by nurse practitioners in management of otitis media. J Am Acad Nurse Pract 13(11):524–529, 2001.

Chapter 20

SIMULATION IN FAMILY PRACTICE AND PUBLIC HEALTH

Gary E. Loyd, MD, MMM

Family practice and public health have been developing simulation as a way to teach decision making. Significant effort is under way to incorporate it into the certification process. DeLia et al. identified how the cost of training primary care physicians is out of balance with the subsidy provided.[1] This imbalance makes the use of cost-effective teaching techniques more important and provides the incentive for primary care specialties to make use of simulation. Procedural simulations are popular with the family practitioner, but the problem-solving enhancements provided by simulation have played a significant role in the literature. This chapter outlines some of the significant findings in simulation as it relates to family and community health.

Physical Examination

In 1994 Campbell, et al. demonstrated that, when using silicone breast models, students taught by female, nonmedical teachers could provide as good an examination as students taught by family medicine faculty. They also demonstrated that students taught with silicone breast models had consistently better examination techniques and significantly higher sensitivity for identifying breast lumps than students who were not taught with the breast models.[2] Benincasa et al. reported that an office-based simulation training program in clinical breast examination could improve the lump-detection skills of primary care physicians. They also found that physicians liked this educational encounter and intended to change their practices to reflect the methods that they were taught.[3] Ferris et al. reported an assessment of three colposcopic models: latex, steak, and bovine cervix. They concluded that each model had strengths and weaknesses. No follow-up performance was reported.[4] Gordon et al. reported that family practice physicians thought that the use of a cardiology patient simulator for continuing medical education was a valuable experience.[5]

Decision Making

Decision making is an essential skill for family physicians. Emery et al. demonstrated during 18 simulated cases that a computerized decision support system for risk and genetic assessment provided superior decision-making support compared with the established pedigree drawing program designed for clinical geneticists.[6] In 1997 Walton et al. described how computer-supported program significantly improved the prescribing of medications during the simulation of 36 cases.[7] Gerritsma and Smal report the development of an interactive, computer-based patient simulation for the study of medical decision- making. When the model was tested with specialists and family practitioners, both groups thought that the realism of the system was good, but the construct validity was confirmed only for the specialist physicians.[8]

There are reports of decision-making support simulation for education of both physicians and patients. Diabetes is a common disease in most family practices. In 2001 Tatti and Lehmann described the usefulness of a virtual diabetes patient simulator called AIDA. Family practice physicians, evaluating the simulator at a conference, found it interesting to interact with and potentially useful in their practice.[9–31]

In 1999 Lyons described the integration of an innovative computer-based physical simulation and Laurillard's conversational framework in the effective teaching of midwifery in Australia.[32] In 1996 Cain and Sharir reported that students who learned how to repair a second-degree perineal birth trauma on a simulator could consistently perform the procedure adequately 8 months after the initial teaching session.[33]

Certification

The development of simulators as assessment tools by the American Board of Family Practice is an advancement in the use of this technology. Several reports describe the American Board of Family Practice's development of computer simulations to facilitate the more comprehensive candidate evaluation for certifying and recertifying family practitioners in the United States.[34] [37] In a related article in 2002, Glavin and Maran outline a system for the development of a tool for assessing clinical competence.[38] Allen et al. reported a new method for assessing the surgical skills of general practice registrars in the United Kingdom by using videotape and simulators. The results of the study indicated that this method consistently identified those who were competent and those who were not competent to be consultants.[39]

Endoscopy

Simulation successfully identified those who already had skills in endoscopy and also demonstrated that simulation skills can be quickly enhanced for beginner endoscopists.[40] Church found that at least 100 colonoscopy cases are necessary to achieve 67% completion and that 125 colonoscopy cases are needed for 75% completion.[41] The Simbionix website demonstrates effective use of the endoscopic simulator in learning endoscopic surgery.[42] Frelitsch demonstrated that a virtual endoscopic simulator improved the performance of novice endoscopists to the point of approaching the scores of experts. The control group did not attain this proficiency.[40] The Medical University of South Carolina's Digestive Disease Center (MUSC-DDC) teaches its Endoscopy Learning Program with simulators.[43] Edmond reported that residents trained on an endoscopic sinus surgical simulator performed consistently better than those not trained on the simulator.[44] Sedlack reported that experienced gastroenterologists thought that computer-based colonoscopy was realistic for basic cases. The computer-based simulation was not able to distinguish between novices and experts.[45]

Ström demonstrated that basic endoscopy can be taught effectively to medical students with significant improvement in performance.[46] In 1998 Rudman et al. described a sinus surgery training simulator that used both individuals and haptic feedback to create a virtual reality environment. They demonstrated that a haptic device was accurate within physical limitations.[47] The Center for Videoendoscopic Surgery at the University of Washington has refined a tissue-realistic physical simulator and virtual reality simulator to assess performance. The center is assessing whether simulator training transfers to clinical practice.[48] In 1998 Tuggy reported that family practice residents who trained to do sigmoidoscopies on a virtual reality simulator improved insertion time by more than 50%, directional errors by 75%, and total time for the examination by 50%; they also increased the percentage of colon viewed by 67% compared with the control group, who performed only on patients.[49] Verma described the development of a virtual reality simulator for vitreoretinal surgery.[50] Pugh reported that data provided by a pelvic simulator were valid and reliable in assessing the performance of the learner.[51]

Cystoscopy

Shah demonstrated that a virtual reality flexible cystoscopy simulator can differentiate between novice and experienced costoscopists.[52] Shah et al. wrote a review about the role of virtual reality in urology, stating the benefits and weaknesses.[53] Watterson et al. reported that the use of a computer-based ureteroscopy simulator allowed residents with no prior surgical training to quickly acquire basic ureteroscopic skills.[54]

Public Health

In 1975 Williams suggested that computer simulation would probably have a future role in the education and training of public health providers.[55] To enhance an interactive simulation program in a community health assessment class for nursing students, videotaped segments of real community situations were added as the students were led through the processes of data collection and evaluation.[56] McLaughlin et al. studied the reliability and validity of two clinical simulation tests and compared the ability of nurses and physicians to assess public health problems. The two groups demonstrated equal proficiency.[57] In Finland, a study involving a computer simulation program designed to assess the decision-making process of public health nurses in children's health found that the nurses' decisions were more closely related to the developmental stage of the child than to the unique needs of each family.[58]

Bioterrorism

Simulation has been in the forefront of developing education and response teams to cope with the growing threat of bioterrorism. Research in the area is now appearing in the literature. Berkenstadt et. al. found that using full protective gear against bioterrorism increased intubation time among experienced anesthesiologists and decreased communication ability during crisis management.[59] Reshetin and Regens reported the results of simulating a dispersion of anthrax spores from a 50-story building and being able to locate where concentrations of such spores should be found afterward.[60] At the University of Louisville, webcast simulations and continuing medical education courses have been developed in mass sarin toxicity, botulism, and anthrax contamination.

References

1. DeLia D, Cantor JC, Duck E: Productivity vs. training in primary care: Analysis of hospitals and health centers in New York City. Inquiry 39:314–26, 2002.

2. Campbell HS, McBean M, Mandin H, et al: Teaching medical students how to perform a clinical breast examination. Acad Med 69:993–995, 1994.

3. Benincasa TA, King ES, Rimer BK, et al: Results of an office-based training program in clinical breast examination for primary care physicians. J Cancer Educ 11:25–31, 1996.

4. Ferris DG, Waxman AG, Miller MD: Colposcopy and cervical biopsy educational training models. Fam Med 26:30–35, 1994.

5. Gordon MS, Ewy GA, Felner JM, et al: A cardiology patient simulator for continuing education of family physicians. J Fam Pract, 1981. 13(3): p. 353–356, 1981.

6. Emery J, Walton R, Murphy M, et al: Computer support for interpreting family histories of breast and ovarian cancer in primary care: Comparative study with simulated cases. BMJ 321:28–32, 2000.

7. Walton RT, Gierl C, Yudkin P, et al: Evaluation of computer support for prescribing (CAPSULE) using simulated cases. BMJ 315:791–795, 1997.

8. Gerritsma, JG, Smal JA: An interactive patient simulation for the study of medical decision-making. Med Educ 22(2):118–123, 1998.

9. Lehmann ED: Preliminary experience with the Internet release of AIDA—an interactive educational diabetes simulator. Comput Meth Progr Biomed 56(2):109–132, 1998.

10. Lehmann ED: AIDA—a computer-based interactive educational diabetes simulator. Diabetes Educ 24:341–346, 348, 1998.

11. Lehmann ED: Experience with the Internet release of AIDA v4.0—http://www.diabetic.org. uk.aida.htm—an interactive educational diabetes simulator. Diabetes Technol Thcr 1:41–54, 1999.

12. Lehmann ED: Interactive educational diabetes simulators: Future possibilities. Diabetes Nutr Metab 12(6):380–387, 1999.

13. Lehmann ED: Short user comments ('sound bites') regarding usage of AIDA v4—http://www.2aida.org—an interactive educational diabetes simulator. Diabetes Technol Ther 2:663–666, 2000.

14. Lehmann ED: User reviews of AIDA online (http://www.shodor.org/aida): A web-based interactive educational diabetes simulator. Diabetes Technol Ther 2:329–342, 2000.

15. Lehmann ED: User experience with the AIDA interactive educational virtual diabetes patient simulator. Diabetes Technol Ther 2:165–171, 2000.

16. Lehmann ED: Spontaneous comments from users of the AIDA interactive educational diabetes simulator. Diabetes Educ 26:633–638, 641–643, 2000.

17. Lehmann ED: Simulating glycosylated hemoglobin (HbA1c) levels in diabetes using an interactive educational virtual diabetes patient simulator. Diabetes Technol Ther 3:517–524, 2001.

18. Lehmann ED, Tatti P: Questionnaires for a randomized controlled trial methodology to evaluate the teaching utility of diabetes simulation programs. Diabetes Technol Ther 3:293–305, 2001.

19. Lehmann ED: The freeware AIDA interactive educational diabetes simulator—http://www. 2aida.org—(2). Simulating glycosylated haemoglobin (HbA1c) levels in AIDA v4.3. Med Sci Monit 7:516–525, 2001.

20. Lehmann ED: The freeware AIDA interactive educational diabetes simulator—http://www. 2aida.org—(1). A download survey for AIDA v4.0. Med Sci Monit 7:504–515, 2001.

21. Lehmann ED: Why are people downloading the freeware AIDA diabetes computing software program: A pilot study. Diabetes Technol Ther 4:793–808, 2002.

22. Lehmann ED, Tatti P: Using the AIDA—www.2aida.org—diabetes simulator. Part 2: Recommended training requirements for health-carers planning to teach with the software. Diabetes Technol Ther 4:717–732, 2002.

23. Lehmann ED: Who is downloading the freeware AIDA v43 interactive educational diabetes simulator? An audit of 2437 downloads. Diabetes Technol Ther 4:467–477, 2002.

24. Lehmann ED: Further user comments regarding usage of an interactive educational diabetes simulator (AIDA). Diabetes Technol Ther 4:121–135, 2002.

25. Lehmann ED: Research use of the AIDA www.2aida.org diabetes software simulation program: a review. Part 2: Generating simulated blood glucose data for prototype validation. Diabetes Technol Ther. 5:641–651, 2003.
26. Lehmann ED: Why people download the freeware AIDA v4.3a diabetes software program: A proof-of-concept semi-automated analysis. Diabetes Technol Ther 5:477–490, 2003.
27. Lehmann ED: Research use of the AIDA www.2aida.org diabetes software simulation program: a review. Part 1: Decision support testing and neural network training. Diabetes Technol Ther 5:425–438, 2003.
28. Tatti P, Lehmann ED: Use of the AIDA diabetes simulation software—www.2aida.org—as an interactive educational tool for teaching student nurses. Diabetes Technol Ther 3:655–664, 2001.
29. Tatti P, Lehmann ED: Utility of the AIDA diabetes simulator as an interactive educational teaching tool for general practitioners (primary care physicians). Diabetes Technol Ther 3:133–140, 2001.
30. Tatti P, Lehmann ED: A randomised-controlled clinical trial methodology for evaluating the teaching utility of interactive educational diabetes simulators. Diabetes Nutr Metab 14:1–17, 2001.
31. Tatti P, Lehmann ED: Using the AIDA—www.2aida.org—diabetes simulator. Part 1: Recommended guidelines for health-carers planning to teach with the software. Diabetes Technol Ther 4:401–414, 2002.
32. Lyons J, Milton J: Recognizing through feeling. A physical and computer simulation based on educational theory. Comput Nurs 17:114–119, 1999.
33. Cain JJ, Shirar E: A new method for teaching the repair of perineal trauma of birth. Fam Med 28:107–110, 1996.
34. Hagen MD, Sumner W, Roussel G, et al: Computer-based testing in family practice certification and recertification. J Am Board Fam Pract 16:227–232, 2003.
35. Sumner W, Hagen MD, Rovinelli R: The item generation methodology of an empiric simulation project. Adv Health Sci Educ Theory Pract 4:27–38, 1999.
36. Sumner W II, Xu JZ: Modeling fatigue. Proceedings of the AMIA Symposium, 2002, pp 747–751.
37. Sumner W II, Truszczynski M, Marek VW: Simulating patients with Parallel Health State Networks. Proceedings of the AMIA Symposium, 1998, pp 438–442.
38. Glavin RJ, Maran NJ: Development and use of scoring systems for assessment of clinical competence. Br J Anaesth 88:329–330, 2002.
39. Allen J, Evans A, Foulkes F, et al: Simulated surgery in the summative assessment of general practice training: results of a trial in the Trent and Yorkshire regions. Br J Gen Pract 48:1219–1223, 1998.
40. Ferlitsch A., Glauninger P, Gupper A, et al: Evaluation of a virtual endoscopy simulator for training in gastrointestinal endoscopy. Endoscopy 34:698–702, 2002.
41. Church J, Oakley J, Milsom J, et al: Colonoscopy training: The need for patience (patients). Aust N Z J Surg 72(2):89–91, 2002.
42. Fresgonese D, Casetti T, Cestari R, et al: Basic Endoscopy Training: Usefulness of a Computer-based Simulator. Atlanta, 2001.
43. Medical University of South Carolina's Digestive Disease Center (MUSC DDC): Endoscopy Learning Program. Available at http://www.ddc.musc.edu/ddc_pro/pro_development/learning. Last accessed 11-2-03.
44. Edmond CV Jr: Impact of the endoscopic sinus surgical simulator on operating room performance. Laryngoscope 112(7 Pt 1):1148–1158, 2002.
45. Sedlack RE, Kolars JC: Validation of a computer-based colonoscopy simulator. Gastrointest Endosc 57:214–218, 2003.
46. Strom P, Kjellin A, Hedman L, et al: Validation and learning in the Procedicus KSA virtual reality surgical simulator. Surg Endosc 17:227–231, 2003.
47. Rudman DT, Stredney D, Sessanna D, et al: Functional endoscopic sinus surgery training simulator. Laryngoscope 108(11 Pt 1):1643–1647, 1998.
48. Center for Videoendoscopic Surgery: http://depts.washington.edu/cves/edu.html. Last accessed 11-2-03.

49. Tuggy ML: Virtual reality flexible sigmoidoscopy simulator training: Impact on resident performance. J Am Board Fam Pract 11:426–33, 1998.
50. Verma D, Wills D, Verma M: Virtual reality simulator for vitreoretinal surgery. Eye 2003. 17:71–73, 2003.
51. Pugh CM, Youngblood P: Development and validation of assessment measures for a newly developed physical examination simulator. J Am Med Inform Assoc 9:448–460, 2002.
52. Shah J, Darzi A: Virtual reality flexible cystoscopy: a validation study. BJU Int 90:828–832, 2002.
53. Shah J, Mackay S, Vale J, et al: Simulation in urology—a role for virtual reality? BJU Int 88:661–66, 2001.
54. Watterson JD, Beiko DT, Kuan JK, et al: Randomized prospective blinded study validating acquistion of ureteroscopy skills using computer based virtual reality endourological simulator. J Urol 168:1928–1932. 2002.
55. Williams AA: Simulation of human behavior: Possibilities for public health education. Health Educ Monogr 3:181–190, 1975.
56. White, J.E. and V.L. Valentine, Computer Assisted Video Instruction & Community Assessment. Nursing and Health Care, 1993. 14(7): p. 349–53.
57. McLaughlin FE, Carr JW, Delucchi KL: Measurement properties of clinical simulation tests: Hypertension and chronic obstructive pulmonary disease. Nurs Res 30:5–9, 1981.
58. Lauri S: Using a computer simulation program to assess the decision-making process in child health care. Comput Nurs 10(4):171–177, 1992.
59. Berkenstadt H, Ziv A, Barsuk D, et al: The use of advanced simulation in the training of anesthesiologists to treat chemical warfare casualties. Anesth Analg. 96:1739–1742, 2003.
60. Reshetin VP, Regens JL: Simulation modeling of anthrax spore dispersion in a bioterrorism incident. Risk Anal 23:1135–1145, 2003.

INTERNAL MEDICINE SIMULATION

Carol L. Lake, MD, MPH, MBA

Training in clinical skills continues to be a challenge for students and medical educators alike. Fewer patients remain in the hospital for a long enough time for medical students to utilize them for learning physical diagnostic techniques. Ambulatory patients are seen in clinics and medical offices, where patient turnover must be rapid and efficient. Patients themselves are becoming more reluctant to have medical students involved in their care. Curriculum reform in many medical schools requires patient contact at an early stage of the second or even first year of medical school. These factors coalesce into a situation in which undergraduate medical education for patient care is compromised by time-effectiveness.

The availability of simulators provides safe, timely, reproducible, and efficient "patient" contact. Even though general physical diagnosis of the head, neck, chest, abdomen, and extremities can be taught using standardized patients, comprehensive examination of the heart, lungs, and gastrointestinal tract using endoscopic techniques or demonstration of a wide variety of heart sounds is not possible except with simulations. Chapter 21 describes one of the earliest and long-standing types of simulator: Harvey, the Cardiology Patient Simulator. Harvey is used by students or residents alone or in groups, with and without mentors, to assess numerous heart and vascular sounds.

Chapter 21 (Simulation in Gastroenterology) and Chapter 22 (Simulation in Pulmonary Medicine) demonstrate methods for learning procedural skills. Procedural training, like surgical training, is focused on safety, outcomes, assessment of competency, and maintenance of skills. Endoscopy is simulated with live animal models, ex vivo animal organ models, and mechanical/computer simulators. However, the logistics of using animal models limits the availability of training to selected times and places. A live animal model or ex-vivo animal organ model is also limited by physical differences from human anatomy, preparation time to simulate the desired pathology, and the need for a facility equipped for animal model training. The animal model cannot recreate the discomfort of a patient during upper and lower gastrointestinal endoscopy or bronchoscopy

The chapter about pulmonary medicine points out that the underutilization of bronchoscopy and transbronchial needle aspiration results from inadequacies in training. New pulmonary medicine technologies, such as bronchial stent placement, laser bronchoscopy, and cryotherapy, are difficult to learn in actual patients. Failure to learn these techniques may result in decreased quality of care. Computer models of pulmonary anatomy permit initial learning of bronchoscopy and its variations, refinements of techniques to mastery, and periodic practice of infrequently used techniques to maintain skills.

The simulators presented in these chapters will continue to be refined and developed. Medical simulation is in its infancy compared with flight simulations and war games. Learning in simulated environments must be validated to ensure that the assessment of trainees is fair, reliable, and reproducible. With improved simulators and validated assessments, training in simulators for cardiologists, gastroenterologists, and pulmonologists will become a standard in training programs and specialty certification rather than an extravagant nicety.

Chapter 21

SIMULATION IN GENERAL CARDIOLOGY

S. Barry Issenberg, MD

Need for Simulation in General Cardiology

Changes in the delivery of health care and the role of the clinician-educator have necessitated a change in the traditional approach to skills training in clinical cardiology. Higher percentages of acutely ill patients and shorter hospital stays have reduced the number of patients as resources for clinical teaching and result in less opportunity for learners to assess adequately patients with a wide variety of diseases and physical findings. Outpatient-based medicine, a significant source of university funding, increases the demands on clinician-educators and limit the time that they can devote to medical education. In addition, recent reform in medical school curricula necessitates patient contact in the early years of the curriculum to provide a clinical context for the basic sciences. As a result, students in all phases of the curriculum are competing for meaningful patient contact at a time when fewer patients are available. Under the present system of medical education, students find it increasingly difficult to keep abreast of topics already included in the curriculum, which itself is overcrowded. Opportunities for student learning need to be readily available to maximize the time-effectiveness of medical training.

These problems have had direct effects on clinical skills training in bedside cardiology. For example, despite evidence that accurate clinical assessment of patients with cardiac signs and symptoms is a cost-effective diagnostic modality,[1,2] direct bedside teaching of these skills takes place with decreasing frequency.[3] The result is a lack of competency in basic bedside skills, as documented in a study demonstrating that house officers have difficulty in identifying common cardiac findings.[4] The same study also stressed the need for structured, supplemental strategies to improve clinical education, including the use of simulation systems for training.

Simulation for Training and Assessment in Clinical Cardiology

Patient simulators can reproduce a wide variety of medical conditions. They are not intended to replace real patients, but they do address the disadvantages inherent in a totally patient-dependent curriculum,[5] including the unavailability of patients with known diseases at a specific time in the curriculum schedule, embarrassment and stress to patients and beginning students, reluctance among patients to participate in an examination that exposes them to large number of learners, unpredictable patient behavior because of changes in the physical signs of disease and overall deterioration, and lack of standardization of patients with unstable disease. As a result of this lack of standardization, students' assessments of one patient may be quite a different experience from than their assessment of others.

There are two requirements for mastery of bedside examination used in patient diagnosis and care. First, skills must be practiced repetitively, and second, trainees must have an orderly examination technique along with knowledge of hemodynamic correlations with bedside findings. Traditional training requires a pool of patients with diverse diseases at different stages of severity as well as observation of treatment combined with instruction by experienced faculty who are motivated to teach. As described above, these requirements have become difficult and often impossible to meet. As a response to these challenges, the MIAMI Group, a consortium of clinicians, educators, and engineers, began work more than 30 years ago to develop a simulator (Harvey, the Cardiology Patient Simulator) that is capable of reproducing—instantly and with high fidelity—the bedside findings of almost all cardiac diseases.

High-fidelity simulators such as Harvey are often seen only as a tool for students to gain experience in psychomotor clinical skills in a nonthreatening environment. Experience with Harvey has shown that it can be used for a much wider range of educational outcomes. Once the psychomotor skills are developed and a given bedside finding is identified, the student may also learn to integrate the pathophysiology, define a differential diagnosis, estimate severity, and make management decisions.

Features of Harvey, the Cardiology Patient Simulator

Harvey provides a comprehensive cardiology curriculum by realistically simulating 27 common and rare cardiac conditions (Table 1). The physical findings programmed for each disease include blood pressure, bilateral jugular venous pulses, bilateral carotid and peripheral arterial pulses, precordial impulse in six different areas, and auscultatory events (Table 2). The auscultatory events are heard in the four classic areas and synchronized with the pulses; they also vary with respiration when appropriate. More than

Table 1.
Harvey Curriculum

Introductory program	Aortic regurgitation, chronic
Normal	Aortic regurgitation, acute
Innocent murmur	Aortic stenosis
Aortic valve sclerosis	Hypertrophic cardiomyopathy
Hypertension	Cardiomyopathy
Angina pectoris	Acute pericarditis
Acute inferior myocardial infarction	Primary pulmonary hypertension
Acute anterior myocardial infarction	Atrial septal defect
Ventricular aneurysm	Ventricular septal defect
Mitral valve prolapse	Patent ductus arteriosus
Mitral regurgitation, chronic	Pulmonary stenosis
Mitral regurgitation, acute	Coarctation of the aorta
Mitral stenosis	Tetralogy of Fallot
Mitral stenosis and regurgitation	

Table 2.
Categories of Findings for Cardiac Conditions

Jugular venous pulse	**First heart sound**
Normal "a" wave larger than "v"wave	Normal single
Giant "a" wave	Normal split
Systolic "cv" wave	Soft
Equal "a" and "v" waves	Loud
Prominent "x" descent	**Systolic sounds**
Carotid arterial pulse	Ejection sound
Normal	Systolic click
Hypokinetic	**Diastolic sounds**
Hyperkinetic	Third heart sound
Bifid	Fourth heart sound
Precordial impulse (location and size)	Opening snap
Normal location and size	**Second heart sound**
Normal location, enlarged	Normal physiologic splitting (NPS)
Inferolaterally displaced, enlarged	NPS and loud P_2
Ectopic location, enlarged	Paradoxic splitting
Left parasternal, enlarged	Persistent expiratory splitting
Pulmonary location, enlarged	Fixed splitting
Absent apical impulse	Single loud A_2
Precordial impulse (contour)	Single loud P_2
Early systolic	**Systolic murmurs**
Early brisk systolic	Early peaking and short
Sustained systolic (SS)	Late peaking and long
Persystolic-early systolic	Holosystolic
Presystolic + SS	Late systolic
SS + early diastolic	**Diastolic murmurs**
Presystolic-SS-early diastolic	Early decrescendo and long
	Early decrescendo and short
	Long diastolic
	Mid diastolic

one example of a particular disease may be represented, simulating the marked differences in the clinical presentation of a particular disease that depend on its chronicity and severity. The curriculum is structured to begin with common, less complex conditions and progress to more complex diseases.

Location of Simulator

One of the most important conclusions of a recent user survey was that the location of the Harvey simulator correlated directly with its use throughout the curriculum. The location should be convenient for both students and the faculty member in charge. Even though Harvey functions as a self-learning device, the availability of knowledgeable faculty and staff ensures a successful program. Locations that contribute to successful use of the simulator include clinical skills centers, a dedicated small classroom in a medical education center, or a dedicated small classroom in the main teaching hospital. The physical location reflects the importance that an institution places on integrating the simulator into its curriculum. Locations that contribute to lack of simulator use include a library setting, an off-site clinic location far from other learning activities, and nondedicated small classrooms in which other educational activities are scheduled.

Most institutions restrict the hours when a simulator may be used. About one-fourth of schools have unrestricted hours. Both approaches have advantages and disadvantages. Restricted use limits the potential off-peak hours for practice and allows a greater degree of control over surveillance of the simulator (damage is less likely to occur when others are around). However, conflicts in scheduling the simulator's use for multiple groups of learners are much more likely. Many schools have found it helpful to implement a "sign-up" schedule for access time when the simulator is not being used as part of a core learning activity. Disadvantages of unrestricted use include an increase in off-peak hours for practice with the simulator (e.g., evenings, weekends) and less control over surveillance. The major advantage is that conflicts in scheduling the simulator's use for multiple groups are less likely. Some schools have found it helpful to implement an electronic access card system to allow entry into the room that houses the simulator.

Suggested Learning Environment

Simulators may be used for teaching in any environment in which a patient may be examined. Individual students or small groups may learn without an instructor by using an accompanying self-assessment computer program. Larger groups may learn in a lecture hall setting by using by infrared stethophones for auscultation and video cameras and a projector for observing other physical findings. The location should be convenient for both students and the faculty member in charge. A dedicated administrator who appropriately represents the faculty member in charge can manage the educational programs associated with simulators.

Allocation of Responsibilities for Simulator Training

It is important to allocate and assign specific responsibilities to integrate, manage, train, and evaluate the simulator's use throughout the curriculum.

Academic Responsibilities

Appoint one faculty member to be responsible not only for use of the simulator in one specific course but also for integration of its use throughout the curriculum. Schools that have been most successful at fully integrating Harvey into the entire curriculum have such a champion of simulator use— typically a clinician who believes in the value of the bedside examination, enjoys the teaching of bedside skills, and often directs a related component of the curriculum.

Administrative Responsibilities

Appoint an administrator of the simulator (often the administrative assistant of the faculty member in charge). Administrative responsibilities relating to simulators include the following:

◆ Briefly orienting students and providing them with appropriate instructions
◆ Scheduling the use of simulators
◆ Serving as a liaison with faculty members to facilitate teaching and learning sessions
◆ Working with the technician to keep records related to maintenance of simulators

Technical Responsibilities

Appoint a technician for the simulator. Anyone who handles the routine maintenance and troubleshooting of technical problems should suffice. If the simulator is used for testing, the technician should be on call in the event that any problems arise.

Use of Cardiology Simulators in Different Contexts

Health Care Professionals

Over many years the following question has been asked: "What population of learners is best suited for training with Harvey?" The answer is simple: the population of learners best suited for training with patients. If a simulator realistically represents patient findings or the patient encounter, it is valid for training many populations of learners. Our worldwide survey of Harvey users confirms that the simulator is currently used in the education of many types of health care professionals at different levels of training, in different settings, in varied contexts, and for different purposes.

The use of simulators is limited more by the instructor's imagination than by the potential of the simulator. It is the responsibility of the instructor to select the findings and/or conditions in each simulator that are most appropriate for training a specific population of learners and to choose the best setting.

Medical Students and Physicians

All institutions with a Harvey simulator use it for training medical students. Seventy-five percent use Harvey for training residents, and 50% use it for continuing medical education.

Physician Assistants and Nurse Practitioners

More than half of physician assistants (PAs) and nurse practitioners (NPs) practice in a primary care setting. In the current era of managed care, PAs and NPs are called on more frequently to conduct initial and follow-up physical examinations. Nearly half of the institutions with a Harvey simulator use it to teach PAs and NPs.

Nurses

About half of the institutions with a Harvey simulator also use it for basic and specialized training of nurses. The simulator has been used successfully to introduce nurses to the clinical examination of cardiology patients and to a wide range of cardiac problems.

Paramedics and Other Health Care Providers

Harvey can contribute to the training programs of other health care providers. Echocardiography technicians can learn the bedside findings of the diseases that they evaluate, and paramedics can learn selected findings that may be important in the acute prehospital setting. Pharmaceutical companies often request training courses that include Harvey for their representatives.

Multiprofessional Education

The importance of teamwork in the delivery of health care is well recognized. One educational implication is an increasing interest in the potential of multiprofessional education. Not uncommonly, the facilities of clinical skills centers, where simulators may be located, are shared among medical students, nursing students, and other health care professionals. It is important that the different users are not seen as competing for the same resources; multiprofessional education should be seen instead an opportunity for shared teaching. Patient management problems can be developed with the simulator as a focus and tackled by a multiprofessional group of students and trainees.

Levels of Education

All institutions with a Harvey simulator use it to train medical students in the later clinical years of their medical school curriculum. The simulator is also used at 75% of institutions during physical diagnosis courses both in the early medical student curriculum and in early postgraduate training. The experiences reflected in our worldwide survey demonstrate that Harvey can be used at any level of medical education.

Early Medical School Training

Harvey can be used throughout the early phases of the curriculum to enrich discussions of the basic sciences. A normal patient can be examined and the findings correlated with normal anatomy and cardiovascular hemodynamics. An example of a patient with abnormal auscultatory events might then be added with a review of the associated pathophysiology.

A clinical example with a problem-based learning approach can also be used so that the students can see what is expected of them in the context of medical practice. A cardiac problem such as myocardial infarction can be used as an example. The learning is made more meaningful for the student when Harvey is used to illustrate the clinical problem.

Later Years of the Medical School Curriculum

Harvey can be used to help students learn clinical skills in cardiology and to strengthen their understanding of the relevant pathophysiology. Harvey and other simulators are not a replacement for contact with real patients, but they can greatly enhance the value of time spent in the clinical context and the overall acquisition by the student of the required competencies. In many centers, Harvey plays a key role in clinical rotations by reinforcing bedside findings elicited from real cases on the wards and in ambulatory care settings. When Harvey is used with the associated computer programs, students also demontrate significant gains in their cognitive knowledge and management skills.

Postgraduate Training

Harvey is of value both for general postgraduate and specialist cardiology training. In generalist training, the device can help postgraduate trainees to learn and/or maintain basic auscultatory skills. It can also be used to develop additional skills and understanding related to more specialized cardiac practice. For example, cardiology fellows must be able to assess the severity of a valvular lesions based on the bedside findings.

At the University of Miami, second- and third-year internal medicine residents have a dedicated teaching ward rotation in which they spend 10 hours over a 4-week period focusing on cardiology clinical skills. In our experience, when residents are taking care of patients in the hospital setting, their focus and time to practice bedside skills on Harvey are limited.

Continuing Medical Education

Maintenance of competence is a continuing challenge facing medical education. The acquisition and retention of basic cardiac bedside skills is becoming a requirement of certification organizations. For example, the American Board of Internal Medicine emphasizes these skills in its Physical Examination Self-Assessment Program as part of its Continuing Professional Development Program.[6]

Simulators such as Harvey provide a convenient and attractive resource for refresher courses for family physicians and hospital doctors. When they are used for this purpose, physicians value the experience and believe that they gain much needed confidence and competence in auscultatory abilities. Simulators can be used as a resource for short continuing professional development courses, in the context of "grand rounds," or at other meetings. A clinical case is presented and the findings demonstrated on the simulator, with the pathophysiologic mechanisms and investigations discussed and explained using the accompanying teaching system. Alternative diagnoses with their associated clinical findings can also be demonstrated on Harvey.

Settings for Simulator Use

Simulators teach best when they are used in a variety of learning environments. The following discussion summarizes several highly effective settings.

Instructor Teaching

Although students learn from Harvey and other simulators with no teacher, it is recommended that the initial session be carried out by the instructor. This arrangement allows an appropriate orientation and the opportunity for the teacher to express his or her curricular goals and to describe firsthand the technique of the bedside examination. Additional sessions with the instructor are scheduled during the course to cover additional disease states and to answer questions about the cases studied during self-learning sessions.

Small Group Instructor Teaching (Bedside Rounds)

A small group is the simplest system for instructor teaching. The instructor should prepare by reviewing the description of the condition that he or she plans to cover during the session. Most elect to start with the normal patient. The instructor can assess the background level of skills and the needs of the students during this interactive session and provide focused teaching. Because these are hands-on, interactive sessions, students maintain a high level of interest for as long as two hours.

Large Group Instructor Teaching (Lecture Hall)

This powerful method of teaching reaches many learners at one time. It also requires additional equipment and a bit of practice by the instructor to demonstrate the findings so that all may share the bedside findings. Harvey is used successfully at medical schools to teach entire classes and at conferences to teach hundreds of learners. Although this format prevents the learner from having direct contact during the session, the use of individual infrared headphones for cardiac auscultation and a video camera and projector for visualization of pulses allows each person to participate in the evaluation of nonauscultatory and auscultatory physical findings. In this way, skillful teachers can incorporate specific clinical findings into lectures about various topics, including anatomy, pathophysiology, clinical diagnosis, and patient management.

Independent Self-Learning (Individual and Small Group)

Most educational use of Harvey falls into this category. Independent learning makes an important contribution to hands-on skills training. Students master the area under study and at the same time develop the ability to work on their own and to take responsibility for their own learning. Because learners can proceed at their own pace, self-learning provides an excellent means of "deliberate practice" of bedside skills.

Peer Teaching (Students Teaching Students)

One student is trained and prepares in advance, assumes the role of the instructor, reviews key findings, and acts as the facilitator during the session. The University of Miami has implemented an Academic Societies program in which senior medical students use Harvey to provide instruction and feedback to first-year medical students about the fundamentals of the cardiac bedside exam. We find this system very exciting. The student-teachers are highly motivated and can become quite skillful. They save instructor time and serve as role models for the students whom they teach.

Range of Learning Outcomes in General Cardiology

In recent years, there has been a growing movement toward outcomes-based education.[7-11] In this performance-based approach, the emphasis is on the product—what sort of practitioner will be produced—rather than on the educational process. Table 3 illustrates the ways in which Harvey has been shown to be a useful tool in aiding educators and students in the teaching and assessing of outcomes.

Table 3.
Use of Simulation in Outcomes-based Education

Outcome	Example of Harvey's Use
Physical examination	Harvey is used to teach fundamentals of cardiac physical examination and to provide opportunity for repetitive practice.
Patient investigation	Harvey's clinical findings can be combined with discussions and management that address diagnostic reasoning, differential diagnosis, and management of condition suggested by findings. This approach is used by some medical teachers in iterative process that allows immediate reprogramming of Harvey to provide different set of "what if" clinical findings to extend discussion to other diagnostic and management possibilities.
Communication skills	Harvey is used in combination with standardized patient scenarios. The learner takes a history from a standardized patient, then examines Harvey (who has findings consistent with the patient presentation), and, finally, verbally communicates findings and their meaning to either the patient or facilitator.
Using basic science in clinical medicine	Harvey is a powerful tool in teaching and reinforcing knowledge and understanding of anatomy and pathophysiology. It allows on-demand access to a wide variety of individual clinical findings and/or patterns of physical findings of specific conditions that may be followed by review of pathophysiology underlying that sign or condition.
Appropriate attitudes and ethical understanding	Harvey is used to frame discussions that relate specific findings to choosing appropriately cost-effective laboratory and imaging investigations. This approach has significant potential to encourage trainees to consider human and societal costs of unnecessary investigations and inappropriate treatments throughout training and in clinical practice.
Clinical reasoning and appropriate decision-making	Harvey often has been used at conferences to present cases that lead to discussions of management by experienced cardiologists and cardiac surgeons. Audience members first become involved with the case by sharing bedside findings and formulating their own diagnoses. They further benefit from the reasoning and decisions made by experienced experts.
Lifelong learning	Harvey provides an opportunity for clinicians to learn and review bedside skills by intermittent repetitive practice. This process is necessary to maintain skills, especially those required to recognize uncommon cardiac conditions.

Use of Simulation for Assessment in General Cardiology

Harvey is an excellent tool for testing bedside cardiovascular examination skills. It is an ideal "standardized patient" for assessment. Patient findings can be presented uniformly, and the process of skills testing thus can be made objective. Harvey is used for formative assessments to monitor a student's progress through a course or a phase of their studies. It is also used for summative assessment at the end of different courses because it meets the fairness criteria that all students can be tested on the same materials and judged by the same standards. Specific areas that can be assessed by Harvey and other simulators are discussed below.

Entire Cardiac Examination

The skills examination covers all significant aspects of the bedside cardiac examination (Table 4). Major categories are vital signs, jugular venous pulse, carotid and peripheral arterial pulses, precordial movement, auscultation, and diagnostic impression. This type of individual testing is time-consuming, but it has high validity and is quite effective.

Auscultation Only

The auscultation-only system focuses on the most important auscultatory findings that should be mastered by all practicing physicians.[3] These findings were chosen by program directors of internal medicine and family medicine residencies, then reviewed and confirmed by our consortium of cardiologists (Table 5).

Bedside Findings Based on Skill/Learner Level

We have also developed a series of questions for different bedside findings based on the expected level of the learner's skills. Table 6 uses the example of a fourth heart sound to demonstrate how the finding may be tested at different levels.

❖ Table 4.
Student Checklist for Normal Physical Examination

No.	Completed	Normal Physical Examination
1		General observation of patient and order of exam
2		*Surface anatomy:* carotid pulses, jugular venous pulsations, palpation, and auscultation areas
3		*Arterial pulses:* rate, rhythm, contour, duration at *brachial, radial,* and *femoral* sites
4		Blood pressure technique
5		*Jugular venous pulsations:* position, timing, contour, central venous pressure
6		Inspection: chest shape and visible impulses
7		Palpation technique
8		Areas of palpation of *apical impulses* (point of maximal impulse) and potential areas for palpable murmurs
9		*Apical impulse* with emphasis on site, size, duration, contour
10		Listening areas and patterns of sound transmission
11		Appropriate use, positioning, and utility of stethoscope; use of bell and diaphragm
12		Normal heart sounds timing in relation to carotid or apical impulse
13		Systole and diastole
14		Normal splitting of the *first heart sound*
15		*Normal inspiratory splitting of the second heart sound*
16		*Third heart sound*

Table 5.
Important Auscultatory Findings

Second sound splitting	Aortic stenosis
Third sound	Aortic regurgitation
Fourth sound	Mitral stenosis
Systolic clicks	Continuous murmur
Innocent murmur	Tricuspid regurgitation
Mitral regurgitation	Pericardial rub

Table 6.
Fourth Heart Sound as Example of Bedside Finding Based on Learner's Skill Level

Difficulty/Learner Level	Variable Tested	Correct Answer
1. First-year medical student	Identify finding	Fourth heart sound (S_4)
2. Second-year medical student	Identify finding and correlate it with underlying pathophysiology	S_4–reduced leftventricular compliance
3. Third-/fourth-year medical student	Identify finding and correlate it with underlying disease and differential diagnosis	S_4–hypertension, aortic stenosis, hypertrophic cardiomyopathy
4. House officer	Identify finding and correlate it with severity of underlying disease process and management	S_4–its presence in "young" patient with aortic stenosis denotes severe disease suggests need for surgery

Self-assessment Exercises with Formative Feedback

A system of self-assessment is an integral part of the Harvey teaching program. Interactive questions embedded in the accompanying computer system provide instant feedback for the learner. Wrong answers result in mandatory remediation with an explanation of why the answer is wrong as well as an explanation of the right answer. If the answer is correct, further explanation is optional. In addition, the system automatically grades each learner's performance, advises the learners what areas to review further, and provides the learner with a record of his or her performance. The instructor is provided with records of both individual and group performance for all categories of learners.

Objective Structured Clinical Examinations

Harvey has also been integrated into OSCE stations covering the cardiovascular system with multiple choice questions, short answer questions, and checklists. Several stations, including one with Harvey may be structured around a "problem of the week" with a series of linked stations testing a range of learning outcomes. Table 7 includes examples of individual stations during a week in which the problem is atherosclerotic heart disease.

> **Table 7.**
> **Examples of Individual Stations When the Problem of the Week Is Atherosclerotic Disease**
>
> 1. Examination of the leg in patient with peripheral vascular disease
> 2. Auscultation of fourth heart sound and mitral regurgitation due to papillary muscle dysfunction in patient with myocardial infarction programmed in Harvey
> 3. Telephone conversation with simulated patient with chest pain
> 4. Advice to simulated patient and his wife on discharge from hospital after myocardial infarction

Learner Portfolios

Students may collect evidence from a variety of sources (personal/small group) of their mastery of the appropriate learning outcomes. This evidence may be in the form of a print-out from the computer program that documents learner use or a logbook documenting the conditions examined and physical findings encountered during exposure to Harvey.

Although it is essential to test students, it takes a long time and some expertise to construct testing instruments that are valid and reliable and to test each student individually by observation of hands-on skills. One should first consider the advantages of systems that are easily administered and automatically graded. Begin by testing:

- The most important findings
- In the most pertinent conditions
- At a basic level of difficulty
- In a group setting
- Using an instrument that can be graded automatically

Conclusion

The purpose of this chapter is to provide an outline for educators interested in the optimal use of simulation to teach and assess clinical cardiology skills with Harvey. New technology and the changing medical education environment are likely to ensure that the use of simulation in cardiology will continue to increase. Cardiology educators need to embrace and harness this potential and use it to enhance the self-directed acquisition of skills for cardiac evaluation throughout the lifelong continuum of medical education.

References

1. Roldan CA, Shively BK, Crawford MH: Value of the cardiovascular physical examination for detecting valvular heart disease in asymptomatic subjects. Am J Cardiol 1996;77:1327–1331.
2. Danford DA, Nasir A, Gumbiner C: Cost assessment of the evaluation of heart murmurs in children. Pediatrics 1993;91:365–368.
3. Mangione S, Nieman LZ, Gracely E, Kaye D: The teaching and pratice of cardiac auscultation during internal medicine and cardiology training: A nationwide survey. An Intern Med 1993;119:47–54.
4. Mangione S, Nieman LZ: Cardiac auscultatory skills of internal medicine and family practice trainees: A comparison of diagnostic proficiency JAMA 1997;278:717–722 [erratum published in JAMA 1998;279:1444].

5. Collins JP, Harden RM: AMEE Medical Education Guide No. 13: Real patients, simulated patients and simulators in medical education. Med Teacher 1998;20:508–521.
6. Norcini J: Perspectives: Computer-based testing will soon be a reality. Am Board Intern Med Newsl Diplom 1999;Summer:3.
7. McNeir G: Outcome-based education, tool for restructuring. Ore School Study Council Bull [Eugene] 1993;36(8).
8. Cohen AM: Relating curriculum and transfer. N Direct Commun Coll 1994;22(2), no. 86.
9. Fitzpatrick KA: Restructuring to achieve outcomes of significance for all students. Educ Leadership 1991;48(8):18–22.
10. Terry PM: Outcome-based education: Is it mastery learning all over again, or is it revolution to the reform movement? Presented at the Seventh Annual Midwest Education Society (CIES) Conference, Indiana, 1996.
11. Harden RM,Crosby JR, David MH: An introduction to outcome-based education. Part 1: AMEE Nol 14: Outcome-based education. Med Teacher 1999;21(1):7–14.

Chapter 22

SIMULATION IN GASTROINTESTINAL ENDOSCOPY

Robert E. Sedlack, MD

Procedural training is coming under increasing scrutiny in all medical specialties, with attention focused on safety, outcomes, and competency assessment. One result of this scrutiny is the growing interest in nonhuman training models and inanimate simulators. The use of simulation as a training tool is not a new concept. It is well documented that the aviation community has successfully used simulators in improving pilot safety and accelerating skill aquisition. The aviation field has accomplished a level of simulation that realistically recreates both basic skill-learning scenarios and rare but dangerous situations in a safe, virtual setting. Similar to aviation, gastrointestinal (GI) endoscopy entails a number of procedural skills that require considerable time to master and are learned with considerable risk to patients' well-being. As a result, it is becoming increasingly necessary to find ways to accelerate the learning curves of trainees in a cost-effective manner that also increases patient safety and satisfaction.[1,2] Advocates speculate that the addition of simulation into the endoscopy training environment can accomplish these goals. In addition, simulation technology has the potential to provide a tool that allows standardized competency assessment.

Over the past decade, endoscopy simulation has progressed primarily along three major pathways: live animal models, ex-vivo animal organ models, and mechanical/computer simulators. Each model has inherent strengths and weaknesses. Which model is the right one for a training program or simulation center depends on the intended role and goals of the simulator's use. This chapter outlines the pros and cons of the various models and attempts to define their best-suited roles in the diverse spectrum of procedures encountered in GI endoscopy.

Live Animal Models

Live animal models have been used in endoscopy for over 30 years. Original work utilized anesthetized dogs and baboons. The canine model was severely limited by its anatomic differences from humans. Although the use of baboons solved this limitation, cost and animal availability made this model undesirable. The optimal animal model should be not only similar to human anatomy but readily available and cost-efficient. Anesthetized juvenile pigs (3–4 months old, weighing 75 lb) were found to satisfy these requirements reasonably well and have been almost exclusively the animal of choice for many years by most institutions.

The use of the live pig model has been well described in procedures involving the upper GI tract.[3] Esophagogastroduodenoscopy (EGD), endoscopic retrograde cholangiopancreatography (ERCP), and endoscopic ultrasound (EUS) can be performed as well as all manners of therapeutics such as deployment of expandable wall stents, papillary sphincterotomy, and fine needle aspirations. It also acts as an excellent model for experimental procedures such as the use of endoscopic fundoplication and mucosal resection devices. Lower endoscopy in live pigs has not been described in the educational setting but certainly has been performed in the research arena for trials of new therapeutic endoscopy equipment and techniques.

The live animal model offers a number of benefits. Probably the most important is the fact that the live tissue looks and behaves the same as live, human mucosa during endoscopy. When tissue is traumatized, edema develops; when a sphincterotomy is performed, bleeding may result; when too much force or coagulation is used, a perforation occurs. In addition, all procedures are performed with traditional endoscopic equipment, thus allowing practice with devices identical to those that eventually will be used to perform procedures on patients.

What role does the pig model currently play in the educational arena? The American Society for Gastrointestinal Endoscopy (ASGE) has frequently used live pig models for many of its hands-on teaching courses—usually at a facility specifically suited for animal model training. An example is the Ethicon Institute in Cincinnati, Ohio, which sponsors numerous hands-on courses for a number of medical organizations each year. Because of the substantial costs involved with live animals, the use of such models has been reserved primarily for training in advanced endoscopic procedures, where the need for simulation realism is greatest and the risk to patient well-being during training would be high. The live porcine model has become the standard for both advanced therapeutic endoscopy training and endoscopic research, especially pertaining to interventional and biliary devices.[4-6] Their use in such procedures has been supported by model comparative studies as well as the ASGE Technology Assessment statement about ERCP simulators, which specifies that the live pig model is "best suited for teaching sphincterotomy, endoprosthesis placement, and manometry" rather than for teaching basic techniques.[7,8]

The live model does have some drawbacks, however. There are anatomic differences of the papilla in pigs and humans. The biliary opening in pigs is very similar to the human papilla, but it is more proximal in the pig model, resting in the distal duodenal bulb. This anatomic difference makes it difficult to teach the proper endoscopic approach for ERCP but enhances training in sphincterotomy. The common bile duct does not merge with the pancreatic duct. Instead, the pancreatic papilla is distal to the biliary papilla. This location makes the live pig an ideal model for training sphincterotomy.[9] Another drawback associated with the pig model is the cost associated with animal purchase, housing facilities, feeding, veterinary staff, and animal disposal. All of these factors add considerable expense to the use of the pig model. In addition, a considerable amount of preparation is involved with live animal models. Preprocedure fasting, anesthesia, and tracheal intubation require substantial time, specialized expertise, and planning prior to model use. In addition, dedicated facilities, equipment, and scopes are necessary for animal endoscopy. Finally, the pig model must adhere to strict animal rights guidelines to ensure the protection of the animals during their use, sacrifice, and disposal. All of these factors make live animal models difficult to support for routine use and are best suited for specialized training and research at facilities that do a large volume of advanced endoscopic education.

Ex-Vivo Animal Organ Models

The impressive realism found in the live pig models led to attempts at developing a model that utilizes porcine tissue but eliminates the expensive and onerous needs for animal care. The models that resulted use a plastic torso or GI tract outline into which harvested porcine GI tracts are placed. The resulting realism is nearly identical to live animal tissue but eliminates all of the costs associated with animal care.

The first model introduced was the Erlanger Endo-Trainer developed at the University of Erlangen-Nürnberg in Germany by Neumann et al.[10] This model uses a large, human-sized torso into which the harvested (ex-vivo) organs (both upper and lower intestinal tracts) are placed (Fig. 1). Not long after the release of the Endo-Trainer, a more portable model was introduced. The Compact Erlangen Active Simulator for Interventional Endoscopy (Compact EASIE) was developed by Hochburger, et al., also in Erlangen, Germany (Fig. 2). Both models have become widely used throughout Europe for advance endoscopy seminars as well as in primary education of trainees at a number of universities. In recent years, these models have been gaining favor in the United States. Many gastrointestinal conventions and endoscopy courses provide demonstrations of these models, even if the course is not based primarily on the use of ex-vivo models. Due to the increasing popularity and demand for these models, a third model entered the market in 2003. The Endo-X Trainer (Medical Innovations, Rochester, Minnesota) was developed at the Mayo Clinic. This model has the advantage of being even more compact and easily transportable than its predecessors (Fig. 3).

The concept of using ex-vivo organs affords not only the retained realism of animal tissue but also the ability to recreate pathology that is not possible with live animals. Simulation of major gastrointestinal bleeding is accomplished by suturing or gluing vessels through the lumen wall and the infusion of artificial blood through these vessels (Fig. 4). The rate of bleeding can be controlled with an infusion pump or simply with a syringe, and the endoscopic results are impressively realistic (Fig. 5). Lumen strictures and masses can be created as well, with the submucosal injection or insertion of different substances or objects. Small objects such as beans or pills can be used to recreate polyps or other submucosal masses (Fig. 6). The reproduction of biliary pathology is also possible with the ex-vivo model. Intraductal biliary stones can be created by the insertion of a small foreign body (such as a baby aspirin or other object) into the harvested bile duct prior to endoscopy. The possibilities of pathology simulation with the ex-vivo model are limitless.

Therapeutic techniques can also be used in the ex-vivo model just as they are in the live porcine model. Despite the fact that the tissue is not living, electrocautery, sphincterotomes, and other devices continue to behave as they would in live tissue. In the ex-vivo models the grounding pad is simply applied to the external surface of the organs.[11]

Clearly the advantages offered by the live animal model are retained with the ex-vivo model but without the cost, facilities, and time commitments. In addition, the added ability to create reproducible pathology at will makes this model particularly attractive as an eventual replacement for the use of live animals in advanced endoscopic teaching.

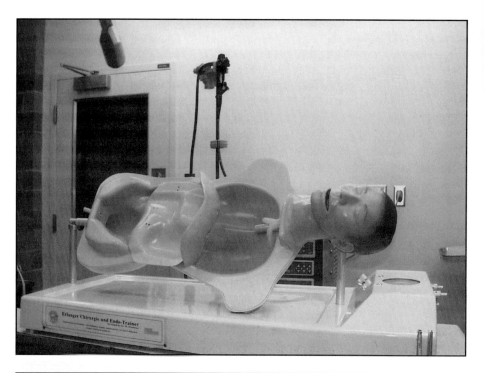

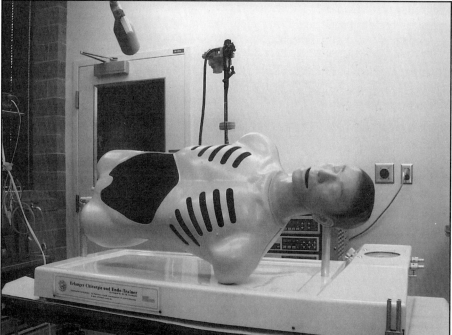

Figure 1. Erlanger Endo-Trainer. The large mannequin allows for ex-vivo organs to be sutured into the internal organ trays **(A)** and can then be covered with the available chest plate **(B)** prior to performing endoscopy.

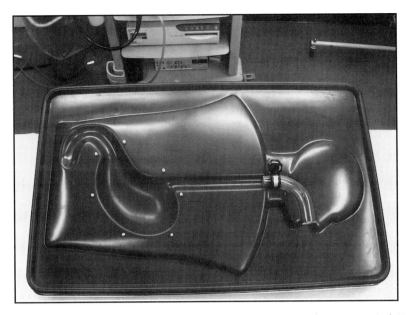

Figure 2. Compact Erlangen Active Simulator for Interventional Endoscopy (Compact EASIE). This ex-vivo model allows porcine organs to be sutured into the trays and offers a more portable model than the larger upper or lower GI tract Erlangen models.

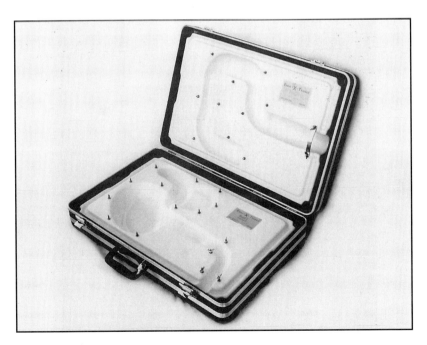

Figure 3. Endo-X Trainer. The Endo-X Trainer is the newest and most compact model available of all of the ex-vivo porcine organ trainers. This compact trainer is shown in its included carrying case, which allows easy and convenient transport.

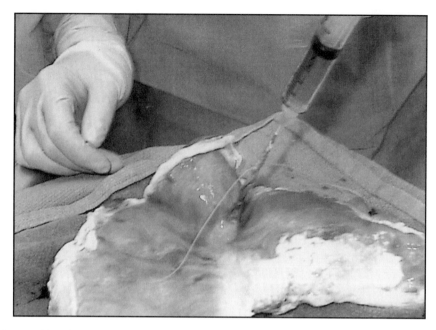

Figure 4. Vessel cannulated with an angiocatheter that has been glued to the external organ surface. The needle of the angiocatheter creates a small hole in the organ wall before it is withdrawn from the catheter. The catheter can then be connected to an infusion pump or syringe by which artificial blood can be infused into the organ's lumen at variable rates.

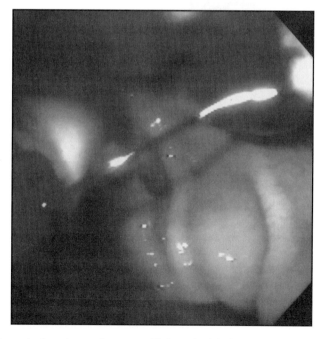

Figure 5. Endoscopic view of an ex-vivo organ with the active infusion of artificial blood via a recreated bleeding vessel.

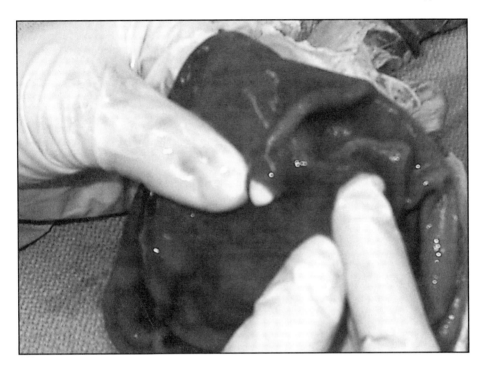

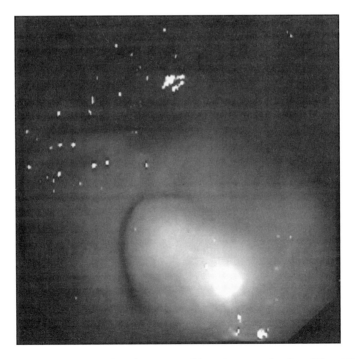

Figure 6. Insertion of a white bean into the organ wall from the external surface (A) and the resulting endoscopic view of the recreated submucosal lesion (B).

Despite these advantages, the ex-vivo model has had some drawbacks. Until recently, organ procurement was the major limiting factor since organs were not commercially available. Traditionally, they were available to institutions only if a nearby meat-processing plant or specialized butcher was hired specifically for this task. Recently, however, the makers of the Endo-X trainer, Medical Innovations, began offering cleaned, prepackaged, frozen organs that can be ordered and shipped overnight. Unlike the juvenile pigs used in live animal models, these prepackaged organs use full-sized adult porcine organs from 200-lb animals, allowing a more accurate facsimile of human anatomy.

Once procurement is accomplished, the frozen organs can be stored until needed. Hours before use, the organs must be thawed. Recreation of any desired pathology can be done at this time. The organs must finally be sutured into place onto the organ platform. The entire process requires a considerable amount of planning prior to organ use. Once in place, however, an individual set of organs can be used by multiple students and requires changing only after a significant number of therapeutic measures have been performed. The Endo-X Trainer model uses a simplistic netting to anchor the organs to the model during use. This technique avoids the time-consuming method of suturing the organ into place and allows rapid changing of organs.

Another drawback of the ex-vivo and live pig models is that colonoscopy is severely limited by the pigs' anatomy. The rectum, sigmoid, and descending colon appear quite natural. Beyond the splenic flexure, however, the organs tend to get quite thin and fragile and typically cannot tolerate the forces associated with endoscopy beyond the distal transverse colon. This model is ideal for flexible sigmoidoscopy, but its use for significant colonoscopy education is precluded.

Certainly, ex-vivo models have already established a role as an ideal replacement for the live model in advanced endoscopy training such as ERCP and upper GI endoscopy.[12] With the affordability of this model, their use for training in even basic endoscopic procedures may be warranted. Early work has validated the model's use in the education of basic endoscopy, suggesting that such a role should be advocated.[13,14] Ex-vivo models eventually may prove to be an ideal training tool for novices prior to beginning patient-based endoscopy. Other educational avenues for these models that have been explored in European training courses are their use in "team training."[15] This concept allows an endoscopist and assistants to learn new procedures or new therapeutic equipment together as a team. Each is taught his or her specific role for any new procedure. This approach allows a seamless integration of new procedures, techniques, or equipment into primary practice. Other obvious potential roles for a model that allows reproducible pathology are its use as a testing tool to assess procedural competence in trainees or possibly for purposes of credentialing or licensing physicians in endoscopic procedures. Due to the many obvious benefits afforded by ex-vivo models, it is likely that they will play an increasingly dominant role in endoscopic education in the near future.

Computer Simulators

Computer-based endoscopy simulators (CBES) are the newest entry into the simulator arena and have received a large amount of attention since their commercial introduction in the late 1990s. Computer simulators have evolved from the mechanical or static simulators such as rubber models of the GI tract. With the commercial introduction of the CBES, the traditional static models have quickly faded from the training environment.

There have been many attempts at computer simulation over the past 15 years.[16,17] The first such model was developed from the work of Williams and Gilles in 1987.[18] The results of this and subsequent early models had been promising, but it was not until the growth of computer technology and graphics during the mid 1990s that a reasonable reproduction of endoscopy was possible.[19] For decades, the aerospace fields have used flight simulation to teach skills and to practice unusual emergency procedures in a safe, controlled environment. Based on simulation successes experienced in the aviation sector, it is tempting to quickly accept an extension of this technology into the mainstream of medical education. The impact of these tools in endoscopic training, however, remains largely untested. Ideally, these tools will be shown to have the ability to teach procedural skills and simulate adverse events without discomfort or risk to patients.

The current commercially available CBESs are limited to two: the AccuTouch simulator (Immersion Medical, Gaithersburg, Maryland) and the GI Mentor II (Simbionix, Cleveland, Ohio). These models consist of a computer model into which a specialized scope is inserted. Simulated endoscopic views are depicted on a monitor resembling a traditional endoscopic display. Resistance to endoscope advancement is transmitted through the scope to the operator's hand to recreate the tactile sensation of navigating luminal angulations or loop formation. In addition, computer voice recordings can simulate different degrees of patient discomfort when internal sensors detect increased force or angulation of the scope. Both models also possess databases for recording trainees' performance on simulated cases. These data can be used to track training progress or for educational research.

The primary difference between these two commercial models is software diversity. The AccuTouch simulator (Fig. 7) currently provides groups of cases (modules) simulating diagnostic flexible sigmoidoscopy and colonoscopy as well as biopsy and polypectomy modules for each of these lower endoscopy procedures. Recently, an endoscopic retrograde cholangiopancreatography (ERCP) module has been developed and was due to be released in 2003. A bronchoscopy module is also available in this platform with added software and special bronchoscope attachment. Each GI module offers approximately six different cases of varying difficulty. In addition to these procedure modules, the simulator provides a multimedia tutorial explaining endoscopic theory and basic procedure techniques as well lessons in anatomy and mucosal pathology. The GI Mentor (Fig. 8), on the other hand, does not offer this useful multimedia training lesson but does offer a much greater variety of procedure software. Available modules offer 10–20 cases each for diagnostic upper GI endoscopy, therapeutic upper GI bleeding, ERCP, and endoscopic ultrasound (EUS) in addition to colonoscopy and flexible sigmoidoscopy.

Another fundamental difference is the mechanism that each manufacturer uses for the force-feedback control. This force-feedback control is the hardware that produces the simulated resistance and tactile sensations transmitted through the scope. The exact mechanics of how each system accomplishes this task is proprietary information. Although both models have been consumer-tested and shown to provide a favorable

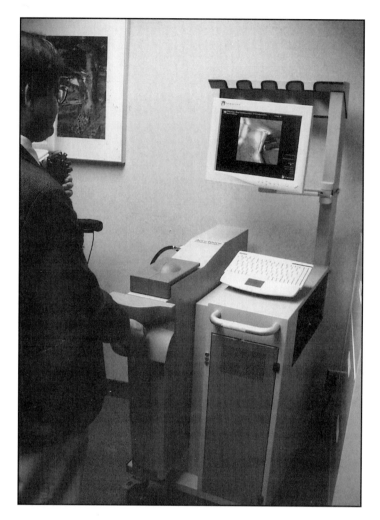

Figure 7. AccuTouch computer simulator (Immersion Medical). This compact, portable computer-based simulator is shown with a trainee performing a lower endoscopy.

degree of overall simulation realism, there are varied opinions between users of each model's force feedback simulation. Currently, direct head-to-head studies are planned to compare the perceived realism between the two models with respect to force feedback as well as many other aspects of simulation realism.

What is the current role for computer simulators in the training environment? Published data and personal work have demonstrated that both commercial models provide endoscopic simulation with a favorable degree of visual and tactile realism.[20,21] One major drawback described in the literature, however, is that endoscopy with either simulator is significantly easier than live endoscopy. [20,21] In these reports, the majority of participants found the simulated colonoscopies to be of excessively low technical difficulty. The fact that an endoscopic novice can complete a CBES colonoscopy on the

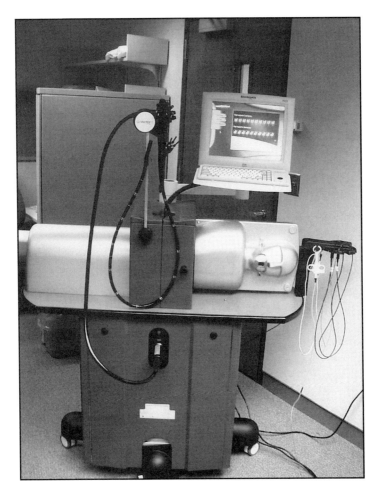

Figure 8. GI Mentor II (Simbionix). This larger computer simulator offers a wider array of endoscopic procedures.

first attempt attests to this procedural ease.[20] In addition, experienced endoscopists have been shown to routinely complete a CBES procedure in one-third of the time required for typical patient-based colonoscopy.[22] Although both models have cases that vary in complexity, the difference is not dramatic enough to have a significant impact on the overall ease of either simulator.

The result of this excessive ease with both simulators gives rise to questions of the ability of computer simulation to teach anything beyond the most basic aspects of endoscopy. This issue was raised in a head-to-head study comparing a computer ERCP simulator with live and ex-vivo porcine ERCP models. The computer's role in ERCP training was believed to be quite limited, and that authors concluded that these models should be relegated to the education of novices in basic endoscopic procedures only.[7] Advanced procedure simulation at this point should be restricted to either the live or ex-vivo animal models.[23]

Certainly, the role of the computer simulator in teaching advanced endoscopy techniques is severely limited, but can it truly be an effective tool for novices? The effectiveness of CBES in basic education has been the focus of numerous studies. Most reports have examined the endpoints of changes in simulator performance by novices. These studies have demonstrated that CBES training results in an improvement in *simulator* skills.[24,25] This outcome seems rather intuitive. The most important unanswered question, however, is whether CBES training can translate into improved *patient-based* endoscopy performance. This issue has only recently been addressed. One report failed to demonstrate any performance advantage in residents receiving CBES training in flexible sigmoidoscopy. The report did demonstrate, however, a statistically significant reduction in patient discomfort during flexible sigmoidoscopy performed by CBES-trained residents compared with procedures by residents who did not undergo simulator training.[26] This report is a significant first step in revealing the clinical benefits of computer training. In addition, pilot data demonstrate that first-year gastroenterology fellows who receive training on a CBES acquire significantly superior patient-based endoscopy skills than fellows who do not undergo the CBES training curriculum.[27] This pilot study demonstrated that during the first 30 colonoscopies performed by each fellow, CBES-trained fellows were able to complete procedures independently (i.e., reach the cecum) in roughly 20% more colonoscopies and to insert the scope 20% further than fellows who did not receive simulator training. If these data can be independently confirmed, CBES may have a strong role in basic endoscopic education for novice trainees. In addition, it has the potential to be used as a measuring tool to determine whether a trainee is ready to begin patient-based training. To accomplish this goal, however, certain basic performance criteria would need to be established first.

Though the current role for CBES may be limited to novice training, it does offer some major advantages over animal models. The computer models are available on demand with no preparation. This feature is certainly highly desirable for most trainees, for whom free time is at a premium. Computer simulators also do not require separate facilities or the dedication of separate endoscopic equipment, as do both live and ex-vivo animal models. In addition, space requirements are minimal for both computer models, which can easily fit in the average trainee's workspaces. Limited space requirements again add to the computer's easy accessibility. Each platform is equipped with wheels to allow mobility between workspaces. The obvious readiness and convenience of CBES make it an ideal training model in the setting of novice education.

Computer models, however, do require a significant financial investment. These simulators cost between $35,000 and $45,000 as an initial investment to purchase the platform, scope, and basic colonoscopy or flexible sigmoidoscopy software. Added modules cost approximately $5,000 each, and additional scopes for ERCP are approximately $10,000. The cost for a full system. including all scopes and software, can be as high as $70,000 to $80,000. These prices vary somewhat between companies and according to the desired software and modules. Although prices may appear prohibitive, the costs need to be put into perspective with the other available training models (Table 1). The costs associated with live porcine models average approximately $700 per animal simulation. This figure includes the costs of animal purchase, veterinary costs, anesthesia, endoscopic supplies (e.g., wires, biopsy cables), endoscope cleaning, and animal disposal. Using this figure, the use of 100 live animals would roughly equal the cost of a

Table 1.
Approximate Costs of Endoscopic Training Models

Expense	Ex-vivo	Live Porcine	Computer Simulation
Initial equipment investment	$3000-$3,500[1]	$0	$35,000-$80,000[2]
Additional costs per simulation set-up	$200[3]	$700[4]	$0

The initial equipment investment costs are one-time expenses and include the purchase of the individual simulator platform. Additional cost per simulation include all costs that recur with each simulation.
1. Cost of the model on which the harvested porcine organs are mounted.
2. Cost consists of $35,000-$45,000 for the base simulator plus $25,000-$35,000 for the optional ERCP and upper GI diagnostic and therapeutic modules.
3. Cost includes organ purchase ($110-$140), preparation, disposal, and scope cleaning (based on our own experience at the Mayo Clinic).
4. Cost includes animal purchase, technician time, preoperative preparation, anesthesia, vivarium costs (housing, feeding, support staff), and animal disposal (based on data provided by the Ethicon Institute, Cincinnati, Ohio).

fully equipped computer simulator. This $700 cost, however, does not include the initial investment of establishing dedicated animal facilities, animal support staff, dedicated endoscopes, and necessary equipment. The ex-vivo models, on the other hand, are somewhat more affordable with the combined costs of animal parts and reusable endoscopic supplies approximating $200 per simulation. At this rate, 250 simulation set-ups could be accomplished at the cost of a single computer simulator. Again this figure does not include the costs of establishing dedicated animal workspaces, simulator model, and separate endoscopic equipment such as endoscopes, light sources, monitors, and scope cleaners. Despite the large initial investment with computer simulator models, it is clear that the cost of any model requires a substantial investment by the training institution.

Despite the initial investment, it has been suggested that computer simulation can provide a significant reduction in the loss of revenue associated with education. It has been reported that training a single fellow in endoscopy can result in a loss of procedure revenue of $500,000 to $1,000,000 per 1000 procedures.[28] This loss is a result of doing one-third fewer procedures due to longer procedure times. With a simulation training curriculum (Table 2), the trainee is removed from the patient endoscopy area, thus allowing a staff endoscopist to operate independently and to perform far more procedures during the time that the student is training on a simulator. In a practice where a staff endoscopist can independently complete 15 procedures per day, a simulator curriculum that removes a trainee from the patient environment for only the first two days translates into the ability to recapture $15,000-$30,000 in lost revenue. Extrapolate this figure out for two days of training for each type of procedure (e.g., colonoscopy, EGD, ERCP), and an institution can quickly recover the initial investment in a computer simulator model.

Although the role of computer simulation may be relegated to basic training at present, the future of computer simulation is limitless. As software and hardware are advanced, this role may eventually expand to allow education for even experienced endoscopists in more advanced procedures. In addition, the computer attractively offers an objective means for measuring endoscopic performance. As the performance evaluation metrics of the computers are improved and validated, it will be possible to establish

◆ Table 2.
Types of Endoscopic Simulation Possible for Each Model

	Colonoscopy	Flexible Sigmoidoscopy	Esophago-duodenoscopy	Upper GI Bleeding[a]	Therapeutic Endoscopy[b]	RCP	US
Live porcine model		✓	✓	✓	✓	✓	✓
Erlanger Endo-Trainer	*	✓	✓	✓	✓	✓	
Compact EASIE			✓	✓	✓	✓	
Endo-X Trainer	*	✓	✓	✓	✓	✓	
AccuTouch	✓	✓			**	✓	
GI Mentor	✓	✓	✓	✓	✓	✓	✓

✓ = capable of performing simulation in that procedure.
[a]Bleeding therapy includes, but is not limited to, epinephrine injection, electro-coagulation, hemo-clip placement, variceal sclerotherapy, and glue injection.
[b]Therapeutic endoscopy includes, but is not limited to, argon plasma coagulation, laser coagulation, expandable metal stent placement, foreign body removal, percutaneous endoscopic gastrostomy (PEG) tube placement, and polypectomy.
*Porcine organs have limited ability to allow endoscopy beyond the extent of a typical flexible sigmoidoscopy.
**The Accutouch and GI mentor are capable of polypectomy only in this category.

working standards of "minimal performance criteria" in endoscopy. These criteria can be applied to the testing of trainees to document basic procedural competencies as outlined by the ASGE or to the credentialing of new staff by medical facilities.[29] Criteria could even conceivably be developed by medical licensing bodies to document competence in various endoscopic procedures. Clearly, current computer simulators are not ready for that kind of responsibility, but technology is certainly advancing in that direction.

Other Training Devices

The ScopeGuide by Olympus is a passive locator device that allows the monitoring of position and orientation of the entire length of the scope throughout live-patient endoscopy. The images are based on the production of magnetic fields by numerous wire coils either embedded down the length of a specialized endoscope or in a simple catheter that is inserted down an endoscope's working channel. The magnetic fields are picked up by a small dish antenna that is part of the main floor unit. Three-dimensional images of the scope are created and displayed in real time, similar to images obtained with fluoroscopy. Unlike fluoroscopy, however, this equipment poses no risks associated with x-ray use.

Clearly colonoscopy can be challenging even in the hands of an experienced endoscopist. The ScopeGuide has been shown to improve insertion times and to reduce the occurrence of loops during colonoscopy. This unique tool has a number of potential training applications as well. Beyond its obvious potential in teaching trainees endoscopic loop recognition and management, it also has the potential to teach endoscopic assistants how to recognize and apply effective external abdominal pressure.

Another tool that has been developed recently is an aid to train EUS endoscopists in fine-needle aspiration techniques.[30] This model is a "phantom" model made up of a modified barium enema bag filled with agar. Within the agar are suspended small foreign bodies such as diced carrots or peas. A linear array echoendoscope and a fine needle can then be used on this bag with the foreign bodies acting as the biopsy targets. Other pathology can also be suspended in the agar, such as saline-filled tips of surgical gloves, which simulate simple cysts.

Conclusion

The advances in all areas of endoscopic simulation have come about due to obvious financial and medicolegal pressures. These forces have demanded that all medical specialties address the cost and safety of procedural education as well as issues of documenting competency. Certainly, each of the models analyzed here has been shown to fulfill the role of safely accelerating endoscopic education. The experience level of the trainee and specific training goals dictate which model is the most appropriate. None of these models, however, have yet been validated for use in the testing of competency. The ultimate goal is the development of an affordable model that is not only a versatile training tool for all levels of experience but also a valid measuring tool. As we advance toward that goal, it is clear that simulators will continue to play an increasingly dominant role in endoscopic education.

References

1. William CB: Endoscopy teaching: Time to get serious. Gastrointest Endosc 1998;47:429–430.
2. Adamsen S: Simulators and gastrointestinal endoscopy training. Endoscopy 2000;32:895–897.
3. Noar MD: An established porcine model for animate training in diagnostic and therapeutic ERCP. Endoscopy 1995;27:77–80.
4. Van Os EC, Petersen BT, Batts KP: Spiral Nitinol biliary stents in a porcine model: Evaluation of the potential for use in benign strictures. Endoscopy 1999;31:253–259.
5. Vorwerk D, Guenther RW, Kuepper W, Kissinger G: Thermal laser-induced stenosis of the common bile duct. An alternative model for experimental research. Invest Radiol 1989;24:758–761.
6. Vorwerk D, Guenther RW, Kuepper W, Kissinger G: Thermal laser-induced stenosis of the common bile duct. An alternative model for experimental research. Invest Radiol 1989;24:758–761.
7. Sedlack RE, Petersen B, Bimoeller K, Kolars JC: A direct comparison of ERCP teaching models. Gastrointest Endosc 2003;57:886–890.
8. ASGE Technology Assessment Committee: New technology status evaluations: Endoscopy simulators. Gastointest Endosc 2000;51:790–792.
9. Parasher VK, Toomey P, Clifton V, Merryman K: Simulated sphincterotomy in a pig model. Gastrointest Endosc 1995;41:240–242.
10. Neumann M, Hochberger J, Felzmann T, Ell C, Hohenberger W: The Erlangen Endo-Trainer. Part 1. Endosc 2001;33:887–890.
11. Parasher VK, Toomey P, Clifton V, Merryman K: Simulated sphincterotomy in a pig model. Gastrointest Endosc 1995;41:240–242.
12. Neumann M, Mayer G, Felzmann T, et al: The Erlangen Endo-Trainer: Life-like simulation for diagnostic and interventional endoscopic retrograde cholangiography. Endoscopy 2000;32:906–910.
13. Neumann M, Siebert T, Rausch J, et al: Scorecard endoscopy: A pilot study to assess basic skills in trainees for upper gastrointestinal endoscopy. Langenbecks Arch Surg 2003;387:386–391.

14. Hochberger J, Neumann M, Maiss J, et al: EASIE- Erlangen Active Simulator for Interventional Endoscopy: A new bio-simulation model. First experience gained in training workshops [abstract]. Gastrointest Endosc 1998;47:AB116.
15. Hochberger J, Maiss J, Magdeburg B, et al: Training simulators and education in gastrointestinal endoscopy: current status and perspectives in 2001. Endoscopy 2001;33:541–549.
16. Williams CB, Baillie J, Gillies DF, et al: Teaching gastrointestinal endoscopy by computer simulation: a prototype for colonoscopy and ERCP. Gastrointest Endosc 1990;36:49.
17. Gerson LB, Van Dam J: The future of simulators in GI endoscopy: An unlikely possibility or a virtual reality? Gastrointest Endosc 2002;55:608–611.
18. Noar MD, Soehendra N: Endoscopy simulation training devices. Endoscopy 1992;24:159–166.
19. Bar-Meir S: Endoscopy simulators: The state of the art, 2000. Gastrointest Endosc 2000;52:701–703.
20. Sedlack RE, Kolars JC: Validation of computer-based endoscopy simulators in training. Gastrointest Endosc 2003;57:214–218.
21. Aabakken L, Adamsen S, Kruse A: Performance of a colonoscopy simulator: Experience from a hands-on endoscopy course, Endoscopy 2000;32:911- 913.
22. Sedlack RE, Kolars JC: Development of a colonoscopy curriculum and performance based assessment criteria on a computer-based endoscopy simulator. Acad Med 2002;77:750–751.
23. Hochberger J, Maiss J, Hahn EG: The use of simulators for training in GI endoscopy. Endoscopy 2002;34:721–726.
24. Ferlitsch A, Glauninger P, Gupper A, et al: Evaluation of a virtual endoscopy simulator for training in gastrointestinal endoscopy. Endoscopy 2002;34:698–702.
25. Tuggy ML: Virtual reality flexible sigmoidoscopy simulator training: Impact on resident performance. J Am Board Fam Pract 1998;11:426–433.
26. Sedlack RE, Alexander J: Computer simulator training enhances patient comfort during endoscopy. Clin Gastroenterol Hepatol 2004;2:348–351.
27. Sedlack RE, Kolars JC: Computer simulator training enhances the competency of GI fellows at colonoscopy: Results of a pilot study. Am J Gastroenterol 2004;99:33–37.
28. McCashland T, Brand R, Lyden E, de Garmo F: The time and financial impact of training fellows in endoscopy. Am J Gastroenterol 2000;95:3129–3132.
29. ASGE Standard of Training Committees: Principles of training gastrointestinal endoscopy. Gastrointest Endosc 1999;49:845–850.
30. Sorbi D, Vazques-Sequeiros E, Wiersema MJ: A simple phantom for learning EUS-guided FNA. Gastrointest Endosc 2003;57:580–583.

Chapter 23

BRONCHOSCOPY SIMULATOR ASSESSMENT

David Ost, MD, FACP

Surveys of fellows and attending physicians demonstrate significant heterogeneity in bronchoscopy experience during training and subsequently during practice.[1–3] Approximately one-fourth of pulmonary fellows perform fewer than 50 bronchoscopies per year.[1] In addition, the number of bronchoscopic exams performed in the United States is decreasing, and this trend can be expected to continue in the future.[4] The lack of adequate exposure during training can lead to underutilization of effective techniques, such as transbronchial needle aspiration (TBNA).[5] This in turn can lead to deficiencies in quality of care.

Concurrent with the decreasing number of standard bronchoscopies is ongoing development of new technologies. Examples include procedures such as bronchial stent placement, laser bronchoscopy, cryotherapy, and electrocautery, to name only a few. These new procedures require physicians to develop methods for continuous education and skill acquisition. Thus, there is a need for improving training and skill acquisition for attending physicians as well as for physicians in training.

Given these constraints, there is an increased need to develop better ways to teach bronchoscopy and assess bronchoscopy skill.[2] Bronchoscopy requires a high degree of manual dexterity and procedural skill as well as an understanding of the anatomy and pathophysiology of the lung. The combination of procedural/physical skills with cognitive skills lends itself well to the application of simulation technology.

The use of simulation technology, although widely accepted in other fields, is only now gaining wider credence in medicine. War games for military use, simulations of nuclear power plants, and management games for executives are routinely used.[6–11] Flight simulators have been among the most widely used and have been shown to improve pilot skills.[12,13] In the medical field, laparoscopic simulators, cardiology patient simulators, and anesthesia simulators are being introduced.[14–23]

Within the field of pulmonary medicine, the application of simulator technology to bronchoscopy offers similar promise. The initial impression of pulmonary fellows suggests that bronchoscopy simulation may prove to be a useful adjunct to traditional training methods.[1,24,25] Bronchoscopy, as the primary procedure performed by pulmonologists, is fundamental to the discipline of pulmonary medicine. Because of its importance to patient care, and because more rigorous standards are being proposed for physician credentialing in general, more attention is being focused on how we teach bronchoscopy and how we can measure quality.[26–29] Potential benefits and applications of simulation include improving health care provider training, performance, and credentialing.

This section focuses on bronchoscopy simulation as one example of medical simulation in pulmonary medicine. Although the cognitive elements are probably more important to doing bronchoscopy, the advantages of simulation technology relate to its ability to teach mechanical and motor skills. This discussion, therefore, is limited to methods of simulation that attempt to teach the mechanical and motor skills necessary for the mastery of bronchoscopy. The initial focus is on how simulator training may be used for different groups and their various training needs. This discussion serves to clarify the objectives that simulators should achieve. Quality performance in real life is determined by the skills that need to be mastered, ideally through bronchoscopy simulation training. A related issue, how to quantify and measure these skills in real life, is also addressed. Finally, to assess the quality of bronchoscopy simulators themselves, validation of simulator training is discussed.

Potential Applications of Bronchoscopy Simulation

Potential applications of simulator technology include training of pulmonary fellows, nonpulmonary physicians, and other health care professionals. It may also be useful for training attending physicians in new procedures, as a method of preparing for complications and rare emergencies, and as a means of physician credentialing.

Training Pulmonary Fellows

Bronchoscopy simulation has the potential to aid in the medical education of pulmonary and anesthesiology residents and fellows.[24,25] Our current paradigm of teaching bronchoscopy has been a replication of the surgical model of teaching, using a "see one, do one, teach one" approach. This approach progresses from cognitive aspects of bronchoscopy to time-limited supervised bronchoscopy, usually in low-risk patients first. More complex procedures in higher-risk patients are added later as skills improve.[30] Other methods, including mechanical and animal models as well as instructional videos, have been used with limited success to supplement this approach.[31-33] Mechanical models are limited by their artificial appearance and the inability to incorporate the appearance of normal and abnormal pathology into the models. Costs, ethical concerns, and anatomic differences between species limit the utility of animal models.[30,34]

The existing system tries to maximize patient comfort, safety, and satisfaction, but there are trade-offs in terms of meeting educational needs. Trainees often have too little exposure to bronchoscopy, and as patients increasingly demand that attending physicians perform the procedures, education and training suffer. Ironically, in the long term, patients suffer most in this arrangement, because future generations of physicians will not have the requisite experience.

Potentially, bronchoscopy simulation can aid by training pulmonary fellows prior to first patient contact. This approach would minimize using patients for practicing basic skills by ensuring that trainees have some degree of skill and knowledge before their first attempt.[25] Bronchoscopy simulation should be able to provide trainees with the fundamental skills necessary to perform a basic bronchoscopy. Ideally the simulator would produce quantitative feedback to trainees about their performance. The simulator also needs to provide data to the educator about whether or not the individual trainee is ready to progress to the next step, namely actual patient care. Presumably the simulator would be integrated into the existing didactic lecture and training programs. The advantage of simulation technology in this setting is that it provides familiarity with the instrument and allows unlimited dedicated practice time. Given the wide variation in natural aptitude between trainees, this arrangement ensures that some basic level of proficiency is achieved prior to first patient contact. It also allows individualization of practice and teaching methods based on aptitude and performance.

Nonpulmonary Physicians and Other Health Care Professionals

The existing system does not allow medical residents to learn by using a hands-on approach. Although residents can observe procedures, they can never do them. This consideration is important because general internists make the initial decision as to whether a pulmonologist should be consulted. Presumably, if physicians are more familiar with a procedure, they can make more appropriate use of it. For medical residents, internists, and oncologists, simulation may help to clarify what bronchoscopy can and cannot do by using a hands-on approach. This approach may help improve the utilization of appropriate bronchoscopic procedures, such as TBNA for lung cancer staging.[5] Thus, consumers of pulmonary services may be able to better decide when a bronchoscopic exam is indicated.

For other health care providers, such as bronchoscopy nurses, respiratory therapists, and intensive care personnel, an accurate simulation may be useful in teaching airway anatomy as well as allow a better appreciation of what is involved in a bronchoscopic exam. The performance of bronchoscopy support personnel and hence team performance may be improved because simulation allows additional practice time and reinforcement. Simulation would be especially helpful in areas such as the intensive care unit, where bronchoscopy, although not an everyday procedure, is frequently required.

New Procedure Training

The ongoing development of new technologies and procedures requires physicians to develop new skills. New developments in bronchoscopy include the placement of bronchial stents and endobronchial ultrasound. Some of these methods are not really "new" but are difficult to learn because most training programs do not have access to them or perform them infrequently. Previous studies have demonstrated that many physicians lack a method to receive formal training in new procedures and techniques, often learning them on their own.[2] The development of training methods that allow physicians to acquire new skills while minimizing patient risk during the learning process is important.

Rare Procedure Maintenance

Simulators may also play an important role in training and preparing for more complex and less common procedures. Skill development and maintenance are difficult in centers where certain procedures are infrequently performed. Ideally all centers would have minimum baseline volume requirements for credentialing physicians to guarantee sufficient experience to maintain skill levels. However, outside referral centers, this ideal may not always be feasible. Complex skill simulation, such as TBNA and interventional pulmonary procedures, can be used to supplement the experience of bronchoscopy teams in these areas.

Rare Complications Preparation

Another area of importance is case management skills. Complications programmed into the simulation train physicians and their team to respond in a timely and appropriate manner. Importantly, it is the performance of the entire team that matters; therefore, training of other health care personnel is an important element in achieving this objective. The most significant bronchoscopy complication, severe pulmonary hemorrhage, is rare, and its rarity limits the ability of the bronchoscopy team to practice and develop expertise. Simulation technology offers the opportunity to prepare for rare but serious complications and gives unlimited practice time. This situation is analogous to using flight simulators to practice the response to unexpected disasters, such as the loss of an engine or power failure in mid air.

Credentialing

Using traditional training methods, it is not clear how best to assess competency and what constitutes an appropriate minimum level of bronchoscopy training. Even the question of how many procedures should be required to complete training is not well studied, with recommendations ranging from 25 to 100.[26,30,35-40] Currently the American Board of Internal Medicine does not specify a minimum number of procedures that need to be done to learn a skill or maintain competence.[1,41] However, hospital credentialing committees want standards that can be readily applied in determining privileges, and the requirement of a minimum number of procedures is a frequently used criterion.[2,3] Evidence-based medicine (EBM) has been used to establish threshold numbers of procedures needed to achieve competence in other fields, such as gastroenterology.[42,43] EBM has led some investigators to recommend that threshold levels be applied for bronchoscopy training as well.[3,26] Unfortunately, there are few data about how to assess clinical competence.[30,35,36]

Simulation has the potential to change the existing paradigm for assessing competence in bronchoscopy.[24] It may provide educators with a more quantifiable means of measuring trainee performance, allowing them to track the progress of trainees in terms of their bronchoscopic skill and readiness to perform independently.[44] Considering that the number of bronchoscopic exams performed in the United States is decreasing, a quantifiable means of measuring performance is important, because it provides an inter-institutional standard of quality rather than a simple measurement of volume.[4] Similarly, it also allows a more objective measurement of performance for credentialing of attending physicians.

What Defines Quality Performance?

Like all simulators, bronchoscopy simulators provide feedback to the participant about decisions, actions, and skills in specific case situations. For simulation purposes, skills may be defined as "actions (and reactions) which an individual performs to achieve a goal."[45] Levels of skill vary along a continuum from none to mastery. Therefore, when testing or teaching a skill, the measures of competence must be based on the training level. The actual skills measured should also discriminate among those with different levels of expertise.

One of the main problems in bronchoscopy training and research is that the set of relevant skills is difficult to define and measure. Similarly, determining the relative importance among skill subsets is highly subjective. For example, how do you balance being fast vs. being accurate in terms of a measurement system for bronchoscopy quality? Similarly, how can we measure and appropriately weight patient comfort, adequate preparation, and theoretical knowledge relative to other performance aspects of bronchoscopy? Although numeric scales have been used to rate some aspects of bronchoscopy training, no validated or standardized instruments are available in this area.

However, given the limited evidence, we can still construct a theoretical framework for assessing bronchoscopy quality. In particular, assessment of bronchoscopy quality needs to take into consideration the dimensions of patient comfort and satisfaction, safety, speed, accuracy, and diagnostic yield.

Patient Comfort and Satisfaction

Patient comfort is related to the adequacy of sedation, properly addressing preexisting patient fears and expectations, providing quality information prior to the procedure, and minimizing the pain of scope insertion.[46–49] In one study of 481 patients, 80% of patients rated physicians as very good or excellent.[47] However, patients were least satisfied with the information that they were provided about bronchoscopy, waiting time before and after bronchoscopy, and the bronchoscopy environment. Factors in the process of care that were identified as potential areas for improvement included providing better information and optimizing the experience of bronchoscope insertion. Indeed, not being bothered by scope insertion was the best predictor of willingness to return for repeat bronchoscopy (Table 1).

Measurement of bronchoscopy quality, viewed from the perspective of patient satisfaction, needs to measure how well the bronchoscope is inserted. Bronchoscopy simulators, therefore, need to provide some corresponding measure of insertion quality to capture this key variable. Similarly, nonmechanical aspects of quality, such as providing quality information, need to be emphasized during training. Providing consistent information to patients may be more a question of process engineering rather than manual dexterity or adequacy of knowledge. These latter aspects of care probably are not as amenable to robotic simulation technology. Therefore, other educational tools should be used to address these issues.

Safety

Patient safety in bronchoscopy primarily relates to the main risks associated with the procedure, including risks from conscious sedation, local anesthetics (toxicity), pulmonary

Table 1.
Factors Determining Patient Satisfaction

Variables	Willingness to have Repeat Bronchoscopy (OR; 95% CI)
Not being bothered by scope insertion	2.0 (95% CI 1.2–3.3)
Better health status	1.4 (95% CI 1.1–1.7)
Better rating of information quality	1.2 (95% CI 1.0–1.3)
Better rating of physician quality	1.1 (95% CI 1.0–1.2)

hemorrhage, and pneumothorax. Thus, any simulator of bronchoscopy needs to provide a corresponding measure of how well each of these risks is minimized. Recognizing that even with optimal performance these complications will occur, simulators also need to be able to measure how well the physician and bronchoscopy team respond to these complications when they do occur. Response to complications constitutes a separate category of quality measurement.

For local anesthetic toxicity, standard guidelines can be used to identify how progressively higher doses of local anesthetics relate to the level of risk.[37] The critical element for simulation is the need to be able to recreate the extrapulmonary symptoms in a realistic manner so that trainees can be made aware and receives useful feedback on their performance. Although most simulators focus on careful simulation of the airway itself, extrapulmonary features are of importance if simulations of complications are to be included.

Similar principles apply to pneumothorax. The symptoms of bronchoscopy-related pneumothorax vary widely, from completely asymptomatic to tension pneumothorax with hypotension and shock. The simulator, therefore, needs to convey this information in a format that mimics actual conditions and allows trainees to get feedback about their decisions, actions, and skills. Thus, vital sign monitoring and elements of the physical exam, such as absence of breath sounds, also need to be modeled.

Pulmonary hemorrhage, although a rare complication, needs to be considered as well. Although pulmonary hemorrhage is much less common than pneumothorax, over 90% of bronchoscopy-related deaths are due to pulmonary hemorrhage. Thus, rapid recognition and an appropriate response are critical for training modules. Simulators need to initially mimic pulmonary hemorrhage and then measure the speed and appropriateness of the response. Appropriate real-life responses will vary with the situation, but certain key principles usually apply. These principles include rapid recognition, tamponade of the bleeding site, access to rapid intubation, and calling for back-up. Although a virtual reality simulator cannot measure all of these factors, some, such as tamponade of the bleeding site, activation of emergency protocols, and intubation, are well suited to simulation technology.

Speed

Rapid completion of all necessary procedures is a practical necessity in the current medical environment. The speed of bronchoscopy is, therefore, a valid measure of one aspect of bronchoscopy quality. To make legitimate comparisons, measurements of speed need to take into account the type of procedure, the number of biopsies, and the amount of time spent in preparation as compared to actual performance of bronchoscopy.

Accuracy

Although speed is important, accuracy is probably more important. Especially for trainees, correct identification of the bronchial segments can be challenging. The standard method of training pulmonary fellows has been to have them identify each bronchoscopic segment as it is visualized, with immediate feedback provided by the instructor. Simulators need to be able to give similar feedback.

Diagnostic Yield

Once the fundamentals are established and basic proficiency is obtained, diagnostic yield is among the most important outcomes to assess. However, it is also the most difficult outcome to measure. Diagnostic yield is highly dependent on case selection and reference standards. The final "correct" diagnosis is often not immediately available at the time of bronchoscopy. The current limitations of the medical record system make compiling such data difficult. For example, if a bronchoscopy to sample mediastinal lymph nodes is negative for evidence of malignancy, is this a false-negative result? Often the answer will not be available for weeks, and when it does become available, the data will not be in a format that is linked to the bronchoscopy data. This situation precludes compilation of meaningful statistical measures of diagnostic yield and quality of performance. The inability to correlate data limits the ability of physicians to measure their own performance and thereby improve the quality of performance in a systematic way.

Simulators need to be able to assess the adequacy and quality of biopsy procedures, such as transbronchial needle aspiration. In this way, a trainee can perform repeated simulations in rapid succession for different types of biopsies and benefit from immediate corrective feedback. Ideally, performance of adequate biopsies on the simulator will improve the probability of obtaining adequate biopsy samples from patients while minimizing complications.

Validation and Assessment of Simulators

The goal of training on the simulator is to improve the probability of quality performance as determined by the outcomes described above. However, there is a paucity of data about bronchoscopy simulation and training. In approaching the problem of simulator validation, it is possible to learn from the methodology of simulator development in engineering fields. In particular, the technical aspects of simulator development for flight simulation may serve as a useful framework. Evaluation of flight simulators demonstrated substantial positive transfer of skills learned on the simulator to the actual task.[12] However, in validating the design and development of flight simulators, it was important first to consider transfer in the other direction. Of note, transfer of skill from simulation to reality is not always equal to transfer of skill from reality to simulation. Although there are no precise quantitative measurements of performance in flight simulators, it has been suggested that, despite a 95% transfer of skills from simulators to aircraft, there is only 5% transfer of skill from aircraft to simulators.[12]

Applying this conceptual framework to bronchoscopy, the simulator validation and assessment process can be divided into two questions. First, does actual bronchoscopy expertise translate into expertise on the simulator? Presumably, if the simulation mimics reality, there will be a high degree of skill transfer. Second, does training on the simulator translate into more rapid acquisition of expertise during actual bronchoscopy?

Skill Transfer from Real Life to Simulation

For design and development of simulators, it is important to try to obtain objective, quantitative measures of skill performance and transfer as well as subjective evaluations. The nature of the measures reflects the purpose of the simulator and the relevant skills that are being taught.[8] Skill transfer can be evaluated in a variety of ways, including both qualitative and quantitative measures.[25]

To demonstrate skill transfer for bronchoscopy, it is necessary to demonstrate that people skilled in bronchoscopy outperform less skilled people when both use the simulator. "Outperform" in this case means both superior mastery of the knowledge base (facts and theory) and superior mechanical skill. Although assessment of facts and theory is standard for medical education, assessment of physical skills is not standardized. However, mechanical/physical skills can still be measured using quantitative methods. Indeed, measurement of mechanical skills in other disciplines is routine. Skills can be ranked in competitive sports based on tournament results and rankings. Differences between novice and champion athletes in measurable skills relevant to the activity are highly reproducible. This difference would be expected in other domains of expertise, such as medicine.[45] A similar methodology can be applied to bronchoscopy training.

Using this approach, the first step in simulator development and testing is to assess how well the simulator distinguishes between novices and experts. A simulator's ability to distinguish novices from experts reflects skill transfer from reality to the simulation. For validation of a simulator, this process helps to address the initial issue of how well the simulator mimics reality.

Most studies of bronchoscopy simulation have not measured this type of skill transfer systematically. However, although rigorous data for older simulators are limited, some preliminary data suggest that skill transfer from reality to modern simulators is indeed very good.[44,50] In one multicenter trial, bronchoscopy simulators were able to distinguish among novice, intermediate, and expert physicians[44] (Figs. 1 and 2). There were clear differences in terms of performance on the simulator between groups when evaluated for speed, number of wall collisions, suction time, and time in red-out (a measure of being too close to the bronchial wall). These observations suggest that skill transfer from actual bronchoscopy to the simulation is accurate and that performance on the simulator, as measured by the above criteria, would be an effective way to assess skill acquisition during bronchoscopy training.

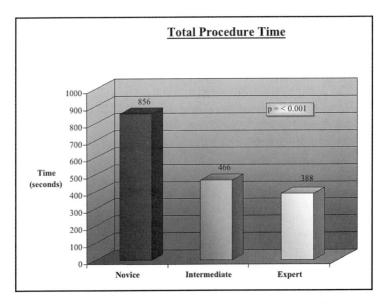

Figure 1. Total procedure time on a bronchoscopy simulator for novice, intermediate, and expert bronchoscopists.

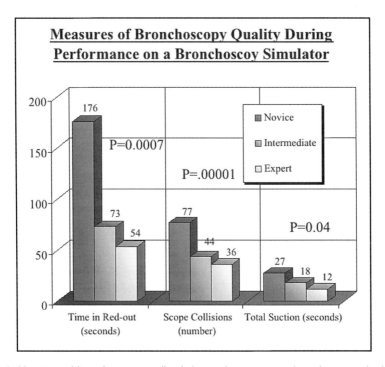

Figure 2. Measures of bronchoscopy quality during performance on a bronchoscopy simulator for novice, intermediate, and expert bronchoscopists.

In addition, when self-study simulation training was integrated into a standard curriculum, the learning curve for novice physicians indicated that skill acquisition using the simulator was practical and actually saved instructional time. There was a demonstrable learning curve for each of the simulated skills, with variation in the rate of skill acquisition depending on the skill (Figs. 3–5). After 20 practice sessions with the simulator there was a significant difference between the self-study group and other novices with respect to procedure time, collisions, and percent of segments entered (Table 2). In addition, there was no significant difference between the self-study group and intermediate-level bronchoscopists with respect to these variables. However, the small sample size limits the statistical power of the analysis, since it is quite possible that beta error occurred. The power of the study to detect a difference between groups at a significance level of 0.05 ranged from 5% to 45% for the variables studied. Thus, although we can say that after 20 sessions the self-study group was superior to novices, we cannot say with confidence, given the sample size, that the self-study group performed as well as intermediates or experts on the simulator because of the high probability of beta error.[44]

Even though the self-study group probably was not the equal of intermediates after 20 practice sessions, a clear learning curve was demonstrated with the simulator (Figs. 3–5). In comparing the average performance of the simulator-trained group in their first five attempts (1–5) vs. subsequent attempts, there was a statistically significant improvement in terms of procedure time, number of collisions, percent of segments entered, and time

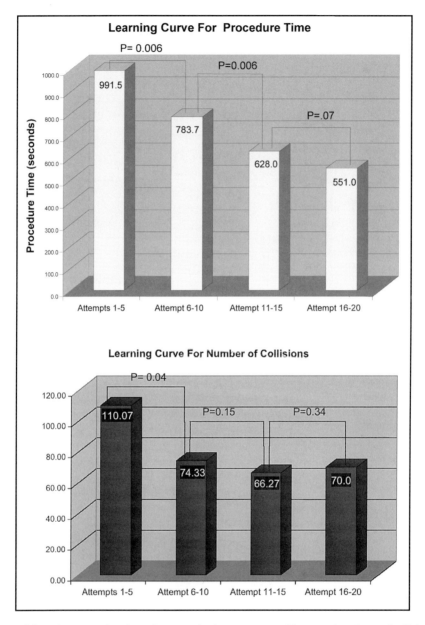

Figure 3. Learning curves for a bronchoscopy simulator as assessed by procedure time and collisions.

in red-out. Linear regression analysis also indicated a significant ($p < 0.0001$) learning effect in terms of total procedure time and bronchoscopy score (Fig. 4).

The type of simulator used in this study was unique compared with older mechanical models used for training.[44,50] The simulator consisted of a proxy flexible bronchoscope, a robotic interface device, and a computer with simulation software and monitor. As shown in Figure 6, the user would insert the proxy bronchoscope into the robotic

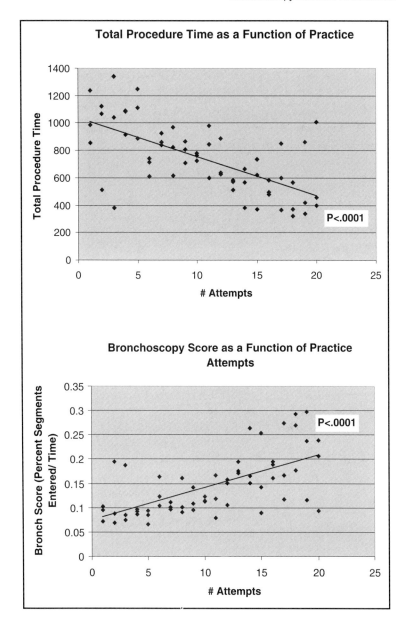

Figure 4. Linear regression analysis of total procedure time and simulation practice. Bronchoscopy score is an aggregate measure of accuracy (percent of segments entered) divided by the amount of time necessary. Therefore, higher numbers reflect improved performance quality.

interface device. The proximal end of the interface was shaped like a human face with a port to insert the bronchoscope through one of the nasal passages. The proxy bronchoscope was supposed to mimic the feel of an actual bronchoscope. The interface device tracked the motions of the bronchoscope and reproduced the forces felt during actual bronchoscopy. The proxy bronchoscope tracked the manipulations of the tip control

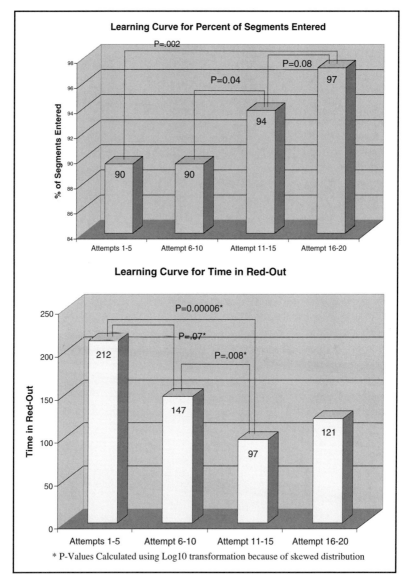

Figure 5. Learning curves for a bronchoscopy simulator as assessed by percentage of segments entered and time in red-out

lever, suction button, and video buttons. In addition, instruments are tracked as they are manipulated in the working channel, allowing biopsies and other diagnostic and therapeutic procedures to be performed on the simulator.

The monitor displays computer-generated images of the airway as the user navigates through the virtual anatomy (Fig. 7). These images change based on the user's actions (as determined by information received from the proxy bronchoscope). The user also feels changes in actual resistance based on the computer's response to user actions. Im-

Table 2.
Comparison of Performance Between Simulator-trained Fellows and Other Bronchoscopists*

Outcome Measure	Bronchoscopy Skill Level			Self-trained with Simulator (n = 3)	p-Value for Simulator-trained Group vs. Other Groups
	Novices (n = 11)	Intermediates (n = 8)	Experts (n = 9)		
Total time (sec)	856 (238)	466 (203)	388 (122)	613 (128)	Novices p 5 0.02 Intermediates p 5 0.12 Experts p 5 0.0008
Time in red-out $\log_{10}$(sec)†	2.083 (0.379)	1.730 (0.396)	1.608 (0.371)	2.051 (.267)	Novices p 5 0.85 Intermediates p 5 0.08 Experts p 5 0.01
Scope collisions	76.9 (30.1)	43.6 (29.1)	36.1 (14.9)	39 (19)	Novices p 5 0.007 Intermediates p 5 0.7 Experts p 5 0.7
Segments entered (%)	75.3 (17.2)	89.9 (11.0)	89.7 (14.9)	98 (3)	Novices p 5 0.004 Intermediates p 5 0.09 Experts p 5 0.04
Suction time (sec)	27.5 (26.9)	18.0 (13.1)	11.7 (7.8)	NA	NA
Lidocaine usage (ml)	12.5 (5.0)	10.2 (2.8)	11.1 (5.4)	NA	NA

NA = not available.
*Values expressed as mean (Standard Deviation) unless otherwise indicated.
†Distribution was skewed, so $\log_{10}$ sec was necessary to compute p-value.

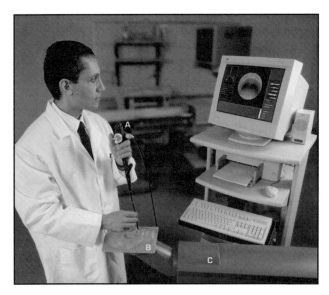

Figure 6. The flexible bronchoscopy simulator (Immersion Medical Systems). A, Proxy FB. B, Mannequin face with port for scope insertion. C, Interface device.

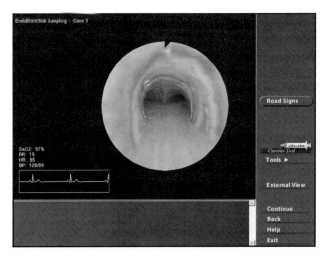

Figure 7. Bronchoscopic view of simulated airway

ages that result from manipulations of the proxy bronchoscope as it "moves" through the virtual patient are displayed for the user in a form similar to actual bronchoscopy.

In addition to being anatomically correct, the virtual patient also behaves in a physiologically realistic manner. The patient breathes, coughs, bleeds, and exhibits changes in vital signs. Proper use of suction allows for a thorough examination of the airway without wall collisions or red-out. Appropriate use of local anesthesia reduces cough and thus wall collisions. Excessive use of local anesthetics results in toxicity, causing the patient to have a seizure or develop a cardiac arrhythmia. Importantly, this information is conveyed as feedback to the user in a realistic manner. For example, the cardiac rhythm strip is visible to users so that they see complications in a manner analogous to actual bronchoscopy rather than getting feedback in a pure textual format.

The critical element is the integration of robotics (to give mechanical force feedback) with computer-generated virtual reality. The virtual reality is generated from a three-dimensional computer-generated model of the airway constructed from the National Library of Medicine's Visible Human male dataset.[51] This dataset consists of digital axial anatomical images at 1.0-mm intervals with associated CT and MRI images. Texture maps based on videotapes of actual bronchoscopic images are then added to give the virtual airway a realistic look. Adjusting the base case virtual airway allows common anatomic variations to be generated, so that a variety of different "patients" can be created. Pathology can be added subsequently.

The simulation software also records all actions of the user and stores this information in a database. Information that is collected and displayed includes time of procedure, time that the bronchoscope is in red-out, number of times that the bronchoscope tip collides with airway walls, percentage of bronchial segments entered, and amount of local anesthetic used. User-specific performance can be tracked so that progress over time can be measured.

Assessing Skill Transfer from Simulation to Real Life

When simulators are used to train students, the ultimate criterion is whether the device allows the student to master the task in less time than would have been required without the simulator (skill transfer from simulator to reality). However, what exactly defines "mastery" of the task of bronchoscopy? As noted above, standardized measures of bronchoscopy quality are lacking and data acquisition is often difficult. Traditionally, qualitative assessment of a student by an accepted expert was used as a measure for assessing trainee progress. Most of the evidence regarding the effectiveness of bronchoscopy simulators has been qualitative in nature, reflecting the traditional method of training and assessment.[23,32–35,43,52–57]

However, with the use of modern simulators, preliminary data indicate that adding combined robotic and virtual reality simulation to a standard curriculum of training improves trainee performance and leads to more rapid skill mastery. In a single-center study of pulmonary fellows, fellows trained with the simulator were able to master basic bronchoscopy skills more rapidly than those trained with traditional methods alone[44] (Table 3). In particular, simulator training improved performance on actual patients in terms of procedure time (speed), number of segments correctly identified (accuracy), number of segments correctly identified per unit time (accuracy/speed), coughing (patient comfort), and the qualitative judgment of bronchoscopy nurse observers.

Other methods of training have included virtual reality simulations combined with didactic testing. In a sense, these are also "simulators," and in such cases simulation technology does improve learning. However, compared with standard didactic methods, the main benefit of simulation technology is its ability to allow trainees to acquire sufficient motor skills prior to first patient contact.

Conclusion

The mastery of procedural skills is critical to many areas of medicine. Bronchoscopy, as a common subspecialty requirement with wide heterogeneity in terms of clinician

Table 3.
Performance of Pulmonary Fellows During Real-life Bronchoscopy

	Control Group*	SIM Group*	p-Value
Total time (sec)	1168 ± 48	815 ± 56	0.001
Number of segments entered (1–18)	12.8 ± 3.5	17.3 + 1.2	0.1
Number of segments correctly identified (1–18)	9.5 ± 6.6	17.3 ± 1.2	0.1
Quality score (% correctly identified/sec)	0.046 ± 0.034	0.119 ± 0.015	0.03
Bronch nurse score (1–10)	3.7 ± 2.5	7.7 ± 0.3	0.05
Lidocaine used (ml)	12.7 ± 4.0	11.7 + 4.5	0.79
Coughing episodes	9.8 ± 1.9	4.3 ± 3.2	0.06
Midazolam used (mg)	2.3 ± 0.5	1.9 ± 0.1	0.25
Meperidine used (mg)	29.2 ± 7.2	45.8 ± 7.2	0.05

*Values are expressed as mean (standard deviation) unless otherwise specified.
Control group: pulmonary fellows trained with conventional methods. SIM group: simulator-trained pulmonary fellows.

experience and mastery, can serve as a useful prototype of how simulation technology can be assessed, validated, and applied in medicine. Previous methods that have been demonstrated to be of benefit in teaching bronchoscopy include mechanical models, instructional videos, and specialized didactic teaching.[25,31–35] Previous models were limited by artificial appearance, the inability to incorporate normal variants into the model, and the inability to have different types of abnormal pathology. The routine use of animal subjects has prohibitive financial costs as well as associated ethical concerns. It is also limited by anatomic differences between species.

The combination of robotic and virtual reality simulation holds promise in addressing many of these problems. Combined robotic/virtual reality simulations can address the problem of acquiring mechanical skills for a wide variety of disciplines. Importantly, this type of mechanical simulation needs to be integrated with concurrent didactic teaching, so that a complete "skill set" is given to the trainee. For bronchoscopy, this skill set would include initial didactic teaching about basic anatomy, indications, risks, complications, and pathology. Simulation technology helps the student to integrate the requisite knowledge of airway anatomy, physiology, and pharmacology while developing the necessary motor skills required for successful bronchoscopy performance. In the future, more complex skills, such as endobronchial biopsy or transbronchial needle aspiration, need to be developed as well. Each of these additions to simulation technology must address the fundamentals of simulator development, assessment, and validation. Quantification of skill transfer, both from reality to the simulator and from simulator to reality, needs to be measured in a systematic manner. Considering the high costs of simulators, this evidence will be needed to convince educational institutions to make the necessary investment in simulator technology.

References
1. Haponik EF, Russell GB, Beamis JF Jr, et al: Bronchoscopy training: Current fellows' experiences and some concerns for the future. Chest 2000;118:625–630.
2. Tape TG, Blank LL, Wigton RS: Procedural skills of practicing pulmonologists. A national

survey of 1,000 members of the American College of Physicians. Am J Respir Crit Care Med 1995;151(2 Pt 1):282–287.
3. Torrington KG: Bronchoscopy training and competency: How many are enough? Chest 2000;118:572–573.
4. Balfe D, Mohsenifar Z: Downward trends in bronchoscopies performed between 1991 and 1997. Chest 1999;116:238–242.
5. Haponik EF, Shure D: Underutilization of transbronchial needle aspiration: Experiences of current pulmonary fellows. Chest 1997;112:251–253.
6. Goodman W: The world of civil simulators. Flight Int Mag 1978;18:435.
7. Rolfe JM, Staples KJ: Flight Simulation. Cambridge, Cambridge University Press, 1986.
8. Ressler EK, Armstrong JE, Forsythe GB: Military mission rehearsal. In Tekian A, McGuire C, McGaghie WC (eds): Innovative Simulations for Assessing Professional Competence. Chicago, University of Illinois Medical Center, 1999, pp 157–174.
9. Keys B, Wolfe J: The role of management games and simulations in education and research. J Manage 1990;16:307–336.
10. Streufert S, Pogash R, Plasecki M: Simulation-based assessment of managerial competence: Reliability and validity. Peron Psychol 1988;41:537–557.
11. Wachtel J: The future of nuclear power plant simulation in the United States. In Waltion DG (ed): Simulation for nuclear reactor technology. Cambridge, Cambridge University Press, 1985, pp 339–349.
12. Office of Naval Research: Visual Elements in Flight Simulation. Washington, DC, National Council of the National Academy of Science, 1973.
13. Dustberry JC: Introduction to Simulation Systems. J Soc Photo-opt Eng 1975;59:141–142.
14. Derossis AM, Bothwell J, Sigman HH, Fried GM: The effect of practice on performance in a laparoscopic simulator. Surg Endosc 1998;12:1117–1120.
15. Melvin WS, Johnson JA, Ellison EC: Laparoscopic skills enhancement. Am J Surg 1996;172(4):377–379.
16. Rosser JC, Rosser LE, Savalgi RS: Skill acquisition and assessment for laparoscopic surgery. Arch Surg 1997;132:200–204.
17. Derossis AM, Fried GM, Abrahamowicz M, et al: Development of a model for training and evaluation of laparoscopic skills. Am J Surg 1998;175:482–487.
18. Gordon MS, Ewy GA, Felner JM, et al: Teaching bedside cardiologic examination skills using "Harvey," the cardiology patient simulator. Med Clin North Am 1980;64:305–313.
19. Ewy GA, Felner JM, Juul D, et al: Test of a cardiology patient simulator with students in fourth-year electives. J Med Educ 1987;62:738–743.
20. Takashina T, Shimizu M, Katayama H: A new cardiology patient simulator. Cardiology 1997;88:408–413.
21. Abrahamson S, Denson JS, Wolf RM: Effectiveness of a simulator in training anesthesiology residents. J Med Educ 1969;44:515–519.
22. Kapur PA, Steadman RH: Patient simulator competency testing: Ready for takeoff? Anesth Analg 1998;86:1157–1159.
23. DeAnda A, Gaba DM: Role of experience in the response to simulated critical incidents. Anesth Analg 1991;72:308–315.
24. Britt EJ, Tasto JL, Merril GL: Assessing competence in bronchoscopy by use of a virtual reality simulator. In Proceedings of the Jubilee 10th World Congress for Bronchology and 10th World Congress for Bronchoesophagology, Budapest, 1998.
25. Issenberg SB, McGaghie WC, Hart IR, et al: Simulation technology for health care professional skills training and assessment. JAMA 1999;282:861–866.
26. Bolliger CT, Mathur PN, Beamis JF, et al: ERS/ATS statement on interventional pulmonology. European Respiratory Society/American Thoracic Society. Eur Respir J 2002;19:356–373.
27. Hildreth EA: A new look at clinical privileges for procedures. Ann Intern Med 1987;107(4):585–587.
28. Roberts JS, Radany MH, Nash DB: Privilege delineation in a demanding new environment. Ann Intern Med 1988;108:880–886.

29. Bruce NC: Evaluation of procedural skills of internal medicine residents. Acad Med 1989; 64:213–216.
30. Shannon JJ, Watts CM, Britt EJ, Lynch JP: Teaching bronchoscopy. In Feinsilver S, Fein A (ed): Textbook of Bronchoscopy. Baltimore, Williams & Wilkins, 1995, pp 133–153.
31. Rayl JE, Pittman JM, Shuster JJ: Preclinical training in bronchoscopic diagnosis of cancer. Chest 1988;93:824–827.
32. King EG, Sproule BJ, Yamamoto I: A teaching model for bronchoscopy. Chest 1976;70: 72–73.
33. Dykes MH, Ovassapian A: Dissemination of fibreoptic airway endoscopy skills by means of a workshop utilizing models. Br J Anaesth 1989;63:595–597.
34. Wood RE, Pick JR: Model systems for learning pediatric flexible bronchoscopy. Pediatr Pulmonol 1990;8(3):168–171.
35. Faber LP: Bronchoscopy training. Chest 1978;73(5 Suppl):776–778.
36. American College of Chest Physicians; Guidelines for competency and training in fiberoptic bronchoscopy. Section on Bronchoscopy. Chest 1982;81:739.
37. American Thoracic Society: Guidelines for fiberoptic bronchoscopy in adults. American Thoracic Society. Medical Section of the American Lung Association. Am Rev Respir Dis 1987;136:1066.
38. Hudson LD, Benson JA Jr: Evaluation of clinical competence in pulmonary disease. Am Rev Respir Dis 1988;138:1034–1035.
39. Prakash UB, Offord KP, Stubbs SE: Bronchoscopy in North America: The ACCP survey. Chest 1991;100:1668–1675.
40. Dull WL. Flexible fiberoptic bronchoscopy. An analysis of proficiency. Chest 1980;77:65–67.
41. American Board of Internal Medicine: Evaluation of Trainees in Pulmonary Medicine. Portland, OR, American Board of Internal Medicine, 1989.
42. Baillie J, Ravich WJ: On endoscopic training and procedural competence. Ann Intern Med 1993;118:73–74.
43. Cass OW, Freeman ML, Peine CJ, et al: Objective evaluation of endoscopy skills during training. Ann Intern Med 1993;118:40–44.
44. Ost D, DeRosiers A, Britt EJ, et al: Assessment of a bronchoscopy simulator. Am J Respir Crit Care Med 2001;164:2248–2255.
45. Ericson KA: The Road to Excellence. Mahwah, NJ, Lawrence Erlbaum Associates, 1996.
46. Lechtzin N, Rubin HR, Jenckes M, et al: Predictors of pain control in patients undergoing flexible bronchoscopy. Am J Respir Crit Care Med 2000;162(2 Pt 1):440–445.
47. Lechtzin N, Rubin HR, White P Jr, et al: Patient satisfaction with bronchoscopy. Am J Respir Crit Care Med 2002;166:1326–1331.
48. Diette GB, Lechtzin N, Haponik E, et al: Distraction therapy with nature sights and sounds reduces pain during flexible bronchoscopy: A complementary approach to routine analgesia. Chest 2003;123:941–948.
49. Poi PJ, Chuah SY, Srinivas P, Liam CK: Common fears of patients undergoing bronchoscopy. Eur Respir J 1998;11:1147–1149.
50. Mehta A, Ost D, Salinas SG, et al: Objective assessment of bronchoscopy skills by a bronchoscopy training simulator. Am J Respir Crit Care Med 2000;161:A234.
51. Ackerman MJ: The visible human project. In Proceedings of the IEEE, 1998, pp 504–511.
52. Beamis JF Jr, Shapshay SM, Setzer S, Dumon JF: Teaching models for Nd:YAG laser bronchoscopy. Chest 1989;95:1316–1318.
53. Colt HG, Crawford SW, Galbraith O III: Virtual reality bronchoscopy simulation: A revolution in procedural training. Chest 2001;120:1333–1339.
54. Cunanan OS, Mazza JE: Integrated electronic display model for teaching bronchoscopy. Chest 1977;72:364–365.
55. Gothe B: Flexible fiberoptic bronchoscopy—an analysis of proficiency. Chest 1980;78:498.
56. Hilmi OJ, White PS, McGurty DW, Oluwole M: Bronchoscopy training: Is simulated surgery effective? Clin Otolaryngol 2002;27:267–269.
57. Rowe R, Cohen RA: An evaluation of a virtual reality airway simulator. Anesth Analg 2002; 95:62–66.

Chapter 24

SIMULATION IN DENTISTRY AND ORAL SURGERY

Judith A. Buchanan, PhD, DMD, and John N. Williams, DMD

Simulation has been a great asset to many fields, perhaps most notably aviation. If simulation is defined as any artificial item or method that mimics in some way a part of the body or a situation in real life, dentistry has been using simulation almost since the inception of the first dental college, chartered in 1840 in the state of Maryland.[1] In the 1890s, shortly after the establishment of dental colleges, G. V. Black, the dentist who brought dentistry into the modern world and put it on the solid, scientific foundation that it now occupies, designed oversized models and instruments to aid in the instruction of dental students.[1] The true power and potential of simulation in health care education have recently been recognized, and simulation has progressed in dental education from oversized models of teeth to simulated patients and the use of virtual reality.[2] This chapter describes some of the steps through that historical progression, focusing on state-of-the-art simulation as it exists today and how it may look in the future.

Importance of Simulation to Dental Education

Although few specialties in medicine, such as surgery, involve substantial expertise in technical or psychomotor skills, virtually all fields of dentistry are highly reliant on well-developed surgical and psychomotor skills. To understand why simulation is of high importance in dental education, a few basic principles should be understood. First, unlike medical school, dental students, over a four-year predoctoral education, spend approximately 50% of their curriculum time in direct patient care.[3] In medicine, faculty deliver the care to patients while students observe; in dentistry, students deliver the care while faculty observe. Hence, dental students must develop minimal psychomotor skills before the initiation of direct patient care.

Second, some appreciation is needed for the type of skills required of a dentist. Caries (frequently called cavities) is one of two major diseases diagnosed and treated in oral health. Caries, a bacterial infection, implies that destruction of tooth structure has taken place. If the disease-caused destruction reaches a certain level, treatment involves surgical removal of the diseased tooth structure and replacement with a metal alloy, precious metal, or plastic material. The removal of the diseased tooth material is a surgical technique performed with a hand-piece (dental drill) and needs to be done in a careful, particular, and precise way, with criteria measured in the tenths of millimeters, while working in an environment with difficult access and less than optimal light that is mobile and often filled with saliva. The surgical removal of the diseased tooth structure according to specific principles is called the **preparation** of the tooth. Once the preparation has been completed, the missing tooth structure is replaced by a **restoration** to re-establish anatomic form and appropriate masticatory function.

Dental students must achieve an acceptable level of surgical competence. However, because surgical procedures on teeth are irreversible, learning these skills on patients is not an acceptable practice. Other dental procedures, such as endodontics (root canal therapy),[4] oral surgery,[5,6] and periodontal surgery are likewise irreversible, and extreme damage to a patient can occur if procedures are not performed by a student with acceptable levels of surgical skills. Some dental techniques, such as suturing,[7] impressions, or calculus removal, can be learned on patients, but for optimal patient care, a certain level of skill should be obtained in almost all clinical procedures before the start of patient care. Hence, most needed psychomotor (or surgical) skills are learned in a simulated manner before students progress to direct patient care. These skills are learned in "preclinical" courses. Because psychomotor and surgical skills represent so much of the actual practice of dentistry, a large portion (in the range of 20–25%[3]) of the dental curriculum is devoted to preclinical coursework. Simulation is essential to developing the minimal level of skill because it allows procedures to be repeated many times until the student shows a consistent, acceptable level of skill before performing them on a patient.

Noncomputerized Simulation

Models of Oral Structures

In the 1870s, photographic slides were not available; hence G.V. Black devised models of treated teeth that were close to three feet high for students to visualize the principles of operative dentistry.[1] The oversized models were helpful in showing various small characteristics of surgically treated teeth that measure in the tenths of millimeters. Models of the dental arches were used as early as the 1920s to help visualize the anatomic structures important to the practice of dentistry and are still helpful today[8] (Figs. 1 and 2). Dental arches are now simulated by plastic constructions of upper and lower arches (complete with teeth) that are called dentoforms (Fig. 3). Although these models are the earliest use of simulation in dental education, it is important to note that all of the mentioned models are still in use today.[8]

Simulation of Teeth and Jaws

Simulations of upper (maxillary) and lower (mandibular) arches, complete with plastic teeth, are used extensively (Fig. 3). The teeth in the arches can be easily removed and replaced as needed. The surgical techniques used in the treatment of diseased teeth can be practiced on plastic teeth, and then the removed tooth structure can be replaced by the addition of the appropriate dental restorative material. Students may use many plastic teeth for each type of preparation in the curriculum and repeat the process until they have shown a level of competency that is determined sufficient by the faculty. Depending on the type of preparation and the innate ability of the student, large numbers of teeth can be used to reach this level of competency. The plastic teeth, however, have some distinct drawbacks.

Natural teeth have distinct anatomic layers, each of varying hardness and with a different tactile sense as it is surgically removed. The most commonly used plastic teeth

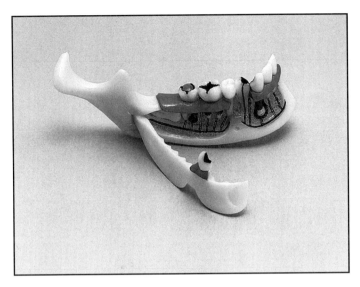

Figure 1. Models demonstrating anatomy of jaw in molar area. (From Frasaco at http://www.frasaco.com.)

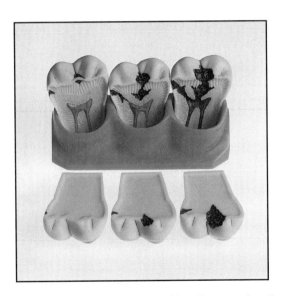

Figure 2. Models showing details of occlusal anatomy. (From Frasaco at http://www.frasaco.com.)

are all of the same consistency; hence students may not learn the feel of the different layers until their first actual experience with patients. Simulated teeth are available with different layers of varied hardness, but still they do not give an identical feel to natural teeth and are highly expensive (Fig. 4).

Specialized teeth or dentoforms are available for all types of restorative dentistry, endodontics (root canals), pediatric conditions, periodontics, oral surgery, and implantol-

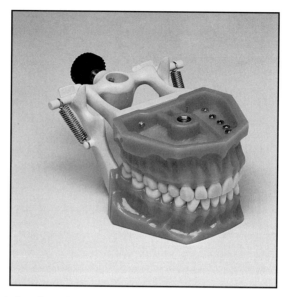

Figure 3. Adult dentoform showing all teeth. (From Frasaco at http://www.frasaco.com.)

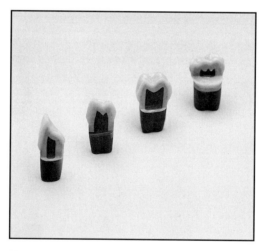

Figure 4. Plastic teeth with simulated enamel, dentin, and pulpal layers. (From Frasaco at http://www.frasaco.com.)

ogy.[9] All of these special simulated oral structures are costly and hence are not in routine use in most dental schools. Rather, they may be used in preparation for specialized examinations, such as clinical board examinations (Figs. 5 and 6).

The proper relationship of the arches and the function of the temporomandibular joint are highly important in the treatment of oral diseases. The physiologic and anatomic relationships of the masticatory system have been simulated in several ways. Arches (or dentoforms) are attached to complicated devices (termed articulators) that simulate the

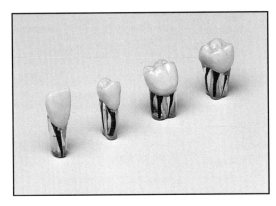

Figure 5. Plastic teeth with smulated pulpal canals. (From Frasaco at http://www.frasaco.com.)

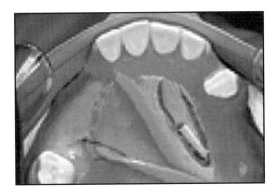

Figure 6. Specialized dentoform with impacted canine for surgical removal exercises. (From Frasaco at http://www.frasaco.com.)

positioning of the arches with relationship to the condyles and temporomandibular joint[9,12] (Fig. 7).The precise and complicated movement of this joint and the corresponding effect on the dental arches are simulated. As a result, these simulated relationships help both with instruction of students and with the actual treatment of patients.

Simulations of Patients

Simulations of patients are a relatively new addition to the armamentarium for teaching dental surgical skills. In order to simulate a patient, mannequins of the head, which include the simulated masticatory system, and sometimes mannequins of the upper torso can be used in conjunction with simulated arches (Figs. 8, 9, and 10) containing plastic teeth (dentoforms).[9,10,13] Students can perform dental procedures in the simulated mouth, and the presence of the head and torso adds much more to the reality of the simulation and is quite helpful in developing good ergonomic skills. Simulation labs of this type are becoming popular in preclinical education in the United States and are often coupled with other technology such as computers. Expansion of this topic can be found in the section about simulation with computers. It is unclear, however, whether the use

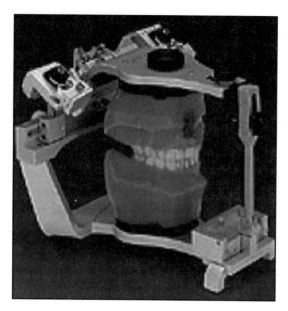

Figure 7. Denar (D5A) Articulator.

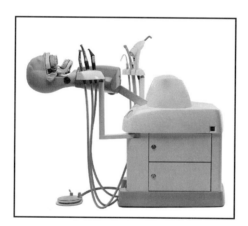

Figure 8. Patient simulator with torso and dental unit. (From Kavo at http://www.kavousa.com.)

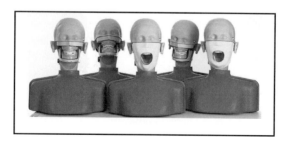

Figure 9. Patient simulators that can attach to a dental chair. (From Kavo at http://www.kavousa.com.)

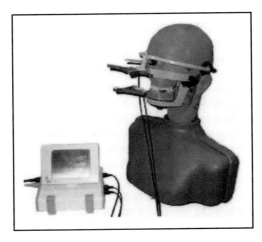

Figure 10. Patient simulator with advanced articulation guides. (From Kavo at http://www.kavousa.com.)

of this type of simulation laboratory improves student learning or prepares students better for direct patient care.[14,15]

For development of nonsurgical skills, people can also act as simulated patients and are termed standardized patients.[16–19] Standardized patients are people, sometimes paid actors, who are carefully coached to present themselves as patients with a set of predetermined characteristics. Standardized patients have been used in medical education since the early 1960s[20] and were first reported in dental education in 1990.[17] Standardized patients help dental students develop appropriate communication and interpersonal skills for such tasks as eliciting a thorough medical and dental history, completing a head and neck exam, and completing accurate and appropriate record keeping. There are many benefits of standardized patients, but this type of instruction is expensive and time-consuming for both students and faculty.[19]

Simulations Using Computers

Cased-based Simulations

Computers can be extremely helpful in simulating patients or presenting case scenarios.[21–29] In case-based computer programs, students are presented with a patient and must respond to a series of questions related to medical history, diagnostic tests, possible diagnoses, appropriate treatment plan, and so forth. Although these programs are interactive, most allow only a limited number of responses, giving some guidance to the student. A recent report describes a computer database that allows free text input in response to a computer-presented clinical case, making the simulation highly realistic.[30]

Computer scenario simulation can facilitate the integration of basic science into the clinical arena, help students in areas of clinical problem solving, allow experience in hard-to-find clinical situations,[21–27] provide opportunities for practice, remediation, and self-assessment, and teach new clinical content.

Computerized business simulations can also be a tool for help in learning practice management skills.[31] Students make decisions in response to various management scenarios (e.g., staffing, location, fees) that simulate a dental practice environment. Each different response has a consequence on the business operation of the simulated dental practice.

In recent years, computer simulations have been discussed for possible use in dental licensure examinations or other evaluation and testing applications. A critical concern, however, is the reliability and validity of computer simulation[32] when it is used for such purposes. Simulations that are used in a teaching environment have as their main priority the improvement of performance. As such, complex situations are often presented in a more simplified manner than found in real life. Simulations that have as their main priority the measurement of performance or the assessment of skills usually occur after the final stage of instruction and as such should present complex systems and images as true to life as possible. Hence, simulations used for dental licensure examinations must meet a higher standard in reliability and criterion validity than those used for performance improvement.

One criticism of simulation is that it is too deterministic. The advantages, however, of using simulation for dental examinations, assuming the level of reliability and validity is sufficient, are compelling. Simulation may have a greater potential validity, is safer in comparison with using live patients, and may be less expensive and easier.[32] As simulations in dentistry become more and more advanced, their use in dental licensure examinations will receive more consideration.

Computer Imaging

Recent advances in computer imaging have allowed the production of highly accurate three-dimensional dental models of the oral apparatus by destructive scanning, laser scanning, or direct imaging of teeth[33–35] (Fig. 11). In addition, imaging systems have been used to capture three-dimensional images of mandibular motion.[34] The technology of computer imaging can be used in the educational component of dentistry,[36] but it is

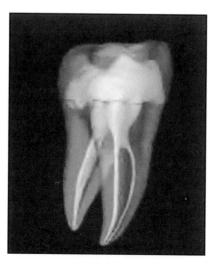

Figure 11. Three-dimensional image of tooth with internal anatomy. (From Simulife Systems, 3D Dental, at http://www.simulife.fr.)

also becoming more important in the practice of dentistry. A dental CAD/CAM unit[37-40] is available that can scan the preparation of a tooth, design the restoration, and mill the restoration from a porcelain block, all in the same unit. The advantage of this technology is that the patient receives a finished crown or porcelain restoration in one visit—a procedure that, without this technology, may take at least two separate visits.

Simulation Labs with Computer Technology

Patient simulation laboratories are becoming more popular in dental education. These labs consist of a large number of simulated patients with instructional media on computer displays (Fig. 12). The computer can display demonstrations by faculty, lesson material, and models of procedures. Hence the computer-supported audiovisual systems add value to the patient simulators by aiding in the transfer of information from instructors, manuals, or reference material directly to the student at chairside.

The computer can "bring life" to the inanimate patient simulator. In early system designs, two different computer systems were used to enhance student instruction. First, a computer monitor linked to a central audiovisual system was used as a presentation system to provide visualization of any teaching material directly to the student's simulated patient station. This arrangement provided the benefit of individualized viewing of any materials and the opportunity for the instructor to enlarge the fine details of oral structures. The subtleties of anatomic details are clearly visible. The second type of computer system is an interactive system in which students have control over access to a wide variety of instructional materials. The interactive computer system using equipment such as a laptop or handheld personal digital assistant provides instant electronic access.

With the development of electronic curricula contained on digital versatile disc (DVD) or CD-ROM as well as the explosive growth in internet web-based materials,[41,42] students have ready access to instructional materials from around the world. VitalSource Technologies[43] originated in higher education of the health sciences as a

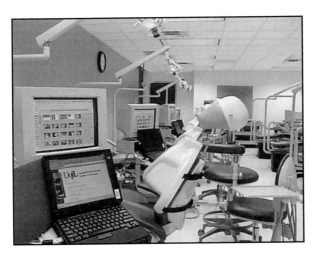

Figure 12. Patient simulator laboratory with computer support. (Courtesy of Dr. John Williams, Dean, University of Louisville, School of Dental Medicine.)

means for enhancing access to digital instructional materials. It was recognized that, while the evolving digital environment created great opportunities for managing, integrating, and accessing educational materials, it also created new challenges in security and effectiveness of access.

As computer technology continues its explosive growth and development, the opportunity exists to combine the presentation and interactive aspects of earlier computer systems into one system. The ability for students to receive detailed real-life visual instructional material is already present and will expand in the future. The expansion of higher broadband widths and wireless technologies will give student access to instructional material not only at the simulated patient station but virtually anywhere.

Simulation with Advanced Technology

Virtual Reality-based Technology

The current stage of development of imaging systems and the techniques of virtual reality have expanded the field of dental education to companies with expertise in virtual reality. The most advanced simulation system in dental education at this time[2,44,45] has been available for only 4–5 years. This unit combines the simulated patient units (described earlier) with sophisticated virtual reality-based technology (VRBT). VRBT allows a computer not only to image the oral structures present in the patient simulator but also to modify the virtual image of the plastic tooth in the computer in real time as it is surgically modified in the dentoform by the student. This process is accomplished by use of infrared emitters on the dentoform and hand-piece (dental drill). An infrared camera can orient the teeth and the hand-piece in space and track in space the resulting surgical removal of tooth structure. The computer can then compare the student-modified tooth to the ideally prepared tooth, previously scanned into the computer. The ideally prepared tooth can be modified by the teaching faculty. The ability of the unit to evaluate a student's preparation against that of a predetermined ideal sets this technology apart from all other simulation technologies. To understand why this ability is so significant, one must consider how students, even in modern simulation laboratories, learn dental procedures.

Students without the availability of VRBT prepare plastic teeth in a dentoform in a laboratory setting. When the student feels that he or she has completed the preparation according to the criteria given, he or she will ask a faculty member for evaluation. Because much of dentistry is art, variability in faculty evaluation is high, and faculty may give students conflicting evaluations. In addition, even the same faculty member may not evaluate student efforts consistently. Students often have to wait for faculty feedback, the feedback is verbal, and it is usually given on the final product—seldom during the process. In VRBT units, the feedback can be given directly by the computer in copious visual detail, always in comparison with the ideal, and at the press of a button (Figs. 13, 14, and 15). There is little apprehension in asking a computer for evaluation or a grade in comparison with requesting the same from faculty. The feedback from the computer is consistent and always immediately available.

The type and number of procedures available on VRBT units have dramatically increased over the past two years. Software is available for all general restorative procedures involving the surgical removal of tooth structure, including simple to complex amalgam preparations, preparations for tooth-colored restorative material, preparations

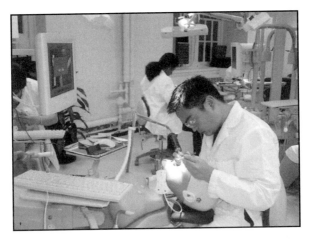

Figure 13. VRBT laboratory. (Courtesy of Dr. Judith Buchanan, Associate Dean, University of Pennsylvania, School of Dental Medicine.)

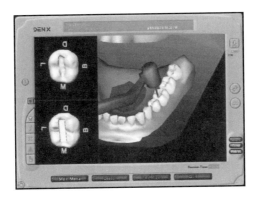

Figure 14. VRBT screen showing student-prepared virtual tooth and ideally prepared tooth. (Courtesy of Dr. Judith Buchanan, Associate Dean, University of Pennsylvania, School of Dental Medicine.)

for posterior teeth or anterior teeth, gold crown procedures, porcelain or porcelain and metal crown procedures, and simple cast gold preparations. For each procedure, several "doctrines" (as termed by the company) or protocols may be available, each with different grading parameters. For instance, one protocol may count any damage to an adjacent tooth as a reason for failure of the procedure, whereas another protocol may not measure this parameter at all. This variation allows certain protocols to be used on more inexperienced students, whereas others can be used at the later stage closer to the time of entry into the clinic. In addition, one protocol may start with a grade of 0. As the student meets certain criteria of the procedure, points can be added. Another protocol can set the grade at 100 at the start and remove points as mistakes are made. Students vary as to which method they prefer. For all procedures, if a student makes a critical error, such as exposing the nerve, the student is notified immediately and fails the procedure.

Research on this type of simulation has shown that students learn dental procedures

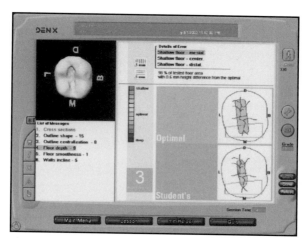

Figure 15. VRBT evaluation screen showing evaluation of depth of preparation of student's tooth compared with the ideal. (Courtesy of Dr. Judith Buchanan, Associate Dean, University of Pennsylvania, School of Dental Medicine.)

faster, are more efficient per unit time, and come to equal or better levels of surgical skill compared with more traditional types of dental education.[2,46,47] VRBT is currently available in 12 of 56 U.S. dental schools and several international schools. The number of units per school ranges from 1 to 40 within the United States and from 4 to 30 internationally. The integration of the technology into the curriculum varies widely among schools. In some schools, the use of VRBT has dramatically influenced educational philosophy and resulted in significant curriculum changes.

Technology with Haptic Focus

The tactile feel associated with surgical dental techniques (such as the surgical removal of different layers of tooth structure and the incision into oral tissues) is an important facet of the practice of dentistry. This skill may be compared to the skill that an anesthesiologist needs to recognize the feel of different layers or structures as a needle is passed through the spine to obtain the proper anesthesia. Simulation of tactile sensations is difficult to obtain but, as in the medical field, several companies are venturing into this arena. At least two companies[48–50] are focusing on this approach to help with dental education.

One system,[48] although still in an early stage, is beginning to market a unit that incorporates the sensation of force feedback, allowing students to perform virtual procedures while preserving the tactile sensations associated with dental procedures. As with most new technology, the system has obvious advantages and disadvantages and a long way to go to achieve an attractive balance between the two. One advantage, of course, is the tactile sensation, which, although some dentists claim that it is not identical to the real-life situation, is definitely a step into the next dimension of simulation. Another advantage is that the oral structures and dental equipment are all virtual and hence do not impose additional costs for the institution or the student. In addition, lesions (e.g., decay, fractures) can be programmed into the unit, allowing a wider variety of simulations in an effort to replicate the plethora of situations seen by practicing dentists.

Programming many different dental conditions into the virtual oral structures is not inexpensive, but once the program is installed, it has unlimited uses. Plastic teeth with oral lesions or root canal systems can cost up to $8 per tooth and, as mentioned before, fall far beyond the practical range for a school that may use thousands of teeth per course. One major disadvantage of this unit is that the operator holds a stylus in the air and looks straight into a computer screen to manipulate the system. This is not the posture or ergonomics exercised in the actual treatment of patients. If the technology could be coupled with the patient simulator, it would be a more powerful tool in dental education.

Advanced Navigational Simulation (Global Positioning Type System)

Just as global positioning systems have been helpful in transportation, the application of similar technology to the human body is helping surgeons from all fields navigate through human structures in a way that has not been feasible in the past.[51,52] In other words, surgeons can visualize directly where they are in the human body, or with the help of advanced technology they can visualize their position by viewing a virtual image of the patient on a computer screen. The virtual image will not only show surgeons where they are in the body but also display a road map showing where the surgeon wants to go. At certain times in a surgical procedure, direct vision may be more helpful; at other times, however, viewing the virtual patient may give the surgeon much more necessary information. In neurosurgery,[51,52] for example, this type of technology has affected the practice of medicine. It also has the potential to affect dentistry in the area of implants.[53]

One of the most invasive treatment options for dentists is the placement of implants. Implants are metal posts of various designs, made from varying materials and surgically inserted into the jaw where teeth are missing. These posts can then be used to attach fixed prostheses made in the image of teeth. Implants have been used for a long time, but only in the past decade or so have they reached a success rate accepted by even the most conservative of dentists. Placement of the implants is extremely important. One must consider both the anatomic structure of the patient and the ease of attaching the prosthesis to the implant after surgery to obtain a functional and esthetic result. A few systems with this type of technology[53] have been tested previously outside the United States, and one[44] recently was approved by the Food and Drug Administration for use with the placement of implants in the United States.

The first step in the use of a unit with this technology is to construct the virtual image of the patient by using CT scans. This information is transferred directly into the unit and can undergo image enhancement to produce a highly accurate virtual image of the patient's jaw. A major advantage of the virtual image is the ability to manipulate and cross-section anatomic areas and accurately measure distances from important anatomic features and landmarks. Different treatment plans can be examined by the extensive manipulations available to the virtual image, and a final optimal treatment plan can be chosen. Software, available to dentists for some time, can be used to establish a patient model sufficient for treatment planning purposes. However, recently developed units allow significantly more than a model for treatment planning, including the stereotactic option and the ability to guide the surgeon during the actual placement of the implants (Figs. 16 and 17). During surgery with an advanced unit, the surgeon who veers from the predetermined treatment plan is immediately notified, and if a critical mistake is imminent, the unit will turn off the dental drill, requiring the surgeon to override the system in

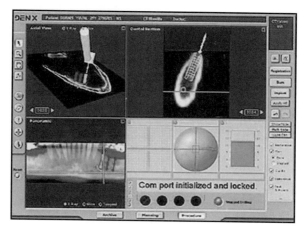

Figure 16. IGI screen demonstrating correct placement of implants. (From DenX, LTD, at http://www. denx.com/company.html.)

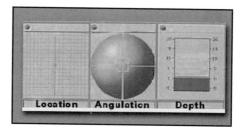

Figure 17. IGI guidance panels for correct surgical placement of implants. (From DenX, LTD, at http://www.denx.com/company.html.)

order to continue on the same path. Hence the use of this system may help to reassure patients (and possibly dentists) of the safety of the procedure. This unit is advantageous both for students learning the surgical procedures and patients undergoing this procedure. However, it appears that the main target audience of this unit and navigational technology is the private practice arena. Since this is one of the first units using navigational technology in dentistry, further experience is needed to determine whether it will be commonly used in dentistry's future.

Simulation and Resources

As discussed previously, the optimal goal of simulation in dentistry is to develop and assess the minimal surgical, psychomotor, and cognitive skills in dental students that must be achieved before the start of direct patient care. Each student must achieve an acceptable level of surgical competence. Additional objectives include improving students' abilities in problem solving, ergonomics, patient rapport, and history taking, establishing differential diagnoses and familiarizing oneself with all dental procedures prior to direct patient care. The resources needed for simulation vary but are extremely important in determining the level of incorporation of various types of simulation. Examples include funds, space, time in the curriculum, staff, and faculty. Part of the equation also includes the attitude of students, faculty, and administration. The field of simulation in dental education is continually under tension. Visionaries recognize the advantages that advanced simulation can bring (especially to dental education). However, the benefit of advanced simulation education cannot be well substantiated, and reluctance to change from more traditional methods may be a barrier in some dental schools. For any simulation to be of great value to a school, it must be shown to be of help in preparation of dental students and at the same time to justify resource demands. Thus, to understand the current status of simulation in dentistry, it is helpful to revisit the types of simulation currently available, evaluate their impact on education when possible, consider the resources needed, and understand the possible attitudes of students, faculty, and administration.

The most popular simulation found in almost every dental school is the simulated teeth and jaws (dentoforms). The dentoform can be mounted simply on a pole in a laboratory or in a more sophisticated simulated patient. Students learn a multitude of procedures on just one or two different types of dentoforms. In most schools, the dentoform is purchased by the student, and after a minimal allocation of teeth by the school, additional teeth, if needed, are usually purchased by the student. The cost of this type of simulation is primarily borne by the student; the school's responsibility is associated with the cost of the laboratory. In schools that have laboratories where students basically mount the dentoform on a pole, the cost of the laboratory is minimal. There is uniform agreement that the educational advantage of the dentoform outweighs the resources needed. If a school has recently invested in a laboratory of simulated patients, the cost to the school can be substantial since simulated patients can be in the range from $5,000 to $10,000 per unit, depending on the type and manufacturer. The optimal number of units for simulated patients is one per student in a class. If the patient simulator laboratory is augmented with computer-assisted instruction, the cost of the laboratory is significantly increased. Patient simulators take up more space than most laboratories without simulators, making space also a resource issue. An important question that is not sufficiently answered is whether the advantages to the educational program offered by patient simulators are worth the expense. It is apparent that patient simulators have not made any drastic change in the way dentistry is taught. In other words, whether students learn procedures on dentoforms on a pole or on dentoforms in a sophisticated patient simulator, the course material and the way in which students are evaluated are very much the same. Faculty members (at a ratio of approximately 1 faculty per 8–10 students) still evaluate students' work during course time. Faculty availability and variability of their evaluations are still problematic with or without patient simulators. Limited studies have addressed the improvement of education with patient simulators, and those that are published are not overwhelmingly supportive.[14,15] Despite little support in the literature, it seems logical that students trained on a unit resembling a real patient will be better prepared, technically, ergonomically, and emotionally, for direct patient care. Additional studies are needed to validate the expense involved in patient simulators.

If patient simulators are equipped with VRBT, the situation changes significantly, both from the standpoint of the cost and the potential impact on the education of students. The cost of VRBT is quite high, around $60,000 per unit (excluding simulated patient);

thus, one unit per student in a class is virtually impossible. However, preliminary data[2,46,47] support the view that the use of VRBT significantly enhances educational objectives. VRBT seems to reduce the time necessary for learning surgical psychomotor skills, improves the efficiency of learning, allows more practice preparations per session, allows students to evaluate their work 3–5 times more often,[46,47] and requires fewer faculty members. It eliminates the inconsistency and variability of faculty evaluations and allows a change in educational philosophy as well as significant changes in curriculum, mainly due to the unlimited availability of the unit. It is common for education in psychomotor instruction to be given in concentrated courses according to specialty area (e.g., restorative, endodontics, periodontics), and the timing of these courses depends on when faculty are available. Thus, some skills may be taught many months or a year before the student actually uses them on a patient. Although this has been the traditional way of teaching dentistry for years, one can easily see that it is not ideal. With the availability of VRBT, students can rotate through a VRBT lab continuously throughout their curriculum to practice their skills in the same way as musicians practice their instruments continuously. They can practice a procedure the night before performing it for the first time on a patient. Learning on VRBT does not depend on the availability of faculty. A point to consider is the shortage of dentists entering the academic field. There are large numbers of vacant dental faculty positions in the United States. Less reliance on faculty in the preclinical courses can be viewed as a significant help with this shortage.

Because students learn psychomotor skills faster with VRBT, the amount of time necessary for preclinical courses can be reduced. Revised curricula with the reduction of time in preclinical courses have been implemented or planned at several dental schools that currently have VRBT. One school is reducing the amount of time in a preclinical course by 25% because of the presence of VRBT.[54]

Attitudes towards advanced simulation, especially VRBT, must also be considered. Teaching methods in surgical psychomotor skills in dental education were mostly static for many years. Some dental faculty members are not comfortable with e-mail, let alone virtual reality. Consider also that simulations such as VRBT can be viewed as decreasing responsibilities of dental faculty and thus reducing the number of required faculty members. One can certainly understand that faculty acceptance may be critical and difficult to obtain in the implementation of advanced simulation. Student acceptance is much less of a problem today. Many students not only feel comfortable with technology; they actually demand it.

Although VRBT seems to meet many educational objectives, the question still remains as to whether it is worth the cost. Besides the direct cost of the units, one must also consider associated costs such as the needs for greater space and excellent technical support. The VRBT contains sophisticated technology that goes beyond the expertise of the average computer technician. Training for faculty, students, and technical support must also be of concern for the successful incorporation of VRBT. Cost/benefit studies that include these parameters are not available and, in any case, may be particular to the needs of individual dental schools. This area requires additional research.

Simulations using haptic or GPS abilities are still in the development stage. It is expected that this technology will also make significant drains on all resources mentioned above. Because they are not yet in use in any dental school, no information is available about their impact on educational objectives. It is clear, however, that the field of simulation is advancing at an increasing rate. Dentistry is certainly not the only health care field investigating and profiting from simulation advances. In fact, advanced technology simulation appears to be on the verge of dramatically affecting all areas of health care education. It seems wise that health care fields could all benefit from the collaboration and sharing of technology, especially in the expensive areas of haptic and navigational simulation.

Future Possibilities of Dental Simulation

Simulation holds the promise of improving the way in which dental students are educated. The sophistication of simulation in the teaching of psychomotor and surgical skills for dental students will continue to be enhanced as dental schools seek alternative ways to educate students more efficiently. Advances in medical simulations offer the opportunity to combine dental VRBT, haptics, or GPS with a medical simulator to present a total simulated patient experience for use in dental education. This technology is currently available for health professions students.

Medical Education Technologies, Inc. (METI) [55] has developed a functional human-like mannequin that exhibits clinical signs. The Human Patient Simulator (HPS)—a computer model-driven, full-sized mannequin—delivers experience in true-to-life scenarios that swiftly change to meet instructors' goals. The ultra-sophisticated and highly versatile HPS blinks, speaks, and breathes, has a heartbeat and a pulse, and accurately mirrors human responses to such procedures as cardiopulmonary resuscitation, intravenous medication, and ventilation. This simulator has several computer-programmed systems (e.g., cardiovascular, pulmonary, pharmacologic, metabolic). These systems utilize computer technology and can be programmed for teaching a variety of basic science concepts and simulated clinical situations. Students can practice repeatedly until the appropriate skills have been mastered (Figs. 18 and 19).

Global Impact

Advanced simulation combining dental and medical systems may also have a significant impact on less developed countries. Many such countries do not have the pre-

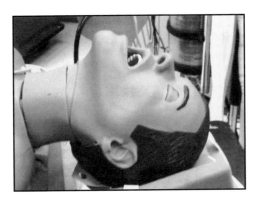

Figure 18. Head of functional human-like mannequin. (From Medical Education Technologies, Inc., at www.meti.com.)

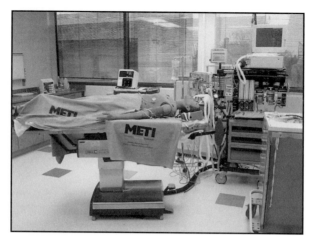

Figure 19. Full figure view of functional human-like mannequin. (From Medical Education Technologies, Inc., at *www.meti.com.*)

professional or professional education opportunities that are available in more developed countries. Many countries do not have a significant number of qualified practitioners to serve as mentors to apprentices. Sophisticated technology that is made portable to facilitate sharing can significantly improve the global education and training of dentists and other oral care professionals. At the same time, the unmet oral health care needs are enormous. Simulation for both education and practice can help countries address these needs and in the long term may be less expensive than acquiring the entire educational infrastructure found in highly developed countries.

Conclusion

Simulation use in dentistry began soon after the establishment of dental education and, because of the nature of the profession and its high dependency on surgical psychomotor skills, one can assume that it will not disappear in the foreseeable future. From all possible indicators, the field of simulation will move forward and adapt to the demands of the profession. The question is not whether VRBT, haptic, and navigational simulation will become part of our professional dental education; the question is only when it will be commonplace. The question of timing may be answered as more information is forthcoming about the impact on educational objectives, the true cost of simulation, and the rate at which faculty can adjust. Since all of the health professions are following similar paths, it seems wise to listen and learn from all and, when possible, to create collaborations. Hopefully, simulations for the entire body, developed collaboratively among health care professions, will be available in the not-too-distant future.

References
1. Ring ME: Dentistry: An illustrated History. New York, Abradale Press, Harry N. Abrams, Mosby-Year Book, 1985, pp 212, 274, 277.
2. Buchanan J: Use of simulation technology in dental education. J Dent Educ 2001;65:1225–1231.

3. Tedesco LA: Issues in dental curriculum development and change. J Dent Educ 1995;59:97–147.
4. Schulz-Bongert U, Weine FS: Method for constructing standardized simulated root canals. J Dent Educ 1990;54:328–330.
5. Liewehr FR, Rouse LE, O'Neill LJ: A preclinical model for exodontia. J Dent Educ 1992; 56:396–398.
6. Whitehead FIH: Models for teaching minor oral surgery. J Dent 1973;2:59–62.
7. Kuba SK, Hoag PM, Rosenfeld LD: A model for the demonstration of suturing techniques. J Periodont 1972;43:573–574.
8. Shillingburg HT, Fisher DW: Use of macro-models in teaching tooth preparations. J Dent Educ 1973;37:39–42.
9. Frasaco at http://www.frasaco.com [accessed November 2, 2003].
10. Kavo at http://www.kavousa.com [accessed November 2, 2003].
11. Denar articulators at http://www.professional.waterpik.com/products_occlusion.CFM [accessed November 2, 2003].
12. Koolstra JH, van Eijden TMGJ: Biomechanical analysis of jaw-closing movements. J Dent Res 1995;74:1564–1570.
13. Patient Simulators at http://www.ohsu.edu/news/archive/2002/102802sim.html [accessed November 6, 2003].
14. Clancy JMS, Lindquist TJ, Palik JF, Johnson LA: A comparison of student performance in a simulation clinic and a traditional laboratory environment: Three-year results. J Dent Educ 2002;66:1331–1337.
15. Chan DC, Pruzler KB, Caughman WF: Simulation with preclinical operative dentistry courses: 3 year retrospective results. J Dent Educ 2000;64:224.
16. Sandoval VA, Dale RA, Hendricson WD, Alexander JB: A comparison of four simulation and instructional methods for endodontic review. J Dent Educ 1987;51:532–538.
17. Johnson JA, Kipp KC, Williams RG: Standardized patients for the assessment of dental students clinical skills. J Dent Educ 1990;54:331–333.
18. Kay CJ, Johnson JA, Kopp KC: Standardized patients for teaching geriatric dentistry. Spec Car Dent 1994;6:229–232.
19. Johnson JA, Kopp KC: Effectiveness of standardized patient instruction. J Dent Educ 1996;60:262–266.
20. Barrows HS: An overview of the uses of standardized patients for teaching and evaluating clinical skills. Acad Med 1993;68:443–453.
21. Finkelstien MW, Johnson LA, Lillie GE: Interactive videodisc patient simulations of oral diseases. J Dent Educ 1987;52:217–220.
22. McGuire CH: Simulation techniques in the teaching and testing of problem-solving skills. J Res Sci Teach 1976;2:89–100.
23. Siegel MA, Firriolo FJ, Finkelstein MW: Computer applications in oral diagnosis. Dent Clin North Am 1993;37:113–131.
24. Mulligan R, Wood GJ: A controlled evaluation of computer assisted training simulation in geriatric dentistry. J Dent Educ 1993;57:16–24.
25. Messer LB, Kan K, Cameron A, Robinson R: Teaching paediatric dentistry by multimedia: A three-year report. Eur J Dent Educ 2002;6:128–138.
26. Fouad AF, Burleson JA: Effectiveness of an endodontic diagnosis computer simulation program. J Dent Educ 1997;61:289–295.
27. Finkelstein MW, Johnson LA, Lilly GE: Interactive videodisc patient simulation of oral diseases. J Dent Educ 1988;52:217–220.
28. Nattestad A, Attstrom R: Information technology in oral health education. Eur J Dent Educ 1997;1:101–107.
29. Abbey LM: Interactive multimedia patient simulations in dental and continuing dental education. Dent Clin North Am 2002;46:575–587.
30. Janda MS, Mattheos N, Nattestad A, et al: A virtual patient for learning periodontal treatment: A simulator for patient encounters by dental students. Design and usability of the software and test of the learning effect for history taking in periodontal patients. Eur J Dent Educ [accepted for publication].

31. Willis DO, Smith JR, Golden P: A computerized business simulation for dental practice management. J Dent Educ 1997;61:821–828.
32. Alessi SM, Johnson LA: Simulations for dental licensure examinations: reliability and validity. Simulations/Games for Learning 1992;22:286–307.
33. Encisco R, Memon A, Mah J: Three-dimensional visualization of the craniofacial patient: Volume segmentation, data integration and animation. Orthop Cranio Res Suppl 2003;6: 66–71.
34. Langenbach GEJ, Ahang F, Herring SW, Hannam AG: Modelling the masticatory biomechanics of a pig. J Anat 2002;201:383–393.
35. Hannam AG: Dynamic modeling and jaw biomechanics. Orthop Cranio Res Suppl 2003; 6:59–65.
36. Suvinen TI, Messer LB, Franco E: Clinical simulation in teaching preclinical dentistry. Eur J Dent Educ 1998;2:25–32.
37. Benjamin SD: CAD/CAM technologies: The future of restorative dentistry. Pract Proced Aesthet Dent 2003;15:308–310.
38. Nakamura TD, Dei N, KojimaT, Wakabayashi K: Marginal and internal fit of Cerec 3 CAD/CAM all-ceramic crowns. Inter J Pros 2003;16:244–248.
39. Kurbad A, Reichel K: All-ceramic primary telescopic crowns with Cerec inLab. Inter J Comp Dent 2003;6:103–111.
40. Touati B: Extensive prosthetic rehabilitation with CAD/CAM generated restorations. Prac Proc Aesthet Dent: 2003;15:293–295.
41. Spallek H, Pilcher E, Lee J, Schleyer T: Evaluation of web-based dental CE-courses. J Dent Educ 2002;66:393–404.
42. Spallek H, Berthold P, Shanley DB, Attstrom R: Distance education for dentists: Improving the quality of online instruction. Am J Distance Educ 2000;14:49–59.
43. Vital Source Technologies VOA article at http://www.voanews.com/article.cfm?objectid=CC2D1706–3433-4F34-A2BE63A8108B6178&title=No%20Textbooks%20Used%20at%20All%2DComputer%20Dental%20School&db=current [accessed November 10, 2003].
44. DenX, LTD at http://www.denx.com/company.html [accessed November 2, 2003].
45. Rose JT, Buchanan JA, Sarret DC: The DentSim system. J Dent Educ 1999;63:421–423.
46. Buchanan J, Gluch J, Stewart D, et al: Use of Virtual reality based technology in teaching dental operative procedures. J Dent Educ 2000:64:227.
47. Buchanan J: Overview of three years' experience with Virtual Reality Based Technology in dental education. J Dent Educ 2001;65:58.
48. Simulife Systems, 3D dental at http://www.simulife.fr [accessed October 27, 2003].
49. Johnson L, Thomas G, Sow S, Stanford D: An initial evaluation of the Iowa dental surgical simulator. J Dent Educ 2000;64:847–853.
50. Thomas G, Johnson L, Dow S, Stanford C: The design and testing of a force feedback dental simulator. Comput Meth Progr Biomed 2001;64:53–64.
51. Speelman JD, Schuurman R, deBie RM, et al: Stereotactic neurosurgery for tremor. Movement Disord 2002;3:S84-S88.
52. Lartinen LV: My 50 years of interest in stereotactic and functional neurosurgery. J Stero Func Neur 2001;77:7–10.
53. Birkfellner W, Solar P, Gahleitner A, et al: In-vitro assessment of a registration protocol for image-guided implant dentistry. Clin Oral Impl Res 2001;12:69–78.
54. Personal communication, Dr. Judith Buchanan, Associate Dean for Academic Affairs, University of Pennsylvania, School of Dental Medicine. November 6, 2003.
55. Medical Education Technologies, Inc., www.meti.com. Accessed November 12, 2003.

Chapter 25

SIMULATION FOR CONSCIOUS SEDATION TRAINING
Basics of Conscious Sedation

Howard A. Schwid, MD, and Brian K. Ross, MD, PhD

Sedation for procedures provides a number of benefits to the patient, including relief of pain, anxiety, and unpleasant memories. Sedation can also facilitate the procedure by preventing patient movement. However, along with the benefits come risks. Sedation of patients is accompanied by loss of airway reflexes and respiratory depression, which predispose to hypoxia and serious complications, including neurologic injury and death.

Patients are sedated for procedures most often during minor surgery in the operating room or emergency department or during radiologic, gastroenterologic, or dental procedures. Sedation is usually administered by personnel other than anesthesiologists or nurse anesthetists, such as nurses, surgeons, emergency physicians, radiologists, gastroenterologists, or dentists. Personnel that administer sedation for procedures should receive specialized training.

Safe administration of sedative agents to facilitate procedures involves a number of skills. These skills include patient evaluation, medication selection and titration, monitoring, management of the airway and emergencies related to administration of sedative agents, and postsedation recovery. A training program for administration of sedative agents for procedures should cover all aspects of care. Understanding the appropriate use of sedative agents and the implications of patient condition is a cognitive skill, whereas airway management is mainly psychomotor. Monitoring of patients and management of emergencies are a mix of cognitive and psychomotor skills. The cognitive skills are best introduced through traditional methods such as classroom lectures, small group discussions, printed materials, and screen-based simulator scenarios. Psychomotor skills can be taught in a clinical environment with real patients and in a mannequin-based simulator. We use both types of simulators for sedation training at the University of Washington Simulation Center because each has its particular applications, advantages, and disadvantages.

Screen-based Simulation for Sedation

The screen-based Sedation Simulator[1] reproduces the cognitive aspects of patient care during procedural sedation. The program presents a patient who is initially anxious and uncooperative (Fig. 1). The user must titrate sedative agents to render the patient in an accommodating state for the procedure. The program has 36 clinical scenarios, including radiology, oral surgery, endoscopy, and minor surgery cases. Many of the simulated patients are quite healthy, whereas some present with acute and chronic illnesses. The ages of the simulated patients vary from 4 years to 82 years. The user can perform his-

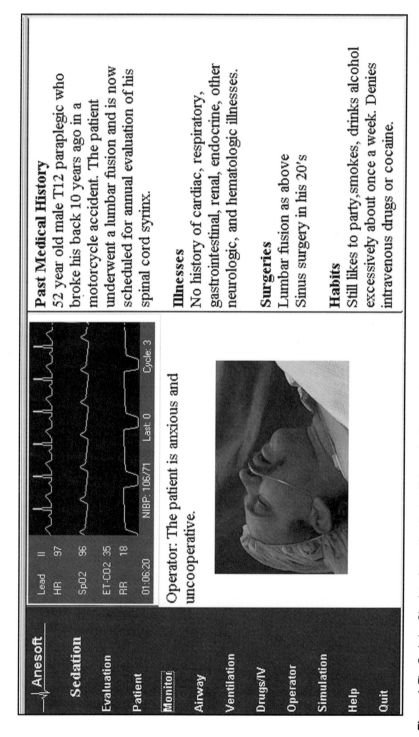

Figure 1. The Sedation Simulator interactive display. Using a simple menu, the trainee can take a history, examine the patient, monitor the patient, administer drugs, and control the airway and ventilation.

tory and physical exam and order laboratory studies while administering sedative agents. A physiologic monitor continuously displays the simulated patient's electrocardiogram, blood pressure, pulse oximetry, and capnogram. Because the Sedation Simulator operates on any Windows computer in a Java-enabled browser, trainees can use the software on their home or office computer in preparation for the formal sedation course.

The Sedation Simulator uses standard two- and three-compartment pharmacokinetic models to predict plasma and effector concentrations during titration of the medications. Different case scenarios use different pharmacokinetic parameters to simulate various groups of patients such as young, elderly, or obese as well as patients with disease states such as renal or hepatic failure. Sedative drugs can be titrated in any combination with bolus doses given at any point in time or as continuous infusions (Table 1). The program calculates the predicted drug concentrations, and the user can view pharmacokinetic plots during the simulated case (Fig. 2). This aspect of the Sedation Simulator program helps trainees learn the proper dosing of sedative agents, including onset times and

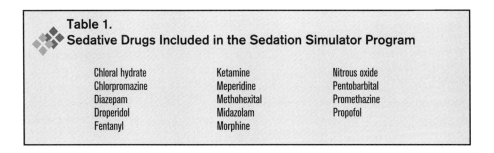

Table 1.
Sedative Drugs Included in the Sedation Simulator Program

Chloral hydrate	Ketamine	Nitrous oxide
Chlorpromazine	Meperidine	Pentobarbital
Diazepam	Methohexital	Promethazine
Droperidol	Midazolam	Propofol
Fentanyl	Morphine	

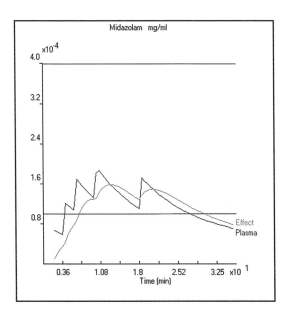

Figure 2. The Sedation Simulator presents a pharmacokinetic plot for multiple bolus doses of propofol plus continuous infusion.

expected duration of action for bolus administration and continuous infusions. Fourteen different sedative drugs are included in the Sedation Simulator (see Table 1), allowing the trainee to sedate the simulated patient with drugs, such as chloral hydrate or promethazine, that have been used historically but are no longer recommended.

The Sedation Simulator is designed for self-study. At our training center, we ask each student to perform a number of simulated sedation cases on the Sedation Simulator during the sedation course. The first case involves a routine sedation for a healthy patient. This case introduces students to the program and allows them to manage a straightforward case. The student learns to administer proper doses of the medications and observe the patient's response. The second simulator case involves sedation of a patient with significant aortic stenosis, providing the opportunity to manage a more complicated patient. The remaining simulator cases involve the management of emergency situations that may occur during sedation (Table 2). The program provides learning objectives and suggested management for each case so that students can review what they should learn from each case simulation (Fig. 3). In addition, if the student ever becomes confused during the simulated case, the program explains the current clinical situation and provides advice about what to do next (Fig. 4). These built-in help features make it possible for the student to achieve a significant learning experience without the presence of an instructor.

The Sedation Simulator also creates a detailed record of each case simulation. The program records the simulated patient's vital signs every 30 seconds and all management options selected by the trainee. The time that incidents occur is also recorded. Response times and management decisions can be reviewed with the student at a later time to reinforce the learning experience. It is not necessary for an instructor to be present during the case simulation, and debriefing for a 30-minute case can be accomplished in just a few minutes, resulting in highly efficient use of instructor time. Typically students use the Sedation Simulator program alone, but feedback from residents indicates that working in pairs or small groups can also provide a favorable training experience.

Strong evidence indicates that use of screen-based simulation programs is an effective training method for medicine. In one study, use of the Anesoft ACLS Simulator software was shown to improve performance during simulated Mega Code management more than review of the ACLS textbook.[3] This study supports the use of the ACLS Simulator to review ACLS guidelines. In another study, the use of the Anesoft screen-based Anesthesia Simulator program was shown to improve response to simulated emergencies in a mannequin-based simulator.[4] Improvement in performance demonstrated in the mannequin-based simulator is predictive of improved response during a real anesthetic critical incident. In a third study, the use of the relatively inexpensive Anesoft screen-

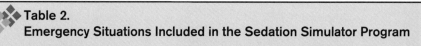

Table 2.
Emergency Situations Included in the Sedation Simulator Program

Agitation	Bradycardia	Hypotension
Anaphylaxis	Bronchospasm	Myocardial ischemia
Apnea	Hypertension	Tachycardia
Aspiration		

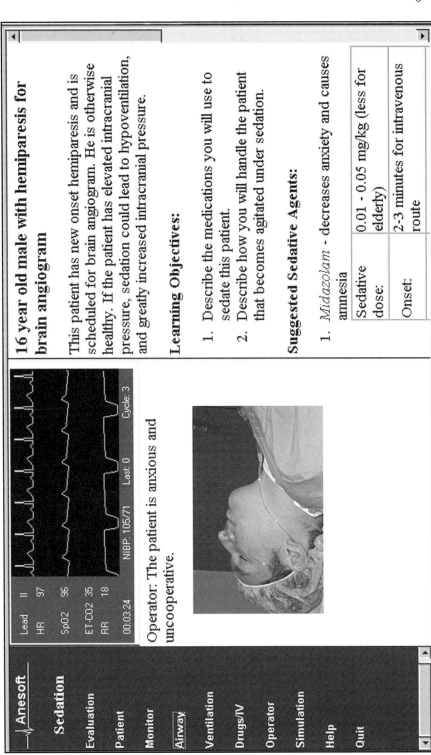

16 year old male with hemiparesis for brain angiogram

This patient has new onset hemiparesis and is scheduled for brain angiogram. He is otherwise healthy. If the patient has elevated intracranial pressure, sedation could lead to hypoventilation, and greatly increased intracranial pressure.

Learning Objectives:

1. Describe the medications you will use to sedate this patient.
2. Describe how you will handle the patient that becomes agitated under sedation.

Suggested Sedative Agents:

1. *Midazolam* - decreases anxiety and causes amnesia

Sedative dose:	0.01 - 0.05 mg/kg (less for elderly)
Onset:	2-3 minutes for intravenous route

Operator: The patient is anxious and uncooperative.

Figure 3. The Sedation Simulator presents learning objectives and suggested case management to inform students what they should be learning from each case.

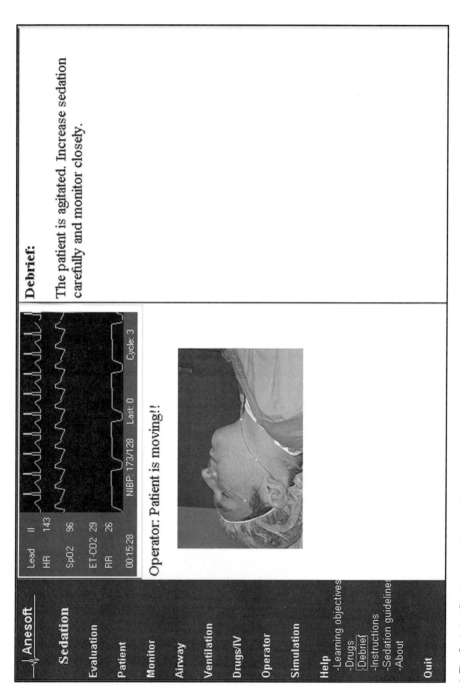

Figure 4. The Sedation Simulator provides a built-in consultant to tell students what they should do next at any point during the simulated case. This technique prevents frustration due to not knowing what to do next, as may occur with other simulation programs.

based Anesthesia Simulator program was shown to improve response to simulated emergencies as much as mannequin-based simulators.[5] The results showed that learning to manage simulated crisis situations such as anaphylactic shock did not vary significantly between mannequin-based simulators and computer screen-based simulators.

Mannequin-based Simulation for Sedation

In the sedation training course at the University of Washington, mannequin-based simulation scenarios are used to reinforce many of the cognitive and psychomotor aspects of patient care for procedural sedation. The cases involve procedures that are commonly scheduled for sedation and are designed to demonstrate general principles that all health care providers administering conscious sedation should know and understand. All of the cases involve issues not only surrounding airway management but also various intraprocedural decisions. Communication between the conscious sedation provider and the procedurist is emphasized. Because the trainees have already learned patient selection and evaluation, drug selection and administration, monitoring skills, and management of emergency situations in lectures and with the screen-based simulator, they can now concentrate on teamwork aspects of care, especially communication with other members of the team.

We use the SimMan simulator (Laerdal Corporation [www.laerdal.com]) in our conscious sedation training course. We selected SimMan over the METI human patient simulator (Medical Education Technologies, Inc. [www.meti.com]) because we were not teaching physiology or pharmacology with the mannequin-based simulator and found SimMan to be easier to program for our sedation scenarios. We believed that the airway and mask ventilation were more realistic with SimMan than with the METI simulator. In addition, SimMan was lighter and more portable and easier to turn on its side for the colonoscopy scenario. Shortcomings of SimMan included lack of voice and nonresponsive eyes. Because voice response is an essential element of conscious sedation, we found it necessary to add a speaker allowing trainees to assess level of response. Mannequin eyelid and pupillary response would significantly improve the quality of the simulation experience for conscious sedation training.

We use four mannequin-based simulation scenarios in our sedation training course. Each scenario is designed to generate a discussion between the person managing the sedation and the person performing the procedure. Decisions must be made whether to continue the procedure and how to manage the patient after the procedure. Four trainees participate in the simulated scenarios. They are trained in groups, with no individual in "the hot seat," to maximize the training experience and minimize stress. One trainee administers the sedative agents and monitors the patient, and the second and third trainees act as assistants. The fourth trainee records the case management, using a checklist designed specifically for that scenario. The simulations are not video-recorded, again to minimize the stress. After each scenario the participants discuss the case, reinforcing the learning objectives provided for each case.

The first simulated case is a 25-year-old man with osteoblastic sarcoma of the cervical vertebrae who is scheduled for Hickman line placement. The patient develops anaphylaxis to antibiotic administration with subsequent tachycardia, hypotension, unconsciousness, and apnea. In this scenario the trainees must develop a differential diagnosis, manage the intraprocedural emergency, handle the airway of an apneic patient, and decide how to manage the patient after the procedure.

The second scenario is a 41-year-old man with cervical disk disease wearing a cervical collar who is scheduled for vasectomy reversal. The patient develops apnea shortly after the surgeon is called from the procedure room. The participants must mange an apneic patient with a difficult airway (cervical collar). The third scenario is a 49-year-old man with multiple hip surgeries, chronic pain, and heavy narcotic use who is scheduled for MRI of an infected hip prosthesis. The trainee must monitor the patient in a difficult situation because the mannequin is placed in a mock-up of the MRI scanner, complete with noise. The simulated patient becomes apneic during the procedure, and the participants must decide whether to abort an expensive procedure before it is completed. The trainees are encouraged to call in a mediator if the radiologist insists on continuing the procedure.

The fourth simulator scenario involves a patient who presents for his procedure in a condition much different from his preprocedure evaluation. A 76-year-old man is scheduled for a follow-up colonoscopy. The patient has been previously "cleared" for the procedure but presents with chest discomfort, mild shortness of breath, and ST segment depression on the electrocardiogram. The trainees must recognize that the procedure should not be started and that the patient needs immediate medical attention. If the participants elect to sedate the patient for the procedure, the chest discomfort progresses to crushing chest pain and cardiac arrest.

We have not formally evaluated the educational impact of the mannequin-based training. Chopra has shown that time spent in a simulator does improve performance,[6] but no studies have been undertaken that demonstrate clear advantages over more traditional teaching methods. On the other hand, the informal feedback provided by the sedation course participants has been highly favorable toward the use of the mannequin-based training.

Conclusion

Many skills are called into play during sedation of patients for procedures. Clearly stating the learning objectives for the course helps define the most efficient training method. Classroom teaching and the screen-based simulator effectively cover cognitive skills such as patient evaluation, drug selection and titration, monitoring, and management of emergencies. Management of the airway in unconscious, apneic patients is best learned in a clinical environment. Training with an anesthesiologist in the operating room or during procedures such as electroconvulsive therapy is an ideal method to learn these skills. Finally, teamwork and communication skills can be honed with the mannequin-based simulator.

Intravenous Conscious Sedation Simulation for Nonphysicians

Gary E. Loyd, MD, MMM

Howard Schwid reviewed the state of the art in computer-assisted and computer-based virtual reality simulation in relation to the teaching of conscious sedation. Other computer-assisted simulations have been reported. In 2000 Medina et al. described the development of a computerized simulator that can reproduce several critical incidents in both pediatric and adult patients receiving sedation for a variety of radiologic procedures.[7] Simulation improved the responses of health care workers as well as the responses of pediatric patients to noisy MRI scanners.[8] Blike et al. also used patient simulators to discover the responses of different personnel to sedation emergencies.[9] Not only have patient simulators been used to address the emergency situations surrounding conscious sedation, but they have also been used to provide instruction in conscious sedation, such as Farnsworth et al. did with nurses.[10] This chapter gives one approach to providing a course in conscious sedation to dental specialists in training at the University of Louisville. There was a perceived need in the School of Dentistry for adequate training in response to evidence that dentists in the community felt inadequate to care for medical emergencies.[11]

Reference texts specifically addressing the administration of sedation are available.[12–14] The initial instruction in conscious sedation for dental students at the University of Louisville is provided by faculty from the School of Dentistry, who themselves provide conscious sedation. Following an outline provided in the reference texts, the subjects taught by faculty include oral sedation, nitrous oxide administration, local anesthetics, and the dentist's approach to pediatric vs. adult patients. These topics are covered in a lecture format (Table 3). The Department of Anesthesiology provides instruction in intravenous (IV) conscious sedation as it relates to cardiovascular physiology, respiratory physiology, basic pharmacology, preprocedure patient evaluation (including physical diagnosis and appropriate patient selection), initiation of intravenous catheters, fluid administration, monitoring complications of IV sedation, common medical emergencies, basic resuscitation, the use of emergent drugs, and patient recovery/discharge.

Table 3.
Topics Covered in Lecture Format

Dental faculty presentations
- Oral sedation
- Nitrous oxide administration
- Local anesthetics
- Pediatric vs. adult patients

Anesthesiology faculty presentations
- Cardiovascular physiology
- Respiratory physiology
- Basic pharmacology
- Preprocedure patient evaluation
- Intravenous catheters cannulation
- IV fluid administration
- Patient monitoring
- Complications of IV sedation
- Common medical emergencies
- Basic resuscitation and complication management
- Emergency drugs use
- Patient recovery/discharge

This is a large list of topics to be covered in the eight hour hours allotted. These topics have evolved from a lecture-based format to a hands-on, active learning experience in the simulation laboratory. Under the lecture format, the students were required to have an anesthesiologist present for the first few cases, in which each student provided conscious sedation. This was a huge waste of nonreimbursable time for the anesthesiologist, and the patient was used as the real learning experience. With the current simulated patient approach, the dental faculty have become comfortable enough with the skills of the students at providing IV conscious sedation that they feel they can adequately and safely supervise the students. This approach frees the teaching time of the anesthesiologist and increases the level of care provided to the patients in the form of fewer IV sticks and a quicker provision of IV sedation without intervention of a teacher to provide coaching along the way. The rest of this chapter outlines the simulation portion of the course as it has been effectively presented to students.

Practical Active Teaching

The goal of the conscious sedation course is to enable the student to provide intravenous conscious sedation to the patient in a safe and professional manner. The course is not intended as a certification course, and no certificate of completion is offered, although it has been requested many times. Usually five to eight students/residents from a combination of general dentistry, periodontics and endodontics are present. Their motivations range from a desire to provide IV conscious sedation to patients in private practice to satisfying the requirements of their residency without any intention of providing IV conscious sedation outside the training environment. After the course, several students from the latter group have changed their attitudes and entertained the possibility of providing conscious sedation to their patients.

The simulation portion of the course is divided into two main sections. The first section is more teacher-centered, with the instructor pushing the agenda and doing much of the talking and simulator interactions. During the second section, the learners provide simulated conscious sedation to simulated patients and practice the skills that they have just learned. The first section begins with an introduction to the high-fidelity simulator, including how to feel for pulses and listen to breath and heart sounds. Students also learn how to work the equipment and monitors. Many of the students have never touched a stopcock or an IV catheter, spiked an intravenous bag of fluid, placed a blood pressure cuff, or attached EKG electrodes. Experience has demonstrated that the instructor should not assume that the student has experience at doing anything. One must inquire. The last portion of the introduction is to the IV conscious sedation documentation form (Fig. 5). This form provides the crux of where discussion and application begin. The sessions are purposely interactive, with the instructor probing for each learner's knowledge and skill baseline and assessing the progress of comprehension throughout the course.

The next part of this first section begins with a demonstration of how to provide uncomplicated IV conscious sedation to a patient without the interview process. Each step is described as it is performed, and each student fills out a dummy sedation form for practice. When sedation drugs are administered, the simulator is put in pause mode while the basic pharmacology of the administered drug is reviewed and the rationale for

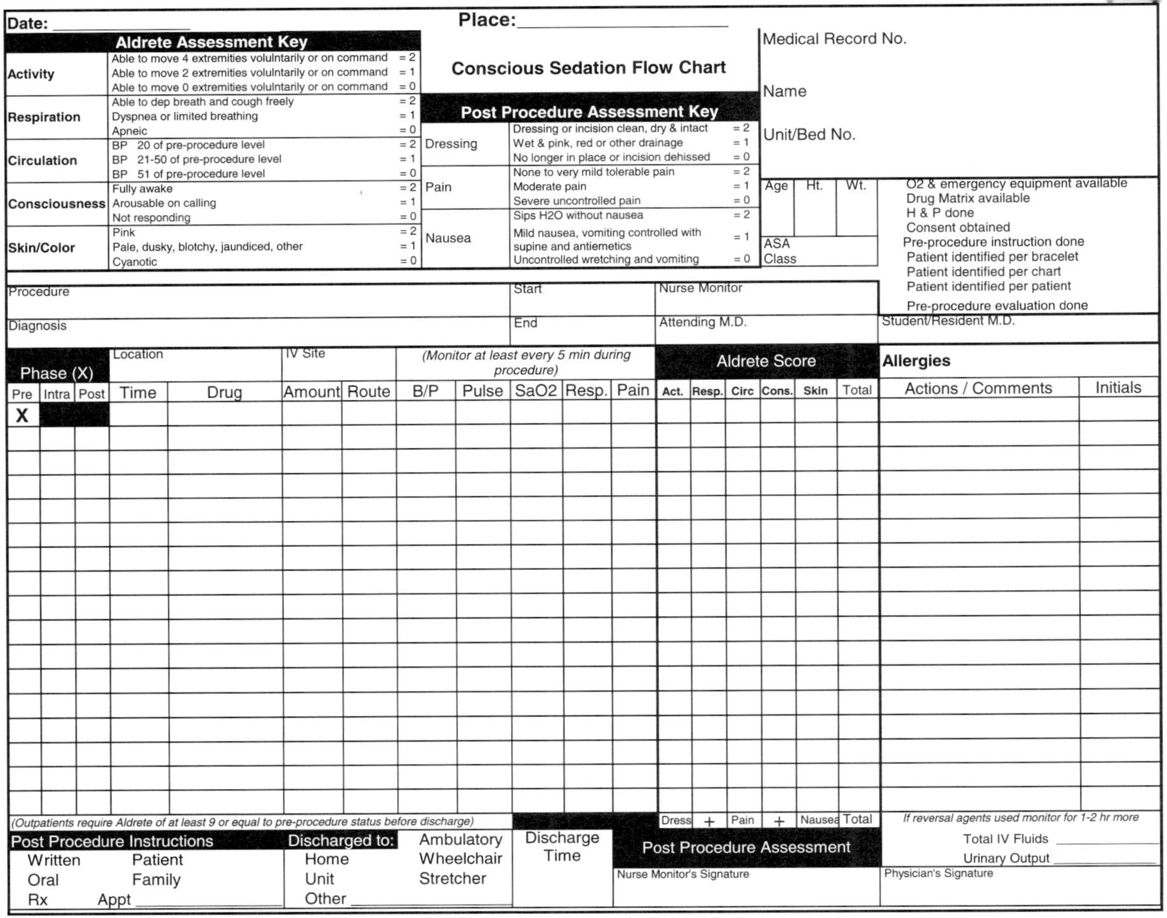

Conscious Sedation Flow Chart

Date: ___   Place: ___   Medical Record No. ___   Name ___   Unit/Bed No. ___   Age ___ Ht. ___ Wt. ___   ASA Class ___

Aldrete Assessment Key

Activity
- Able to move 4 extremities voluntarily or on command = 2
- Able to move 2 extremities voluntarily or on command = 1
- Able to move 0 extremities voluntarily or on command = 0

Respiration
- Able to dep breath and cough freely = 2
- Dyspnea or limited breathing = 1
- Apneic = 0

Circulation
- BP 20 of pre-procedure level = 2
- BP 21-50 of pre-procedure level = 1
- BP 51 of pre-procedure level = 0

Consciousness
- Fully awake = 2
- Arousable on calling = 1
- Not responding = 0

Skin/Color
- Pink = 2
- Pale, dusky, blotchy, jaundiced, other = 1
- Cyanotic = 0

Post Procedure Assessment Key

Dressing
- Dressing or incision clean, dry & intact = 2
- Wet & pink, red or other drainage = 1
- No longer in place or incision dehissed = 0

Pain
- None to very mild tolerable pain = 2
- Moderate pain = 1
- Severe uncontrolled pain = 0

Nausea
- Sips H2O without nausea = 2
- Mild nausea, vomiting controlled with supine and antiemetics = 1
- Uncontrolled wretching and vomiting = 0

Procedure ___   Diagnosis ___

Start ___ End ___   Nurse Monitor ___   Attending M.D. ___   Student/Resident M.D. ___

O2 & emergency equipment available / Drug Matrix available / H & P done / Consent obtained / Pre-procedure instruction done / Patient identified per bracelet / Patient identified per chart / Patient identified per patient / Pre-procedure evaluation done

Allergies ___

(Monitor at least every 5 min during procedure)

Phase (X) Pre	Intra	Post	Location	Time	Drug	Amount	Route	IV Site	B/P	Pulse	SaO2	Resp.	Pain	Actions / Comments	Initials
X															

Aldrete Score
Act.	Resp.	Circ	Cons.	Skin	Total

Post Procedure Assessment
Dress + Pain + Nausea = Total
Nurse Monitor's Signature ___

(Outpatients require Aldrete of at least 9 or equal to pre-procedure status before discharge)

Post Procedure Instructions: Written / Oral / Rx
Patient / Family / Appt

Discharged to: Home / Unit / Other
Ambulatory / Wheelchair / Stretcher

Discharge Time ___

If reversal agents used monitor for 1-2 hr more
Total IV Fluids ___   Urinary Output ___
Physician's Signature ___

Figure 5. Conscious sedation flow chart.

selection is provided in a mini-didactic. In addition to textbooks, each student is provided a supplemental packet of information covering all areas presented during the simulation sessions. The written test is derived from the textbook and handouts. After each mini-didactic, the sedation case proceeds. The simulator is again activated, and the evidence of the sedation is manifested in the simulator. At this point, basic cardiac and respiratory physiology is reviewed, since all of the students had these courses early in their training. When the procedure is finished, the recovery phase and discharge criteria are covered.

After the uncomplicated case, the more challenging patients and events are introduced. It has been reported that in general dentistry practices, the most common medical emergencies are vasovagal syncope, hypoglycemia, angina, seizure, choking, asthma, hypertensive crisis, anaphylaxis, myocardial infarction, and cardiac arrest.[11] The cardiovascular cases (myocardial ischemia with ACLS intervention, hypertensive crisis, hypotension, anaphylaxis) are presented first, because they are most likely to cause the patient's demise. ACLS is not covered as a didactic in the simulation, since all students must be certified in ACLS before they begin the IV conscious sedation course. With little history, a simulated sedation case is started. As the EKG begins to demonstrate ST depression, the case is paused, and discussion centers on basic EKG reading, preoperative history taking, differential heart sounds, the American Heart Association algorithm for cardiac work-ups, and the American Society of Anesthesiologists' physical classification system. Then the case is allowed to progress intermittently while treatment modalities and clinical correlations to the basic physiology and pathophysiology are presented. This portion of the course tends to be the most intense and takes the longest.

The anaphylaxis cases make a nice bridge into the respiratory cases. The same simulation format as with the cardiovascular cases is followed for the respiratory and neurologic cases. The respiratory cases include anaphylaxis, asthma attack, and oversedation. The oversedation case also makes a nice transition into the neurologic cases, which also cover hypoglycemia, seizures, and stroke. During the respiratory cases, airway management skills are taught, including intubation.

Basic portions of the preoperative evaluation, covered in the cardiovascular, respiratory, and neurologic portions of the course, are now pulled together with the addition of other data gathering as well as interpersonal communication. A sample of a form used is presented in Figure 6. The students learn how to obtain the information quickly while relieving as much of the patient's anxiety with interpersonal skills as possible. Patient selection is an important part of providing a safe, sedated experience. The learners are allowed to practice history taking and basic physical examinations on either the instructor or standardized patients. The interpersonal experience does much to relieve the anxiety of the students in preparation for their real experience.

After the practice of the preoperative evaluation, the students obtain hands-on practice at providing the entire IV conscious sedation experience. The instructor removes him- or herself from the scene (behind a one-way mirror is best, but a corner of the room can work) so that students can gain experience in simulation. The different cases are randomly presented so that the students are challenged to detect and treat. While two or three students are acting out the functions of the sedation team, the other students are practicing IV catheter skills on mannequins. The simulation portion of this course has

Sedation Pre & Postoperative Evaluation

Proposed Procedure

Patient Identification

Preoperative Diagnosis

Date Scheduled | **Date Assessed**

Student/resident | **Attending faculty for the case**

Allergies

NKDA ☐

Sex M ☐ F ☐ **Age:** **Height:** **Weight:**

NPO Status:

Medical Problem List / Status

	Y	N	Systems Review
			Smoking History
			ETOH History
			Drug Abuse
			Neuro/Seizure
			Respiratory
			Cardiovascular
			Renal
			Endocrine
			Contag. Dz
			Bleeding Disorder
			GI/Reflux
			Preg/LMP

CXR

EKG

Physical Exam

Neuro

Oral

Neck

Lungs

Heart

Other

Medications

Past Surgeries / Anesthetics

Vital Signs			
Date / Time			
B / P			
Pulse			
Resp			
Temp			

Laboratory Data			
Date / Time			
Hgb			
Hct			
Platelets			
WBC			
NA			
K			
Cl			
CO2			
Glucose			
BUN			
Creatinine			
Ca / Mg			
PT / PTT			
INR			
ACT			
Beta HCG			
ABG PH			
ABG PCO2			
ABG PO2			
FiO2			
Vent TV			
Vent Rate			
Vent Peep			
Vent PSV			
Vent PIP			

IV Access

Bld/FFP Type & Avail

Prior Positioning Problems Y ☐ N ☐ N/A ☐

Family Hx of Anes Comp Y ☐ N ☐ N/A ☐

ASA Physical Status

1 2 3 4 5 6 E

Sedation Plan

Informed Consent Obtained

Y ☐ N ☐ N/A ☐

Preoperative Evaluation Reviewed by:

Attending Faculty Signature:

Date: **Postoperative Note**

Time:

Signature:

Figure 6. Sedation pre- and postoperative evaluation form been performed at the University of Louisville in a total of eight hours. One anecdotal attempt was made at shortening the learning experience to six hours, but the students were not able to adequately perform the IV sedation in the simulated cases and required an additional two hours of practice.

Conclusion

The value of patient- and computer-assisted simulations is being discovered in many arenas. They have been used to identify the weaknesses in health care providers' responses to emergencies related to conscious sedation, the training of personnel in providing conscious sedation, and the alleviation of much of the anxiety that patients feel about the procedures. The outline of a course proven to produce health care providers capable of administering conscious sedation safely has been described. Much work still remains to be done, and the best methods of providing the optimal education and training in conscious sedation still need to be elucidated.

References

1. Schwid HA, Miller K: Sedation Simulator. Anesoft Corporation. Issaquah, WA, 2002. Available at www.anesoft.com. Last accessed 11/3/03.
2. Medina LS, Racadio JM, Schwid HA: Computers in radiology. The sedation, analgesia, and contrast media computerized simulator: A new approach to train and evaluate radiologists' responses to critical incidents. Pediatr Radiol 2000;30(5):299 305.
3. Schwid HA, Rooke GA, Ross BK, Sivarajan M: Use of a computerized ACLS simulator improves retention of ACLS guidelines better than textbook review. Crit Care Med 1999;27:821–824.
4. Schwid HA, Ross BK, Rooke GA, Michalowski P: Screen-based anesthesia simulator with debriefing improves performance in a mannequin-based anesthesia simulator. Teach Learn Med 2001;13:92–96.
5. Nyssen AS, Larbuisson R, Janssens M, Pendeville P, Mayne A: A comparison of the training value of two types of anesthesia simulators: Computer screen-based and mannequin-based simulators. Anesth Analg 2002;94:1560–1565.
6. Chopra V, Gesink J, de Jong J, et al: Does training on an anesthesia simulator lead to improvement in performance? Br J Anaesth 1994;73:293–297.
7. Medina LS, Racadio JM, Schwid HA: The sedation, analgesia, and contrast media computerized simulator: A new approach to train and evaluate radiologists' responses to critical incidents. Pediatr Radiol 2000;30:299–305.
8. Rosenberg DR, et al: Magnetic resonance imaging of children without sedation: Preparation with simulation. J Am Acad Child Adolesc Psychiatry 1997;36(6):853–859.
9. Blike G, Cravero J, Nelson E: Same patients, same critical events—different systems of care, different outcomes: Description of a human factors approach aimed at improving the efficacy and safety of sedation/analgesia care. Qual Manag Health Care 2001;10:17–36.
10. Farnsworth ST, et al: Teaching sedation and analgesia with simulation. J Clin Monit Comput 2000;16(4):273–285.
11. Girdler NM, Smith DG: Prevalence of emergency events in British dental practice and emergency management skills of British dentists. Resuscitation 1999;41:159–167.
12. Malamed SF: Sedation: A Guide to Patient Management, 4th ed. St. Louis, Mosby, 2002, p 608.
13. Malamed SF: Medical Emergencies in the Dental Office, 5th ed. St. Louis, Mosby, 2000, p 529.
14. Park R, Sladen RN: Sedation and Analgesia in the Critically Ill. London: Blackwell Science, 1995, p 216.

Chapter 26

SIMULATION FOR CONTINUING HEALTH PROFESSIONAL EDUCATION

Adam I. Levine, MD

Maintaining medical competence requires a lifelong commitment to learning. The exponential rise of medical knowledge and technology heightens the demand that practicing health care providers continuously acquire and master new information and skills throughout their careers or risk becoming clinically obsolete. The Association of American Medical Colleges recognizes that "continuing medical education (CME) is the predominant mechanism by which health-care providers maintain their clinical competence."[1] Specialty boards use the certification and recertification process to acknowledge and verify clinical competence. For practitioners deemed clinically incompetent, evaluation and remediation processes exist.

Since their inception, medical simulators have been eagerly and successfully incorporated into continuing education (CE) activities. This enthusiasm has led the way to dedicated simulator meetings, integration of simulation into established CE forums and workshops, traveling and mobile simulator-based CE activities, and expansion of regional simulator centers devoted to conducting CE courses. The eagerness of the health care community to use simulations for CE has not been mirrored in their use for evaluation, certification, and remediation of the practicing health care provider. This chapter discusses continuing education, certification, and remediation as well as the present and future roles of simulation for such activities.

Continuing Health Care Education

Oversight
Accreditation Council for Continuing Medical Education (ACCME)
The ACCME is the prevailing accrediting body governing CME activities.[2] Through a voluntary self-regulated system of accreditation, the ACCME carries out its mission to "identify, develop, and promote standards for quality CME" (Table 1). The ACCME identifies and sets standards for appropriate CME content, providers, activities, and educational modalities. CME, as defined by the ACCME, is the process of lifelong learning that serves to maintain, develop, or increase the knowledge, skills, professionalism, and relationships used by physicians in the care of patients. Such activities support physicians' learning and improvement, which contribute to their maintenance of competence, licensure, certification, and privileges. According to the ACCME:

> [T]he content of accredited CME must be the body of knowledge and skills generally recognized and accepted by the profession as facilitating the delivery of effective health care. The content must also be based on sound scientific

> ### ◆ Table 1.
> ### Primary Responsibilities of the ACCME
>
> 1. Set and administer standards and criteria for providers of quality CME for physicians and related professionals.
> 2. Certify that accredited providers are capable of meeting the requirements of the ACCME.
> 3. Relate CME to medical care and the continuum of medical education.
> 4. Evaluate the effectiveness of its policies.
> 5. Assist providers in continually improving their programs.
> 6. Assure physicians, the public, and the CME community that CME programs meet the ACCME's criteria for compliance.

evidence generally accepted within the profession of medicine. The ACCME recognizes that CME activities will take many forms, including lecture, workshop, printed and computer-based materials. Such activities can be conducted through person-to-person encounters, electronically mediated activities or any combination of the aforementioned.

American Medical Association (AMA)

The AMA is the other organization responsible for CME oversight. The AMA also provides definitions of CME and guidelines for acceptable courses, educational content, and providers.[3] The AMA established a nationally recognized CME credit system and a means to recognize CME accomplishments. In 1968, the AMA established an AMA Physician's Recognition Award (PRA) category 1 CME credit system. A physician can receive the PRA by obtaining a specific amount of AMA PRA category 1 credits. Receiving the PRA demonstrates the physician's dedication to continuing clinical competency and satisfies many states' requirements of CME for relicensure. The AMA also established guidelines for CME training designed to teach new skills and procedures. Four levels of training achievements have been defined and must be verified by the CME provider and used for certification[3] (Table 2).

Requirements for Participation in CME

International, national, state, and local institutions require health care providers to participate in a minimum number of CME credit hours per year to maintain certification, licensure, and clinical privileges. In the United Kingdom physicians are required to participate in continuing professional development.[4] Twenty-three of the 24 American medical specialty boards have time limits on specialty certification and require re-

> ### ◆ Table 2.
> ### Levels of Training Achievement
>
> Level 1: Verification of attendance
> Level 2: Verification of satisfactory completion of course objectives
> Level 3: Verification of proctor readiness (can perform procedure under supervision)
> Level 4: Verification of physician competence to perform the procedure (perform procedure without supervision)

certification every 7–10 years.[5] Required recertification moves participation in CME toward a mandatory process.[6] Two-thirds of all states and U.S. territories require participation in a minimum of 12 to 50 CME credit hours per year for state licensure renewal,[7] and many hospital medical boards require CME for continuing privileges and staff reappointment.

Like physicians, dentists and nurses have continuing education requirements. The opportunities for the use of simulation in dentistry and nursing education are detailed in other chapters. For example, requirements for dental continuing eductation and nursing continuing education in the commonwealth of Kentucky are summarized in Tables 3 and 4, respectively. Similar requirements are found in the statutes of other states and provinces.

Goals and Objectives

Continuing medical education is the mainstay by which health care professionals retain and review previously mastered material, learn new and current standards of care, and develop and practice new skills. For CME to be relevant, it is expected to initiate a change in behavior and to enhance physician performance, resulting in improved patient outcome.[8]

In an attempt to reform and improve CME, the American College of Obstetricians and Gynecologists organized a conference in 1997 to discuss and outline principles for effective CME. The conference produced eight principles for CME that can serve as a guide to CME providers across all specialties for improvement in their CME activities:[9]

1. CME planning and program development should be based on needs assessment including outcome data.

2. The goals of CME should include the development of skills necessary for lifelong learning, the exercise of clinical reasoning, an understanding of the decision-making process, and the specific content acquisition.

3. The multiple goals of CME should be reinforced by the appropriate choice of learning method.

4. Incorporation of new instructional technologies for CME should be based on their intrinsic strengths as learning tools after thorough evaluation.

5. Faculty development is important within CME and should include exposure to new learning methods (theory and application), enabling faculty to translate their content expertise into formats more appropriate to learners' needs.

6. Professional and, whenever possible, interdisciplinary interaction should be given priority in CME programming.

7. Educational activities should be supportive of and coordinated with the transition to evidence-based medicine.

8. Outcomes-based measures of CME effectiveness and research should be introduced into the determinants of physicians' practice behaviors.

Continuing Professional Development

The Standing Committee on Postgraduate Medical and Dental Education (SCOPME) in the United Kingdom, in an effort to expand the scope of CME, recommended that CME include management, teaching, and research concepts that more appropriately reflect the roles of modern physicians (Table 5). SCOPME's recommendations led to the development of continuing professional development (CPD).[10]

Table 3.

Requirements for Dental Continuing Education in Kentucky

KRS 313.080 and 313.305 require a dentist to accumulate continuing education credits as a condition of license renewal. Each licensed dentist requesting renewal of license shall fulfill requirements for three categories.

Category A

1. Complete a two-hour course on HIV/AIDS every ten years.
2. Complete a basic life support (BLS) course certified by the American Heart Association or a cardiopulmonary resuscitation CPR course certified by the American Red Cross and maintain certification.

Category B: Complete 20 hours of scientific dental-based courses given in a classroom presentation format.

Category C: Complete 10 hours of CE from scientific dental-based courses given in a classroom presentation format, business, home study, magazine/journal articles, computer or video articles, or non-dental health-related courses.

Sixty minutes of participation in a classroom presentation course equals one point. Sixty minutes of participation in a business course shall receive one point, or one business point shall be approved for attendance at the following types of meetings: local dental, regional dental, national dental, dental specialty, study club dental, hospital staff, or nursing home meetings. Two business points shall be granted for attendance at an annual state meeting.

Table 4.

Requirements for Nursing Continuing Education in Kentucky

Registered nurse continuing education requires one of the following:

1. Proof of earning 30 approved contact hours—two of the 30 must be an approved HIV/AIDS course or
2. A national certification or recertification related to the nurse's practice role (in effect during the entire period or initially earned during the period), plus two contact hours of an approved HIV/AIDS course or
3. Proof of earning 15 approved contact hours, including two contact hours of an approved HIV/AIDS course, plus at least one of the following: completion of a nursing research project as principal investigator, coinvestigator, or project director; publication of a nursing-related article in a refereed professional publication; a professional nursing educational presentation that is made to other health professionals, at least one hour in length, not part of the licensee's primary job function, and evidenced by a program brochure, course syllabi or letter from the offering provider documenting licensee's presentation; a nursing employment evaluation that is satisfactory for continued employment (must be signed by supervisor with the name, address, and phone number of the employer); a successfully completed nursing employment competency validation (validated by employer with the name, address, and phone number of employer).

Table 5.

Continuing Professional Development Principles

1. Patient care
2. Teaching
3. Communication
4. Team working
5. Familiarity with the law
6. Knowledge of relevant ethical issues
7. Management
8. Information techology
9. Audit
10. Research

Effectiveness of Continuing Education

The cost devoted to producing CE activities in the United States approaches one billion dollars a year.[11] This enormous investment pales in comparison with the incalculable cost to society if CE fails to meet its goals. Guaranteeing CE effectiveness is essential to the well-being of the health-care system. Despite this fact, the majority of the 2500 accredited CE providers in the United States still utilize traditional learning activities, such as grand rounds and lectures,[12] which generally fail to significantly affect clinical practice or health care outcome.[13] How, then, can CE maintain its relevance and achieve the desired goals of improved health care? Many CE providers have questioned the effectiveness of their CE activities and in doing so have sought solutions to improving CE outcomes. Understanding and incorporating learning theory into CE activities as well as assessing CE outcome have taken center stage in the attempt to improve CE effectiveness.

Learning Theory and CME

Since its inception, adult learning theory, introduced by Knowles,[14] has been a key component of CE design. Although never validated, the concepts of Knowles' theory are used in an attempt to develop effective CE programs. Knowles suggested that people learn differently throughout their lives. He asserted that adults are self-directed, problem-based learners who rely on previous experience to learn from and to determine what they need to know. He assumed that adult learners are self-motivated and self-directed and can readily assess their own strengths and weakness[14] (Table 6).

Factors Influencing CE Effectiveness.

What factors determine CE effectiveness? To answer this question, a review of the CE literature was conducted by Davis and associates to determine whether formal CE is effective and under what conditions formal CE can initiate a change in performance and patient outcome. The studies reviewed included a wide range of CE formats, such as conferences, refresher courses, seminars, lectures, and workshops, and explored the effect of formal CE on American, Canadian, and French internists, pediatricians, and family practitioners. The authors concluded that "interactive CME sessions that enhance participant activity and provide the opportunity to practice skills can effect change in professional practice and, on occasion, health care outcome." They also concluded that "didactic sessions alone do not appear to be effective in changing physician performance."[15]

Not surprisingly, increased learner participation and interaction between educator and student also increased overall satisfaction with the teaching program.[16] Cantillion and Jones determined that, although interactive experience is important, it is much more effective for the adult learner when it is accompanied by feedback, suggesting

---

◈ Table 6.
Adult Learning Theory Principles

1. Adults are self-directed in the planning and evaluation of their learning.
2. Adults learn through experience.
3. Adults have a problem-solving approach to learning.
4. Adults learn best what is relevant and useful.

that effective CE should contain feedback.[17] The concept of feedback was supported by Reiter and associates, who determined that adults are not innately self-directed learners who can accurately assess their own strengths and weakness.[18] Smith et al. examined whether interactive didactic sessions, such as problem-based learning sessions, were more effective than traditional activities. The authors concluded that problem-based learning is no more effective for increasing physician performance than other educational strategies.[19]

Why, then, does traditional didactic-based CE persist, despite the knowledge that hands-on, interactive sessions with feedback appear to be the most effective format for initiating behavioral change and resulting in improved performance and possibly improved patient outcome? Several answers have been suggested including, ease of course design, cost, and dependence on traditional undergraduate models of education.[15]

Simulation for Continuing Education

Simulator-based, interactive, hands-on educational experiences are ideal vehicles to ensure CE effectiveness. It is not surprising, therefore, that the medical community has embraced the use of simulation for CE activities. Since their inception, anesthesia simulators have been adopted by many specialties. As technology improves and more and more specialties incorporate simulation into their undergraduate education, it is likely that simulator use will play a major role in the future of CE and CPD. This enthusiasm has also led the way to the development of an international simulator meeting dedicated to disseminating information about medical simulators. Currently numerous simulator products are commercially available, ranging from full-scale human simulators to part-task surgical and procedure-based products. This section presents the history of medical simulation-based meetings. Simulator use for the continuing education of practicing heath care providers is also discussed, along with the advantages and disadvantages for incorporating such simulators into CE activities.

Dedicated Simulator Meetings

In 1995, the Department of Anesthesiology at the University of Rochester hosted the First Conference on Simulators in Anesthesiology Education, which was the first meeting developed and organized for the sole purpose of discussing and disseminating information about anesthesia simulators.[20] The second such conference, also hosted by the University of Rochester, took place in the spring of 1996. The goals and objectives for this meeting were similar to those of the first. Due to the ever-increasing interest in simulation, the third annual Rochester simulator meeting took place in the winter of 1998 as a joint meeting with the Society for Technology in Anesthesia (STA).[21] Broadening the goals and objectives, the meeting was intended to expand the target audience beyond anesthesiology and to include simulators and simulation applications from other medical fields. In 1999, the first International Meeting on Medical Simulation (IMMS) was launched as a component of the STA's annual meeting. Now in its fourth year (2003), the IMMS is the preeminent international simulator meeting designed to accommodate a broad target audience from academic medicine, private clinical practice, and industry. The meeting, which grants up to 16 hours of CME credit sponsored by the STA, serves to provide an educational and research forum for the medical simulator community; to offer opportunities for hands-on learning using various simulators; to present current research in the use of simulators for medical education; to provide a forum to learn about future simulator technologies; and to provide a forum for industry to try new simulator products.[21]

Use of Simulation in Established Anesthesiology Conferences

In addition to dedicated simulator-based meetings, simulator use and discussion have been incorporated into pre-existing national and local meetings. Most notably, the Society for Education in Anesthesia (SEA) conducted a dedicated simulator meeting of its own and since has periodically included simulator-related workshops and discussion during its broader educational meetings.[22] For years simulator utilization has been incorporated into established workshops on thoracic anesthesia and airway management at the American Society of Anesthesiology's annual meetings[23] and the Post-Graduate Assembly of the New York State Society for Anesthesiology.[24] Although conducting hands-on, individual simulator sessions at a large conference can pose significant logistic problems, with proper planning it has been demonstrated to be highly successful.[25] International meetings such as the South African Congress of Anesthesiologists and the Association of Southeast Asian Nations (ASEAN) Congress of Anesthesiologists have provided simulator-based management training for several years.

Use of Full-scale Patient Simulators for Continuing Education

Originally known as anesthesia simulators, full-scale, mannequin-based patient simulators have since been incorporated into a variety of medical specialty CE programs, including emergency medicine, intensive care, radiology, and obstetrics/gynecology. Understandably, anesthesiologists have led the way to readily incorporate patient simulators into educational endeavors, including undergraduate and CE activities. There are numerous CE applications for full-scale simulators. Of particular interest is the use of full-scale simulators to allow practicing health care providers the opportunity to use new pharmacologic agents, to learn and perfect clinical skills and techniques not available or not mastered during training, and to refresh crisis management techniques.

Introduction of New Drugs into Practice

In a novel application, patient simulators were successfully used to introduce and educate practicing anesthesiologists about remifentanil, a newly developed, potent, ultra-short-acting narcotic.[26] Due to remifentanil's unique characteristics, the Food and Drug Administration (FDA) strongly recommended that the manufacturer make an effort to introduce the agent to practicing anesthesiologists prior to its use in the clinical setting. From 1996 through 1997, a "traveling simulator course" was developed to educate 836 practitioners in 58 cities. With a technically challenging and impractically expensive mobile unit of equipment, simulators, technicians, and educators, practitioners were able to participate in hands-on, interactive simulator sessions that illustrated remifentanil's unique characteristics in their hometown or local hospital. The simulated environment gave participants the ability to use an agent with which they had little, if any, clinical experience before using it on actual patients. The simulator also gave participants the ability to experiment with new techniques or try different techniques on the same patient. Due to the abilities of the simulator, participants could also obtain information that would otherwise not be available in real clinical situations, such as visual outputs of plasma and effector site drug levels. During and immediately after the sessions, participants were able to ask questions and receive timely feedback about the drug and their own performance. The overwhelming response from the practitioners was positive; with 81% stating that the simulator environment was an excellent means to learn about a new agent. Seventy-three percent of the responders reported that the simulator experience changed their perception of remifentanil. Unfortunately, follow-up surveys to assess actual clinical impact from the educational experience were not obtained.

Anesthesia Crisis Resource Management (ACRM)

The use of full-scale simulators for training practicing anesthesiologist in the skills associated with ACRM has received much attention. These skills are undoubtedly new to many practicing anesthesiologists because there is little formal education in resource management and decision-making during crises in anesthesia residency training. Holzman and associates demonstrated that ACRM skills could be taught to practicing anesthesiologists using a full-scale simulator.[27] They also demonstrated that the anesthesiologists viewed the experience favorably. In addition, it has been shown that, despite being intimidated and anxious, practicing anesthesiologists overwhelmingly viewed the experience as rewarding and said that it contributed to their education.[28] To date, however, it has yet to be shown whether attending ACRM courses improves physician performance or patient outcome. CRM course are currently available at many dedicated simulator centers throughout the country, offering sessions for anesthesiologists as well as surgeons, critical care physicians, emergency medicine physicians, radiologists, and obstetricians -gynecologists.

Miscellaneous Use of Full-scale Patient Simulators for Continuing Education

Not surprisingly, full-scale patient simulators have been adopted by an ever-increasing number of medical specialties to successfully educate physicians in a variety of courses, including advanced trauma life support (ATLS),[29] neonatal resuscitation,[30] combat warfare readiness,[31] and intensive care training.[32] As more specialty educators see the benefit and adoptability of full-scale simulation in their own educational programs, more and more practicing physicians, from a variety of specialties, will have the benefit of exposure to simulator-based education during CE activities.

Limitations to the Use of Full-scale Simulation for Continuing Education

Unproven Technology

The widespread use of simulation in the medical community may be limited by several factors, such as the current lack of evidence for clinical transference of skills and abilities learned in a simulator. Such factors will affect other considerations, such as cost and inconvenience. It needs to be determined whether the cost of such CE activities is warranted. Although it seems logical that small group interactive simulator sessions would be the ideal mechanism for continuing medical competence,[15] research demonstrating that simulator-based CE is superior to other formats has not been done.

Logistics and Expense

Several venues for full-scale simulator-based CE have been discussed, including dedicated mobile units,[26] temporary simulator laboratories set up at major conferences,[25] and permanent dedicated simulator centers.[27] Each of these options possesses unique and common advantages and logistical and economic concerns. Each requires the presence of a full-scale simulator; ancillary equipment to run the simulator, such as gas and power supplies; and clinical equipment, such as ventilators and monitors. Each also requires the presence of skilled simulator educators and supporting staff and technicians.

Establishing a dedicated center avoids the logistics of moving the equipment, but the participants must be willing to pay for and take time out to travel. In addition, dedicated centers must consider their start-up and operating costs; devoted simulator sessions for a small group of participants can be expensive (see Chapter 5). Mobile units are certainly convenient for participants and allow a significant number of health care providers to be exposed to simulation, but in logistic terms arriving at new, unfamiliar sites with expensive delicate equipment is extremely difficult and expensive. Temporary simulator set-ups at established conferences involve the same logistic issues as the mobile option but allow exposure of the greatest number of participants to simulator-based education in the shortest time span. Guaranteeing individual, high-quality time on the simulator unfortunately can be difficult without proper planning,[25] but participants can also take advantage of the other learning opportunities at the conference while waiting their turn. Simulator-based CE is currently expensive and logistically difficult compared with traditional CE formats. Overhead expenses are not discussed in existing literature, nor are the costs per student to execute these programs. Studies to explore financial issues are warranted at this time.

In an attempt to maximize participant numbers and reduce cost, Cooper and associates explored the use of telecommunications to transmit a simulated scenario from a dedicated simulator center to several remote locations.[33] Although the participants viewed the experience as extremely positive, further study is needed to determine whether this format has any educational benefit over traditional methods.

As technology improves and becomes less expensive, mobile full-scale simulators will become commercially available, and as more health care providers become interested in participating in simulator CE activities, the cost of such activities will undoubtedly decrease.

The "Oscopies" Surgical and Procedural Part-task Trainers

During the past two decades rapidly expanding technology has rendered the ability to learn and master new surgical techniques and complex procedures after residency training paramount in the maintenance of clinical surgical competence. Due to this rapid expansion, many practicing surgeons were not exposed to minimally invasive surgical techniques during their residency training. Unlike open procedures, minimally invasive techniques, used by many surgical disciplines, require proficiency in ambidextrous maneuvers with unique instruments, enhanced hand-eye coordination, and depth perception.[34] In the past traditional methods for teaching minimally invasive techniques to practicing physicians have included apprenticeships with other certified laparoscopic surgeons and attending courses involving practice with animal models.[35] Perhaps the parallel advances in computer technology and capabilities that have enabled a rapid development in virtual reality visualization and simulation technology may be the answer[36] to creating a more efficient and effective means to help current and future surgeons learn new technology.

Currently, procedural and surgical simulators are commercially available for a variety of medical, dental, and nursing specialties.[34–38] What roles do minimally invasive surgical simulators play in CME? Can these simulators be used to train novice as well as experts in new and challenging surgical procedures? Although the data are promising and many investigators have demonstrated that using simulators gives the novice the dexterity skills of a more proficient operator[39–41] that may, in fact, be transferable to the clinical environment,[42–44] to date no commercially available laparoscopy simulator has been developed that teaches complete surgical procedures. The future and CE application of virtual reality simulators is wide open. Based on the rapid development of these high-fidelity, compact, relatively inexpensive devices, one may postulate that in the near future full and interactive procedures will be available and apprenticeship and animal utilization will be modalities of the past.

Combining Simulator Technology for Enhanced Experiences in Continuing Education

Incorporation of several simulator technologies into CE courses can be highly successful and effective. Using specialty-specific part-task trainers (e.g., intravenous, endoscopy, and bronchoscopy simulators) that have adult and pediatric capabilities in combination with full-scale simulators, one can create an entire simulated clinical environment specifically targeted to the needs of pediatrics, pediatric and adult critical care, pulmonary medicine, and GI physicians. Training of nurses and technicians to assist with these procedures can also be accomplished in the simulated environment.

Computer- and Internet-based Simulation for Self-directed Continuing Education

There are many opportunities to satisfy CE obligations via computer-based educational programs. Many companies offer such simulator-based products for CE credit for a variety of specialties and formats. These products typically include a didactic as well as a scenario section for participant interaction. One merely needs to query an Internet search engine to find numerous opportunities to participate and receive credit in self-directed, Internet-based CE courses. Several companies accredited by the ACCME offer software-based courses in areas such as ACLS, anesthesia, bioterrorism, critical care, hemodynamics, and sedation. Participants can receive credit hours in category 1 of the Physician's Recognition Award of the AMA. Computer-based simulation is a cost-effective, efficient means to educate and has been shown to improve retention compared with printed material.[47]

Certification and Recertification of Health Care Providers

The process of certification and recertification serves to acknowledge and document the maintenance of clinical competency. The ACGME defines six areas of competency: patient care (including clinical reasoning), medical knowledge, practice-based learning (including information management), interpersonal and communication skills, professionalism, and systems-based practice (including health economics and teamwork).[48] Assessment of these domains, however, is complex and imperfect.

The three most commonly used assessment methods are subjective evaluations by supervising clinicians, multiple choice examinations to evaluate factual knowledge, and abstract problem-solving.[49] Most specialty boards rely on written multiple choice exams with or without an additional oral examination. Although multiple choice examinations offer excellent reliability in the evaluation of knowledge and problem-solving,[50] clinical skills and application cannot be assessed. Slogoff and associates suggest that the certification by the American Board of Anesthesiology is valid because certification rates correlated positively with subjective assessment of resident abilities by program directors.[51]

Simulation for Certification and Recertification

Is there a role for medical simulation in the certification process of heath care providers? Can the addition of simulation to the process improve assessment of practicing physicians? In an attempt to validate the use of simulation for assessment, research has established the reliability of evaluating performance in a simulator[52–55] and the ability of performance in a simulator to predict the participant's level of training.[38, 39,56] Although the feasibility of evaluating resident and medical student performance with simulation[57,58] has been explored, to date there is a dearth of material examining the use of simulators for certification and recertification of practicing health care providers.

Although the American Society of Anesthesiology appointed an ad hoc committee to examine the use of simulators for a number of functions,[23] the use of simulation for certification and recertification has gained little momentum. Lampe stated that the use of simulators to assess performance is in its infancy,[59] and in 1998 Kapur and Steadman suggested many reasons why full-scale simulation was not ready to be incorporated into the certification process.[60] The authors concluded that "the role of such patient simulators in clinical competency evaluation, insofar as performance in the simulator environment predicts future patient outcome, is not at all clear." They add that "much research is needed for the development of appropriate scenarios with objective and unbiased testing and scoring strategies." Studies are ongoing to establish validity and reliability for certification/recertification use.

For the medical community to embrace simulation for certification, many events must first take place, including development of cost-effective simulators with improved physical signs, validation of simulated scenarios and physiologic responses, and the widespread adoption of simulation for medical education. Given the rate of technologic development, societal demand for improved health care and reduced medical errors, and the broad acceptance of simulation for education by health care providers, it is highly likely that practitioners some day will have to demonstrate and maintain their competence via simulation.

Evaluation and Remediation of Incompetent Health Care Providers

Rapidly emerging medical technology and innovations require practicing health care professionals to continuously maintain clinical competence. Those who do not keep pace with the exponential rise in medical knowledge may find themselves to be judged as clinically incompetent, posing a risk to patients and society. Peer-reviewed incidents, continuing quality assurance, and litigation have created the need for evaluation and assessment of incompetent practitioners. Many states have mechanisms to evaluate and mandate remediation of incompetent health care providers through mandatory CE.[61] It has been observed that moderately to severely incompetent physicians did not improve after traditional remedial continuing medical education.[62] Perhaps there is a superior evaluation and screening process for physicians, dentists, or nurses who may be better candidates for remediation?

Simulation in the Evaluation and Remediation of Incompetent Practitioners

Can simulation improve the evaluation and screening of incompetent health care providers and predict which practitioners will have success in remediation programs?

Rosenblatt et al. determined that using a full-scale simulator to evaluate an anesthesiologist with lapsed medical skills facilitated the decision to recommend and prescribe a remedial program for the practitioner.[63] Based on traditional methods of assessment, such as written and oral examinations, the physician was determined to have such a severe lapse of medical knowledge that the evaluators initially believed that he was not a candidate for remediation. Incorporating a simulator into the assessment process proved valuable because the evaluators could see firsthand that, despite his severe knowledge deficiencies, he was able to safely identify and correct major hemodynamic and respiratory problems in a timely and correct manner. The evaluators were able to determine that the best remediation process for this physician would encourage and support the acquisition of up-to-date medical knowledge. Although a follow-up on the success of the remediation process for this physician is not available, incorporating simulation into the process added to the total assessment of his skills.

The simulated environment offers many advantages over traditional assessment tools. Practicing physicians, dentists, and nurses do not take written and oral exams frequently (although hospital nurses often are required to demonstrate competencies using brief written tests). Because of this lack of familiarity, using only these modalities for evaluation should be considered inadequate, and even competent physicians may have difficulties. The simulator allows the practicing physician an opportunity to be in a familiar environment, where preparation, approach to clinical situations, technical abilities, knowledge application, judgment, response to clinical problems, problem-solving abilities, and accuracy in record-keeping can be assessed.[63] Although simulator use may not be ready for the certification and assessment of clinical competence, full-scale simulators can aid in the evaluation of practicing physicians being considered for retraining and remediation due to incompetence. Likewise, dental simulators can be used to judge the clinical performance of the incompetent dentist or oral surgeon, and nursing techniques and competencies can be assessed in the patient simulator.

Simulator Use for the Rehabilitation of Impaired Physicians, Dentists, or Nurses

Incompetence is not limited to lapses in medical skills or knowledge; it can also result from chemical dependency. In another unique application, Levine and Goldiner report their success in using a simulator laboratory as a component of the rehabilitation process for the impaired practicing health-care provider.[64] They suggest that working in a simulator laboratory facilitates the rehabilitation of the impaired health-care provider by offering an opportunity to have a sense of structure and responsibility, develop teaching and communication skills, develop a sense of worth and respect, and learn unique skills in the use of medical simulation. In addition, the simulator allowed the unique opportunity to maintain clinical skills and judgment during the rehabilitation process without being in an actual clinical environment.

Conclusion

Continuing medical education, certification, recertification, and, if necessary, remediation are essential to the well-being of patients, society, and the health care industry. Evaluating and assessing the effectiveness of these processes to ensure clinical competence are paramount. The use of medical simulation for these processes is in its infancy, but already it has had—and will continue to have—a major role in the improvement of the educational process for practicing health care providers.

References

1. Association of American Medical Colleges website at http://www.aamc.org.
2. Accreditation Council for Continuing Medical Education website at http://www.accme.org.
3. American Medical Association website at http://www.ama.org.
4. Weindling AM: Education and training: Continuing professional development. Curr Paediatr 2001;11:369–374.
5. State Medical Board Regulations on continuing medical education for licensure reregistration. E Medicine web site at http://cme.emedicine.com/cmebystate.html.
6. Misra S, Robertson WO: CME needs assessment: A statewide survey. J Contin Educ Health Profess 1994;14:119–125.
7. Peck C, McCall M, McLaren B, Rotem T: Continuing medical education and continuing professional development: International comparisons. BMJ 2000;320:432–435
8. Barnes BE: Creating the Practice-Learning Environment: using technology to support a new model of continuing medical education. Acad Med 1998;73:278–281.
9. Abrahamson S, et al: Continuing medical education for life: Eight principles. Acad Med 1999;74:1288–1294.
10. SCOPME: Continuing Professional Development for Doctors and Dentists. London, SCOPME, 1998.
11. Richards T: Continuing medical education. BMJ 1998;316:246.
12. Lewis CE: Continuing medical education: Past, present, future. West J Med 1998;168:334–340.
13. Davis DA, Thompson MA, Oxman AD, Haynes RB: Changing physician performance: A systematic review of the effect of continuing medical education strategies. JAMA 1995;274:700–705.
14. Knowles M, et al: Andragogy in Action. Houston, Gulf Publishing, 1984.
15. Davis D, et al: Impact of formal continuing medical education: Do conferences, workshops, rounds and other traditional continuing education activities change physician behavior or health care outcome? JAMA 1999;282:867–874.
16. Gercenshtein L, Fogelman Y, Yaphe J: Increasing the satisfaction of general practitioners with continuing medical education programs: A method for quality improvement through increasing teacher-learner interaction. BMC Fam Pract 2002;3:15–19.
17. Cantillion P, Jones R Does continuing medical education in general practice make a difference? BMJ 1999;318:1276–1279.
18. Reiter HI, Eva KW, Hatala RM, Norman GR: Self and peer assessment in tutorials: Application of a relative-ranking model. Acad Med 2002;77:1134–1139.
19. Smits P, Verbeek J, Buisonje C: Problem based learning in continuing medical education: a review of controlled evaluation studies. BMJ 2002;324:153–156.
20. Lampotang S, Good M, Westhorpe R, et al: Logisics of conducting a large number of individual sessions with a full-scale patient simulator at a scientific meeting. J Clin Monit 1997; 13:399–407.

21. University of Rochester Department of Anesthesiology website at http://web.anes.rochester.edu/index.htm.
22. Society for Technology in Anesthesia website at http://www.anestech.org.
23. Society for Education in Anesthesia website at http://www.seahq.org.
24. American Society of Anesthesiologists website at http://www.asahq.org.
25. New York State Society for Anesthesiologists website at: http://www.nyssa-pga.org.
26. Murray BW, Good ML, Gravenstein JS, et al: Learning about new anesthetics using a model driven, full human simulator. J Clini Monit 2002;17:293–300.
27. Holzman RS, Cooper JB, Gaba DM, et al: Anesthesia crisis resource management: Real-life simulation training in operating room crises. J Clin Anesth 1995;7:675–687.
28. Kurrek MM, Fish KJ: Anesthesia crisis resource management training: An intimidating concept, a rewarding experience. Can J Anaesth 1996;43:430–434.
29. Block EF, Lottenberg L, Flint L, et al: Use of a patient simulator for the advanced trauma life support course. Am Surg 2002;68:648–651.
30. Halamek LP, et al: Time for a new paradigm in pediatric medical education: Teaching neonatal resuscitation in a simulated delivery room environment. Pediatrics 2002;106:e45.
31. Vardi A, Levin I, Berkenstadt H, et al: Simulation-based training of medical teams to manage chemical warfare causalities. Isr Med Assoc J 2002;4:540–544.
32. Hegarty MK, Bloch MB: The use of simulators in intensive care training. Curr Anesth Crit Care 2002;13:194–200.
33. Cooper JB, Barron D, Blum R, et al: Video teleconferencing with realistic simulation for medical education. J Clin Anesth 2000;12:256–261.
34. Derossis AM, Fried GM, Abrahamowicz M, et al: Development of a model for training and evaluation of laparoscopic skills. Am J Surg 1998;175:482–487.
35. Bockholt U, Ecke U, Muller W, et al: Real time simulation of tissue deformity for the nasal endoscopy (NES) In Westwood JD, Hoffman HM, Robb RA, et al (eds): Medicine Meets Virtual Reality. Studies in Health Technology and Infomatics, vol 62. Amsterdam, IOS Press, 1999, pp 74–75.
36. Bro-Nielson M, Tasto JL, Cunningham R, Merrill GL: PreOP™ endoscopy simulator: PC-based immersion training system for bronchoscopy. In Westwood JD, Hoffman HM, Robb RA, et al (eds): Medicine Meets Virtual Reality. Studies in Health Technology and Infomatics, vol 62. Amsterdam, IOS Press, 1999, pp 76–82.
37. Shah J, Darzi A: Virtual reality flexible cystoscopy: A validation study. BJU Int 2002;90:828–832.
38. Ferlitsch A, Glauninger P, Gupper A, et al: Evaluation of a virtual endoscopy simulator for training in gastrointestinal endoscopy. Endoscopy 2002;34:698–702.
39. Colt HG, Crawford SW, Galbraith O: Virtual reality bronchoscopy simulation: A revolution in procedure training. Chest 120:1333–1339.
40. Issenberg SB, McGaghie WC, Hart IR, et al: Simulation technology for health care professional skills training and assessment. JAMA 1999;282:861–866.
41. Gorman PJ, Meier AH, Krummel TM: Simulation and virtual reality in surgical education. Arch Surg 1999;134:1203–1208.
42. Ahlberg G, Heikkinen T, Iselius L, et al: Does training in a virtual simulator improve surgical performance? Surg Endosc 2002;16:126–129.
43. Hamilton EC, Scott DJ, Kapoor A, et al: Improving operative performance using a laparoscopic hernia simulator. Am J Surg 2001;182:725–728.
44. Scott DJ, Bergen PC, Euhus DM, et al: Intense laparoscopic skills training improves operative performance of surgery residents. Surg Forum 1999;50:670–671.
45. Schwid HA, Odonnell D: The Anesthesia Simulator-Recorder: A device to train and evaluate anesthesiologists' response to critical incidents. Anesthesiology 1990;72:191–197.
46. Schwid HA: Computer simulation and management of critical events. Acad Med 1994;69:213.
47. Schwid HA, Riike, GA Ross BK, et al: Use of computerized advanced life support simulator improves retention of advanced cardiac life support guidelines better than a textbook review. Crit Care Med 1999;27;821–824.

48. ACGME outcome project. Accreditation Council for Graduate Medical Education website at http:// www.acgme.org.
49. Newble D, Dawson B, Dauphinee D: Guidelines for assessing clinical competency. Teach Learn Med. 1994;6:213–220.
50. Norcini JJ, Swanson DB, Grosso LJ, et al: A comparison of knowledge synthesis and clinical judgment: multiple-choice questions in the assessment of physicians. Eval Health Prof 1984;7:485–499.
51. Slogoff S, Hughes FP, Hug CC, et al: A demonstration of validity for certification by the American Board of Anesthesiology. Acad Med. 1994;69:740–746.
52. Morgan PJ, Cleave-Hogg D, Guest CB: A comparison of global ratings and checklist scores from an undergraduate assessment using an anesthesia simulator. Acad Med. 2001;76:1053–1055.
53. Devitt H, Kurrek M, Cohen M, et al: Testing the instrument: Internal consistency during evaluation of performance in an anesthesia simulator. Anesthesiology 1996;85(3A):A931.
54. Devitt JH, Kurrek MM, Cohen MM, Fish K: Testing the raters: Inter-rater reliability of standardized anaesthesia simulator performance. Can J Anaesth 1997;44(9):924–928.
55. Gaba DM, Botney R, Howard S, et al: Interrater reliability of performance assessment tools for the management of simulated anesthetic crisis. Anesthesiology 1994;81(No 3A):A-A.
56. Devitt JH, Kurrek MM, Cohen MM, et al: Testing internal consistency and construct validity during evaluation of performance in a patient simulator. Anesth Analg 1998;86:1157–1159.
57. Devitt JH, Kurrek M, Cohen M: Can medical students be evaluated by a simulator based evaluation tool developed for practicing anesthesiologists? Anesthesiology 1997;87(3A):A947-A947.
58. Schwid HA, Rooke GA, Carline J, et al: Evaluation of anesthesiology residents using mannequin-based simulation: A multiinstitutional study. Anesthesiology 2002;97:1434–1444.
59. Lampe M: Appraisal and reassessment of the specialist in anesthesia. Best Pract Res Clin Anesth. 2002;16:391–400.
60. Kapur PA, Steadman RH: Patient simulator competency testing: Ready for takeoff? Anesth Analg 1998;86:1157–1159.
61. Rosner F, Balint JA, Stein RM: Remedial medical education. Arch Intern Med. 1994;154:274–282.
62. Hanna E, Premi J, Turnball J: Results of remedial continuing medical education in dyscompetent physicians, Acad Med. 2000;75:174–176.
63. Rosenblatt MA, Abrams KJ, et al: The use of a human patient simulator in the evaluation of and development of a remedial prescription for an anesthesiologist with lapsed medical skills. Anesth Analg. 2002;94:149–153.
64. Levine AI, Goldiner PL: The novel use of a human patient simulator laboratory as a unique environment for the successful rehabilitation of the impaired anesthesiologist. Poster presentation at the 2001 International Meeting on Medical Simulation, 2001.

Chapter 27

SIMULATION IN RESPIRATORY THERAPY

Viva Jo Siddall, MS, RRT, RCP, CCRC

As the number of educational facilities that acquire human patient simulators increases, so does the diversity of their use. Written documentation of what is believed to be successful utilization of high-fidelity patient simulation in various educational settings is scattered throughout medical and educational journals.[1–4]

The field of anesthesiology is a forerunner in utilizing high-fidelity patient simulation in education and training programs.[5,6] In a nonthreatening educational setting, clinicians can experience unusual situations such as malignant hyperthermia, anaphylaxis, or the "can't ventilate, can't intubate" scenario without the possibility of harming a real patient. Repeated exposures to these types of rare but real patient scenarios allow the clinician to bridge the gap between theory and clinical practice.

A simulator is defined as an apparatus that generates test conditions approximating actual or operational conditions.[7] In medical training, a human patient simulator can represent an actual patient surrounded by various scripted story elements, allowing the student to practice what has been introduced in textbooks as theory (passive learning) in the clinical setting (active learning) without placing patients at risk. One of the advantages of bridging the gap between passive and active learning with a recreation of the clinical setting is the ability to expose the learner to actual equipment used during patient care and to the daily interactions among patients, themselves, and machines. A second advantage is the ability to control repeated practice of rare clinical events, which allows the learner to gain the experience necessary to build confidence as a practitioner before first-time exposure to patients and families. Even more importantly, learners have the means to work through various plans of care for given patient scenarios and actually witness the fruits of their labor in real time.

Application of High-Fidelity Patient Simulators to Respiratory Therapy

The Human Patient Simulator (HPS) Version 6.1 (Medical Education Technologies, Inc., Sarasota, Florida) provides a strong platform for training allied health practitioners such as respiratory therapists. This high-fidelity mannequin has the physical characteristics of an adult male/female or pediatric patient and manifests various clinical signs and characteristics, including EKG readings, self-regulated spontaneous respiratory rate, audible heart/breath sounds, palpable pulses, chest excursion, and airway patency. Various vital signs that are computer model-driven are available for display: oxygen saturation (SaO_2), end-tidal carbon dioxide ($EtCO_2$), invasive arterial blood pressure and noninvasive cuff blood pressures, central venous pressure (CVP), pulmonary artery pressure (PAP), and intracranial pressure (ICP). The ability to simulate a patient's vital signs and physical attributes serves as an important enhancement to the educational process focused on teaching core assessment skills, which serve as a foundation for respiratory therapy practitioners.

The aspects of the HPS mannequin that allow training in simple and complex airway management skills include an anatomically realistic representation of the upper airway (oropharynx, nasopharynx, and larynx) of an adult or pediatric patient. These features enable the respiratory practitioner to gain exposure to the skills required to facilitate artificial airway placement through direct laryngoscopy or blind nasal intubation, as well as to recognize the hazards of esophageal intubation and incorrect placement of an endotracheal tube into the right or left bronchus. Finally, exposure to simulation of the "can't ventilate, can't intubate" patient allows the practitioner to work through various plans of action to achieve the best-case scenario.

The pharmacology feature in the HPS supports interventions with over fifty medications through preprogrammed pharmacokinetic and pharmacodynamic parameters. Enhancing a simulated patient scenario with appropriate medication responses and reactions to various disease processes allows the respiratory care practitioner to come one-step closer to the true patient experience. Medications are administered to the human patient simulator in a number of ways with the help of a computer and a bar code reader. The purpose of this feature is to allow the mannequin to react to the medication like a real patient. The practitioner may administer simulated nebulized respiratory medications, and the HPS will manifest the desired patient effects for that scenario through manipulation of various computerized variables.

Applications of Adult Learning Principles

Conventional pedagogic methods are based on preparatory training or instruction through the transfer of knowledge and skills from teachers to students, whereas andragogy examines the art and science of helping adults learn.[8] Together, pedagogy and androgony represent a continuum that ranges from teacher-directed to self-directed learning. Adults are viewed as independent; therefore, they are classified as self-directed learners by Merriam and Caffarela.[9] An adult learner may move across this continuum at any time during his or her life and require the transmission of knowledge and skills from various perspectives. When an adult is learning a new task, she or he may learn most effectively when traditional didactic pedagogies are used, as is the case with first-year respiratory therapy students. In contrast, an adult who is practicing a previously learned skill and wishes to expand his or her knowledge base—for example, by pursuing continuing education units to maintain qualification for a state licensing requirement—may learn more efficiently in an environment that emphasizes andragogic methods of knowledge transfer. Adult education is not simply a process of transmitting what is known; it may be defined rather as a lifelong process of continuing inquiry.[10]

New students, novice practitioners, and seasoned veterans can benefit from time engaged in deliberate educational exercises.[10] Human patient simulators can accommodate individuals or teams of people with a wide range of experience levels; combined with a strong educational program, this approach creates a solid forum for adult learning.

A facilitator of adult learning experiences needs to be aware of the concept of learning curves in developing programs that introduce a new skill.[11] Success at learning a new skill improves with repeated practice; moreover, learners reach a plateau of success after attaining initial competency but differ in the number of attempts required to reach the success plateau. Finally, performance may fade without regular repeated practice.[10,12] The HPS can prove to be of invaluable service to both the educator and the learner by allowing repeated, deliberate practice for skill sets without the need to wait for the ideal patient situation to present itself.

Instructional Design of a Respiratory Therapy-Focused Simulator Session

After a needs assessment is done, a focus topic should be identified. The focus topic guides the instructional design process and serves as a blueprint for the educational sessions. The blueprint for designing a simulation session maps the flow of events that act upon and involve the learner. A structure of interwoven communication among learners, instructors, session facilitators, and the mannequin interacts with the sole purpose of aiding in the process of learning, ultimately moving the participant from one state of mind to another. Thus, a sound foundation of adult learning theory is appropriate for mapping out the instructional events that should be in place to support the acquisition and retention of the focus topic.[13] The events incorporated in the instructional design set a course for the learner to move from a starting point to the desired educational outcome by way of predefined target objectives through interaction with the simulated surroundings. The various events related to the session should be clearly scripted in the instructional design to enable the facilitator and the learner to maintain focus on the desired educational topic.

When new learning takes place, previously acquired cognitive and psychomotor capabilities need to be readily available for instant recall and application. An advanced simulator session such as the one presented in this chapter assumes that the learner has previously mastered component ideas (concepts, rules) of respiratory therapy. Evaluation of the educational experience for the focus topic is easier to accomplish without the "noise" produced by inadequately mastered foundation skills. Immediate indication that the desired learning has occurred is supplied when the appropriate performance is evoked. The level of the learner's performance, which is defined by a pre-established criterion, can be considered an immediate learning outcome.

The instructional design of sessions should be tempered with a broad approach to practice, based on best-practice methods and standard guidelines and grounded in established literature.[14] If a developed session has this framework as its foundation, the question of reliability and validity of the learning outcomes will be easier to establish. Repeated measures of the educational outcomes for identical sessions will demonstrate the reliability concerning the learner's capability beyond that of the level of chance.[13] Development of criteria-based outcome measures addresses issues surrounding validity. Criteria-based measures describe the level of performance by the learner that is necessary to be considered acceptable for the focus topic of the session.[15]

Evaluation methods should be applied to the entire educational program as well as the individual learner's performance. An evaluation process should be ongoing to establish the appropriateness and effectiveness of the educational intervention. Two evaluation methods, formative and summative, lead to decisions guiding program revision and continuation. A formative evaluation gathers evidence used during the development phase of the program to address the feasibility and effectiveness of the lesson design.[16] Summative evaluation is undertaken when the program development is considered complete rather than ongoing. Its purpose is to draw conclusions concerning the effectiveness of the executed educational intervention. The primary concern with this type of evaluation is that learning outcomes are primarily assessed by observations or tests of human capabilities as reflected in the objectives stated in the learning objectives. Learning outcomes based on stated objectives take into consideration the mastery of intellectual skills, problem-solving abilities, psychomotor skills, attitudes, and whether facts or generalizations have been learned.

Debriefing the Educational Experience

Formal debriefing or feedback of an educational experience with the learner sets the stage for the exchange of information between participants of the session and should have a focus on performance improvement. Feedback is a continuous process, and the milieu in which it is given may affect both quantity and quality of the learner's performance.[17] Feedback may be incidental (spontaneous) or intentional (deliberate) and should come from trained evaluators or facilitators.[18]

After the scenario is concluded, the session is not complete unless adequate quality time is set aside for feedback concerning the degree of correctness of the learner's performance. In the session included in this chapter (Appendix), the learner knows up front the intent of the session (from the criterion-based objectives) and the level of acceptable performance (from the stated evaluation criteria and competencies). The debriefing period allows a constructive exchange of thoughts between the learner and facilitator, setting the stage for the learner to self-correct clinical or behavioral performance.

The level of debriefing used in the session involves mutual cooperation between a knowledgeable facilitator and a practicing respiratory therapy clinician. Both participants must have expertise in the subject matter. The motive for the session must be non-threatening to gain the trust of the learner; only in an atmosphere of mutual trust and respect can high-quality learning be fostered.

Formal education sessions are videotaped and archived at our institution. Included in the scenarios are situations in which the learner must document the course of care for the simulated patient on an institution flow sheet or a patient chart. All of the information provided by the audiovisual equipment, written documentation, computerized tracking through data logs, and evaluations/checklists completed by the facilitator are available at the time of the debriefing.

The session described in this chapter (Appendix) addresses clinical competencies or technical clinical skills performance. However, it may be used to focus on behavioral interactions between the learner and other members of the health care team or the patient's family. How much time is available must be considered in deciding what will be evaluated during a single session. In fact, one well-constructed scenario may be used many times, each time with a different declared focus topic—for example, resource allocation, interpersonal communication skills, ethics, professionalism, or leadership development.

Simulation for Teaching in Respiratory Therapy

As respiratory therapy techniques and expertise have changed drastically over the years, so too must the educational strategies used to train people to become the respiratory care practitioners of the future. The integration of a high-fidelity human patient simulator into an existing respiratory therapy curriculum allows students to enhance technical skills and apply those skills in patient care scenarios. The scenario outlined in the Appendix is an example of an educational session (facilitator's perspective) developed for use with a high-fidelity human patient simulator.

Before attending the simulator session, the student receives a lesson packet with the following materials: suggested readings, outline of the session, evaluation criteria, selected competencies, proficiency evaluation forms, and clinical simulation evaluation forms. The simulation session includes (1) an orientation to the simulator center and competencies, (2) the simulation, and (3) formal debriefing. The session is videotaped for use during the debriefing process.

Conclusion

High-fidelity human patient simulators are effective tools that can be used to enhance the educational experience at all levels of respiratory care practice. The level of simulation fidelity is matched to the task requirements necessary to meet the technical expertise and clinical demands required of respiratory therapy practitioners. Practitioners may be observed as individuals or as members of a health care team.

Appendix: Respiratory Therapy Simulation Sessions

Topic: Patient management training session

Target population: Respiratory therapists (RRT) and students

Goal: Introduction to critical care patient management

Setting: Critical care unit

Focus:

1. Theory application to patient after open heart surgery/ventilator management scenario

2. Proficient use of equipment used to monitor patients in critical care

3. Competencies, including intubation/extubation, suctioning, A-line blood draw, spontaneous ventilatory parameters, ventilator management

Approximate time: 2.0 hours (includes orientation to simulator center, simulation, competencies, debriefing)

Objectives (upon completion of the session)

1. The participant will be able to identify the indications and hazards of continuous mechanical ventilation.

2. The participant will perform the tasks required to set up a ventilator, make parameter changes, and discontinue a ventilator for simulated patient use.

3. The participant will formulate and execute a plan of care focused on a patient after open-heart surgery through critical care management of a simulated patient.

Facilitator instructions to participant:

The scenario starts with the participant being asked to come in to help out with the increased work load 2 hours early for her scheduled 12-hour night shift; the assignment is to take care of the third open-heart patient of the day. This is no problem for you because you want extra money for the vacation you will be taking in a few weeks at the end of March. The participant will care for a 63-year-old man who has undergone open-heart surgery involving four vessels. ABGs are assessed to prompt desired ventilator changes.

I. Report to ICU and prepare for patient arrival.

1. Set up room for open heart patient.

    Ventilator

    Monitors

    Additional equipment necessary for patient care

    [Part I and II of Ventilator Management Competency]

2. Get report from assigned patient care team.

    Anticipated time of patient arrival to unit

    Progress of surgery

Patient history:

Don is a retired man who works 3 or 4 days a week at a golf course during the summer and spends his winters in Florida. He recently has not had much energy and felt chest pain after a meal severe enough to drive himself to a small hospital in Florida near his campground. Diagnosis: myocardial infarction (MI). Emergent heart catheterization is ordered, which cannot be done at this hospital. After 5 days of not being able to receive treatment, Don signs out against medical advice and flies to Chicago, where he gets in a car and travels to his home hospital for treatment. He presents to the emergency department, where he is admitted and scheduled for heart catheterization on the following morning. The heart catheterization reveals 4 severe blockages, and surgery is scheduled for later that day. It is March 15.

Patient physical exam:

Height: 5 ft 9 in	No diabetes mellitus	Positive for seasonal allergies
Weight: 275 lb	Knee replacement	No medications at this time
Nonsmoker	No baseline pulmonary	Preoperative arterial blood
Nondrinker	function tests ordered	gases: 7.42/52/95/RA

II. Patient arrives in ICU (hour 0).

 1. Assume care of patient from transport team.

  [Part III of Ventilator Management Competency]

Status after surgery:

 Baseline vitals: heart rate, 105; respiratory rate, spontaneous 0; blood pressure, 135/70 mmHg; SvO_2, 66%; SaO_2, 97%; temperature, 34° C; PIP, 50 cm H_2O.

Report from transport team:

 Don 65 Y M S/P CABG x 4, internal mammary, saphenous vein, difficult intubation with fiberscope size 6 ETT 23 at lips, vitals stable, no blood given. Only problem: "He was difficult to close. I have never seen so much wire to close a chest. The doctor had to do it two times, even needed help to hold the chest closed" MD (surgeon) Orders: slow wean, am extubation, don't let him cough. Patient is arousable, cooperative. "Oh yeah, the daughter is a RRT."

 2. Assist patient care team with patient.

  a. Watch airway during removal of wet blankets, placement of dry blankets, EKG patch removal, RN assessment, and visual exam. Chest x-ray, warming blanket

 3. Assess patient.

Patient drops SaO_2 to 89%, SVO_2 to 57% with activity. Vitals otherwise stable. Chest x-ray fluffy, and chest tube has 500 cc blood from rolling. Patient stabilizes; 30 minutes have passed.

 4. Send arterial blood gases (ABG)

  [A-line Aspiration Competency]

 5. Review, chart, and respond to ABG results.

III. Ventilator check (hour 4)

 1. Perform routine ventilator check

  [Part IV of Ventilator Management Competency]

Patient is arousable, cooperative, does not complain of pain, appears puffy, and coughs hard when moved. SATs fall, but recovery is complete in 10 minutes with help of increased oxygen. Breath sounds: rhonchi; thick yellow mucus with suctioning; copious thick clear mucus with oral suctioning; vital signs stable; temperature normalizing.

IV. Weaning patient (hour 12)

 1. Discuss weaning of patient in anticipation of an early am extubation with patient care team.

Patient is awake, alert, cooperative, complains of endotracheal tube; breath sounds: occasional rhonchi that clear with suctioning. However, patient remains diminished on left; vital signs stable; no pressors; minimal blood in chest tubes.

V. Prepare for extubation (hour 16)

 1. Obtain spontaneous ventilatory parameters.

  [Ventilatory Parameters Competency]

 2. Extubate patient.

  [Intubation/Extubation Competency—Part B]

   3. Discontinue ventilator.

   [Part V of Ventilatory Management Competency]

Patient is stable, vital signs are good; breath sounds: rhonchi that clear with strong splinted cough, slight wheeze bilateral, diminished on left; thick yellow sputum produced. Morning chest x-ray reveals haziness (left > right); NC, 4 lpm with bubble bottle; IS at bedside, Swan-Ganz catheter and $EtCO_2$ discontinued.

   4. Write orders for patient plan of care after extubation.

   5. Attend shift report.

Facilitator instructions to participant:

   The therapist returns 48 hours later for her next 12-hour shift. The assignment is the high end of ICU and the third-floor telemetry unit. The therapist checks the two ventilator patients in the ICU and heads up to telemetry to give the last 4 times/day treatments that are due. It is 20:00, and you realize you are going to see Don, the patient you had earlier in the week immediately after open heart surgery. He is in a room by himself, with no fan. His dinner tray is untouched, and he is sitting up in a chair.

Patient status:

   Heart monitor shows atrial fibrillation; SaO_2 of 90–91% on a 50% venti-mask (nasal cannula 6 lpm with bubble bottle for meals and ambulation); respiratory rate is 20–24, with pursed lipped breathing; diaphoretic; no complaints of shortness of breath. Breath sounds are diminished bilaterally (left > right) with scattered wheeze, weak cough. Chest x-ray shows pleural effusion on left, bilateral fluffiness, elevated diaphragm on left. Patient states, "I am not hungry, it is hot in here. I am tired, I have been up in a chair for a long time."

VI. Assume care of telemetry patient.

   1. Assess patient.

   2. Administer breathing treatment.

   3. Encourage to deep-breathe and cough (DB&C).

   4. Identify causes of deterioration over the past 48 hours.

   5. Chart.

   6. Report/discuss patient status with patient care team.

Facilitator instructions:

   The therapist is called to the ICU to help with suctioning another patient. He gets very busy in the unit and since the 4 times/day, 3 times/day, and twice-daily treatments are finished, there is no need to go back to the telemetry unit. Things quiet down in the ICU around 0300, and the therapist has checked with everyone else. None of the other therapists need help so he or she decides to go check on the patients upstairs. As the therapist enters the telemetry unit, only the unit clerk is visible and the monitor shows atrial fibrillation for Don's heart rate. When the therapist enters the room, it is noted that a roommate has been added and all the contents of the room have been shoved right next to each other. It is very hot in the room. and the curtain is pulled to divide the room in half. Don is lying flat in bed supine with his NC running. The nurse who has been on break shows up and asks what is going on.

Patient status:

   Heart rhythm: atrial fibrillation; respiratory rate, 6; labored paradoxical breathing; no use of accessory muscles noted, just abdominal movement; SaO_2, 63%; the patient is nonresponsive to verbal or physical stimuli.

VII. Telemetry unit
    1. Assess patient breathing
    2. Call code
    3. Bag mask ventilate with 100% O_2
    4. Place oral airway
    5. Instruct help to prepare for intubation
    6. Perform intubation
       [Intubation/Extubation Competency—Part A]
    7. Prepare for transport to ICU
       a. Monitor
       b. Oxygen tank
       c. Resuscitation bag with reservoir
       d. Mask
    8. Give report to ICU therapist.

Topic: Evaluation criteria
Goal: Evaluation of introduction to critical care patient management training
Evaluation of procedures: In addition to clinical skills, the evaluator should note the interpersonal skills, effective communication, and professionalism of the participant.

Performance	Essential Task	Evaluation Criteria
A. Prepare ICU room for open heart patient	Set up necessary equipment	Ventilator Management Competency Part I and II
	Ventilator, monitor (i.e., $EtCO_2$, POX, SX, IS, blanket (splinting), clip board, flow sheet, endotracheal tube, resuscitation bag/mask, oxygen flow meters	
	Obtain necessary patient information	
B. Patient transfer from operating room	Assume responsibility for airway/ventilatory management	Ventilator Management Competency Part III
	Assess patient	Appropriate charting
	Obtain ABG	A-line Aspiration Competency
	Necessary ventilator parameter changes in response to patient status	Appropriate ventilator changes and charting
C. Ventilator management	Perform routine ventilator check	Ventilator Management Competency Part IV
	Perform appropriate patient care	ETT Suctioning Competency
D. Wean patient	Discuss plan of care for weaning patient	Interaction with facilitator/teaching if necessary
E. Prepare for extubation	Establish readiness for extubation with patient care team	Gathers appropriate information
	Obtain spontaneous ventilatory parameter values	Ventilatory Parameter Competency
F. Discontinuance of mechanical ventilation	Extubate patient	Intubation/Extubation Competency Part B
	Discontinue ventilator	Ventilator Management Competency Part V
	Develop ongoing POC for patient transferring out of ICU	Write verbal order in patient chart
G. Establish patient airway	BLS-ABC	AHA BLS algorithm
	LOOK, LISTEN, FEEL, 2 breaths, check pulse-initiate rescue breathing	
	Perform Intubation	Intubation/Extubation Competency Part A
	Prepare for transport to ICU	Appropriate report to ICU day shift RRT
	Transport patient to ICU	

Topic: Ventilator management competency
Purpose: To demonstrate the ability to perform all tasks associated with providing ventilatory support for a patient.
Focus skills: Ventilator set-up
Monitor(s) set-up
Ventilator parameter changes
Ventilator discontinuance

I. Gather/assemble equipment.

1. Ventilator/disposables
2. $EtCO_2$/disposables
3. POX
4. Suction equipment/disposables
5. Stethoscope
6. Charting documents
7. HME or equivalent
8. Test lung
9. Temperature probe
10. Water traps
11. Resuscitation bag
12. Blanket

II. Perform ventilator/room set-up.

1. Wash hands
2. Assemble ventilator according to manufacturer specifications for specific type and current hospital/department P&P
3. Connect test lung to patient circuit maintaining asepsis
4. Prepare equipment for patient arrival
5. Set appropriate ventilator settings and alarm parameters for specified patient
6. Turn ventilator on
7. Set-up additional monitoring equipment

III. Receive patient from transport team.

1. Wash hands
2. Don gloves
3. Attach patient to ventilator
4. Ensure monitors are turned on
5. Assess baseline patient status (i.e., BS, HR, RR, SaO_2, $EtCO_2$, B/P, PIP, ETT placement)
6. Receive report form anesthesiologist
7. *Obtain ABG/correlate with POX and $EtCO_2$
8. Make necessary ventilator changes
9. Ensure airway device is secure
10. Chart postoperative baseline ventilator check
11. Review postoperative chest x-ray

IV. Execute ventilator check/parameter change.

1. Address/inform patient of activity
2. Wash hands
3. Don gloves

4.   Assess patient
     i.   Breath sounds
     ii. Vital signs: $EtCO_2$, POX, HR, B/P, SvO_2
     iii. ETT placement/tape
     iv. * Suction if necessary ETT/oral
5.   Chart necessary ventilator information (See specific department P&P)
     i.   Mode
     ii. Vt spontaneous/machine
     iii. Respiratory spontaneous/machine
     iv. FiO_2
     v.   PIP
     vi. Check other parameters ie PEEP, PS, Pause
6.   Wean patient if appropriate using POX and $EtCO_2$ monitors and vital signs. Confirm with patient care team as appropriate.
7.   Monitor patient for change in vitals
8.   Chart necessary patient information
9.   Position patient if necessary
10. Drain condensation from tubing/drain cups or check HME
11. Wash hands
12. Report any patient changes/observations to the patient care team

V. Discontinue ventilator support.
1.   Address/inform patient of activity
2.   Wash hands
3.   Don gloves
4.   Assess patient
     i.   Breath sounds
     ii. Vital signs: $EtCO_2$, POX, HR, B/P, SvO_2
     iii. ETT placement/tape
     iv. Suction if necessary ETT/oral
5.   *Check spontaneous ventilatory parameters
6.   *Extubate patient
7.   Turn off ventilator
8.   Discontinue $EtCO_2$ monitor
9.   Strip ventilator of disposables and discard. Check hospital P&P for appropriate method
10. Wipe down equipment
11. Remove gloves
12. Wash hands
13. Remove equipment from room

VI. Chart.
*Reference to other competencies.

Please circle appropriate response.

Completed

| Acceptable |
| Unacceptable |

Evaluator's Name (Print) _____

Signature _____

Date _____   Participant Name (Print) _____
                                     Signature _____

If unacceptable, please explain why.

_____
_____
_____
_____
_____

Suggested plan to improve performance if unacceptable:

_____
_____
_____
_____

Topic: Arterial line aspiration competency
Purpose: Sampling arterial blood from an indwelling pressure line for the purposes of blood gas analysis
Focus skill: Arterial blood acquisition
I.   Gather/assemble equipment.
1. Arterial blood gas kit for arterial lines (3-cc syringe)
2. Waste syringe if not in arterial line kit (10-cc syringe)
3. Alcohol pads
4. Gauze
5. Gloves
6. Towel/protective pad
7. Goggles
8. Mask
9. Appropriate paperwork (i.e., ABG requisition)
II.   Confirm order/inform patient.
III. Perform procedure.
1. Wash hands
2. Place towel/protective pad under arterial line sampling port
3. Put on gloves
4. Place gauze directly under sampling port
5. Remove waste syringe from protective covering
6. Remove cap from sampling port and swab with alcohol
7. Attach waste syringe to sampling port
8. Silence monitor
9. Note SaO_2 and $EtCO_2$ readings for ABG correlation
10. Turn stopcock off to pressure line
11. Gently aspirate 10 cc of blood
12. Remove and discard waste syringe
13. Turn stopcock arrow to midway point between pressure line and patient
14. Attach small syringe to sampling port
15. Turn stopcock off to pressure line

16. Gently aspirate 2 cc of blood (Avoid air bubbles)
17. Turn stopcock off to sampling port
18. Remove syringe
19. Express air bubbles and cap syringe
20. Turn stopcock off to patient
21. Clear stopcock port by pulling pigtail on transducer, flushing with pressure bag solution into a gauze
22. Turn stopcock off to the sampling port
23. Clear distal pressure line by pull pigtail on transducer
24. Swab sampling port with alcohol
25. Replace dead ender on sampling port
25. Assess arterial line for frequency response and line patency
26. Clean up supplies
27. Remove protective gear: gloves, mask, goggles
28. Wash hands
29. Document ABG: time, site, FiO2, method of delivery, ventilator setting, RR
30. Process blood

IV. Report/chart results.

Please circle appropriate response.

Completed | Acceptable |
               | Unacceptable | Evaluator's Name (Print) _____
                                 Signature _____

Date _____   Participant Name (Print) _____
                                 Signature _____

If unacceptable, please explain why.

_____
_____
_____
_____
_____

Suggested plan to improve performance if unacceptable:

_____
_____
_____
_____

Topic: Endotracheal suctioning competency
Purpose: The removal of accumulated secretions from the airway of a patient with an endotracheal (ETT) or nasotracheal (NTT) tube in place
Focus skill: Sterile technique
        Endotracheal/nasotracheal suctioning

I.   Gather/assemble equipment.

1. Suction machine/regulator
2. Connective tubing
3. Sterile suction catheters

    4. Sterile gloves
    5. Stethoscope
    6. Goggles
    7. Mask
    8. Resuscitation bag
II. **Confirm/inform patient.**
III. **Employ universal precautions.**
     Gloves, mask, goggles
IV. **Perform sterile suction procedures.**
    1. Wash hands
    2. Position patient in upright position (45° to 90°).
    3. Confirm need for suctioning
    4. Assess vital signs: HR, RR, B/P, SaO_2
    5. Preoxygenate with 100% O_2
    6. Request/prepare patient to "splint" if capable
    7. Drape patient (chest/incision area)
    8. Put on sterile gloves
    9. Attach sterile tip of catheter to connective tubing.
       Note: 1 hand sterile, 1 hand clean
    10. Disconnect patient from circuit/O_2 device
    11. Without applying suction place sterile catheter into ETT/NTT
    12. While removing catheter apply intermittent suction by occluding port on suction catheter for no longer than 15 seconds
    13. Attach patient to circuit/O_2 device or give positive pressure breaths
    14. Note vital signs
    15. Repeat 9 through 13 if necessary
    16. Wipe off catheter
    17. Suction mouth
    18. Aseptically remove/dispose gloves, catheter, mask
    19. Position patient
V.   **Record/report results: color, consistency, patient response to procedure**

Please circle appropriate response.

Completed | Acceptable |
             | Unacceptable | Evaluator's Name (Print) _____
                              Signature _____

Date _____   Participant Name (Print) _____
                          Signature _____

If unacceptable, please explain why.
_____
_____
_____
_____
_____

Suggested plan to improve performance if unacceptable:

_____
_____
_____
_____

Topic: Intubation/extubation competency
Purpose: The process of insertion and removal of an oral endotracheal tube
Focus skills: Direct visual oral laryngoscopic ETT insertion
               Removal of ETT
A.   Intubation Procedure
I. Check and assemble all necessary equipment for endotracheal intubation.
     1. Laryngoscope and blade
     2. Suction equipment/supplies
     3. 10-cc syringe
     4. Stylet
     5. Tape
     6. Lubricant
     7. Endotracheal tubes
     8. Stethoscope
     9. Tongue blade (wooden)
     10. Adhesive (benzoin)
     11. Resuscitation bag/mask
II.   Confirm orders/verify patient/inform patient.
III. Employ universal precautions.
     1. Wash hands
     2. Gloves, mask goggles
IV. Perform intubation
     1. Inform patient of procedure
     2. Position patient
     3. Oxygenate patient with 100% O_2
     4. Introduce laryngoscope into oropharynx (Miller vs. McIntosh)
     5. Under direct laryngoscopy visualize cords
     6. Insert ETT through vocal cords (note distance marker)
     7. Remove laryngoscope
     8. Remove stylet
     9. Inflate cuff
     10. Verify ETT placement 5 point BS, $EtCO_2$, condensation
     11. Connect ETT to breathing circuit or maintain positive pressure breaths
     12. Secure ETT
     13. Request chest x-ray
     14. Clean up supplies
     15. Wash hands
V.   Chart appropriate information

Please circle appropriate response.

Completed   Acceptable
                 Unacceptable   Evaluator's Name (Print) _____
                                     Signature _____

Date _____   Participant Name (Print) _____
                                     Signature _____

If unacceptable, please explain why.

_____
_____
_____
_____
_____

Suggested plan to improve performance if unacceptable:

_____
_____
_____
_____

B. Extubation Procedure

I.   Check and assemble all necessary equipment for extubation procedure and possible reintubation.
1. Laryngoscope and blade
2. Suction equipment/supplies
3. 10-cc syringe
4. Stylet
5. Tape
6. Lubricant
7. Endotracheal tubes
8. Stethoscope
9. Scissors
10. Tissues/towels
11. Resuscitation bag/mask

II.   Confirm orders/verify patient/inform patient.

III. Employ universal precautions.
1. Wash hands
2. Gloves, mask, goggles

IV. Perform extubation.
1. Inform patient
2. Position patient
3. Suction trachea and oropharynx
4. Preoxygenate with 100% O_2
5. Remove ties/tape while stabilizing ETT
6. Deflate cuff

7. Remove ETT:
   a. Insert a sterile suction catheter into ETT
   b. Apply suction on removal
   c. Remove suction catheter and ETT simultaneously

   OR

   d. Ask patient to take a deep breath and quickly remove ETT
8. Encourage patient to speak, deep breath and cough
9. Administer O_2 via the appropriate device
10. Note vital signs: HR, RR, B/P, SaO_2, BS
11. Position patient, place incentive spirometer at bedside
12. Clean up supplies/equipment
13. Wash hands

V. Chart appropriate information

Please circle appropriate response.

Completed | Acceptable / Unacceptable

Evaluator's Name (Print) _____
Signature _____

Date _____

Participant Name (Print) _____
Signature _____

If unacceptable, please explain why.

_____
_____
_____
_____
_____

Suggested plan to improve performance if unacceptable:

_____
_____
_____
_____

Topic: Ventilatory parameters competency
Purpose: The assessment of a patient's ventilatory reserve by means of tidal volume (V_T) determination, minute volume (V_E), negative inspiratory force (NIF), and slow vital capacity (SVC)
Focus skill: Obtaining above noted parameters from vented patient for purpose of extubation
I. Gather equipment.
   1. Negative pressure manometer with patient attachment
   2. Wright's respiratometer
II. Confirm/inform patient.

III. **Employ universal precautions.**
   Gloves, mask, goggles
IV. **Perform SVC, V_T, V_E procedures.**
   1. Position patient in upright position (45° to 90°).
   2. Inform patient of task (SVC)
   3. Connect patient to Wright's
   4. Instruct patient to take a big breath in and exhale long and slow
   5. Repeat if necessary
   6. Note results
   7. Inform patient of task (V_E)
   8. Connect patient to Wright's
   9. Instruct patient to breathe normally for 60 seconds
   10. Determine the respiratory rate and total minute volume and calculate the patient's average tidal volume
   11. Note results
V. **Perform NIF procedure.**
   1. Position patient in upright position (45° to 90°).
   2. Inform patient of task
   3. Connect patient to negative pressure manometer
   4. Instruct patient to take deep breath in
   5. Repeat if necessary
   6. Note results
VI. **Record results/report observations.**

Please circle appropriate response.   Complete Checklist   Acceptable   Unacceptable
If unacceptable, please explain why.

_____
_____
_____
_____

Suggested plan to improve performance if unacceptable:

_____
_____

Evaluator's Name (Print) _____
                  (Sig) _____

Date _____

Participant's Name (Print) _____
                   (Sig) _____

Proficiency Evaluation Form

Name _____   Date _____

Evaluation Results

Evaluator Name (Print)_____   Signature _____

Key: A Acceptable   U Unacceptable   N Not Applicable

Performance	Results	Comments
A. Prepare ICU room for patient	A U N	
B. Patient transfer of care from OR transport team	A U N	
C. Ventilator Management	A U N	
D. Wean Patient	A U N	
E. Prepare for extubation	A U N	
F. Discontinuance of mechanical ventilation	A U N	
G. Establish patent airway	A U N	
Comments:		
Student	Date	Evaluator

Follow-Up: _____

_____

_____

_____

Final Clinical Simulation Evaluation

The purpose of this evaluation is to assess the overall performance of students in the clinical simulation setting. Use the following definitions; please rate your perception of the student's capability in each area listed below.

Scale: 3   Exceptional-Behavior or ability appears to be outstanding

2   Satisfactory-Behavior or ability appears to be acceptable

1   Unsatisfactory-Behavior or ability appears to be unacceptable

0   No opinion-Insufficient opportunity to observe the student in this area

Cognitive-Knowledge and Intellectual Functioning

In my opinion, the student's

1. Knowledge of respiratory therapy procedures is   3 2 1 0
2. Knowledge of respiratory therapy is   3 2 1 0
3. Ability to transfer information from clinical situation to another is   3 2 1 0
4. Ability to integrate and transfer theory to specific clinical activities is   3 2 1 0
5. Ability to adapt to changing situation is   3 2 1 0
6. Ability to problem solve is   3 2 1 0
7. Ability to make decisions is   3 2 1 0

For any of the preceding items marked "1," please explain.

Psychomotor-Technical and Clinical Proficiency

In my opinion, the student's:

8. Ability to apply monitoring devices is   3 2 1 0
9. Ability to troubleshoot equipment is   3 2 1 0

10. Ability to prepare appropriate equipment is   3 2 1 0
11. Ability to secure and maintain an appropriate airway is   3 2 1 0
12. Ability to perform procedures within the allotted timeframe is   3 2 1 0
13. Overall quality of work is   3 2 1 0
For any of the preceding items marked "1," please explain.

Affective-Professional Attitude and Behavior

In my opinion, the student's:

14. Compliance with hospital and program policies is   3 2 1 0
15. Communication with patients is   3 2 1 0
16. Communication with patient care team is   3 2 1 0
17. Cooperation with peers is   3 2 1 0
18. Response to supervision is   3 2 1 0
19. Attitude to clinical setting is   3 2 1 0
20. Organizational skills are   3 2 1 0
21. Response to criticism is   3 2 1 0
22. Initiative to ask questions and seek help when needed is   3 2 1 0
For any of the proceeding items marked "1," please explain.

Summary

In general, I consider:

23. The student's knowledge to be   3 2 1 0
24. The student's technical ability to be   3 2 1 0
25. The student's professional behavior to be   3 2 1 0
For any of the proceeding items marked "1," please explain.
Please indicate whether or not you agree with the following statements by responding yes or no.

26. Overall the student delivers safe and effective anesthesia patient care.   yes no
27. I believe that I conducted a fair and impartial evaluation.   yes no
28. I feel confident about the accuracy of the evaluation results.   yes no
For any of the proceeding items marked "no," please explain.

Evaluator comments and recommendations:

Evaluator Name (Print)_____

Signature _____

Date_____

References

1. Bond WF, Kostenbader M, McCarthy JF: Prehospital and hospital-based health care providers' experience with a human patient simulator. Prehosp Emerg Care 2001;5:284–287.
2. Bond WF, Spillane L: The use of simulation for emergency medicine resident assessment. Acad Emerg Med 2002;9:1295–1299.
3. Euliano TY: Teaching respiratory physiology: Clinical correlation with a human patient simulator. J Clin Monit Comput 2000;16(5–6):465–470.
4. Gorman PJ, Meier AH, Rawn C, Krummel TM: The future of medical education is no longer blood and guts, it is bits and bytes. Am J Surg 2000;180:353–356.
5. Denson JS, Abrahamson S: A computer-controlled patient simulator. JAMA 1969;208:504–508.
6. Abrahamson S, Denson JS, Wolf RM: Effectiveness of a simulator in training anesthesiology residents. J Med Educ 1969;44:515–519.
7. Morris W (ed): The American Heritage Dictionary of the English Language. Boston, Houghton Mifflin Company, 1981.

8. Merriam SB: An Update on Adult Learning Theory. San Francisco, Jossey-Bass Publishers, 1993.
9. Merriam SB, Caffarella RS: NetLibrary Inc. Learning in Adulthood AComprehensive Guide, 2nd ed. San Francisco, Jossey-Bass Publishers, 1999.
10. Shysh AJ: Adult learning principles: You can teach an old dog new tricks [comment]. Can J Anaesth 2000;47:837–842.
11. Shysh AJ, Eagle CJ: The characteristics of excellent clinical teachers [comment]. Can J Anaesth 1997;44:577–581.
12. Konrad C, Schupfer G, Wietlisbach M, Gerber H: Learning manual skills in anesthesiology: Is there a recommended number of cases for anesthetic procedures? Anesth Analg1998;86: 635–639.
13. Gagné RM, Briggs LJ, Wager WW: Principles of Instructional Design, 4th ed. Fort Worth, Harcourt Brace Jovanovich College Publishers, 1992.
14. Salas E, Burke CS: Simulation for training is effective when. . . . [comment]. Qual Safe Health Care 2002;11:119–120.
15. Mager RF: Preparing Instructional Objectives. Palto Alto, CA, Fearon, 1962.
16. Dick W, Carey L: The Systematic Design of Instruction, 3rd ed. Glenview, IL, Scott Foresman Little Brown Higher Education, 1990.
17. Smith M (ed): Introduction to Performance Technology. Washington, DC, National Society for Performance and Instruction, 1986.
18. Rothwell WJK: Mastering the Instructional Design Process: A Systematic Approach, 2nd ed. San Francisco, Jossey-Bass, 1998.

Chapter 28

COMMUNITY AND LEGAL SERVICES

Martin P. Eason, MD, JD

The primary use of human patient simulators has been to train medical personnel; however, as more simulators become available, innovative nonmedical uses will be developed. Some of those nonmedical uses are currently in place. To illustrate, simulators may be used as part of a party's evidence in a legal action, in primary education to teach basic scientific principles, in outreach programs to inform the public on public health and safety issues, and to aid engineers in designing more ergonomic operating room and health facility environments. Examples of these uses and possible limitations are discussed in this chapter. In discussing these issues, it should be noted that because these uses are so novel, there is a paucity of directly relevant literature.

Simulators Used in the Courtroom

As the sophistication of simulators increases, the more realistic the simulations become. Thus, as the output of the simulators approaches real life, there is a greater push to use that output to represent actual events. This principle is particularly true in the legal arena. The courts in the United States are now faced with the difficult question of whether to allow simulations, also called computer-generated evidence (CGE), to be admitted into evidence. In one case, simulation provided by a human patient simulator was admitted into evidence as a representation of the actual events that occurred in an operating room during a crisis. The central questions facing the courts currently are whether simulator-generated evidence should be admitted as evidence and, if so, whether it is simply a demonstration of events as testified to by a witness, defined as demonstrative evidence, or whether it can by itself be admitted as evidence of actual events, defined as substantive evidence.

To illustrate the use of CGE as evidence, we can posit a situation in which the simulation could be introduced into evidence. Let us assume a medical malpractice case in which a patient died. The cause of death was cardiac arrest. The plaintiffs allege that the death was caused by an overdose of an induction agent during anesthesia. They wish to introduce into evidence a simulation of the hemodynamic effects of a given dose of propofol on a simulator mannequin programmed with the physiologic parameters similar to those of the decedent. The simulation shows severe hypotension leading to myocardial ischemia, which results in a malignant rhythm leading to death. The plaintiffs wish, therefore, to show that, based on the simulation, the administration of the propofol was causative in the patient's death. Because the uses of simulation in current society are ubiquitous, the simulation illustrated above could be easily used in the courtroom as evidence of liability.

However, for any exhibit to be admitted as evidence in a legal case, it must conform to certain rules. In the federal courts these rules are dictated by the federal rules of evidence. In state courts, admissibility of evidence must also follow evidentiary rules, which, in most cases, are modeled after the federal rules. The rules of evidence dictate that, in order for evidence to be admissible, it must meet the following criteria: (1) it must be relevant—that is, it tends to prove or disprove something that is at issue in a case; (2) even if it is relevant, the probative value of the evidence cannot be outweighed by the risk of "unfair prejudice," it cannot mislead or confuse the jury, and it cannot waste time or be unnecessarily cumulative; (3) it must be authenticated—that is, it must be what it purports to be; (4) it must not contain hearsay, and, if it does, it must fit into a category of an exception that would make it admissible; and (5) if it is offered as scientific evidence, it must conform to the special rules that regulate the admissibility of scientific evidence. Although other rules may be applicable, the rules discussed above are the most germane in the discussion of the admissibility of computer-generated evidence. They are discussed in more detail below.

For an exhibit to be admissible as evidence in a case, it must be relevant. Evidence is relevant if it can help a trier of fact, the jury in a jury trial or the judge in a nonjury trial, determine whether a fact is more or less likely to have occurred. That is, it helps the trier determine whether there existed or did not exist a fact that is germane to the dispute between the parties. In the illustrative case, the simulation would be relevant if it showed that the cardiac arrest was more likely to have occurred due to the administered dose of the induction agent. Admissibility would not be difficult if there were other evidence of the actual events and the simulation was used solely to illustrate the events as they happened (for example, if there were records of hypotension and cardiac ischemia that led to the dysrythmia and an expert then testified to these facts). The simulation would therefore be merely a clarification of the expert's testimony. All that would be necessary for admissibility is for the expert to authenticate the evidence. That is, he or she would have to state that the simulation is a "fair and accurate" illustration of his testimony. If instead of using the simulation to demonstrate a witness' testimony, the exhibit itself were used to demonstrate what in fact occurred, the hurdle for admissibility would be greater. For example, if there were no records of what happened, the plaintiffs could use the simulation to show that, based on the patient's physiology and the dose of induction agent given, hypotension would occur, leading to myocardial ischemia and death. Rather than being used as demonstrative evidence, the evidence is now used as evidence in and of itself.

In order for the evidence to be admissible in this form, the courts apply another test for relevancy. To be relevant, conditions demonstrated by the simulation must be "substantially similar" to the actual conditions as they occurred. Why is there a different relevancy standard for substantive versus demonstrative evidence? When the evidence is used for demonstrative purposes, a witness is relating his or her opinion of the sequence of events based on the evidence presented. The relevancy of the evidence is based on the jury's acceptance of the witness' credibility in linking the simulation to the actual events. In contrast, when a simulation is used as substantive evidence, the simulation is being presented as a representation of what actually occurred in the absence of any other evidence. Therefore, in order for the evidence to be a valid representation of the actual events, the model must be similar to the actual object to establish the requisite link. The only way to establish that link is for the conditions portrayed in the simulation to be substantially similar to those that actually existed. In our example, the physiology programmed into the mannequin must be similar to that which existed in the patient at the time of the adverse event. If not, then the simulation, no matter how precise, cannot be relevant. Just how similar the simulation must be remains open to question. One court has held that the simulation must be nearly identical to be relevant. One legal commentator has suggested that, rather than having the more stringent standard of substantial similarity, a more lenient standard of general similarity should be applied. He argues that, rather than having a judge decide whether a piece of evidence should be allowed, it should be left to the jury to determine the validity of the simulation. If a simulation has weaknesses in its approximation of the actual environment, the opponents of the evidence can challenge its validity to the jury. In cases in which simulations have been admitted as substantive evidence, the simulations have been those in which the conditions have been relatively simple and followed easily reproducible formulas. Examples include accident reconstructions in which velocity, friction, and surface conditions are easily reproducible. In the use of the medical simulator, however, reproduction of the physiologic environment of the patient may be more difficult, and, as such, the simulation may be not be substantially similar enough to meet the standard for relevancy. Whether these simulations are determined to be relevant depends on the sophistication of the technology in approximating more closely actual human physiology and whether the courts are more or less stringent in defining "substantially similar."

Even if the court determines that the evidence is relevant, it may still be excluded if it is determined that its probative value—that is, its value in helping the jury determine an issue—is outweighed by unfair prejudice, leads to confusion of the issues, or is misleading to the jury. Unfair prejudice may be exemplified by the presentation of a bloody crime scene. While it would be probative, there is the danger that the jury will respond with emotion rather than logic. The same can be said with a simulation. Its precision and presentational strength may cause the jury to give it more credence that it should. In the case of medical simulators, there is a danger that the technologic "gee-whiz" character of the simulation may give it more evidentiary value than another type. The jury may believe that since the "evidence" is computer-generated, it must therefore be true. Because simulated depictions may be so realistic, judges may disallow such evidence for fear that the jury may give it undue weight. Moreover, the evidence may be disallowed because it may be considered prejudicial and misleading. A simulation, because of its realistic character, may unfairly boost the testimony of an expert that may otherwise be questionable. In one case, the judge disallowed a simulation because it was so effective that he feared that it would remove the jury from its fact-finding role.

Another hurdle that simulations must overcome before being admitted as evidence is that they must be authenticated. That is, there must be some threshold finding that the exhibit is what it purports to be. For example, if a plaintiff claims that he tripped on a sidewalk because there was a hole in the concrete, a photograph of the sidewalk showing the hole must be authenticated as being the sidewalk where the person tripped. This authentication can be made if the photographer testifies that the picture was taken at that particular location. Similarly, with a simulation offered as evidence, the proponent of the evidence must demonstrate that the data presented by the simulator "fairly and accurately" represent the conditions that existed when the patient was injured. The standard for authentication varies with the purpose for the evidence. If the simulation is offered as demonstrative evidence, the requirements are not as stringent.[3] For example, if the plaintiff were only trying to illustrate the opinions of an expert or to represent data from an anesthesia record, the only requirement would be that the simulation fairly and accurately demonstrated the opinion. The expert would need only to testify that the evidence does so. On the other hand, if the simulation were to be used as substantive evidence, the hurdle would be much higher. In contrast to demonstrative evidence, in which the software of the simulator is used merely to represent known facts, to be used as substantive evidence, the software in the simulator actually would be "creating" the facts. To authenticate the evidence, therefore, the proponent of the evidence needs to show that the software contains all relevant data and algorithms, that such information is accurate, and that the data and algorithms interact in such a way that has accurately represented the real-world interactions. For a particular simulation, the proponent must show that under particular conditions, a particular intervention will result in a predictable event. For example, if the proponent wants to show that a particular drug caused hypotension, which led to cardiac arrest, he or she must demonstrate that the simulated physiology of the mannequin is substantially similar to the patient's physiology and the simulated result is what would have actually occurred when the drug was given, based on calculated interactions. For situations in which simple mathematical formulas can be used to simulate a particular event, such as an auto accident reconstruction, this goal may be easy. For the human body, however, because the input factors are multifactorial and their interactions so complex, it may be very difficult to demonstrate that the simulated physiology accurately represents that of the patient and that the simulated result is the only one that could have occurred. To be authenticated, therefore, the proponent must show that all input data are complete and accurate, the software is an accurate representation of realty, and the results are predictable and reliable.

Another hurdle facing the admission of simulation as evidence is the issue of hearsay. According to the federal rules of evidence, hearsay is defined as an out-of-court statement offered to prove the matter asserted. For example, if a witness testifying in an auto accident, in order to show that the defendant is liable, states that someone told him that the defendant ran a red light, the statement that "the defendant ran a red light" was made out of court and is being used to prove that the defendant did in fact run a red light. That statement would be considered hearsay. If evidence is determined by the court to be hearsay and does not fit into an exception under which it may be allowed, it will not be admitted as evidence. The reason for this prohibition lies in the court's belief that it is unfair to admit a statement into evidence if the opponent of the statement cannot cross-examine the declarant of the statement. In the example above, if the witness stated that he saw the defendant run the red light, the opposing counsel can cross-examine the witness about such issues as his or her personal knowledge of the accident, his or her motive for making the statement, and poor memory. However, if the witness said that his or her friend Sam had told him or her that he (Sam) had seen the car run the red light and Sam cannot be cross-examined as a witness, it would be unfair to the opposing party to admit Sam's statement into evidence; thus, that statement would be considered hearsay. With computer simulations, the analysis of whether the evidence is hearsay or not again depends on whether it is being presented as demonstrative or substantive evidence. In the case of a simulation presented as demonstrative evidence, it is essentially a pictorial representation of an expert's opinion or verbal testimony. The expert can be cross-examined and the reliability of the evidence tested. It is not, therefore, an out-of-court statement whose declarant cannot be questioned.

However, if the simulation is not used as a display of a witness' statement but is used to prove the truth of the matter asserted, it may be considered hearsay and not be admissible. For example, if a simulator shows that the only possible cause of a patient's hypotension was an overdose of a drug without any extrinsic evidence as to that assertion, the simulation is, in effect, making the statement. When a computer is inputted with data to generate a result, an opponent can argue that the result generated by the computer's program is hearsay because the result is simply a computer programmer's assumption of how the event must have or would have occurred, given those particular input variables. Because the computer generates the evidence, there is no one that the opposing party can cross-examine about the validity of the computer's output.[4] Of course, the proponent of the evidence may always counter that the response is not actually hearsay but merely a preprogrammed response to a set of admissible variables. For example, if the output of the equation is $3 + 3 = 6$, is this answer generated by the computer hearsay, or is it a preprogrammed answer performed by a device? In this example, the answer is simple: $3 + 3$ always yields 6 and is not disputable. In the physiologic example, however, the response is not as predictable and may vary depending on the data inputted in the computer or the underlying software algorithms. Thus, the argument that the computer-generated result is merely an invariable preprogrammed result of a device would probably not be successful. Nevertheless, the proponent may argue that the result should be admissible based on an exception to the hearsay rule.

This exception states that an expert may rely on evidence that is hearsay for his or her opinion if that evidence is "reasonably relied upon by experts in the particular field in forming or inferences upon the subject." To be admissible under this rule, however, the expert must be familiar with the software program used to generate the result. An Ohio court has determined that for computer-generated evidence to be used as substantial evidence, the expert must (1) be qualified in the particular field and (2) be "qualified in the field or at least, the technique of generating a computer simulation or re-creation, based on certain input data." Thus, if the proponent of evidence generated by the human patient simulator can demonstrate that it is the type generally relied upon by experts for their opinions and that their witness is qualified as an expert in the use of human patient simulators, this exception may allow the admission of simulator evidence as substantive evidence. Because this technology is so new, however, the proponent may have difficulty showing that experts in the field rely on the data generated by the simulators to form their opinions, thus failing to meet the requirement for the hearsay exception. The use of simulators in the teaching and research arenas is increasing, however, and in the near future experts in the field may indeed rely on simulated results to demonstrate physiologic and pharmacologic principles. If a court determines that this is so, this exception to the hearsay rule would permit admission of computer-generated results as substantive evidence. The test above has been used in an Ohio court to admit computer-generated evidence.

Another exception to the hearsay rule is the "catch-all" exception. Under this exception, hearsay evidence may be admitted, even if it does not fit under accepted exception, if it has strong "probative value," is considered "trustworthy," and serves the "interests of justice" by being admitted. The proponent may argue that because the creators of the software have no incentive to "lie" about the accuracy of their software and because these simulations are based on scientific principles, they are inherently trustworthy. As to the probative value of a simulation, because on many occasions it is unknown how an event occurred, thus necessitating a simulation, the simulation is highly probative in regard to the resolution of the issue. Finally, whether the evidence serves the interest of justice by being admitted is left to the discretion of the judge.

Even if the evidence may be admissible for the reasons discussed above, another admissibility hurdle that a proponent of the simulation as evidence must pass is the "scientific evidence" under the rules of evidence. That is, if evidence is considered scientific, it must meet more stringent criteria to be considered admissible. Because computer simulations are generated using computer science, they may be considered scientific evidence. The criteria for admissibility of scientific evidence are described in *Daubert v. Merrell Dow Pharmaceuticals*. In that case, the Supreme Court elucidated four factors that must be met in order for scientific evidence to admissible: (1) whether the evidence can be (or has been) tested; (2) whether the theory or technique has been subjected to peer review and publication; (3) whether the technique has a known or potential rate of error; and(4) whether there has been particular degree of acceptance within the relevant scientific community. With respect to simulators such as the human simulators, the first factor may be met with random tests of input data or presentation of evidence of manufacturer research indicating the reliability of the simulation. If the simulation can be reliably tested and shows consistent responses, this first requirement may be sufficient for the court. As for the last factors, because the technology is so new, it may prove difficult to meet the Daubert criteria. However, as more simulations are used and more research is done using this technology, it will be subject to peer review, rates of error will be known, and simulations will be widely accepted by the scientific community. Once this acceptance occurs, the hurdle imposed by the Daubert criteria will be easily overcome and simulations will be deemed admissible scientific evidence.

Computer-generated evidence is finding its way into the courtrooms. Currently, however, it is used mostly as demonstrative evidence. However, many evidentiary rules form obstacles that prevent the simulations from being admitted as substantive evidence. Simulations that follow simple physical rules, can predictably simulate actual environmental conditions, and are relied on by experts in the field to formulate their opinions are being admitted as substantive evidence. Physiologic simulators probably have not attained the level of sophistication to be deemed acceptable by most courts as substantive evidence. As technology improves, however, that status may change, and more simulations will be used as substantive evidence.

Simulators Used for Public Education

As an educational tool, human patient simulators are not limited to medical training institutions. They may be used to educate the public at large on a variety of topics.

At the University of Louisville, the human patient simulators have been used in community outreach programs to educate the public about bioterrorism. Case scenarios involving nerve gas, botulism, and anthrax have been designed to increase public awareness of these potential disasters. To illustrate, the public is invited to a lecture session, which is then followed by a demonstration with standardized patients trained and moulaged to mimic the physical findings of these pathologic states. A demonstration of the physiologic effects of these conditions is then presented using the human patient simulator. The combination of these simulation techniques adds a degree of reality that otherwise could not be appreciated. Participants in these outreach programs reported that the simulations were very successful in educating them about these conditions and have increased their awareness of bioterrorism.

Another public use of the simulations has been in the arena of drug abuse prevention. Some institutions have used human patient simulators to demonstrate the negative physiologic changes associated with drug abuse (e.g., dysrythmia with cocaine). Another related use has been the use of simulators to educate teenagers about the harm from cigarette use and to discourage smoking. In these simulations, the participants are shown the gradual decline in physiologic function and the harm to the pulmonary and cardiovascular systems with increasing years of cigarette use.

Human patient simulators have also been used to teach basic scientific concepts to middle and high school students. By providing a hands-on approach and demonstrating real-world application of scientific principles, these simulators allow active learning of abstract concepts and make learning a more enriching and effective experience.

Other Uses

In addition to their use as a teaching tool, simulators have also been used to improve operating room equipment design. Engineers have used mannequins to improve the ergonomic design and layout of operating equipment. By having the ability to simulate realistic medical conditions, the designers have a more accurate picture of the motions and activities of health care personnel as they manage various clinical situations. This knowledge is therefore helpful in designing equipment that promotes ergonomic efficiency. With this improved design, less motion is wasted and corrective measures taken in emergency situations may be taken more quickly and effectively.[5]

Finally, the simulator can be used as a recruitment tool. Because a simulator can be a state-of-the-art educational tool for an institution, the presence of this equipment can elevate the status of an institution. As such, the simulator can be used to recruit prospective medical students, house staff, and attending staff. At our institution, the simulators are extensively used in the facility tour for prospective educational and professional applicants. Many of the applicants cite the presence of the simulators as a significant reason why they would choose to attend or work at our institution. Until more institutions acquire simulators, facilities that are fortunate enough to have them can use them to recruit desirable applicants.

Conclusion

As simulator technology improves, more nonmedical uses for simulators will be found. Although their use in the legal arena may be currently limited, as the technology becomes more sophisticated and the courts become more aware of their evidentiary potential, their use will most likely increase. Additonally, there are many uses other than for training of medical personnel. As the public becomes more aware of the existence and impact of these devices, more uses will probably be found.

Bibliography
1. Federal Rules of Evidence.
2. Kofke WA, Rie MA, Rosen K: Acute care crisis simulation for jury education. Med Law 2001;20 (1): 79–83.
3. Butera KD: Seeing is believing: A practitioner's guide to the admissibility of demonstrative evidence. Cleve State Law Rev 1998.
4. Galves F: Where the not-so-wild things are: Computers in the courtroom, the federal rules of evidence and the need for institutional reform and more judicial acceptance. Harvard J Law Technol Winter, 2000.
5. Personal conversation with J.S. Gravenstein, MD, University of Florida.

SIMULATION: THE FUTURE

Chapter 29

TECHNOLOGY-ENHANCED SIMULATION: LOOKING AHEAD TO 2020

Ruth Greenberg, PhD

Practical Health Care Simulation begins with two chapters that provide a detailed history of technology-enhanced simulation in health care education and an overview of its current status. At the conclusion of his chapter, "The Current Status of Simulation Education in Health care," Martin Reznek, Wayne State University, comments, "It is remarkable to consider that this technology is just in its infancy." Despite its current sophistication, health care simulation is, indeed, still in its infancy and likely to become more specialized—and more available—during the next two decades.

Thus, we conclude our discussion of practical health care simulations with an examination of three questions:

1. What will be the role of simulation in training health care professionals in 2020?

2. As simulation technologies mature, what types of new simulations might health care educators expect to use to teach their students?

3. What barriers might prevent the expansion of simulation technology, and how might these barriers be overcome?

The responses to these questions, in most cases, are those of the clinical educators whose advice and simulation scenarios are included in *Practical Health Care Simulation*. Naturally, their predictions are personal and reflect their own experiences with technologically enhanced simulations. Taken together, however, they represent a thoughtful overview of what we might expect to witness as simulation education progresses during the first quarter of the twenty-first century.

The Role of Simulation in Health Care Education in 2020

At the International Meeting on Medical Simulation (IMMS) in January of 2003, David Gaba, considered by many to be the father of technology-enhanced health care simulation, spoke of two possible scenarios:

1. Despite its early promise, simulation dies out; no one is able to show that it is worth the money and better than anything else; training is a low priority in health care budgets.

Or

2. Simulators become totally embedded in the fabric of health care, not just medicine, and are used throughout one's career for testing new medical equipment; researching issues on human performance in health care; and training, certification and recertification. This chapter focuses on the second, more optimistic scenario.[1]

Several chapter authors believe, as Gaba does, that "by 2020, simulation will be totally embedded in the fabric of health care."[2] James Gordon, Harvard University, postulates that simulators will become "more common, more mainstream across all health care domains."[3] This will occur because more schools will purchase simulators to support their educational programs. As Gordon stated, "Three years ago, there was very limited interest in simulation; now everyone wants to start a center."[4] There is no doubt that interest in simulation in health care education is growing. To illustrate, the November 2003 issue of *Medical Education* contains at least nine articles on simulation-related topics. Moreover, the number of institutions building new simulation centers is expanding, as is the number of simulators sold each year.

What factors will grow the interest in and use of technology-enhanced simulation in health care education programs? Gordon suggests three factors: (1) simulators will provide safer, risk-free training experiences; (2) simulators will allow educators to control clinical education experiences and thus standardize training; and (3) simulations will enable educators to address issues of decreasing availability of patient contact efficiently and appropriately.[5]

The view that simulation education will expand is shared by other chapter authors. Craig Roberts, University of Louisville, predicts that simulation will be used to recertify and test the proficiency of surgeons in terms of the procedures that they perform (e.g., total hip and total knee replacement).[6] Kathy Rosen, West Virginia University, predicts that health care educational programs will experience a paradigm shift toward a "mastery learning" model in which model students will be "forced to document knowledge and skills competency in a simulated environment before being allowed to practice on humans."[7] In this system, training is skill-limited, not time-limited, and simulation is one of the cornerstones of this process; students are not permitted to practice on patients until they have demonstrated mastery in a simulated environment.[8] David Ost, North Shore Hospital, believes that simulation's ability to provide unlimited, unsupervised practice time will be a major force in expanding its role in health care training. Since most clinical training occurs in small groups with only a few students per attending physician, simulation will increase the efficiency of learning, lower costs, and improve performance.[9]

One final factor may contribute to the expansion of simulation in health care education. Mike Olympio, Wake Forest University, predicts that we will see "discrete objectives, many of which are proven valid for simulation, and a lot less haphazard simulation."[10] Gary Loyd, University of Louisville, echoes this viewpoint: "Simulation, over the next 20 years, will expand as the validity and reliability of simulation as a superior teaching and assessing tool becomes established."[11] Finally, Amitai Ziv, Chaim Sheba Medical Center, Israel; Paul Roote Wole, University of Pennsylvania; Stephen Small, University of Chicago; and Shimon Glick, Ben-Gurion University of the Negev, Israel, suggest that simulators, used properly, have the potential to make medical training more humanistic. Although we do not yet have sufficient "proof" that simulation-based medical education actually improves skills, Ziv and his colleagues suggest that it may provide an important tool for addressing concerns about patient safety and error reduction.[12]

New Simulations on the Horizon

As the role of simulation in health care education expands, so too will the sophistication of the simulations available for purchase: as technology advances, so too will simulators. What will patient simulators and simulations look like in 2020? Kirsti Lonka, Karolinska Institute, predicts that we will see more simulators and more realistic environments as technology proceeds—simulations that are not just three-dimensional but that actually take place in three-dimensional space. Moreover, these environments will mix simulations and real-word objects; for example, operating room equipment and simulators will create a real-world environment for training.[13] Kathy Rosen, West Virginia University, dreams about a more totally immersive environment in which trainees will be able to converse and touch a simulated patient and its family members. She believes that advances in plastics should allow skin color and temperature to change. In addition, new simulators will be based on better physiologic modeling, and various simulation technologies will be integrated, much like the "cave" environment created at the University of Michigan. Rosen would also like to see a combination of haptics and virtual reality replace the unisex mannequins in current use.[14]

Elizabeth Sinz, West Virginia University, predicts that simulation will go in the direction of full-scale simulation and virtual reality. She envisions the development of more advanced partial-task trainers, using haptics that will allow medical trainees of all types to learn procedures and management strategies before they actually take care of patients.[15] Mike Olympio, Wake Forest University, adds that more robust surgical simulators and improvements in airway simulators will be developed. He predicts that more sophisticated skin simulations will be available that will allow the simulators to exhibit various types of rashes and discolorations; he believes also that simulators will mimic spontaneous movements of the extremities and that trainees will one day use simulators that offer central access to the subclavian or carotid artery with blood return and infusion capability.[16]

Haptics and virtual reality will have an enormous impact on the nature of simulations used by trainees in 2020. David Seligson, University of Louisville, suggests that haptics gives us the possibility to transfer robot-assisted surgery from the simulator directly into real life, which will increase accuracy and patient safety. For example, surgeons are now doing more complicated fracture fixation with implants, using more exacting tools that must be used in a prescribed sequence; if future surgeons use haptic-enhanced simulations to learn what the tools are, how to use them, and the exact steps in the procedure, meaningful process improvement will be achieved.[17] Craig Roberts, University of Louisville, predicts that we will see more portable simulation technology—for example, portable CD or PDA programs with training for future surgeons in three-dimensional thinking, visual acuity, spatial relationships, three-dimensional anatomy, and triangulation with instruments, especially for arthroscopic/minimally invasive procedures.[18] Pam Morgan, University of Toronto, believes that pediatric simulators will become far more realistic, comparable to adult simulators, and that we will witness the introduction of baby simulators.[19] David Ost, North Shore University Hospital, expects that simulated bronchoscopies will become more sophisticated, which will result in improved trainee performance at first patient contact and will allow faculty to focus their teaching efforts on higher level without getting bogged down in the mundane aspects of simple bronchoscopy.[20]

Medical Education Technologies, Inc. (METI) is currently working toward the development of a virtual hospital concept and seeking medical school partners to achieve its vision. METI's virtual hospitals will have the capacity to "replicate any health care delivery setting, for both typical and unconventional medical operations. It can be used as an integrated system or with each of its components operating independently."[21] These virtual hospital will rely on various types of simulators and simulations, resulting in more realistic representations of patients and health care systems.

Another initiative that will affect the future of simulation in health care education is the National Center for Collaboration in Medical Modeling and Simulation (VMASC), a joint effort of Eastern Virginia Medical School and Old Dominion University. The ultimate goal of the center is to create a paradigm shift in medical education "to shift from the traditional apprenticeship training model to a model based predominantly upon modern modeling and simulation technologies." That model will require the development of virtual patients and complete human simulations.[22]

James Gordon, Harvard University, summarizes the changes that we may witness: robust integration of full body and procedural simulation. What we need hardware for now may become a virtual reality holadex by 2020. The hardware will become less important while the software engineering becomes more important. Simulation will involve more complicated procedures, and procedures and total body experiences will become totally integrated.[23] David Gaba, Stanford University, concurs that trainees will use better, denser models and software in virtual realities and virtual words—fully immersible virtual reality with virtual patients, virtual people, and virtual settings. Indeed, virtual reality may one day entirely replace simulators.[24]

Will We Get There: Barriers to Overcome

The most often cited barrier to realizing the predictions described in this chapter is cost. Simulators are expensive, simulation development is expensive, and health care education funding is rapidly decreasing. As David Ost, North Shore University Hospital, explains, medical education has no income stream that pays for capital investment such as simulation technology, nor are there any incentives for buying this equipment. It rarely generates revenue and is extremely costly.[25] Pam Morgan, University of Toronto, suggests that some centers are moving toward multidisciplinary uses to increase utilization and decrease costs. However, these centers must also purchase a variety of equipment and simulators as well as recruit faculty from various disciplines to meet the training needs of each user group. Funding to create and sustain these centers can be quite high.[26]

Elizabeth Sinz, West Virginia University, suggests another approach to funding, one that involves a major shift in philosophy. She predicts that simulation centers will need to employ "simulation experts" rather than medical experts to run the simulators and teach trainees. In addition, Sinz believes that making residency a one-year experience, with trainees being permitted to "work" as doctors at an earlier point and having to perform procedures only after they have demonstrated mastery on a simulator, would re-establish the apprentice model used during the nineteenth century to train physicians and, in turn, create a new revenue stream that could be used to support simulation training.[27]

Another barrier is knowledge. Pam Morgan, University of Toronto, believes that faculty need to be educated about the existence of technology-enhanced simulation and its uses in education.[28] James Gordon, Harvard University, echoes this statement. He believes that faculty who have not seen simulation in practice do not believe that it will be useful to them as teachers. Gordon believes that we need to get faculty in a room and show them how to do an entire encounter (history, physical exam, procedure); this approach might demonstrate to nonbelievers that simulation can be an excellent adjunct to the training process.[29] Mike Olympio, Wake Forest University, suggests one approach to overcoming this barrier: department chairs could mandate simulation training and mandate that people teach in simulation centers.[30] Although Olympio's solution is unlikely to be popular, the role of administration in encouraging and offering faculty exposure to the potential educational benefits of patient simulations is likely to be critical to expanding the use of simulation.

According to Kirsti Lonka, Karolinska Institute, the worst barrier is that educators, technology experts, and clinical faculty work independently of one another; she believes that these three groups need to be integrated.[31] Brian Felice, University of Rhode Island, believes that the most challenging barrier to overcome relates to determining how to integrate simulation into an existing curriculum. In his case, integrating the simulator into pharmacology education was very time-consuming and challenging. He emphasizes the role of continuous assessment and refining of simulations in overcoming this challenge.[32]

Related to this barrier is the challenge of validity. According to David Gaba, Stanford University, faculty are searching for evidence-based medical approaches and outcomes approaches. We need to demonstrate that the simulators save lives or money. Proving that they improve performance is difficult but not impossible. But these studies are expensive, and one test may not be enough to demonstrate validity.[33] Mike Olympio, Wake Forest University, agrees that a major barrier to the expansion of technology-enhanced simulation in health care education is the validation that simulation is effective (not "my teaching is effective") as well as the need for peer-analyzed curriculum development and consensus around the learning objectives appropriate for simulation-enhanced education.[34]

R. Bowen Loftin, Old Dominion University, identifies what he believes are the five "grand" challenges facing medical simulation: tissue modeling, multimodal simulation, transfer of training to the clinical environment, seamless integration of the virtual and real, and the potential of simulation as a recertifying tool for practicing physicians. These challenges, in addition to other less grand challenges—for example, fidelity, data representation, and cost—will be the focus of the Virginia Modeling, Analysis and Simulation Center, of which Loftin is the executive director.[35]

This chapter has focused primarily on the more positive of the two possible scenarios presented by David Gaba at IMMS—that is, simulation will become totally embedded in the training of future health care professionals.[36] The educators who currently use technology-enhanced simulation to train medical, dental, nursing, and allied health professionals believe in and are committed to the role patient simulation does play and can play in the future to enhance teaching and learning. However, as Gaba suggested, it is also possible that, despite its early promise, simulation in health care education may not exist in 2020. If researchers fail to validate its benefits, administrators may conclude that simulation is not worth funding.

My own view lies somewhere between Gaba's two possible scenarios for simulation's future. I believe that simulation technology will undoubtedly advance. New, more sophisticated simulators will become available, but they will be expensive. Simulation-based education will be used more extensively to train, certify, and recertify health care professionals. Virtual reality, haptics, and simulation will become integrated at a few high-end centers, but these will be few. Individuals and institutions that are able to identify funds—through generous alumni, private industry, or federal agencies—will build state-of-the-art centers that will attract many visitors and enhance the training of health care professionals able to access their facilities. However, the biggest obstacle to translating our vision of a simulation embedded training system into reality will be, I predict, the need to motivate and convince the current generation of clinical educators that simulation-based education will produce better educated trainees. Validation studies will help, but, in the end, it will fall upon the current simulation users to "convert" the nonusers—a formidable task.

Practical Health Care Simulation was written to help achieve that goal. We hope that the strategies and scenarios collected from around the country can provide a useful tool for current and prospective simulation users. Our commitment to expanding the base of faculty users drove us to produce this book and will continue to drive our efforts to increase use at our own institution and at institutions around the world.

References

1. Gaba D: Telephone conversation, 18 Feb. 2003.
2. Gaba D: Telephone conversation, 18 Feb. 2003.
3. Gordon J: Telephone conversation, 4 Mar. 2003.
4. Gordon J: Telephone conversation, 4 Mar. 2003.
5. Gordon J: Telephone conversation, 4 Mar. 2003.
6. Roberts C: E-mail correspondence, 25 Nov: 2003.
7. Rosen K: E-mail correspondence, 21 Nov. 2003.
8. Rosen K: E-mail correspondence, 21 Nov: 2003.
9. Ost D: E-mail correspondence, 21 Nov. 2003.
10. Olympio M: E-mail correspondence, 13 Apr. 2003.
11. Loyd G: E-mail correspondence, 25 Nov. 2003.
12. Ziv A, Wolpe PR, Small SD, Glick S: Simulation-based medical education: An ethical imperative. Acad Med 2003;78(8):783–788.
13. Lonka K: E-mail correspondence, 14 Apr. 2003.
14. Rosen K: E-mail correspondence, 18 Apr. 2003.
15. Sinz E: E-mail correspondence, 21 Nov. 2003.
16. Olympio M: E-mail correspondence, 13 Apr. 2003.
17. Seligson D: E-mail correspondence, 11 Apr. 2003:
18. Roberts C: E-mail correspondence, 25 Nov. 2003.
19. Morgan P: E-mail correspondence, 16 Apr. 2003.
20. Ost D: E-mail correspondence, 21 Nov. 2003.
21. Medical Education Technologies, Inc: METI virtual hospital: Concept paper, Nov. 2003.
22. Loftin B: Med school 1:0: Can computer simulation aid physician training? Available at http://www:odu:edu/ao/instadv/quest/MedSchool:html. Accessed 21 Apr. 2003.
23. Gordon J: Telephone conversation, 4 Mar. 2003.
24. Gaba D: Telephone conversation, 18 Feb. 2003.
25. Ost D: E-mail correspondence, 21 Nov. 2003.
26. Morgan P: E-mail correspondence, 16 Apr. 2003.
27. Sinz E: E-mail correspondence, 21 Nov. 2003.
28. Morgan P: E-mail correspondence, 16 Apr. 2003.
29. Gordon J: Telephone conversation, 4 Mar. 2003.
30. Olympio M: E-mail correspondence, 13 Apr. 2003.
31. Lonka K: E-mail correspondence, 14 Apr. 2003.
32. Felice B: E-mail correspondence, 9 Apr. 2003.
33. Gaba D: Telephone conversation, 18 Feb. 2003.
34. Olympio M: E-mail correspondence, 13 Apr. 2003.
35. Loftin RB: Grand challenges in medical modeling and simulation. Presented at the Western MultiConference (WMC), Orlando, FL, 2003.
36. Gaba DM: Simulation in health care: Two retrospective histories? Presented at the International Meeting on Medical Simulation (IMMS), San Diego, CA, 2003.

Index

Numbers in **bold face** indicate entire chapter.

Critical care, simulation in *(cont.)*
  in respiratory therapy, 542–545
  in shock management, 288
  for teamwork development, 288–289
  testing and assessment applications of,
    292
  in use and interpretation of invasive moni-
    tors, 281–282
  in use of vasoactive medications and
    inotropes, 282–283
  in ventilation management, 284–286
Critical Care Simulator (Anesoft), 13
Critical Concepts, Inc., 13
Critical events, in virtual hospital experience,
  172
Cyanosis simulation, 284
Cystoscopy simulation, in family practice
  instruction, 435

D
da Vinci Robotic Surgical System, 381
"Death" scenarios
  in critical care training, 289
  in emergency medicine training, 299
Debriefing
  in Advanced Cardiac Life Support simula-
    tion, 196
  in anesthesiology simulation
    in abdominal aneurysm repair scenario,
      259, 261
    in cerebral aneurysm scenario, 256,
      257–258
  in crisis management simulation, 221
  in disaster response simulation, 306
  in emergency medicine simulation, 187,
    297, 298, 299–300
  in nursing education simulation, 191
  in pulmonary simulation, 183
Debriefing rooms, in simulation centers
  floor plans of, 68–69, 71, 72
  space requirements for, 55–56
Decision making
  in combat, 157, 161, 223, 245
  in crisis management, 215–220
  in critical care, 279
  effect of cognitive dispositions to respond
    on, 298
  in family practice, 433–434
  with interactive, computer-based patient
    simulators, 433–434

Decision making *(cont.)*
  naturalistic, 215–217
  in pediatrics, 430
  by public health nurses, 435
  virtual reality simulator use in, 223
Decontamination, as disaster response skill,
  306, 329–330
Defibrillation simulation
  in emergency medicine training, 298
  ventricular/fibrillation/pulseless ventricular
    tachycardia algorithm in, 153
Defibrillators, 393
  development of, 7–8
  programmable, 395
  simulated (low-voltage), 393
Demand-and-supply curves, 90–92, 93, 94
Denar Articulator, 492
Dental education, simulation in, 487–506
  computer-based simulation, 493–500
    business practice simulation, 493–494
    case-based simulations, 493–494
    computer imaging in, 494–495
    navigational simulation, 499–500
    simulation laboratory with computer
      technology, 495–496
    simulation with advanced technology,
      496–500
    technology with haptics focus, 498–499
    virtual reality-based technology, 496–498
  future possibilities of, 503
  global impact of, 503–504
  with human patient simulators, 491–492,
    501
  importance of, 487–488
  in intravenous conscious sedation training,
    514–520
  noncomputerized simulation, 488–493
    dentoforms, 488, 489–491, 496, 500
    models of oral structures, 488, 489
    simulation of teeth and jaws, 488–491,
      492
  in practice management, 493–494
  psychomotor skills development in, 487,
    488, 500
  resources needed for, 500–503
  surgical skills development in, 488, 500
Dental implants placement, 489–490
  navigational simulation of, 499–500
Dental licensure examination, simulation in,
  494